AF667856

# Clinical Guide to Heart Transplantation

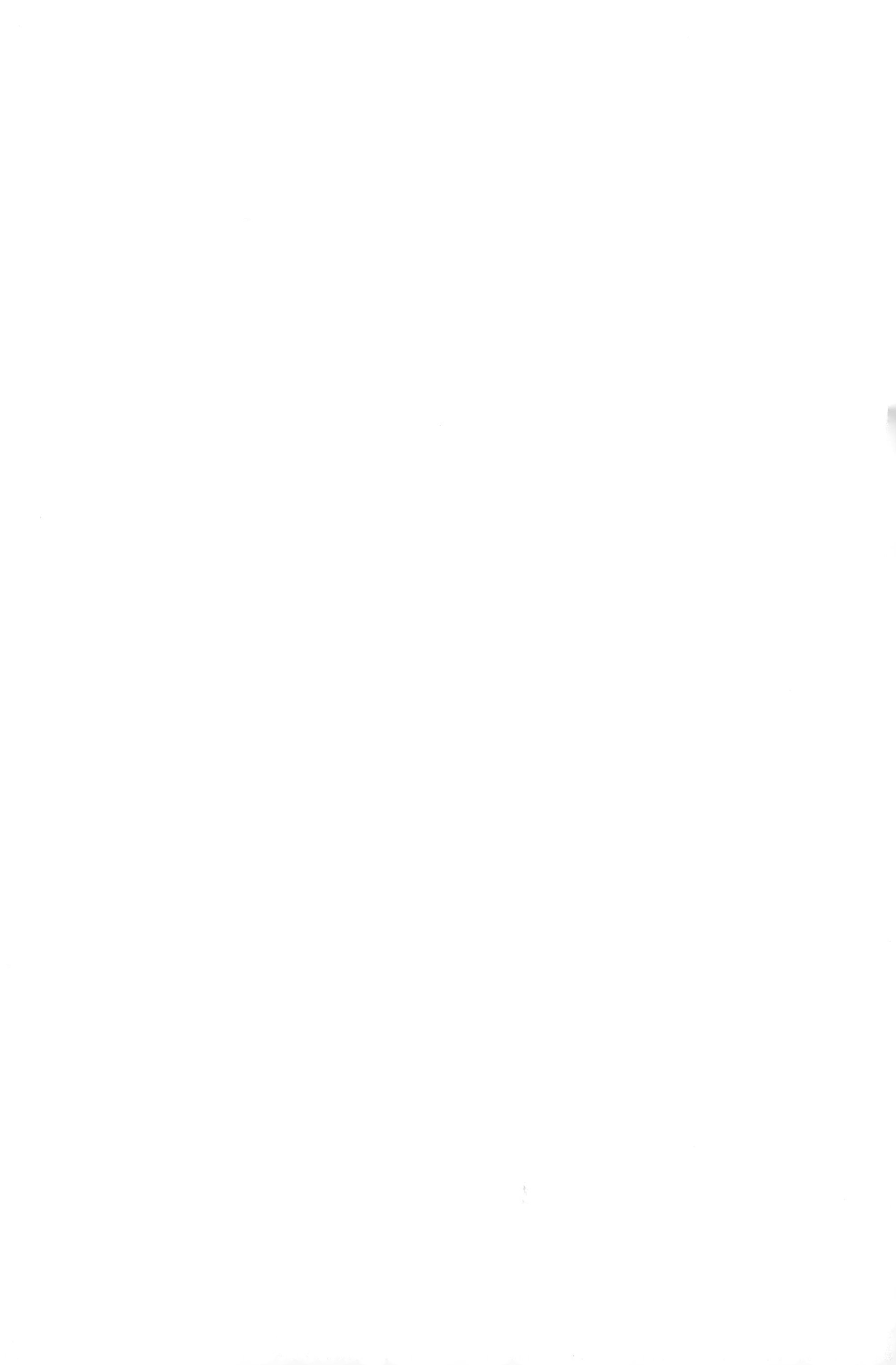

Jon Kobashigawa
Editor

# Clinical Guide to Heart Transplantation

Second Edition

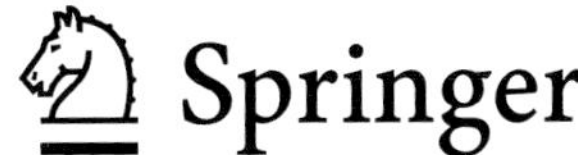

*Editor*
Jon Kobashigawa
DSL/Thomas D. Gordon Professor
of Medicine
Director, Advanced Heart Disease
Division
Director, Heart Transplant Program
Associate Director, Smidt Heart Institute
Associate Director, Comprehensive
Transplant Center
Cedars-Sinai Medical Center,
Los Angeles, CA, USA

ISBN 978-3-031-88289-0 ISBN 978-3-031-88290-6 (eBook)
https://doi.org/10.1007/978-3-031-88290-6



This Springer imprint is published by the registered company Springer Nature Switzerland AG
The registered company address is: Gewerbestrasse 11, 6330 Cham, Switzerland

*This edition of Clinical Guide to Heart Transplantation is dedicated to the memory of our dear colleague and co-author, Jignesh Patel M.D. Ph.D.*

# Introduction

In the 8 years since the first edition of this *Clinical Guide to Heart Transplantation* was published, the field of cardiac transplantation has evolved significantly. Innovations in donor procurement and preservation are being deployed, including the use of donors who suffer circulatory death, expanding the availability of hearts for patients who need them. New biomarkers and diagnostic tools are being leveraged to better assess risk and to calibrate monitoring and early intervention. New concepts in immunotherapy are being explored as we get closer to the goal of personalized medicine. The technology for both artificial and bio-engineered hearts is advancing at a previously unimagined pace and xenotransplantation as a viable therapeutic option is now within our reach. Machine learning is being used to power diagnostics, including the use of big data to improve pathology assessments by leveraging information at the molecular level. The advent of virtual visits, virtual crossmatching, and virtual reality have propelled our field into a new era. Indeed, transplantation medicine remains a fertile frontier for translational research.

This 2nd Edition incorporates emerging science in the field and provides updates on evidence-based management strategies for patients both pre- and post-heart transplantation. This includes the unexpected and hard-earned knowledge of how to manage immunocompromised patients during a pandemic, the management of sensitized patients awaiting heart transplantation, and the complexities of patients who require dual-organ transplantation.

Though the science, medicine, and practice of heart transplantation has entered a new and exciting phase, the *art* of heart transplantation remains the same. The art of caring for a patient, of listening to their story, of understanding their goals and their fears, of shaping a course of treatment with them rather than for them, remains the hallmark of good medicine. "What is the right thing for this patient?" This is still the question that drives our work, even as we strive to break new ground and cross old barriers.

As practitioners in this field, we are charged with making critical determinations in the management of patients, donor organs, and the transplant process itself in order to achieve the greatest benefit in the utilization of a scarce resource, including the hard task of addressing equity and access. This handbook is designed to be a reference for those on the front lines. While this compilation of best practices cannot address the complexity of the individual patients we care for on a daily basis, it is my hope that it will serve to help us ask the right questions, access the best evidence, and ultimately make the best decisions for the patients we are privileged to serve.

Los Angeles, USA
October 2024

Jon Kobashigawa M.D.

# Contents

# Editor and Contributors

## About the Editor

**Jon Kobashigawa** MD, is the DSL/Thomas D. Gordon professor of Medicine, director of the Advanced Heart Disease Section, director of the Heart Transplant Program and the associate director of the Cedars-Sinai Smidt Heart Institute as well as the associate director of the Comprehensive Transplant Center of the Cedars-Sinai Medical Center.

He received his undergraduate degree at Stanford University and earned his medical degree at Mount Sinai School of Medicine in New York. He is a past president of the International Society of Heart and Lung Transplantation, past chair of the American College of Cardiology Committee on Heart Failure and Transplantation, and past member of the United Network of Organ Sharing National Thoracic Committee and President of the American Society of Transplantation.

Dr. Kobashigawa is recognized nationally and internationally as a leader in heart transplantation. He has published more than 400 peer-reviewed articles, chapters and monographs in the field of heart failure and transplantation and has chairedseveral multicenter clinical studies. Dr. Kobashigawa has organized and chaired numerous International Consensus Conferences to discuss pertinent questions regarding heart failure and heart transplant. He lectures at universities around the world and has mentored many young physicians who have ascended to important academic positions throughout the country.

## Contributors

**Juan C. Alejos** UCLA Mattel Children's Hospital, Los Angeles, CA, USA

**Yevgeniy Brailovsky** Thomas Jefferson University, Philadelphia, PA, USA

**Pedro Catarino** Cedars-Sinai Smidt Heart Institute, Los Angeles, CA, USA

**David H. Chang** Cedars-Sinai Smidt Heart Institute, Los Angeles, CA, USA

**Robert M. Cole** Cedars-Sinai Smidt Heart Institute, Los Angeles, CA, USA

**Howard J. Eisen** Thomas Jefferson University, Philadelphia, PA, USA

**Fardad Esmailian** Cedars-Sinai Smidt Heart Institute, Los Angeles, CA, USA

**Michele Hamilton** Cedars-Sinai Smidt Heart Institute, Los Angeles, CA, USA

**Majid Husain** UCLA Mattel Children's Hospital, Los Angeles, CA, USA

**Michelle M. Kittleson** Cedars-Sinai Smidt Heart Institute, Los Angeles, CA, USA

**Jon Kobashigawa** Cedars-Sinai Smidt Heart Institute, Los Angeles, CA, USA

**Evan Kransdorf** Cedars-Sinai Smidt Heart Institute, Los Angeles, CA, USA

**Andrew Lin** Aurora St. Luke's Medical Center, Milwaukee, WI, USA

**Yosef Manla** Cedars-Sinai Smidt Heart Institute, Los Angeles, CA, USA

**Jaime D. Moriguchi** Cedars-Sinai Smidt Heart Institute, Los Angeles, CA, USA

**Emily Newman** Thomas Jefferson University, Philadelphia, PA, USA

**Andriana P. Nikolova** Cedars-Sinai Smidt Heart Institute, Los Angeles, CA, USA

**Jillian Oft** Division of Infectious Diseases, Cedars-Sinai Medical Center, Los Angeles, CA, USA

**Jignesh Patel** Cedars-Sinai Smidt Heart Institute, Los Angeles, CA, USA

**Krishan Patel** Cedars-Sinai Smidt Heart Institute, Los Angeles, CA, USA

**Yael Peled** Leviev Heart and Vascular Center, Sheba Medical Center, Tel Hashomer, Ramat Gan, Israel; Faculty of Medical and Health Sciences, Tel Aviv University, Tel Aviv, Israel

**Indranee Rajapreyar** Tufts Medical Center, Philadelphia, PA, USA

**Lily Stern** Cedars-Sinai Smidt Heart Institute, Los Angeles, CA, USA

**Rose Tompkins** Cedars-Sinai Medical Center, Guerin Congenital Heart Program, Smidt Heart Institute, Los Angeles, CA, USA

**Phillip Zakowski** Division of Infectious Diseases, Cedars-Sinai Medical Center, Los Angeles, CA, USA

**Xiaohai Zhang** HLA and Immunogenetics Laboratory, Comprehensive Transplant Center, Cedars-Sinai Medical Center, Los Angeles, CA, USA

# Part I
# Advanced Heart Failure Treatments

# Medical Therapy for Patients with End-Stage Heart Failure

1

Michele Hamilton and Yosef Manla

**Abstract**

Medical and device therapy for heart failure (HF) has evolved substantially over the past decade. This has changed the landscape not only towards improved survival and quality of life for all HF patients but also resulted in more appropriate and efficient utilization of advanced HF therapies, including heart transplantation and mechanical support in those with end-stage HF. This chapter provides a comprehensive guide to navigating the evolving therapeutic options for HF patients, focusing on the four pillars of guideline-directed medical therapy for heart failure with reduced ejection fraction. The chapter also explores device therapies and highlights the need for patient-centered care.

**Keywords**

Heart failure · Inotropes · Implantable cardioverter-defibrillator · Cardiac resynchronization

M. Hamilton (✉) · Y. Manla
Cedars-Sinai Smidt Heart Institute, Los Angeles, CA, USA
e-mail: michele.hamilton@cshs.org

Y. Manla
e-mail: Yosef.manla@cshs.org

## Clinical Pearls

- For patients presenting with advanced HF, whenever possible, the goal is to further optimize medical therapy and lifestyle opportunities, with ultimate referral for heart transplantation or durable mechanical support if the patient's condition does not stabilize.
- Established "pillars" of guideline-directed medical therapy (GDMT) include renin-angiotensin system (RAS) inhibitors, betablockers, mineralocorticoid receptor antagonist (MRAs), and sodium-glucose cotransporter 2 (SGLT-2) inhibitors. These GDMTs have been demonstrated to reduce heart failure hospitalizations and mortality. Systematic upward titration to maximally tolerated doses of all of these agents is key to improving patient outcomes.
- Diuretics continue to be central to reducing congestion in patients with volume overload.
- Sacubitril/ valsartan (an angiotensin receptor and neprilysin inhibitor, ARNI) is indicated as the first-line RAS inhibitor therapy for patients with class II/III heart failure, with careful monitoring of renal function and BP during titration. A 36-h wash-out period is needed during any change to or from an ACEI and ARNI.
- SGLT2 inhibitors are indicated for all symptomatic heart failure patients, with or without diabetes, across all left ventricular



J. Kobashigawa (ed.), *Clinical Guide to Heart Transplantation*, https://doi.org/10.1007/978-3-031-88290-6_1

ejection fractions, as long as renal function is not severely impaired (eGFR less than 20–30 ml/min).

- The implantable cardioverter-defibrillator is a suitable option for primary prevention in patients with LVEF ≤ 30% at least 40 days after myocardial infarction, and in patients with symptomatic ischemic and non-ischemic heart failure (NYHA Class II-III, LVEF < 35%) despite optimization of medical therapy.
- Cardiac resynchronization therapy is also appropriate for heart failure patients (NYHA class II-ambulatory IV, LVEF ≤ 35%) who demonstrate substantial prolongation of the QRS interval on ECG (≥150 ms) and are in sinus rhythm.
- Other medications, including vericiguat and ivabradine, and interventions such as transcatheter mitral valve repair or implantable pulmonary artery pressure sensors may also be considered for patients with persistent HF symptoms despite maximally tolerated GDMT.
- Type IC antiarrhythmics and dronedarone, as well as the non-dihydropyridine calcium channel blockers, diltiazem and verapamil, and the diabetes medications (thiazolidinediones and DPP-4 inhibitors) are contraindicated in patients with HFrEF. NSAIDs may also lead to worsening renal function and fluid retention in this population.

## Introduction

Heart Failure (HF) continues to impose a significant burden on patients and healthcare systems worldwide. In the United States, HF prevalence continues to rise, largely because of the increasing age of the population and improved post-myocardial infarction survival. In 2020, there were over 6.7 million HF patients, leading to over 1 million hospitalizations. HF was a contributing cause to at least 400,000 deaths [1, 2]. Multiple classification systems have been developed to precisely characterize the extent of disease progression in patients with HF patients, including the American College of Cardiology (ACC)/American Heart Association stages of HF progression and the New York Heart Association (NYHA) functional classification of HF symptoms and functional capacity [3, 4] (Table 1.1).

Medical and device therapy for HF has evolved substantially over the past decade. This has changed the landscape not only towards improved survival and quality of life for all HF patients but also resulted in more appropriate and efficient utilization of advanced HF therapies, including heart transplantation and mechanical support in those with end-stage HF [3]. Unfortunately, significant racial and ethnic disparities persist in both survival and access to care, including access to advanced therapies, with non-Hispanic Black patients having the highest mortality rate [5]. Somewhat counterintuitively, despite improvements in post-myocardial infarction survival and HF therapy, demographic rise in overall life expectancies has contributed to an actual increase in the advanced HF population [6].

Most of the pharmacological therapies discussed below are usually initiated in patients in the earlier stages of HF; however, in the evaluation of patients with advanced HF, we should attempt to maximize any indicated medical and device therapies to stabilize them, which can potentially delay or avoid the need for transplantation. Though approximately half of HF patients have preserved systolic function (HFpEF), those with reduced systolic function—LVEF < 40% (HFrEF)—are generally younger and have fewer comorbidities, comprising the majority of those eligible for transplantation and mechanical circulatory support; consequently, the focus of this discussion will be on HFrEF [3]. However, some patients with HFpEF, including those with refractory arrhythmias or ischemia and restrictive and hypertrophic cardiomyopathies, may also be appropriate transplant candidates.

**Table 1.1** Comparison of classifications of heart failure disease progression and symptoms

| ACC/AHA stages of HF [3] | | NYHA functional classification 2013 [4] | |
|---|---|---|---|
| Stage A: at risk for HF | At risk for HF but without symptoms, structural heart disease, or cardiac biomarkers of stretch or injury | – | |
| Stage B: pre-HF | No symptoms or signs of HF with evidence of 1 of the following<br>– Structural heart disease<br>– Increased filling pressures or<br>– Risk factors and increased levels of biomarkers* | I | No limitation of physical activity. Ordinary physical activity does not cause symptoms of HF |
| Stage C: symptomatic HF | Structural heart disease with current or previous symptoms of HF | I | No limitation of physical activity. Ordinary physical activity does not cause symptoms of HF |
| | | II | Slight limitation of physical activity. Comfortable at rest, but ordinary physical activity results in symptoms of HF |
| | | III | Marked limitation of physical activity. Comfortable at rest, but less than ordinary activity causes symptoms of HF |
| | | IV | Unable to carry on any physical activity without symptoms of HF, or symptoms of HF at rest |
| Stage D: advanced HF | Marked HF symptoms that interfere with daily life and with recurrent hospitalizations despite attempts to optimize GDMT | IV | Unable to carry on any physical activity without symptoms of HF, or symptoms of HF at rest |

* or Persistently elevated cardiac troponin in the absence of competing diagnoses resulting in such biomarker elevations
ACC, indicates American College of Cardiology; AHA, American Heart Association, GDMT, guideline-directed medical therapy; and HF, heart failure, NYHA: New York Heart Association

## Medical Therapy for Heart Failure with Reduced Ejection Fraction HFrEF

The importance of a diligent approach to the prevention of HF in Stage A (risk factors only) and Stage B (structural cardiac disease without HF) patients cannot be overemphasized [3]. For patients who have developed HF symptoms (Stages C and D), our medical therapy has evolved to include diuresis for congestive symptoms and fluid retention, in conjunction with four "pillars of therapy" with Level 1 indications, together referred to as "guideline-directed medical therapy "(GDMT). These include renin-angiotensin system inhibitors, beta-blockers, mineralocorticoid inhibitors (MRA), and, most recently, sodium-glucose cotransporter-2 inhibitors (SGLT2i) (Fig. 1.1).

In addition, lifestyle changes, including smoking cessation, avoidance of alcohol for some patients, healthy diet, as well as increasing exercise and outpatient cardiac rehabilitation programs (Level 1A and 2A indications), can contribute to improved survival, functional capacity, and quality of life [3, 7–9].

One of the major interventions to improve outcomes in HF patients is an emphasis on maximizing the number and target doses of the GDMT. The studies for each element of our therapy have shown the greatest benefit for those achieving target doses [10–22]. There are also registry data demonstrating substantial improvement in outcomes for each additional element. Despite this information, only approximately 40% of outpatients appear to be on each of the appropriate medications, and very few are on target doses of all medications [23]. Though there are individual-specific contraindications to achieving some of these goals (such as renal insufficiency and hypotension), other barriers, such as high cost, poor access to care, and incomplete medication education, need to be addressed to maximize GDMT for all our patients.

From a practical standpoint, in a stable, chronic HF patient, a ladder-type approach with alternating, steady upward titration of each family of medications every 1–2 weeks, with close monitoring of symptoms, vitals, and laboratory studies, can efficiently achieve the optimal regimen. A specialized, multidisciplinary program may facilitate this process for complex patients. Patients with persistent symptoms with minimal activity (NYHA Class III) or at rest (Class IV) despite maximally tolerated GDMT or who demonstrate progressive HF with worsening end-organ damage or intolerance to prior GDMT are classified as Stage D and often labeled "advanced" or "end-stage." Regardless of etiology, stage D HF patients have a high 5-year mortality rate and warrant referral to a specialized center. If the patient fails

**Fig. 1.1** Treatment recommendations for patients with HFrEF are displayed. Step 1 medications may be started simultaneously at initial (low) doses recommended for HFrEF. Alternatively, these medications may be started sequentially, with sequence guided by clinical or other factors, without need to achieve target dosing before initiating next medication. Medication doses should be increased to target as tolerated (Adapted with permission from: Heidenreich et al. 2022). ACEi, indicates angiotensin-converting enzyme inhibitor; ARB, angiotensin receptor blocker; ARNi, angiotensin receptor-neprilysin inhibitor; COR, Class of Recommendation; CRT, cardiac resynchronization therapy; GDMT, guideline-directed medical therapy; ICD, implantable cardioverter-defibrillator; hydral-nitrates, hydralazine and isosorbide dinitrate; HFrEF, heart failure with reduced ejection fraction; LBBB, left bundle branch block; MCS, mechanical circulatory support; LVEF, left ventricular ejection fraction; MRA, mineralocorticoid receptor antagonist; NSR, normal sinus rhythm; NYHA, New York Heart Association; and SGLT2i, sodium-glucose cotransporter 2 inhibitor. as a footnote or in a reference list at the end of your publication, as follows. Reprinted from Journal of the American College of Cardiology, 79 (17), Paul A. Heidenreich, Biykem Bozkurt, David Aguilar, Larry A. Allen, Joni J. Byun, Monica M. Colvin, Anita Deswal, Mark H. Drazner, Shannon M. Dunlay, Linda R. Evers, James C. Fang, Savitri E. Fedson, Gregg C. Fonarow, Salim S. Hayek, Adrian F. Hernandez et al. 2022 AHA/ACC/HFSA Guideline for the Management of Heart Failure A Report of the American College of Cardiology/American Heart Association Joint Committee on Clinical Practice Guidelines, e263–e421. Copyright (2020), with permission from Elsevier ▶

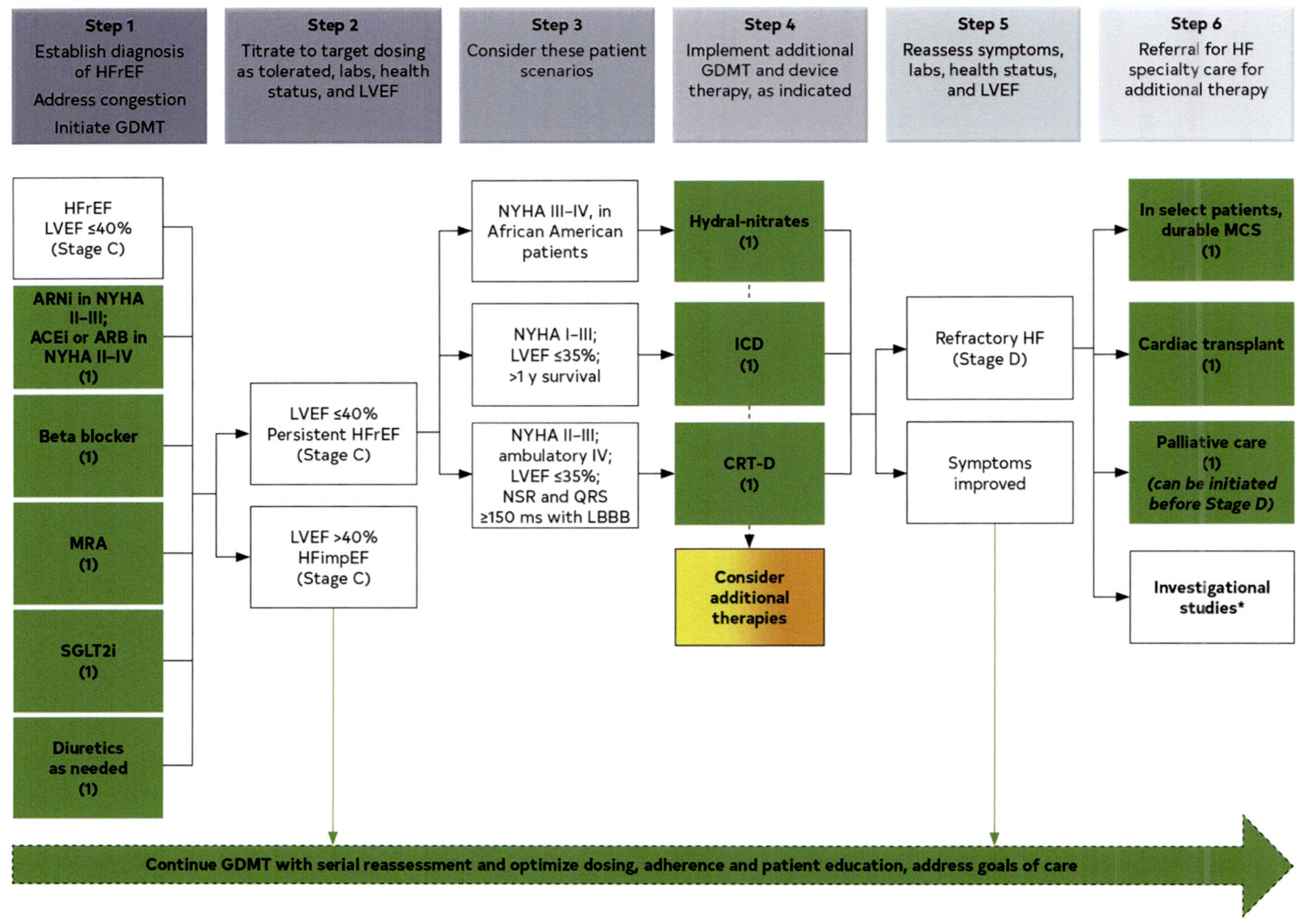
Step 1
Establish diagnosis of HFrEF
Address congestion
Initiate GDMT
Step 2
Titrate to target dosing as tolerated, labs, health status, and LVEF
Step 3
Consider these patient scenarios
Step 4
Implement additional GDMT and device therapy, as indicated
Step 5
Reassess symptoms, labs, health status, and LVEF
Step 6
Referral for HF specialty care for additional therapy
HFrEF LVEF ≤40% (Stage C)
ARNi in NYHA II–III; ACEi or ARB in NYHA II–IV (1)
Beta blocker (1)
MRA (1)
SGLT2i (1)
Diuretics as needed (1)
LVEF ≤40% Persistent HFrEF (Stage C)
LVEF >40% HFimpEF (Stage C)
NYHA III–IV, in African American patients
NYHA I–III; LVEF ≤35%; >1 y survival
NYHA II–III; ambulatory IV; LVEF ≤35%; NSR and QRS ≥150 ms with LBBB
Hydral-nitrates (1)
ICD (1)
CRT-D (1)
Consider additional therapies
Refractory HF (Stage D)
Symptoms improved
In select patients, durable MCS (1)
Cardiac transplant (1)
Palliative care (1) (can be initiated before Stage D)
Investigational studies*
Continue GDMT with serial reassessment and optimize dosing, adherence and patient education, address goals of care

oral medical therapy, the medical treatment may shift to hemodynamically guided therapy with an indwelling pulmonary artery catheter and intravenous vasodilator and/or inotropic agents or possible temporary mechanical devices, in conjunction with evaluation for cardiac transplantation and/or durable mechanical support (see Chaps. 2 and 3). For patients not felt to be appropriate candidates for advanced therapies, palliative options, including home inotropic support or hospice care, may be considered. Palliative and supportive care discussions to assist with symptom management, caregiver support, goals of care, etc. should be incorporated throughout the course of HF illness by all levels of care providers [24].

## Diuretics/Fluid Management

Diuretics, most commonly loop diuretics such as furosemide, bumetinide, and torsemide, are recommended across all HF populations with symptoms and signs of fluid retention and are integral to the care of advanced HF patients. They have a Class 1 indication, with only level of evidence C due to their importance for symptom management and improving exercise tolerance [3], but lack of data demonstrating survival benefit. For patients with right ventricular failure and presumed intraperitoneal fluid and bowel edema, bumetanide and torsemide may have better relative absorption than furosemide. In cases of treatment-refractory fluid overload, loop diuretic effect may be effectively "boosted" when these diuretics are used in combination with a thiazide such as metalazone [25]. In hospitalized patients with refractory fluid overload and worsening hyponatremia, vasopressin antagonists (tolvaptan) may be temporarily effective, but, like the addition of a thiazide diuretic, they have not proven to improve outcomes. Controversy exists regarding the benefit of dietary salt and fluid restriction [26]; in general, salt restriction to less than 2–3 gm/day is felt to be prudent for patients with congestive symptoms (Class 2A recommendation), with fluid restriction reserved for those with more refractory volume management issues [3].

## Renin-Angiotensin Inhibitors: ACE Inhibitors (ACEi), Angiotensin Receptor Blockers (ARB), and Combined ARB/Neprilysin Inhibitors (ARNi)

Angiotensin-converting enzyme inhibitors (ACEi) were considered the first-line treatment for chronic symptomatic heart failure with reduced ejection fraction (NYHA Class II/III), based on studies demonstrating improved survival [19], and ARBs remain a reasonable alternative for ACEi intolerant patients (due to cough or angioedema) [27]. However, the development of the ARNis has changed this paradigm. Sacubitril/valsartan is a combination of a neprilysin inhibitor which reduces breakdown of natriuretic peptides, and an ARB. The sacubitril entity provides additional diuresis and vasodilation (including in the pulmonary circuit). PARADIGM-HF, a randomized trial of sacubitril/valsartan compared to the ACE-inhibitor, enalapril, in HFrEF, showed evidence at 27 months of reduction in a combined endpoint of HF admissions and mortality in the sacubitril/valsartan study arm, with the primary benefit related to reduced hospitalizations [14]. Based on these data and studies showing safety of initiating ARNIs in hospitalized and ACEI -naïve patients [28], ARNIs are now recommended as first line therapy for NYHA Class II/III HFrEF patients (Class1A). It is also recommended that patients on ACEi/ARB should be switched to an ARNi when possible, but there must be at least a 36-h hiatus between doses for any change to/from ARNi and ACEi due to angioedema risk. From a practical standpoint, especially in advanced HF patients, ARNIs may lead to a greater drop in blood pressure due to the additional diuretic and vasodilatory properties, so ACEis and ARBs may be initiated instead in patients with marginal initial blood pressures (less than 90–100 mmHg) or those previously intolerant of an ARNI due to an unacceptable hypotensive response. Blood pressure and renal function must be monitored regularly for any of these medications, and none of them should be used concurrently. Notably, sacubitril/valsartan is contraindicated in patients with any history of angioedema or other adverse reactions to ACEi.

## Beta-Blockers

In combination with ARNIs or ACE inhibitors, beta blockers should be prescribed to all patients with stable heart failure (NYHA II–IV) with reduced ejection fraction. Large, international multicenter trials demonstrated that carvedilol, bisoprolol and metoprolol succinate are effective in reducing the risk of death and combined risk of death or hospitalizations [29]. The COPERNICUS trial specifically demonstrated their safety in the NYHA Class IV population [11]. Initiation of beta-blockers should be avoided in patients with substantial volume overload or on inotropic support within the past 48 h, due to the potential for exacerbating HF in those situations. Carvedilol is considered the first-line betablocker due to an incremental survival benefit over metoprolol in the COMET trial [30]; however, metoprolol, a more cardioselective agent without additional alpha-blockade properties, may be preferrable for patients with relatively low blood pressure or a history of bronchospasm. All betablockers need gradual upward titration to monitor for bradycardia and hypotension, and minimize worsening fatigue symptoms.

## Mineralocorticoid-Receptor Antagonists

Aldosterone-receptor antagonists, including spironolactone and eplerenone, have survival benefit in immediate post-MI patients with HF and LVEF<40% as well as NYHA Class II-IV chronic HFrEF patients, when added to other medical therapy [15, 31]. These agents have only mild diuretic properties with potassium sparing, but their survival benefit is felt to be related to avoidance of adverse remodeling. Renal function must be monitored closely upon initiation and upward titration of MRAs, with concomitant reduction in replacement potassium dosing. MRAs should be avoided in patients with renal insufficiency (eGFR less than 30 mL/min/1.73m2) and hyperkalemia (>5.0 mEq/dl). Patients should also be advised of the approximately 10% risk of breast tenderness and/or gynecomastia.

## SGLT2 Inhibitors

SGLT2i's inhibit glucose reabsorption in the kidney and are known to reduce HF admissions in diabetic patients with cardiovascular disease (or at high risk). More recently, multiple trials, including DAPA-HF and EMPEROR-Reduced, have consistently shown reduction in a combined endpoint of HF admissions and mortality (related primarily to HF hospitalizations) from SGLT2i in symptomatic HF patients, in diabetics and non-diabetics, and across all LVEF groups [32, 33]. Diuretic dosing should usually be reduced and renal function monitored closely when SGLT2i are initiated due to the glucosuria-related diuresis caused by these medications. They should be avoided in patients with eGFR less than 20–30 mL/cc/min/1.73 $m^2$.They often lead to a small rise in creatinine when initiated, but actually provide renal protection over 1 year follow up (34). Hypotension, euglycemic ketoacidosis, and peroneal infections are additional potential risks, but overall consideration has led to a Class 1A indication for the addition of SGLT2i to the other GDMT in all symptomatic HF patients. Thiazolidinediones and DPP-4 inhibitors should be avoided in HF patients [3].

### Hydralazine and Isosorbide Dinitrate

The combination of hydralazine and isosorbide dinitrate (arterial and venodilators respectively) is recommended, in addition to other GDMT, for African Americans with NYHA Class III-IV HFrEF, having demonstrated improved mortality and quality of life in the A-HeFT Trial. The benefit in non-African Americans is unclear, but there is evidence to suggest that these vasodilators are useful in reducing morbidity and mortality in symptomatic HF patients who are unable to tolerate ACEi or ARBs, or those with persistent HF symptoms and adequate blood pressure despite maximal titration of the other GDMT [3].

### Additional Medications

The role of **digoxin** in the care of HF patients has diminished, now with only a 2B indication for symptomatic patients to reduce hospitalizations [3]. Since it has a narrow therapeutic window, with increased mortality at serum levels > 1.0 ng/mL, it should be used cautiously in patients with advanced HF and fluctuating renal function. ***Ivabradine,*** a selective inhibitor of the cardiac pacemaker "funny" current $I_f$ that lowers heart rate without affecting contractility; in a European 6558-patient multicenter study—the SHIFT TRIAL [35], it was found among patients in sinus rhythm with a heart rate > 70 bpm on maximally tolerated beta-blocker dosage to reduce the risk of HF hospitalization. This has led to a 2A recommendation, but it is important that beta blockade dosing has truly been maximized prior to considering Ivabradine. It is not indicated in atrial fibrillation since it only acts on the sinus node and actually increases the risk of de novo atrial fibrillation. ***Vericiguat,*** an oral soluble guanylate cyclase stimulator with vasodilatory properties and potential for fibrosis reduction has a 2B indication for HFrEF patients with worsening HF, based on the VICTORIA trial in which it led to a small reduction in hospitalizations in this high risk population [36]. Its ultimate role for our advanced HF patients is not yet clear. Other medications currently with 2B indications include the **potassium binders** to allow upward titration of ACEi/ARNI/MRA in patients with hyperkalemia, and **Omega-3 PUFA** which showed a 10% reduction in mortality in one trial [37, 38]. Non-dihydropyridine calcium channel blockers (dilitiazem and verapamil) and non-steroidal anti-inflammatory agents should be avoided in HF patients due to risk of worsening symptoms.

## Device Management of Advanced Heart Failure

### Cardiac Resynchronization Therapy

Approximately one-third of HF patients demonstrate substantial prolongation of the QRS interval on ECG, which is associated with dyssynchronous left and right ventricular contractility leading to further increased oxygen demand, LV dilation and reduced contractility, and ultimately worse outcomes [39]. In these patients, left ventricular pacing (termed cardiac resynchronization therapy (CRT) or biventricular pacing) can improve ventricular contractile function, diminish secondary mitral regurgitation, reverse ventricular remodeling, and provide sustained improvement in LVEF [40].

Thus, in patients with reduced LV function (EF ⩽35%), sinus rhythm, left bundle branch block and a QRS width ⩾150 ms, who display NYHA class II, III or ambulatory IV symptoms despite optimal medical treatment, cardiac resynchronization therapy (CRT) is recommended (Class 1A) to improve symptoms and exercise capacity while decreasing hospitalizations and mortality [3]. For those patients who meet all the aforementioned categories except for a shorter QRS width within the 120–149 range, or without a typical LBBB pattern, CRT may also be considered, although evidence for a benefit is less clear

(Class2A and 2B).CRT is also appropriate for those patients with reduced LVEF and >40% RV pacing which can further impair contractility [3]. Importantly, CRT should not be considered a "rescue therapy" and is not indicated for patients who are functionally stage IV and not ambulatory, are requiring inotropic support, or have an expected life-expectancy of <1 year due to comorbidities or frailty.

## Implantable Cardioverter-Defibrillator (ICD)

Patients who have systolic dysfunction are at risk of sudden cardiac death (SCD) due to ventricular tachyarrhythmias. For secondary prevention of SCD, ICD implantation has been demonstrated to reduce mortality in cardiac arrest survivors and in patients with sustained symptomatic ventricular tachyarrhythmias [41]. For primary prevention of SCD in HF patients with optimal pharmacological treatment, guidelines [3] specify a 1A indication for ICD therapy in selected patients with LVEF ⩽35% at least 40 days after myocardial infarction and in patients with ischemic and non-ischemic HF (NYHA class II–III) with LVEF ⩽35% to reduce mortality [42]. ICDs also have a 1A indication for patients with an ischemic cardiomyopathy with LVEF less than 30%, even if asymptomatic. The data supporting primary prevention ICDs is strongest in those with an ischemic etiology. The DANISH Trial demonstrated a reduction in cardiac, but not overall, mortality, in patients with nonischemic cardiomyopathy, which was seen primarily in younger patients [43]. Primary prevention of ICD, therefore, requires shared decision-making on an individual basis for patients with dilated cardiomyopathy and reduced LVEF. ICDs may be considered (2A indication) now for high risk genetic arrhythmogenic cardiomyopathy patients with LVEF as high as 45%, and we can likely anticipate further changes in guidelines for primary prevention as our genetic understanding of cardiomyopathies becomes more refined. Subcutaneous defibrillators rather than transvenous devices may also be considered in younger patients for whom anti tachycardia or bradycardia pacing is not anticipated, avoiding vascular and endocarditis risks [44].

Since many patients with HFrEF have indications for both CRT and ICD, these devices are often implanted together, sharing a generator (CRT-D). Similar to CRT, ICD's should not be implanted in patients with Class IV symptoms and/or predicted survival of less than 1 year. Other implantable electrical devices are under investigation, including baroreceptor and vagal nerve stimulation and His and left bundle pacing [3]. Cardiac contractility modulation, in which an impulse is applied to the RV septal wall during the refractory period to improve contractility, has been FDA approved for Class III HFrEF patients to improve quality of life, but does not yet have positive outcomes data [45]. Class 1C antiarrhythmics and donadrenone should be avoided in HF patients due to increased risk of sudden death and worsening HF.

## Transcatheter Mitral Valve Edge-To-Edge Repair (TEER)

Functional secondary mitral regurgitation (MR) in HF patients can contribute to worsening symptoms, left ventricular dilation and contractility, as well as pulmonary hypertension. In the COAPT Trial [46], patients with LVEF as low as 20%, NYHA Class III symptoms, with persistent severe MR despite maximally tolerated GDMT, had a significant reduction in mortality and hospitalizations after TEER. Of note for the advanced HF population, there was also a reduction in need for cardiac transplantation. A trial of TEER in HF patients with relatively less MR compared to the degree of left ventricular dilation (MITRA-FR) did not show similar benefits, suggesting optimal candidates for the procedure are those with disproportionately more MR [47]. Since functional MR can be dynamic, TEER should only be considered if it remains severe after GDMT has been optimized and CRT performed (if indicated).

## Indwelling Pulmonary Artery Pressure Sensors

The CardioMEMS implanted pulmonary artery (PA) sensor was shown to reduce hospitalizations in Class III HFrEF and HFpEF patients in the Champion Trial [48], but was not confirmed in the Guide-HF Trial [49], leaving this device with a 2B indication. Other remote monitoring devices are being investigated, awaiting the findings.

## Treatment of the Hospitalized Patient with Acute Decompensation

As stated in the guidelines, the goal of treatment for patients hospitalized with decompensated HF (Class 1C indication) should address reversible factors, establish optimal volume status, and advance GDMT toward targets for outpatient therapy. Unless the patient has cardiogenic shock or substantial creatinine rise, withholding GDMT during a hospitalization for decompensated HF may be detrimental, and both initiation and upward titration of GDMT during a HF admission appear to have long-term benefits [50]. Diuresis should be complete and not be withheld for small increases of creatinine (<0.3), as persistent congestion at discharge is a poor prognostic factor. Bedside ultrafiltration and addition of low dose dopamine to iv diuresis have not improved outcomes [51]. Persistent hypotension or hypoperfusion require administration of inotropic support; management of cardiogenic shock is reviewed in Chap. 2.

## References


1. Members WC, Bozkurt B, Ahmad T, Alexander KM, Baker WL, Bosak K, et al. Heart failure epidemiology and outcomes statistics: a report of the Heart Failure Society of America. J Card Fail. 2023;29(10):1412.
2. Tsao CW, Aday AW, Almarzooq ZI, Anderson CAM, Arora P, Avery CL, et al. Heart disease and stroke statistics—2023 update: a report from the American Heart Association. Circulation. 2023;147(8):e93-621.
3. Heidenreich PA, Bozkurt B, Aguilar D, Allen LA, Byun JJ, Colvin MM, et al. 2022 AHA/ACC/HFSA guideline for the management of heart failure: a report of the American College of Cardiology/American Heart Association Joint Committee on Clinical Practice Guidelines. J Am Coll Cardiol. 2022;79(17):e263-421.
4. Yancy CW, Jessup M, Bozkurt B, Butler J, Casey DE, Drazner MH, et al. 2013 ACCF/AHA guideline for the management of heart failure: a report of the American College of Cardiology Foundation/American Heart Association Task Force on Practice Guidelines. J Am Coll Cardiol. 2013;62(16):e147-239.
5. Lewsey SC, Breathett K. Racial and ethnic disparities in heart failure: current state and future directions. Curr Opin Cardiol. 2021;36(3):320–8.
6. Savarese G, Lund LH. Global public health burden of heart failure. Card Fail Rev. 2017;3(1):7.
7. Folsom AR, Shah AM, Lutsey PL, Roetker NS, Alonso A, Avery CL, et al. American Heart Association's Life's Simple 7: avoiding heart failure and preserving cardiac structure and function. Am J Med. 2015;128(9):970–6.
8. Aggarwal M, Bozkurt B, Panjrath G, Aggarwal B, Ostfeld RJ, Barnard ND, et al. Lifestyle modifications for preventing and treating heart failure. J Am Coll Cardiol. 2018;72(19):2391–405.
9. Lara KM, Levitan EB, Gutierrez OM, Shikany JM, Safford MM, Judd SE, et al. Dietary patterns and incident heart failure in US adults without known coronary disease. J Am Coll Cardiol. 2019;73(16):2036–45.
10. Simon T, Mary-Krause M, Funck-Brentano C, Jaillon P. Sex differences in the prognosis of congestive heart failure: results from the Cardiac Insufficiency Bisoprolol Study (CIBIS II). Circulation. 2001;103(3):375–80.
11. Packer M, Fowler MB, Roecker EB, Coats AJS, Katus HA, Krum H, et al. Effect of carvedilol on the morbidity of patients with severe chronic heart failure: results of the carvedilol prospective randomized cumulative survival (COPERNICUS) study. Circulation. 2002;106(17):2194–9.
12. Investigators* S. Effect of enalapril on survival in patients with reduced left ventricular ejection fractions and congestive heart failure. N Engl J Med. 1991;325(5):293–302.
13. Garg R, Yusuf S. for the Collaborative Group on ACE Inhibitor Trials. Overview of randomized trials of angiotensin-converting enzyme inhibitors on mortality and morbidity in patients with heart failure. JAMA. 1995;273(18):1450–6.
14. McMurray JJV, Packer M, Desai AS, Gong J, Lefkowitz MP, Rizkala AR, et al. Angiotensin–neprilysin inhibition versus enalapril in heart failure. N Engl J Med. 2014;371(11):993–1004.
15. Pitt B, Zannad F, Remme WJ, Cody R, Castaigne A, Perez A, et al. The effect of spironolactone on

morbidity and mortality in patients with severe heart failure. N Engl J Med. 1999;341(10):709–17.
16. Zannad F, McMurray JJV, Krum H, van Veldhuisen DJ, Swedberg K, Shi H, et al. Eplerenone in patients with systolic heart failure and mild symptoms. N Engl J Med. 2011;364(1):11–21.
17. McMurray JJV, Solomon SD, Inzucchi SE, Køber L, Kosiborod MN, Martinez FA, et al. Dapagliflozin in patients with heart failure and reduced ejection fraction. N Engl J Med. 2019;381(21):1995–2008.
18. Packer M, Anker SD, Butler J, Filippatos G, Pocock SJ, Carson P, et al. Cardiovascular and renal outcomes with empagliflozin in heart failure. N Engl J Med. 2020;383(15):1413–24.
19. Flather MD, Yusuf S, Køber L, Pfeffer M, Hall A, Murray G, et al. Long-term ACE-inhibitor therapy in patients with heart failure or left-ventricular dysfunction: a systematic overview of data from individual patients. The Lancet. 2000;355(9215):1575–81.
20. Pitt B, Remme W, Zannad F, Neaton J, Martinez F, Roniker B, et al. Eplerenone, a selective aldosterone blocker, in patients with left ventricular dysfunction after myocardial infarction. N Engl J Med. 2003;348(14):1309–21.
21. Cr M. Effect of metoprolol CR/XL in chronic heart failure. Lancet. 1999;353:2001–7.
22. Ezekowitz JA, McAlister FA. Aldosterone blockade and left ventricular dysfunction: a systematic review of randomized clinical trials. Eur Heart J. 2009;30(4):469–77.
23. McCullough PA, Mehta HS, Barker CM, Van Houten J, Mollenkopf S, Gunnarsson C, et al. Mortality and guideline-directed medical therapy in real-world heart failure patients with reduced ejection fraction. Clin Cardiol. 2021;44(9):1192–8.
24. Braun LT, Grady KL, Kutner JS, Adler E, Berlinger N, Boss R, et al. Palliative care and cardiovascular disease and stroke: a policy statement from the American Heart Association/American Stroke Association. Circulation. 2016;134(11):e198-225.
25. Friedrich EB, Böhm M. Management of end stage heart failure. Heart. 2007;93(5):626–31.
26. Mahtani KR, Heneghan C, Onakpoya I, Tierney S, Aronson JK, Roberts N, et al. Reduced salt intake for heart failure: a systematic review. JAMA Intern Med. 2018;178(12):1693–700.
27. McMurray JJV, Östergren J, Swedberg K, Granger CB, Held P, Michelson EL, et al. Effects of candesartan in patients with chronic heart failure and reduced left-ventricular systolic function taking angiotensin-converting-enzyme inhibitors: the CHARM-added trial. The Lancet. 2003;362(9386):767–71.
28. Velazquez EJ, Morrow DA, DeVore AD, Duffy CI, Ambrosy AP, McCague K, et al. Angiotensin–neprilysin inhibition in acute decompensated heart failure. N Engl J Med. 2019;380(6):539–48.
29. Brophy JM, Joseph L, Rouleau JL. β-Blockers in congestive heart failure: a Bayesian meta-analysis. Ann Intern Med. 2001;134(7):550–60.
30. Poole-Wilson PA, Swedberg K, Cleland JGF, Di Lenarda A, Hanrath P, Komajda M, et al. Comparison of carvedilol and metoprolol on clinical outcomes in patients with chronic heart failure in the Carvedilol Or Metoprolol European Trial (COMET): randomised controlled trial. The Lancet. 2003;362(9377):7–13.
31. Pitt B, Remme W, Zannad F ft, Neaton J, Martinez F, Roniker B, et al. Eplerenone post-acute myocardial infarction heart failure efficacy and survival study investigators. Eplerenone, a selective aldosterone blocker, in patients with left ventricular dysfunction after myocardial infarction. 2003.
32. Zannad F, Ferreira JP, Pocock SJ, Anker SD, Butler J, Filippatos G, et al. SGLT2 inhibitors in patients with heart failure with reduced ejection fraction: a meta-analysis of the EMPEROR-reduced and DAPA-HF trials. The Lancet. 2020;396(10254):819–29.
33. Butler J, Packer M, Filippatos G, Ferreira JP, Zeller C, Schnee J, et al. Effect of empagliflozin in patients with heart failure across the spectrum of left ventricular ejection fraction. Eur Heart J. 2022;43(5):416–24.
34. Zelniker TA, Braunwald E. Mechanisms of cardiorenal effects of sodium-glucose cotransporter 2 inhibitors: JACC state-of-the-art review. J Am Coll Cardiol. 2020;75(4):422–34.
35. Swedberg K, Komajda M, Böhm M, Borer JS, Ford I, Dubost-Brama A, et al. Ivabradine and outcomes in chronic heart failure (SHIFT): a randomised placebo-controlled study. The Lancet. 2010;376(9744):875–85.
36. Armstrong PW, Pieske B, Anstrom KJ, Ezekowitz J, Hernandez AF, Butler J, et al. Vericiguat in patients with heart failure and reduced ejection fraction. N Engl J Med. 2020;382(20):1883–93.
37. Tavazzi L, Maggioni AP, Marchioli R, Barlera S, Franzosi MG, Latini R, et al. Effect of n-3 polyunsaturated fatty acids in patients with chronic heart failure (the GISSI-HF trial): a randomised, double-blind, placebo-controlled trial. Lancet. 2008;372(9645):1223–30.
38. Pitt B, Anker SD, Bushinsky DA, Kitzman DW, Zannad F, Huang IZ. Evaluation of the efficacy and safety of RLY5016, a polymeric potassium binder, in a double-blind, placebo-controlled study in patients with chronic heart failure (the PEARL-HF) trial. Eur Heart J. 2011;32(7):820–8.
39. Young JB, Abraham WT, Smith AL, Leon AR, Lieberman R, Wilkoff B, et al. Combined cardiac resynchronization and implantable cardioversion defibrillation in advanced chronic

heart failure: the MIRACLE ICD trial. JAMA. 2003;289(20):2685–94.

40. Bristow MR, Saxon LA, Boehmer J, Krueger S, Kass DA, De Marco T, et al. Cardiac-resynchronization therapy with or without an implantable defibrillator in advanced chronic heart failure. N Engl J Med. 2004;350(21):2140–50.
41. Lee DS, Green LD, Liu PP, Dorian P, Newman DM, Grant FC, et al. Effectiveness of implantable defibrillators for preventing arrhythmic events and death: a meta-analysis. J Am Coll Cardiol. 2003;41(9):1573–82.
42. Bardy GH, Lee KL, Mark DB, Poole JE, Packer DL, Boineau R, et al. Amiodarone or an implantable cardioverter–defibrillator for congestive heart failure. N Engl J Med. 2005;352(3):225–37.
43. Køber L, Thune JJ, Nielsen JC, Haarbo J, Videbæk L, Korup E, et al. Defibrillator implantation in patients with nonischemic systolic heart failure. N Engl J Med. 2016;375(13):1221–30.
44. Al-Khatib SM, Stevenson WG, Ackerman MJ, Bryant WJ, Callans DJ, Curtis AB, et al. 2017 AHA/ACC/HRS guideline for management of patients with ventricular arrhythmias and the prevention of sudden cardiac death: a report of the American College of Cardiology/American Heart Association Task Force on Clinical Practice Guidelines and the Heart Rhythm Society. J Am Coll Cardiol. 2018;72(14):e91-220.
45. Abraham WT, Kuck KH, Goldsmith RL, Lindenfeld J, Reddy VY, Carson PE, et al. A randomized controlled trial to evaluate the safety and efficacy of cardiac contractility modulation. Heart Fail. 2018;6(10):874–83.
46. Stone GW, Lindenfeld J, Abraham WT, Kar S, Lim DS, Mishell JM, et al. Transcatheter mitral-valve repair in patients with heart failure. N Engl J Med. 2018;379(24):2307–18.
47. Grayburn PA, Sannino A, Packer M. Proportionate and disproportionate functional mitral regurgitation: a new conceptual framework that reconciles the results of the MITRA-FR and COAPT trials. JACC Cardiovasc Imaging. 2019;12(2):353–62.
48. Givertz MM, Stevenson LW, Costanzo MR, Bourge RC, Bauman JG, Ginn G, et al. Pulmonary artery pressure-guided management of patients with heart failure and reduced ejection fraction. J Am Coll Cardiol. 2017;70(15):1875–86.
49. Lindenfeld J, Zile MR, Desai AS, Bhatt K, Ducharme A, Horstmanshof D, et al. Haemodynamic-guided management of heart failure (GUIDE-HF): a randomised controlled trial. The Lancet. 2021;398(10304):991–1001.
50. Tran RH, Aldemerdash A, Chang P, Sueta CA, Kaufman B, Asafu-adjei J, et al. Guideline-directed medical therapy and survival following hospitalization in patients with heart failure. Pharmacother J Hum Pharmacol Drug Therapy. 2018;38(4):406–16.
51. Wan SH, Stevens SR, Borlaug BA, Anstrom KJ, Deswal A, Felker GM, et al. Differential response to low-dose dopamine or low-dose nesiritide in acute heart failure with reduced or preserved ejection fraction: results from the ROSE AHF Trial (Renal Optimization Strategies Evaluation in Acute Heart Failure). Circ Heart Fail. 2016;9(8):e002593.

# Mechanical and Surgical Options for Patients with End-Stage Heart Failure

2

Robert M. Cole, Jaime D. Moriguchi, and Yosef Manla

**Abstract**

While the introduction of novel heart failure (HF) therapeutics has improved the quality of life and survival in advanced HF patients, overall morbidity and mortality are still high. Patients with refractory end-stage HF may ultimately require either short or long-term mechanical circulatory support (MCS) or heart transplantation. Once the patient is deemed to have advanced HF and likely to benefit from advanced therapies, the optimal strategy for implantation should include selecting the most appropriate MCS device with the best durability and lowest incidence of adverse events and which provides adequate cardiac output for either one or both failing ventricles. This chapter provides an overview of the current indications and outcomes of MCS devices used in patients with advanced HF.

R. M. Cole (✉) · J. D. Moriguchi · Y. Manla
Cedars-Sinai Smidt Heart Institute, Los Angeles, CA, USA
e-mail: Robert.Cole@cshs.org

J. D. Moriguchi
e-mail: MoriguchiJ@csmns.org

Y. Manla
e-mail: Yosef.manla@cshs.org; Yosef.manla1@gmail.com

**Keywords**

Heart failure · Mechanical circulatory support · Ventricular assist devices · Heart transplantation

## Clinical Pearls

- General indications for referral for advanced heart failure therapies include left ventricular ejection fraction ≤ 25%, persistent New York Heart Association class III or IV symptoms, recurrent atrial fibrillation or ventricular tachycardia with implantable cardioverter defibrillator shocks, and inotrope dependence.
- Patient selection for mechanical circulatory support should be a multidisciplinary decision involving advanced heart failure/transplantation cardiologists, cardiothoracic surgeons, nurses, social workers, and palliative care clinicians, amongst others.
- Ventricular assist devices may be used as bridge-to-transplant, bridge-to-candidacy, bridge-to-recovery, or as a destination therapy.
- Relative contraindications to left ventricular assist device implantation include acute cardiogenic shock with uncertain neurological status, active severe bleeding, uncontrolled systemic infection, severe right ventricular



J. Kobashigawa (ed.), *Clinical Guide to Heart Transplantation*, https://doi.org/10.1007/978-3-031-88290-6_2

dysfunction, severe uncorrected aortic insufficiency or mechanical aortic valve.

- The INTERMACS profile is useful for perioperative risk assessment and stratification for future outcomes post-implant, including mortality and complications. INTERMACS 1–3 may be considered for bridge-to-transplant or destination therapy using a durable, long-term continuous flow device.
- Mechanical circulatory support device-related adverse events include device thrombosis, driveline infection, stroke, and gastrointestinal bleeding.
- Short-term mechanical circulatory support methods are indicated in the setting of acute refractory cardiogenic shock, including intra-aortic balloon pump, Impella, TandemHeart and veno-arterial extracorporeal membrane oxygenation support.

## Introduction

While the introduction of novel heart failure (HF) therapeutics has improved the quality of life and survival in advanced HF patients, overall morbidity and mortality are still high [1]; refractory end-stage HF patients may ultimately require either short or long-term mechanical circulatory support (MCS) or heart transplantation (HTx) [1, 2]. The paucity of available donor hearts and the prevalence of significant comorbidities, which may be contraindications to transplantation, has led to the increasing use of MCS devices [3]. Furthermore, patients with advanced HF considered too unstable to await a suitable donor organ may require univentricular or biventricular ventricular assist devices as bridge-to-transplantation therapy, and have been shown to improve quality of life, survival-to-transplantation rates, and post-transplant survival [4, 5].

Numerous clinical clues can help identify patients with advanced HF and trigger consideration of referral for evaluation of advanced therapies, including but not limited to inotrope dependence, left ventricular ejection fraction ≤ 25%, persistent New York Heart Association class III or IV symptoms, and recurrent atrial fibrillation or ventricular tachycardia with implantable cardioverter defibrillator shocks (Table 2.1) [6]. Generally, patient selection for MCS should be a multidisciplinary decision involving advanced HF/transplantation cardiologists, cardiothoracic surgeons, advanced practice providers, nurses, social workers, and palliative care clinicians, amongst others. Once the patient is determined to have advanced HF, the likelihood of benefit from referral to advanced therapies should also be assessed. For instance, advanced therapies could be less beneficial in patients whose goal of care is to avoid a multipart medical or surgical regimen, as well as in those with a severely limited lifespan or functional status due to other non-cardiac conditions [6]. Contemporary MCS includes both temporary and durable (long-term) forms. Durable support primarily consists of ventricular assist devices (VADs) and total artificial hearts (TAHs), the latter of which will be discussed in Chap. 28. Overall, the optimal strategy for implantation should include selecting the most appropriate MCS device with the best durability and lowest incidence of adverse events and which provides adequate cardiac output for either one or both failing ventricles. This chapter provides an overview of MCS devices and indications for their usage in end-stage HF patients.

## Ventricular Assist Device Categories: A Generational History

More than 50 years ago, the first successful VAD was implanted by Dr. Michael DeBakey with the aim of acting as a bridge to cardiac recovery [8]. VADs are mechanical circulatory pumps that partially or completely take over ventricular function in order to assist systemic circulation and improve end-organ perfusion. A VAD may be used as a left ventricular (LVAD), right ventricular (RVAD), or as a biventricular assist device (BiVAD).

Initially introduced in the 1980s, the first generation of long-term LVADs consisted of large para-corporeal devices such as the

**Table 2.1** Clinical clues to help identify patients with advanced HF

| |
|---|
| • Inotrope dependence |
| • LVEF ≤ 25%, particularly with high-risk features on echocardiogram (grade III or IV diastolic dysfunction; significant RV dysfunction; high pulmonary artery pressures or severe MR despite attempts at decongestion) |
| • ≥2 Hospitalizations or emergency department visits for decompensated HF in 12 month |
| • Persistent NYHA class III or IV symptoms, including fatigue and confusion |
| • High-risk biomarker profile (e.g., hyponatremia, very elevated natriuretic peptides or troponin) |
| • Escalating doses of diuretics (e.g., >160 mg/d furosemide) or persistent edema despite escalating diuretic doses |
| • Down titration of GDMT as a result of hemodynamic intolerance such as hypotension (SBP < 90 mm Hg), dizziness, excessive fatigue, or nausea |
| • Discontinuation of ACE inhibitor/ARB/ARNI because of hypotension or renal intolerance |
| • Progressive renal failure with rising creatinine/BUN |
| • Recurrent atrial fibrillation or VT with ICD shocks |
| • Nonresponse to cardiac resynchronization therapy |
| • Cardiac cachexia (i.e., unintentional loss of >5% of body weight attributable to HF) |
| • High mortality risk from validated risk prediction models or calculators |

ACE indicates angiotensin-converting enzyme; ARB, angiotensin II receptor blocker; ARNI, angiotensin receptor–neprilysin inhibitor; BUN, blood urea nitrogen; GDMT, guideline-directed medical therapy; HF, heart failure; ICD, implantable cardioverter defibrillator; LVEF, left ventricular ejection fraction; MR, mitral regurgitation; NYHA, New York Heart Association; RV, right ventricular; SBP, systolic blood pressure; and VT, ventricular tachycardia. Reprinted with permission: Alanna A. Morris, Prateeti Khazanie, Mark H. Drazner, Nancy M. Albert, et al., Guidance for Timely and Appropriate Referral of Patients With Advanced Heart Failure: A Scientific Statement From the American Heart Association, Circulation, 144 (7), e238–e250. https://doi.org/10.1161/CIR.0000000000001016; American Heart Association

Thoratec PVAD and Abiomed BVS 5000 (and subsequently the AB 5000). Intracorporeal devices included the HeartMate I IP/VE (Thoratec Inc., Pleasanton, California, USA) and the Novacor N100 (WorldHeart Inc., Salt Lake City, Utah, USA). All of these functioned on the basis of pulsatile systemic perfusion, otherwise known as "pulsatile-flow" devices. However, their bulkiness, lack of durability, and proclivity to malfunction and complications meant that patients were often bedridden and had less than optimal outcomes, including high stroke rates [9]. Subsequent miniaturization of the control and power-supply components resulted in smaller versions of these first-generation pulsatile VADs that could be implanted intra-abdominally [10, 11]. While these enabled patients to mobilize, these devices still remained restricted to patients with a large body surface area; device failure rates remained high, infections continued to be problematic, and durability remained poor [12].

The second generation of LVADs consisted of smaller, continuous axial flow pump systems that allowed considerably less extensive surgery (thus reducing the risk of complications, see Fig. 2.1) and conferred improved durability, the ability to use in a wider range of patients due to smaller size, and reduced thrombogenicity. The increase in durability arose in part from the fact that there was only one moving part. The prototypic second-generation LVAD is the HeartMate II (HM II; Thoratec Inc., Pleasanton, California, USA) (Fig. 2.2). Second-generation VADs successfully demonstrated superior survival and less organ failure in patients when compared to patients on first-generation pulsatile VADs. The 1-year survival for these more modern devices has been reported at 81% for bridge-to-transplantation and 73% for destination therapy [13, 14], which was significantly improved from the first generation of LVADs. Furthermore, the introduction of continuous flow devices led to significantly improved quality of life, general

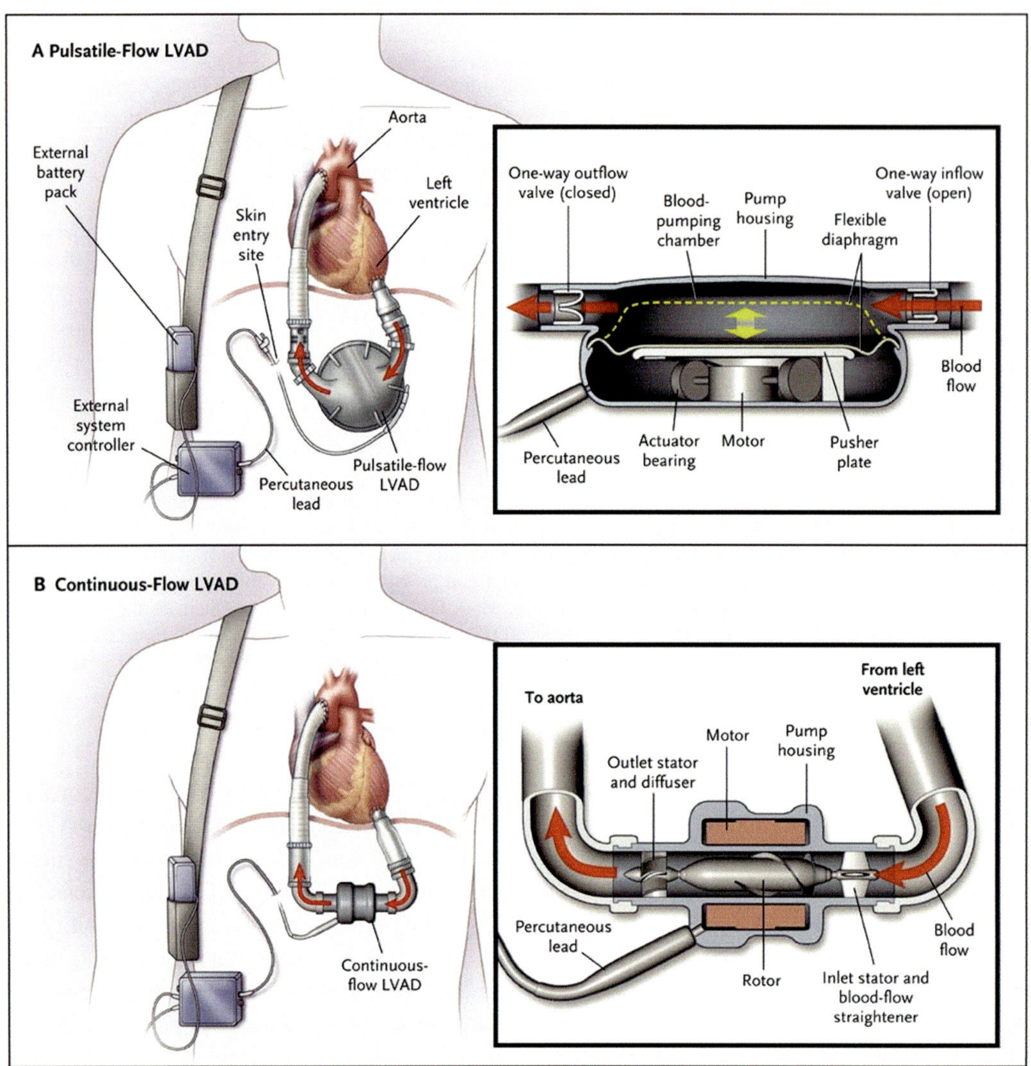


**Fig. 2.1** A visual overview of left ventricular assist devices (LVAD). Panel **a** shows a first-generation pulsatile flow left ventricular assist device (LVAD). Panel **b** shows a second-generation continuous flow LVAD. Both mechanical pumps are placed in the abdominal wall. The inflow cannula of the LVAD is placed in the apex of the left ventricle. The outflow cannula is subsequently anastamosed with the ascending aorta. A percutaneous lead connects the LVAD pump with an external system controller and the battery pack. From [The New England Journal of Medicine, Mark S. Slaughter, Joseph G. Rogers, Carmelo A. Milano, et al., Advanced Heart Failure Treated with Continuous-Flow Left Ventricular Assist Device, 361 (16), 2241–2251, Copyright © (2009) Massachusetts Medical. Reprinted with permission from Massachusetts Medical Society

well-being, and ability to perform self-care post-LVAD implantation [14, 15]. This improvement meant that LVAD patients were able to engage in daily life as outpatients relatively unperturbed.

The subsequent and most contemporary third generation of LVADs have sought to further refine the continuous-flow concept, typically utilizing centrifugal rather than axial flow through the device. There have also been continued improvements in pump technology to optimize hemocompatibility and minimize adverse events through the development of hydrodynamic or magnetic levitation technology and programmed pulsatility. Furthermore,

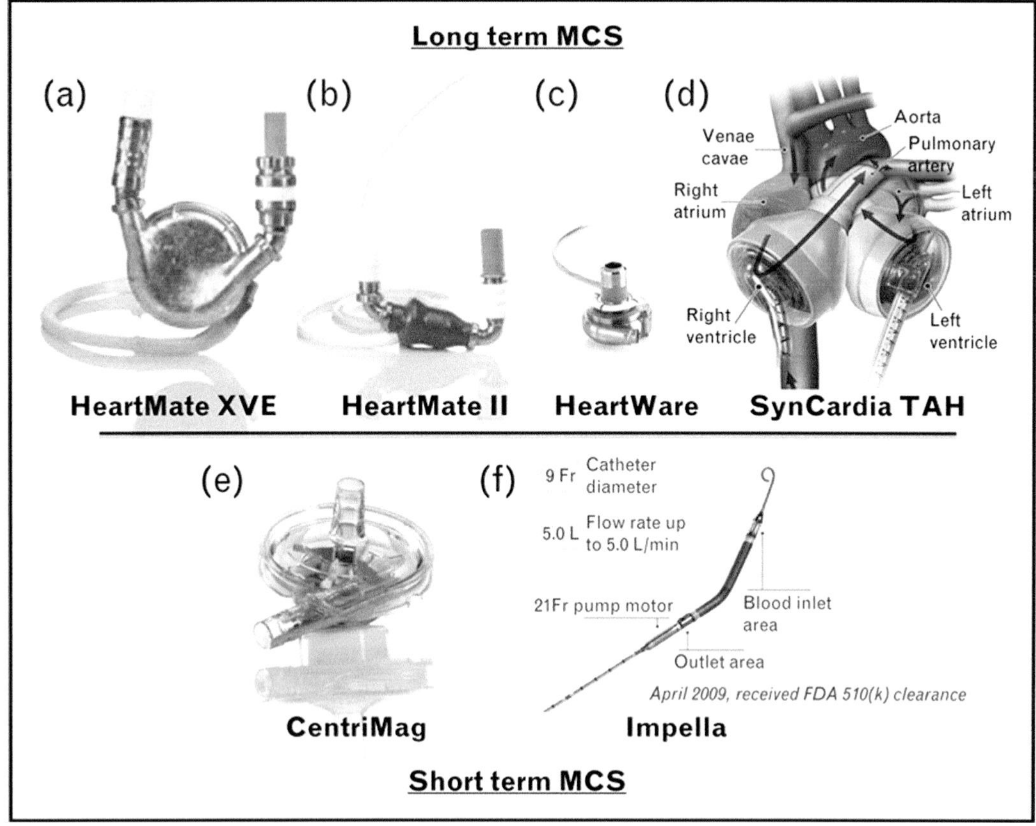


**Fig. 2.2** Overview of commonly used mechanical circulatory support devices. First-generation device **a** Thoratec HeartMate XVE: pulsatile flow LVAD (left ventricular assist device) (reprinted with the permission of Thoratec Incorporation). Second-generation LVAD **b** Thoratec HeartMate II (reprinted with the permission of Thoratec Incorporation). Third-generation LVAD **c** HeartWare HVAD (reprinted with the permission of HeartWare). Approved TAH **d** SynCardia CardioWest TAH (courtesy: SynCardia.com). Short-term MCS devices with **e** Levitronix CentriMag extracorporeal RVAD (reprinted with the permission of Thoratec Incorporation), and the **f** AbioMed Impella 5.0 (reprinted with the permission of Abiomed). RVAD, right ventricular assist device; TAH, total artificial heart. Reprinted with permission from Hadi Toeg, Talal Al-Atassi, Jose Garcia, et al., An update on mechanical circulatory support for heart failure therapy, Current Opinion in Cardiology, 29, 2, 167–173; https://doi.org/10.1097/hco.0000000000000037

smaller pumps can be implanted within the pericardium, thus further reducing postoperative complications. The most prominent examples of third-generation LVADs include the HeartWare HVAD centrifugal pump (HeartWare International Inc., Framingham, Massachusetts, USA) (Fig. 2.1) and the HeartMate 3 LVAD (Abbott, St Paul, MN, USA). However, it should be noted that the HeartWare LVAD system has been discontinued due to significant adverse events and inferior clinical outcomes [7].

The five-year follow-up to the MOMENTUM 3 trial evaluated the composite endpoints of survival to transplant, cardiac recovery, or LVAD support free of debilitating stroke or need for reoperation to replace the pump by comparing patients who had received HeartMate II and HeartMate 3 LVAD devices. The 5-year Kaplan–Meier estimate of these endpoints was 54.0% in the HeartMate 3 group versus 29.7% in the HeartMate II group. Furthermore, serious adverse events, including stroke, bleeding,

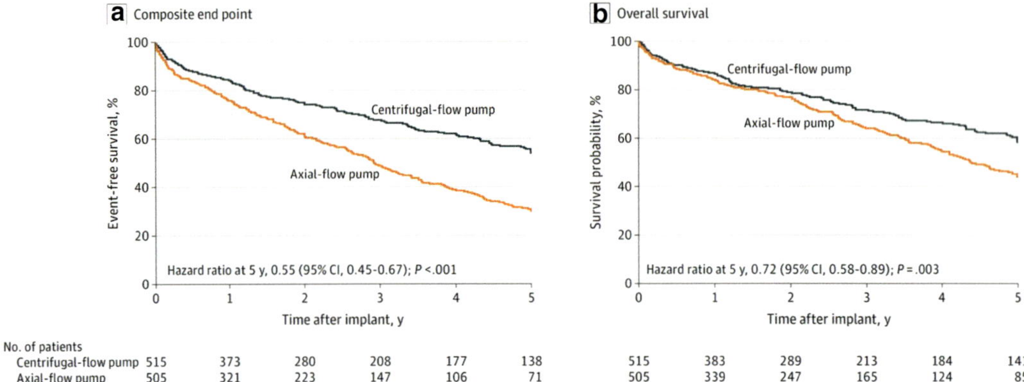


**Fig. 2.3** composite end point and overall survival in a study of 5-year outcomes in patients with fully magnetically levitated versus axial-flow left ventricular assist devices. Reproduced with permission from [JAMA. 2022. 328 (13): 1233–1242. doi: https://doi.org/10.1001/jama.2022.16197]. 

and pump thrombosis, were found to occur less frequently in the centrifugal flow (HeartMate 3) LVAD group (Fig. 2.3) [17]. At the time of this writing, the HeartMate 3 LVAD system is indicated as a bridge to transplantation or myocardial recovery or as destination (long-term) therapy.

## Total Artificial Heart (TAH)

As an emerging alternative to VADs in patients with biventricular failure or anatomy unsuitable for univentricular support, TAHs will be discussed in Chap. 28

## Trends in Ventricular Assist Device Use: Strategies and Outcomes

Ventricular assist devices are typically intended for use as either short or long-term therapy. Short-term therapy refers to utilization as a bridge-to-transplant or stabilization of the patient with an anticipated possibility of future listing for transplant, known as bridge-to-candidacy. It can also refer to utilization as a possible bridge to cardiac recovery. Long-term therapy is also known as destination therapy and refers to patients in whom a HTx is not intended in the future; thus, the VAD is the terminal treatment. It is important to note that patients who receive VAD therapy may subsequently shift between short and long-term therapy categorizations depending on clinical outcomes and transplant candidacy, which may alter future intentions, particularly as survival in destination therapy has improved (Fig. 2.4) [18, 19].

In rare cases (<5% of implants), LVADs have acted as a bridge to myocardial recovery, the theory being that unloading of the ventricle leads to reverse ventricular remodeling and subsequent functional improvement [20], in combination with time and administration of optimal guideline-directed medical therapies. While this appears more likely to occur in myocarditis and other recoverable etiologies of HF, there are currently no reliable parameters with which to predict those patients who will demonstrate substantial myocardial recovery.

The Interagency Registry for Mechanically Assisted Circulatory Support (INTERMACS) represents the largest registry of MCS device utilization in the world, with more than 150 participating hospitals across the US and Canada. Its purpose is to collect MCS-related data and assess trends in survival, device strategy, and risk factors for poor outcomes. The most recent

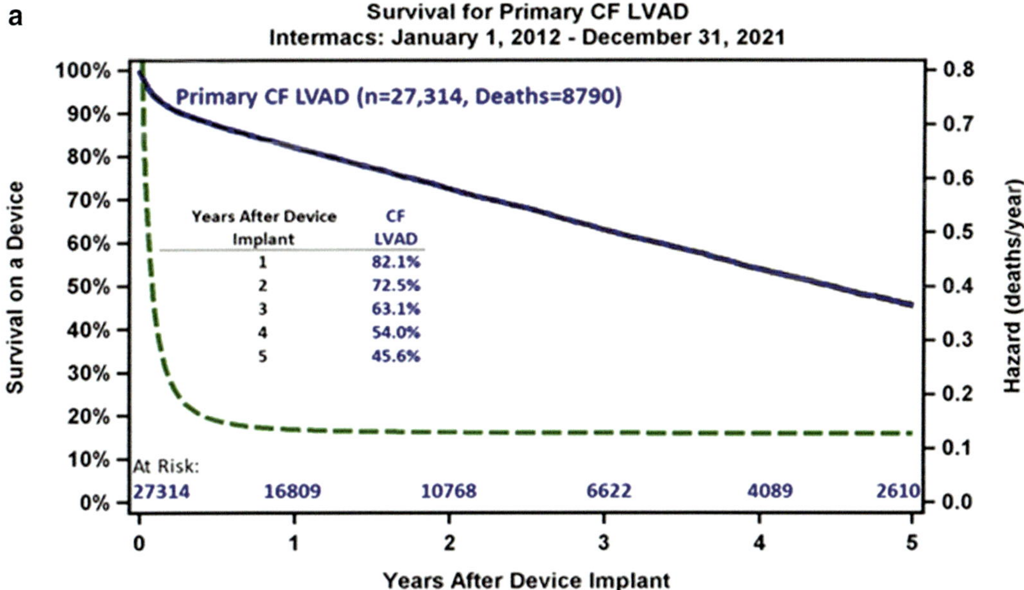


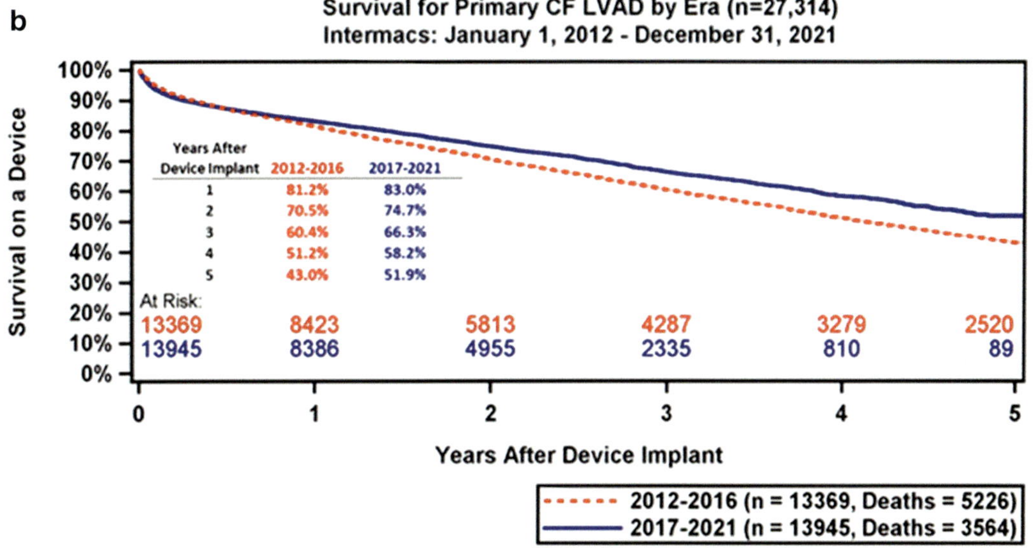


**Fig. 2.4** Kaplan–Meier survival analysis for all patients and by continuous flow left ventricular assist device (CF LVAD) era. **a** Kaplan–Meier estimated survival after CF LVAD implantation for the past decade. Hazard rates are depicted by dashed red line. **b** The estimated survival is compared between the previous era (2012–2016) and the current era (2017–2021). Intermacs, Interagency Registry for Mechanically Assisted Circulatory Support. Reprinted from The Annals of Thoracic Surgery, 115 (2), Melana Yuzefpolskaya, Sarah E. Schroeder, Brian A. Houston, Monique R. Robinson, Igor Gosev, Alex Reyentovich, Devin Koehl, Ryan Cantor, Ulrich P. Jorde, J ames K. Kirklin, Francis D. Pagani, David A. D'Alessandro, The Society of Thoracic Surgeons Intermacs 2022 Annual Report: Focus on the 2018 Heart Transplant Allocation System, 311–327., Copyright (2023), with permission from Elsevier

INTERMACS 2022 annual report highlights MCS data from 2012 to 2022, including outcomes data for 27,314 patients who have undergone continuous flow LVAD therapy [18]. Of note, the 1-year and 5-year survival of patients who underwent LVAD implantation between 2017 and 2021 was 83.0 and 51.9%, respectively. This improvement from the prior decade is likely multifactorial and likely reflects improvement in device technology, patient selection, and patient management [18]. In recent years, with the growing development and improvement of temporary MCS devices as a bridge to transplant in combination with changes in the US HTx allocation system in 2018, there has been an overall decline in utilization of short-term (bridge-to-transplant) LVADs, with destination-therapy devices being the predominantly intended implant strategy, representing 81.1% of implants in 2021 compared to 56.5% in 2018 [18].

## Contraindications to LVAD Insertion

Relative, but not absolute contraindications to LVAD insertion include acute cardiogenic shock with uncertain neurological status, active severe bleeding (as patients on VAD require anticoagulation), active uncontrolled systemic infection, severe right ventricular dysfunction, severe uncorrected aortic insufficiency or mechanical aortic valve that will not be converted to a bioprosthesis [12]. Furthermore, patients who would be unable to physically operate their pump and would not respond to device alarms may also be considered unsuitable candidates [21]. Irreversible end-organ damage other than cardiac also poses a potential contraindication to VAD therapy. An inability to take anticoagulant therapy is an absolute contraindication to LVAD support. Management guidelines for LVAD patients are continually being updated and assessed, with increasing numbers of centers reporting their data [15, 21]; as such, it is anticipated that these contraindications will change with improvements in LVAD technology, surgical methods, and postoperative management.

## INTERMACS Profile and Risk Factors for Mortality Post-Implant

The INTERMACS profile [22] assigns patients with advanced HF into seven different classifications according to clinical status, hemodynamic profile, and level of end-organ damage (Table 2.2). The lower the number, the more gravely ill the patient; for example, an INTERMACS 1 patient will demonstrate hemodynamic instability and cardiogenic shock despite increased inotropic doses and/or MCS; in contrast, an INTERMACS 7 patient is a functional, ambulatory NYHA class IIIa patient with no fluid overload. Such a scale was designed for the purposes of perioperative risk prediction and stratification for future outcomes post-implant, including mortality and complications. The major risk factors for mortality following continuous-flow device implantation include patients on hemodialysis, patients who represent INTERMACS 1 and 2 levels at the time of LVAD implant, advanced age, history of stroke, previous ICD placement, increased bilirubin and requirement for RVAD implant in the same operation [18].

## Potential Adverse Events with Left Ventricular Assist Devices

The most common adverse events after LVAD therapy include stroke, bleeding, infection, device malfunction, arrhythmia, and renal dysfunction. In the contemporary era of LVAD therapy, major adverse events typically occur most frequently in the first 90 days from LVAD implantation, except for MCS-related infection, which typically occurs after the first 90 days. Fortunately, the most recent era of LVAD support (2017–2021) has shown significant improvement in rates of adverse events when compared to the prior era. More specifically, 1-year freedom from gastrointestinal bleeding improved from 74.9 to 82.1%, and 1-year freedom from device malfunction/pump thrombosis improved from 80.7 to 92.9%. 1-year freedom from a first stroke has improved to 88.7% [18].

**Table 2.2** INTERMACS (Interagency Registry for Mechanically Assisted Circulatory Support) scale for classifying patients with advanced heart failure

| Profiles | Definition | Description |
|---|---|---|
| INTERMACS 1 | *Crash and burn* | Hemodynamic instability in spite of increasing doses of catecholamines and/or mechanical circulatory support with critical hypoperfusion of target organs (severe cardiogenic shock) |
| INTERMACS 2 | *Sliding on inotropes* | Intravenous inotropic support with acceptable blood pressure but rapid deterioration of kidney function, nutritional state, or signs of congestion |
| INTERMACS 3 | *Dependent stability* | Hemodynamic stability with low or intermediate, but necessary due to hypotension, doses of inotropics, worsening of symptoms, or progressive kidney failure |
| INTERMACS 4 | *Frequent flyer* | Temporary cessation of inotropic treatment is possible, but the patient presents frequent symptom recurrences and typically with fluid overload |
| INTERMACS 5 | *Housebound* | Complete cessation of physical activity, stable at rest, but frequently with moderate water retention and some level of kidney dysfunction |
| INTERMACS 6 | *Walking wounded* | Minor limitation on physical activity and absence of congestion while at rest. Easily fatigued by light activity |
| INTERMACS 7 | *Placeholder* | Patient in NYHA functional class II or III with no current or recent unstable water balance |

Reprinted from The Journal of Heart and Lung Transplantation, 28 (6), Lynne Warner Stevenson, Francis D. Pagani, James B. Young, Mariell Jessup, Leslie Miller, Robert L. Kormos, David C. Naftel, Karen Ulisney, Patrice Desvigne-Nickens, James K. Kirklin, INTERMACS Profiles of Advanced Heart Failure: The Current Picture, 535–541, Copyright (2009), with permission from Elsevier

Despite the improved morbidity and adverse event profile in the modern era of third generation LVADs, rehospitalization rates still remain high, with one study demonstrating an average of $1.64 \pm 1.97$ admissions per patient-year follow-up [23]. The most common reasons for readmission are infection and gastrointestinal bleeding resulting from anticoagulation.

## Left Ventricular Assist Device Selection

Ventricular assist device selection is generally tailored according to the patient's expectations and clinical status, using a multidisciplinary approach. Hemodynamically stable patients who are typically classified as INTERMACS 1–3 may be considered for bridge-to-transplant or destination therapy using a durable, long-term continuous flow device such as those already mentioned. However, in the hemodynamically unstable or deteriorating patient (i.e., INTERMACS 1 or 2), short-term MCS therapy should be immediately considered (see next section). Such a measure provides the patient with essential circulation and allows the medical team more time to optimize clinical status, perform neurologic assessment, and decide on further management (LVAD, transplant, etc.). Pertinently, in regard to the timing of assist device therapy, reports have shown that the survival of patients undergoing bridge-to-transplantation therapy is improved when assist devices are implanted electively, as compared to implantations for urgent or emergency indications [16]. Of note, there may be a further benefit from the implantation of LVAD therapy in patients who are INTERMACS profile 4 when compared to the continuation of optimal medical therapy, as seen in the 2-year follow-up to the ROADMAP trial [24].

## Short-Term Options for Mechanical Circulatory Support

### Intra-Aortic Balloon Pump

The intra-aortic balloon pump is a mechanical device that increases myocardial oxygen perfusion while simultaneously increasing cardiac output and decreasing afterload. Typically inserted via the femoral artery, it consists of a cylindrical polyethylene balloon that sits in the aorta, approximately 2 cm (0.79 in) from the left subclavian artery and counter pulsates. This method is often used as the first mechanical support treatment in efforts to improve coronary perfusion in the setting of refractory cardiogenic shock. Absolute contraindications include severe aortic valve insufficiency and severe aortic pathology, including dissection, while relative contraindications include aortic aneurysm and the presence of any aortic vascular grafts. Possible complications include ischemic leg, cerebral embolism, aortic dissection, and mediastinal bleeding.

### Extracorporeal Membrane Oxygenation

Veno-arterial extracorporeal membrane oxygenation (VA-ECMO) is a rapid mode of emergency biventricular support typically used as a last resort salvage therapy in the setting of cardiogenic shock, where implanting durable mechanical device is not possible/feasible (Fig. 2.5). Acting essentially as a form of cardiopulmonary bypass, VA-ECMO provides excellent hemodynamic support via a non-pulsatile (often centrifugal) pump connected in-line to a membrane oxygenator that receives blood via inflow venous cannulas, commonly inserted into the femoral vein, and which returns oxygenated blood via an outflow arterial cannula, commonly inserted into the femoral artery. Survival rates in refractory cardiogenic shock patients with ECMO vary by clinical indication, with survival to discharge varying from 39 to 80% [25, 26]. The main disadvantages of ECMO are the relative lack of durability (mean of 4 days), the inability to unload the left ventricle, and the potential hemocompatibility issues, including

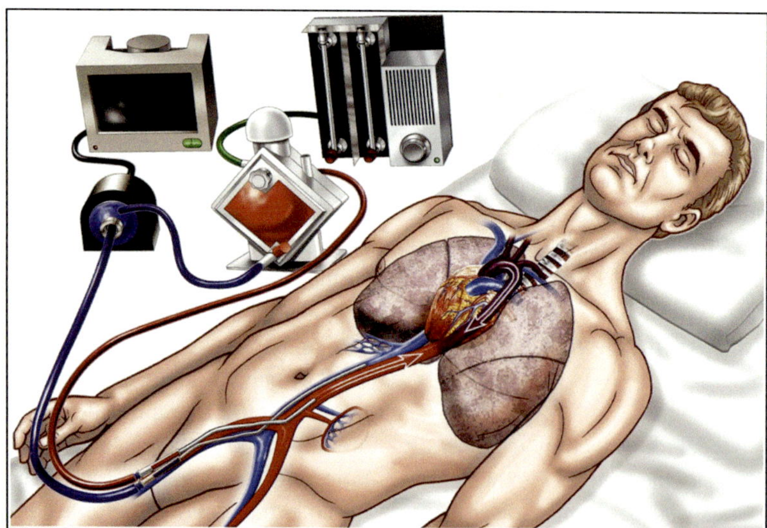

**Fig. 2.5** Functional diagram of femoral venoarterial ECMO in a patient. Reprinted from Journal of the American College of Cardiology, 63/25, Darryl Abrams, Alain Combes, Daniel Brodie, Extracorporeal Membrane Oxygenation in Cardiopulmonary Disease in Adults, 2769–2778, Copyright (2014), with permission from Elsevier

bleeding related to vascular access [25, 26]. Patients who survive are typically subsequently transitioned to a VAD, TAH, or, less commonly, to a transplant.

## Percutaneous Mechanical Circulatory Support

Continued advances in temporary MCS technology have resulted in new devices such as the Impella (Abiomed, Danvers, MA, USA) (Fig. 2.1); the Impella is a micro axial catheter-based percutaneous ventricular assist device, which can be inserted in either venous or arterial access configurations to support the right and left ventricle, respectively. In the left-sided support configuration, the catheter is inserted via the femoral or axillary/subclavian artery and directed retrograde across the aortic valve to provide adequate perfusion in hemodynamically unstable patients. Impella catheters can be considered for support during high-risk percutaneous coronary interventions, cardiogenic shock, and as a bridge to myocardial recovery or transplant/LVAD, amongst other indications. As of the time of writing, the surgically implanted Impella 5.5 offers the most significant left ventricular support, up to 6 L per minute of flow. Impella devices are more frequently utilized as a bridge to HTx and are currently prioritized over durable LVADs under the current US heart allocation policy. In a study of the UNOS database from 2010 to 2021, waitlist and post-transplant outcomes were assessed for patients bridged to HTx with Impella 5.0 and 5.5 devices. It showed that bridging with these devices was safe, with low overall rates of waitlist mortality or clinical deterioration. These patients also had excellent 1-year post-transplant outcomes [27]. The TandemHeart® (Cardiac Assist, Inc., Pittsburgh, Pennsylvania, USA) is another percutaneous LVAD that requires a trans-septal puncture [28]. In a contemporary cohort of 50 patients presenting with cardiogenic shock enrolled in the THEME registry (a multicenter, prospective, observational study), the use of TandemHeart® was associated with a 74% 30-day survival and a 66% 180-day survival [29].

## Heart Transplantation

HTx remains the gold-standard surgical option for refractory end-stage HF. Chaps. 3 and 4 will detail indications and evaluation criteria.

**In summary**, despite improved outcomes of the novel HF therapeutics, morbidity and mortality rates remain excessively high for patients with advanced HF. In these cases, MCS, including temporary and durable devices, are imperative in their management. Once the patient is deemed to have advanced HF and likely to benefit from advanced therapies, the optimal strategy for implantation should include selecting the most appropriate MCS device with the best durability and lowest incidence of adverse events and which provides adequate cardiac output for either one or both failing ventricles.

## References


1. Members WC, Bozkurt B, Ahmad T, Alexander KM, Baker WL, Bosak K, et al. Heart failure epidemiology and outcomes statistics: a report of the Heart Failure Society of America. J Card Fail. 2023;29(10):1412.
2. Heidenreich PA, Bozkurt B, Aguilar D, Allen LA, Byun JJ, Colvin MM, et al. 2022 ACC/AHA/HFSA guideline for the management of heart failure. J Card Fail [Internet]. 2022;28(5):e1-167. https://doi.org/10.1016/j.cardfail.2022.02.010.
3. Zhou AL, Etchill EW, Giuliano KA, Shou BL, Sharma K, Choi CW, et al. Bridge to transplantation from mechanical circulatory support: a narrative review. J Thorac Dis. 2021;13(12):6911.
4. Copeland JG, Smith RG, Arabia FA, Nolan PE, Sethi GK, Tsau PH, et al. Cardiac replacement with a total artificial heart as a bridge to transplantation. N Engl J Med. 2004;351(9):859–67.
5. Holley CT, Harvey L, John R. Left ventricular assist devices as a bridge to cardiac transplantation. J Thorac Dis. 2014;6(8):1110.
6. Morris AA, Khazanie P, Drazner MH, Albert NM, Breathett K, Cooper LB, et al. Guidance for timely and appropriate referral of patients with advanced heart failure: a scientific statement from the American Heart Association. Circulation. 2021;144(15):e238-50.

7. Kuehn BM. FDA: stop using Medtronic's heartware ventricular assist device. JAMA. 2021;326(3):215.
8. Hetzer R, del Maria Javier MF, Dandel M, Loebe M, Delmo EMJ. Mechanical circulatory support systems: evolution, the systems and outlook. Cardiovasc Diagn Ther. 2021;11(1):309.
9. Rose EA, Gelijns AC, Moskowitz AJ, Heitjan DF, Stevenson LW, Dembitsky W, et al. Long-term use of a left ventricular assist device for end-stage heart failure. N Engl J Med. 2001;345(20):1435–43.
10. Goldstein DJ, Oz MC, Rose EA. Implantable left ventricular assist devices. N Engl J Med. 1998;339(21):1522–33.
11. Christiansen S, Klocke A, Autschbach R. Past, present, and future of long-term mechanical cardiac support in adults. J Card Surg. 2008;23(6):664–76.
12. Toeg HD, Al-Atassi T, Garcia JP, Ruel M. An update on mechanical circulatory support for heart failure therapy. Curr Opin Cardiol. 2014;29(2):167–73.
13. Lok SI, Martina JR, Hesselink T, Rodermans BFM, Hulstein N, Winkens B, et al. Single-centre experience of 85 patients with a continuous-flow left ventricular assist device: clinical practice and outcome after extended support. Eur J Cardiothorac Surg. 2013;44(3):e233-8.
14. Park SJ, Milano CA, Tatooles AJ, Rogers JG, Adamson RM, Steidley DE, et al. Outcomes in advanced heart failure patients with left ventricular assist devices for destination therapy. Circ Heart Fail. 2012;5(2):241–8.
15. Kirklin JK, Naftel DC, Kormos RL, Stevenson LW, Pagani FD, Miller MA, et al. Fifth INTERMACS annual report: risk factor analysis from more than 6,000 mechanical circulatory support patients. J Heart Lung Transplant. 2013;32(2):141–56.
16. Deng MC, Weyand M, Hammel D, Schmid C, Kerber S, Schmidt C, et al. Selection and management of ventricular assist device patients: the Muenster experience. J Heart Lung Transplant. 2000;19(8):S77-82.
17. Mehra MR, Goldstein DJ, Cleveland JC, Cowger JA, Hall S, Salerno CT, et al. Five-year outcomes in patients with fully magnetically levitated vs axial-flow left ventricular assist devices in the MOMENTUM 3 randomized trial. JAMA. 2022;328(12):1233–42.
18. Yuzefpolskaya M, Schroeder SE, Houston BA, Robinson MR, Gosev I, Reyentovich A, et al. The Society of Thoracic Surgeons Intermacs 2022 annual report: focus on the 2018 heart transplant allocation system. Ann Thorac Surg. 2023;115(2):311–27.
19. Varshney AS, DeFilippis EM, Cowger JA, Netuka I, Pinney SP, Givertz MM. Trends and outcomes of left ventricular assist device therapy: JACC focus seminar. J Am Coll Cardiol. 2022;79(11):1092–107.
20. Mancini DM, Beniaminovitz A, Levin H, Catanese K, Flannery M, DiTullio M, et al. Low incidence of myocardial recovery after left ventricular assist device implantation in patients with chronic heart failure. Circulation. 1998;98(22):2383–9.
21. Feldman D, Pamboukian SV, Teuteberg JJ, Birks E, Lietz K, Moore SA, et al. The 2013 International Society for Heart and Lung Transplantation Guidelines for mechanical circulatory support: executive summary. J Heart Lung Transplant. 2013;32(2):157–87.
22. Stevenson LW, Pagani FD, Young JB, Jessup M, Miller L, Kormos RL, et al. INTERMACS profiles of advanced heart failure: the current picture. J Heart Lung Transplant. 2009;28(6):535–41.
23. Hasin T, Marmor Y, Kremers W, Topilsky Y, Severson CJ, Schirger JA, et al. Readmissions after implantation of axial flow left ventricular assist device. J Am Coll Cardiol. 2013;61(2):153–63.
24. Starling RC, Estep JD, Horstmanshof DA, Milano CA, Stehlik J, Shah KB, et al. Risk assessment and comparative effectiveness of left ventricular assist device and medical management in ambulatory heart failure patients: the ROADMAP study 2-year results. JACC Heart Fail. 2017;5(7):518–27.
25. Paden ML, Conrad SA, Rycus PT, Thiagarajan RR. Extracorporeal life support organization registry report 2012. ASAIO J. 2013;59(3):202–10.
26. Prodhan P, Bhutta AT, Gossett JM, Dodgen AL, Seib PM, Imamura M, et al. Comparative effects of ventricular assist device and extracorporeal membrane oxygenation on renal function in pediatric heart failure. Ann Thorac Surg. 2013;96(4):1428–34.
27. Hill MA, Kwon JH, Shorbaji K, Kilic A. Waitlist and transplant outcomes for patients bridged to heart transplantation with Impella 5.0 and 5.5 devices. J Card Surg. 2022;37(12):5081–9.
28. Kar B, Adkins LE, Civitello AB, Loyalka P, Palanichamy N, Gemmato CJ, et al. Clinical experience with the TandemHeart® percutaneous ventricular assist device. Tex Heart Inst J. 2006;33(2):111.
29. Megaly M, Gandolfo C, Zakhour S, Jiang M, Burgess K, Chetcuti S, et al. Utilization of TandemHeart in cardiogenic shock: insights from the THEME registry. Catheter Cardiovasc Interv. 2023;101(4):756–63.

# 3 Evaluation for Heart Transplant Candidacy

Michele Hamilton and Yosef Manla

**Abstract**

Evaluation for heart transplant (HTx) candidacy necessitates a multidisciplinary effort to integrate medical, and psychosocial parameters and work in concert with the patient's care goals, considering the full complement of individually appropriate options. This chapter summarizes HTx indications and pretransplant evaluation.

**Keywords**

Heart failure · Heart transplantation · Cardiopulmonary exercise testing

## Clinical Pearls

- Evaluation for heart transplantation candidacy necessitates a multidisciplinary effort to integrate medical and psychosocial parameters and work in concert with the patient's care goals.
- General indications for evaluation for transplant listing include cardiogenic shock requiring continuous intravenous inotropic support or mechanical support, refractory NYHA class III-IV/AHA stage D heart failure, recurrent sustained ventricular arrhythmias, severe untreatable angina and end-stage congenital heart disease.
- Evaluation for heart transplantation includes assessment of heart failure severity, immuno-compatibility, evaluation of multi-organ function, infectious serology and vaccinations, malignancies, as well as a psychological, social, and financial assessment (including insurance coverage).
- Cardiopulmonary exercise testing (CPET) provides an objective measure of cardiac impairment and prognosis via measurement of oxygen consumption at peak exercise (peak VO2).
- Heart failure patients on beta-blockers with a VO2max ≤ 12 ml/kg/min or younger patients with less than 50% of predicted VO2max, considered in conjunction with other evidence of functional impairment and clinical course, may be appropriate for transplant.
- Hemodynamic assessment with right heart catheterization also is important for assessment of the level of cardiac impairment and confirm there is no evidence of irreversible pulmonary hypertension.
- The Heart Failure Survival Score (HFSS) and Seattle Heart Failure Model (SHFM)

M. Hamilton (✉) · Y. Manla
Cedars-Sinai Smidt Heart Institute, Los Angeles, CA, USA
e-mail: michele.hamilton@cshs.org

Y. Manla
e-mail: Yosef.manla@cshs.org



J. Kobashigawa (ed.), *Clinical Guide to Heart Transplantation*, https://doi.org/10.1007/978-3-031-88290-6_3

are multifactorial scores that may be helpful in guiding decisions on listing for heart transplantation.

## Introduction

As the outcomes for both heart failure (HF) therapy and heart transplantation (HTx) have improved, and the field of durable mechanical circulatory support (MCS) is maturing, the risk/benefit ratio for medical therapy and HTx has evolved [1]. It is appropriate to consider HTx for patients with advanced heart disease and, despite maximal medical therapy, a poor quality of life related to HF symptoms [New York Heart Association (NYHA) Class III/IV) or high risk of sudden death—in the absence of life-limiting non-cardiac illnesses. Intensive care unit patients in cardiogenic shock are now the substantial majority of patients who receive HTx [2]. Evaluation for HTx candidacy necessitates a multidisciplinary effort to integrate medical and psychosocial parameters and work in concert with the patient's care goals, considering the full complement of individually appropriate options [3]. An additional layer of complexity in determining candidacy for HTx is the scarcity of donor organs, so we need to consider not only providing the best treatment for each patient but also responsible allocation of this scarce resource. Though there has been some recent increase in HTx, due in part to the use of donation after circulatory death, there have been only approximately 4,000 HTx annually in the US, with many more in need [4].

## Indications for Heart Transplantation

The most common indications for transplantation include refractory cardiogenic shock requiring continuous intravenous inotropic or temporary MCS, followed by progressive NYHA class III-IV/AHA stage D HF, refractory ventricular arrhythmias, severe untreatable angina, and end-stage congenital heart disease [5]. Also, patients on a durable ventricular assist device may be eligible for transplant, and HTx patients who develop significant cardiac allograft vasculopathy, often with restrictive cardiac physiology, may be considered for redo-transplant (Table 3.1).

For the patient in irreversible cardiogenic shock, the options include transplantation, durable left ventricular assist devices (LVAD), total artificial heart, or palliative care. The role of durable MCS has been discussed in the previous chapter; short-term (1 year) survival with the HeartMate III device now rivals transplant at 85–90%, but transplant remains the gold standard for long-term survival and functional capacity [6, 7]. For ambulatory patients with progressive stage D HF and NYHA Class IIIb/IV symptoms, a combination of clinical

**Table 3.1** General indications for cardiac transplantation

- Refractory cardiogenic shock requiring intra-aortic balloon pump counterpulsation or mechanical circulatory support (i.e., left ventricular assist device (LVAD), total artificial heart)
- Cardiogenic shock requiring continuous intravenous inotropic therapy (i.e., dobutamine, milrinone, etc.)
- Cardiopulmonary exercise testing demonstrating $V_{O2}$max ≤ 14 mL/kg/min in patients not on beta-blockers, or $V_{O2}$max ≤ 12 mL/kg/min in patients on beta-blockers
- Persistant NYHA class of III or IV heart failure symptoms despite maximized medical, surgical and/or resynchronization therapy
- Recurrent life-threatening left ventricular arrhythmias despite an implantable cardiac defibrillator, maximal pharmacological antiarrhythmic therapy, or catheter-based ablation
- End-stage congenital HF with no evidence of pulmonary hypertension
- Refractory angina despite maximal medical therapy and not amenable to percutaneous or surgical revascularization
- Severe hypertrophic or restrictive cardiomyopathy, with NYHA Class IV symptoms
- Transplanted patients who develop significant cardiac allograft vasculopathy with refractory cardiac allograft dysfunction

NYHA: New York Heart Association

parameters, hemodynamics, and functional status are used to determine if patients are likely to have improved outcomes with transplantation. The need for LVAD as either a destination alternative or bridge to transplant is also considered as part of the evaluation for this population.

## The Evaluation

An evaluation usually consists of consultations from a multidisciplinary team, including HF /transplant cardiology specialist, cardiothoracic surgeon, and other medical specialties as needed, as well as transplant coordinators, social workers, pharmacists, and dieticians. Evaluation for HTx includes assessment of HF severity, immuno-compatibility, evaluation of multi-organ function, infectious serology and vaccinations, malignancies, as well as a psychological, social, and financial assessment [8] (Table 3.2).

## Assessment of Heart Failure Severity

All patients undergo an echocardiogram to identify structural and hemodynamic parameters, providing prognostic factors and potential alternatives to transplant. A left ventricular ejection fraction (LVEF) of <25% has been shown to be associated with increased mortality and morbidity compared to an ejection fraction>35% [9]. However, low LVEF alone within a cohort of patients with advanced HF has been shown to be poorly predictive of short-term or medium-term mortality. An echocardiogram may identify valvular abnormalities, such as severe functional mitral regurgitation or aortic stenosis, with potential for transcatheter devices or severe RV dysfunction, making LVAD unacceptably high risk.

Right heart catheterization (RHC) measurement of hemodynamics is an important test as part of the initial assessment for HTx candidacy both to assist in the optimization of current therapy and assess prognosis and potential contraindications to HTx. RHC will also need to be repeated in some patients periodically while waiting if there was initially reversible pulmonary hypertension or if there has been subsequent worsening of HF symptoms [10]. Higher right atrial, pulmonary capillary wedge and pulmonary artery systolic pressures, lower mean arterial pressure, and lower cardiac index have all been variably associated with increased mortality, with pulmonary capillary wedge pressure after maximal hemodynamically guided therapy being the optimal target to predict survival [10–14].

Cardiopulmonary exercise testing (CPET), a bicycle or treadmill-based exercise test with gas exchange measurements via a mouthpiece, is considered the best means to objectively determine if a patient's severity of functional impairment merits listing for transplantation [10]. One of the key measurements in CPET that provides prognostic information is oxygen consumption at peak exercise or peak VO2. This measure is a reflection of the maximal amount of oxygen the heart can deliver to the peripheral tissues at a sufficient rate for aerobic respiration. The ISHLT guidelines state that a cut-off for peak VO2 of 12–14 ml/kg/min in HF patients should be used to guide which patients are sufficiently impaired for transplantation since studies have demonstrated that patients with preserved exercise capacity ($V_{O2}$max > 14 mL/kg/min) despite severe resting hemodynamic impairment, have survival and functional capacity equal to those afforded by HTx [3, 15, 16]. In view of improved survival in patients on beta-blockers, these patients should be generally considered at increased risk only at the low end of this peak VO2 range. Since peak VO2 is also affected by age and weight, it is helpful to adjust peak VO2 to lean body weight in obese patients and to use a percentage of predicted peak VO2 for each individual patient, with <50% predicted considered sufficiently impaired for transplantation [17–19]. It must be emphasized that the decision to list must not be made on peak VO2 measurement on CPET alone; many other factors, including pulmonary, peripheral vascular, pulmonary vascular, or musculoskeletal disease, may also reduce the peak VO2. These can often be differentiated by other parameters

**Table 3.2** Recommended tests for initial evaluation of heart transplant candidacy

| Recommended tests |
| --- |
| • Weight/body mass index<br>• Immuno-compatibility<br>– ABO typing<br>– Human leukocyte antigen tissue typing<br>– Panel reactive antibodies and flow cytometry<br>• Assessment of severity of heart failure<br>– Cardiopulmonary exercise test<br>– Echocardiogram<br>– Right heart catheterization<br>• Evaluation of multi-organ function<br>– Routine laboratory work (basic metabolic profile, complete blood count, liver function tests)<br>– Urinalysis with toxicology screen<br>– 24-h urine collection for protein and creatinine<br>– Pulmonary function tests<br>– Chest radiograph<br>– Abdominal ultrasonography<br>– Carotid Doppler (if >50 years or with ischemic heart disease)<br>– Ankle-brachial indices (if >50 years or with ischemic heart disease)<br>– Dental examination<br>– Ophthalmologic examination (if diabetic)<br>– Chest and abdomen/pelvic CT scans (if indicated)<br>• Infectious serology and vaccination<br>– Hepatitis B surface, core, envelope antigen, antibody (IgG/IgM)<br>– Hepatitis C Ab<br>– Human immunodeficiency virus (HIV)<br>– Rapid plasma reagin<br>– Immunoglobulin G for herpes simplex virus<br>– Cytomegalovirus, toxoplasmosis, Epstein-Barr virus, varicella<br>– Purified protein derivative<br>– If from Latin American: Chagas screen<br>– Immunizations: influenza, pneumovax, hepatitis B, COVID<br>• Preventive and malignancy<br>– Stool for occult blood × 3<br>– Colonoscopy (if indicated or if >50 years)<br>– Mammography (if indicated or if >40 years)<br>– Papanicolaou smear test<br>– Prostate-specific antigen and digital rectal examination (men >50 years)<br>• General consultations<br>– Social assessment<br>– Psychiatry<br>– Financial<br>– As indicated: pulmonology, nephrology, infectious disease, endocrinology, hematology |

Abbreviations: IgG: immunoglobulin G; IgM: immunoglobulin M

incorporated in the CPET test. Surpassing anaerobic threshold (AT) defines a maximal CPET test from a cardiac standpoint. AT is defined as the point during exercise at which oxygen delivery to exercising muscles is insufficient to sustain aerobic respiration, so anaerobic pathways are predominantly utilized. Exercise beyond this threshold, identified by respiratory exchange ratio (RER) > 1.05, helps differentiate true cardiac limitation from poor effort or potentially confounding pulmonary or musculoskeletal limitations. Ventilatory efficiency ($V_E/V_{CO2}$) on CPET testing, defined as the ratio of minute ventilation ($V_E$) to the rate of carbon dioxide production ($V_{CO2}$), maybe a more powerful prognostic factor than $V_{O2}$max and is independent of body mass index [20, 21]. Stability or improvement on serial CPET testing is also a useful finding for identifying patients who, in conjunction with clinical stability, may be safely removed from the transplant waiting list.

## Models to Predict Survival in Advanced HF Patients

While certain measurements, such as LVEF, are poor prognostic indicators by themselves, the combination of multiple measures, including hemodynamics and peak VO2, can improve prognostic value. Several broader models have been developed to provide further predictive value, but they are of variable use in individual decision-making. Since 1- and 3-year transplant survival is approximately 90% and 85% respectively, the ISHLT guidelines recommend HTx only for patients with predicted survival on medical therapy significantly less than these values. The HF Survival Score (HFSS) is a risk model derived from a multivariable analysis of 268 ambulatory patients referred for consideration of cardiac transplantation initially from 1986 to 1991 and subsequently validated in a population of 199 similar patients from 1993 to 1995, with further modifications since then [22]. The component predictors of survival in the HFSS included the following: presence or absence of coronary artery disease; resting heart rate; LVEF by echocardiography; mean arterial blood pressure; presence or absence of an intraventricular conduction delay on electrocardiogram; serum sodium; and peak VO2 as determined by CPET. Using this analysis, patients can be categorized into low risk, with a one-year survival of 93%, for whom transplant can generally be safely deferred, or medium and high risk, with a 1-year survival of 72% and 43%, respectively [22], warranting consideration for HTx.

The Seattle HF Model (SHFM) is another scoring tool derived from a cohort of 1125 HF patients and subsequently validated in 9942 patients [12]. It is most useful for estimating the prognosis of ambulatory patients with advanced HF. The SHFM incorporates more clinical and laboratory variables. Most pertinently, the model is able to assess the impact of newer HF therapies and devices (including implantable cardioverter-defibrillators and cardiac resynchronization therapy) on predicted survival. The primary limitation of the SHFM is that it was derived from an ambulatory HF population and thus may overestimate survival in the overall advanced HF population [23, 24].

## Psychosocial Evaluation

Psychosocial assessment should be performed on all candidates prior to listing for transplantation to make sure they have the support, understanding, and commitment needed to have a successful transplant. This involves compliance with the complex medical regimen, as well as the social support needed to assist with personal care, meals, and transportation to follow-up appointments or emergency care. This usually requires both primary and secondary dedicated caregivers. Isolated, stable cognitive impairment is not a contraindication to transplant if the social support structure is strong, but dementia would not be acceptable, owing to its progressive nature and overall poor prognosis.

Psychiatric evaluation should also be incorporated into the overall evaluation process for HTx listing to identify any active psychiatric illness that may negatively affect adherence to care regimens and would need to be stabilized and monitored longitudinally before transplant listing. Since depression is common in HF patients and can adversely affect post-transplant outcomes, it should be addressed and treated both pre and post-transplant. Evaluation by palliative or support care teams is required for consideration of durable mechanical support and should be considered for transplant evaluations as well.

## References


1. Reed SD, Yang JC, Rickert T, Johnson FR, Gonzalez JM, Mentz RJ, et al. Quantifying benefit-risk preferences for heart failure devices: a stated-preference study. Circ Heart Fail. 2022;15(1):e008797.
2. Varshney AS, Berg DD, Zhou G, Sinnenberg L, Hirji S, DeFilippis EM, et al. Bridging strategies and

cardiac replacement outcomes in patients with acute decompensated heart failure-related cardiogenic shock. Eur J Heart Fail. 2023;25(3):425–35.
3. Peled Y, Ducharme A, Kittleson M, Bansal N, Stehlik J, Amdani S, et al. International society for heart and lung transplantation guidelines for the evaluation and care of cardiac transplant candidates—2024. J Heart Lung Transplant. 2024.
4. Barboza AB, Dhanani NH, Browning K, Wood RP, Hall DR. Trends in donation after circulatory determination of death donor utilization: Lessons from Houston. Transplant Rep. 2023;8(2):100135.
5. Mancini D, Lietz K. Selection of cardiac transplantation candidates in 2010. Circulation. 2010;122(2):173–83.
6. Hanke JS, Dogan G, Zoch A, Ricklefs M, Wert L, Feldmann C, et al. One-year outcomes with the HeartMate 3 left ventricular assist device. J Thorac Cardiovasc Surg. 2018;156(2):662–9.
7. Velleca A, Shullo MA, Dhital K, Azeka E, Colvin M, DePasquale E, et al. The International Society for Heart and Lung Transplantation (ISHLT) guidelines for the care of heart transplant recipients. J Heart Lung Transplant. 2023;42(5):e1-141.
8. Mehra MR, Kobashigawa J, Starling R, Russell S, Uber PA, Parameshwar J, et al. Listing criteria for heart transplantation: international society for heart and lung transplantation guidelines for the care of cardiac transplant candidates—2006. J Heart Lung Transplant. 2006;25(9):1024–42.
9. Miller LW, Kubo SH, Young JB, Stevenson LW, Loh E, Costanzo MR. Report of the consensus conference on candidate selection for heart transplantation-1993. J Heart Lung Transplant. 1995;14(3):562–71.
10. Mehra MR, Canter CE, Hannan MM, Semigran MJ, Uber PA, Baran DA, et al. The 2016 international society for heart lung transplantation listing criteria for heart transplantation: a 10-year update. J Heart Lung Transplant. 2016;35(1):1–23.
11. Keogh AM, Baron DW, Hickie JB. Prognostic guides in patients with idiopathic or ischemic dilated cardiomyopathy assessed for cardiac transplantation. Am J Cardiol. 1990;65(13):903–8.
12. Levy WC, Mozaffarian D, Linker DT, Sutradhar SC, Anker SD, Cropp AB, et al. The Seattle heart failure model: prediction of survival in heart failure. Circulation. 2006;113(11):1424–33.
13. Rickenbacher PR, Trindade PT, Haywood GA, Vagelos RH, Schroeder JS, Willson K, et al. Transplant candidates with severe left ventricular dysfunction managed with medical treatment: characteristics and survival. J Am Coll Cardiol. 1996;27(5):1192–7.
14. Kittleson MM, Kobashigawa JA. Management of advanced heart failure: the role of heart transplantation. Circulation. 2011;123(14):1569–74.
15. Mancini DM, Eisen H, Kussmaul W, Mull R, Edmunds LH Jr, Wilson JR. Value of peak exercise oxygen consumption for optimal timing of cardiac transplantation in ambulatory patients with heart failure. Circulation. 1991;83(3):778–86.
16. Goda A, Lund LH, Mancini D. The Heart Failure Survival Score outperforms the peak oxygen consumption for heart transplantation selection in the era of device therapy. J Heart Lung Transplant. 2011;30(3):315–25.
17. Yancy CW, Jessup M, Bozkurt B, Butler J, Casey DE, Drazner MH, et al. 2013 ACCF/AHA guideline for the management of heart failure: a report of the American College of Cardiology Foundation/American Heart Association Task Force on Practice Guidelines. J Am Coll Cardiol. 2013;62(16):e147-239.
18. Committee 2009 Writing Group to Review New Evidence and Update the 2005 Guideline for the Management of Patients with Chronic Heart Failure Writing on Behalf of the 2005 Heart Failure Writing, Jessup M, Abraham WT, Casey DE, Feldman AM, Francis GS, et al. 2009 focused update: ACCF/AHA guidelines for the diagnosis and management of heart failure in adults: a report of the American College of Cardiology Foundation/American Heart Association Task Force on Practice Guidelines: developed in collaboration with the International Society for Heart and Lung Transplantation. Circulation. 2009;119(14):1977–2016.
19. O'Neill JO, Young JB, Pothier CE, Lauer MS. Peak oxygen consumption as a predictor of death in patients with heart failure receiving β-blockers. Circulation. 2005;111(18):2313–8.
20. Ferreira AM, Tabet JY, Frankenstein L, Metra M, Mendes M, Zugck C, et al. Ventilatory efficiency and the selection of patients for heart transplantation. Circul Heart Fail. 2010;3(3):378–86.
21. Bard RL, Gillespie BW, Lange DC, Nicklas JM. Improving prognostic assessment of patients with advanced heart failure using ventilatory efficiency. J Heart Lung Transplant. 2010;29(5):589–91.
22. Aaronson KD, Schwartz JS, Chen TM, Wong KL, Goin JE, Mancini DM. Development and prospective validation of a clinical index to predict survival in ambulatory patients referred for cardiac transplant evaluation. Circulation. 1997;95(12):2660–7.
23. Gorodeski EZ, Chu EC, Chow CH, Levy WC, Hsich E, Starling RC. Application of the Seattle heart failure model in ambulatory patients presented to an advanced heart failure therapeutics committee. Circul Heart Fail. 2010;3(6):706–14.
24. Kalogeropoulos AP, Georgiopoulou VV, Giamouzis G, Smith AL, Agha SA, Waheed S, et al. Utility of the Seattle heart failure model in patients with advanced heart failure. J Am Coll Cardiol. 2009;53(4):334–42.

# 4 Potential Contraindications to Heart Transplantation

Michelle M. Kittleson

**Abstract**

Heart Transplantation (HTx) is considered the gold standard for the treatment of refractory end-stage heart failure. Due to the scarcity of available donor hearts, careful evaluation for HTx candidacy is warranted. Thus, the goal of a HTx evaluation is to determine if: the patient's cardiac status is limited enough, on optimal medical therapy, to benefit from HTx; the patient does not have co-morbidities that would preclude HTx; and the patient demonstrates compliance and possesses adequate social support. Finding a balance between maximal individual survival benefit and maximal utility will always remain a complex issue requiring frequent reassessment. Ultimately, the decision to list a patient for transplantation is not based on any one test or factor but acknowledges multiple factors, including indicators for poor prognosis without transplant as well as potential contraindications that may cause suboptimal outcomes post-transplant. This chapter will summarize the contraindications to HTx as well as psychological and financial considerations.

M. M. Kittleson (✉)
Cedars-Sinai Smidt Heart Institute, Los Angeles, CA, USA
e-mail: michelle.kittleson@cshs.org

**Keywords**

Heart failure · Heart transplantation · Contraindications · Evaluation · Psychological · Financial

## Clinical Pearls

- Potential relative contraindications include age > 70 years, obesity (BMI > 35 kg/m2), pulmonary hypertension, primary pulmonary disease, poorly controlled diabetes (HbA1C > 7.5%) or diabetes with end-organ damage, renal dysfunction (eGFR < 30 ml/min/1.73 m$^2$), and any active infection excluding left ventricular assist device -related infections.
- Absolute contraindications include severe or multiple of the above relative contraindication factors, metastatic malignancy, severe cerebrovascular disease, strong indicators for non-compliance, and a lack of social/caregiver support.
- Ultimately, the decision to list a patient for transplantation is not based on any one test or factor but acknowledges multiple factors, including indicators for poor prognosis without transplant as well as potential contraindications that may cause suboptimal outcomes post-transplant.


J. Kobashigawa (ed.), *Clinical Guide to Heart Transplantation*, https://doi.org/10.1007/978-3-031-88290-6_4

## Introduction

Despite advances in pharmacological and device treatment of chronic heart failure (HF), long-term morbidity and mortality remain unacceptably high; the 5-year mortality rate for patients with symptomatic HF approaches 50% and may be as high as 80% at 1 year for end-stage patients [1]. For those patients in whom these therapies (as detailed in Chaps. 1 and 2) have been attempted without success, heart transplantation (HTx) may be a suitable option and is considered the gold standard for the treatment of refractory end-stage HF. Evaluation for transplant candidacy and transplant indications have been described in Chap. 3. This chapter will summarize the contraindications to HTx. Due in part to the scarcity of available donor hearts, careful evaluation for candidacy is warranted. Thus, the goal of a HTx evaluation is to determine if: (1) the patient's cardiac status is limited enough, on optimal medical therapy, to benefit from HTx (i.e., "sick enough"); (2) the patient does not have co-morbidities that would preclude HTx (i.e., "well enough"); and (3) the patient demonstrates compliance and possesses adequate social support ("can adapt to a transplant lifestyle"). Finding a balance between maximal individual survival benefit and maximal utility will always remain a complex issue requiring frequent reassessment. A limited number of established contraindications are described in Table 4.1. Many of these factors are not absolute and need to be considered in the context of the severity of the patient's heart disease and associated co-morbidities. The degree to which they are interpreted and applied may vary considerably among transplant programs.

A useful rule is that the presence of any non-cardiac condition that would substantially increase the peri- or postoperative risks of the transplant or itself shorten life expectancy would represent a medical contraindication. Similarly, any psychosocial issues that would increase the risk of death from rejection due to medical non-adherence would also place the patient at a prohibitively high risk for transplant.

## Heart Transplant Contraindications

### Age

As life expectancy continues to increase, traditional age limits for HTx may be expanded in select cases. Generally, patients are considered for HTx if they are 70 years of age or less, since advances in post-transplant care have shown that survival in the older age group is comparable to that of younger recipients [2]. Older age does confer more risk of certain post-transplant complications; compared to recipients under the age of 60 years of age, older transplant recipients have more infections, renal dysfunction, and malignancy, but less rejection [3, 4]. Increasing recipient age is associated with an increase in post-transplant mortality, particularly in patients aged ≥ 70 years at the time of transplant, with the incidence of specific causes of post-transplant mortality varying widely with recipient age [3, 4]. Thus, patients over the age of 70 years may have acceptable outcomes, but careful consideration of associated co-morbidities is essential. At some centers, such patients are offered nonstandard donor hearts, including those with coronary artery disease, mildly decreased left ventricular ejection fraction, left ventricular hypertrophy, or donor age older than 55 years old. This practice allows older patients to undergo HTx without denying the scarce resource to younger candidates, with comparable outcomes [5]. However, while older donors may be considered for older HTx candidates, this practice is of uncertain value given the observation that older donors are associated with worse post-transplant survival both in young and old recipients [6]. This issue raises the ethical question of using the scarce resource of young donor hearts for older recipients, further exacerbated by the potential need for dual organ transplantation [7]. Physiologic age may be more important than chronologic age with respect to survival and rehabilitation potential. As a result, many programs focus less on fixed upper age limits and instead assess the patient's functional status, integrity of major organ systems, and the

**Table 4.1** Summary of potential contraindications to cardiac transplantation

| Potential contraindication | Comments |
|---|---|
| Age | >70 years old is a relative contraindication depending on associated comorbidities |
| Obesity | BMI < 35 kg/m$^2$ is recommended |
| Malignancy | Active or metastatic neoplasms are an absolute contraindication |
| Pulmonary Hypertension | TPG > 15 mmHg, PVR > 5 Wood units or pulmonary artery pressure > 60 mmHg with one of the above, or the inability to achieve PVR < 2.5 Wood Units with vasodilator or inotropic therapy, are relative contraindications; such patients may benefit from long-term unloading with ventricular assist device followed by reassessment |
| Primary Pulmonary Disease | In the presence of known primary lung disease, e.g. emphysema or fibrosis, in combination with impaired pulmonary function tests, defined as $FEV_1$ < 40% of predicted, FVC < 50% of normal, $DL_{CO}$ < 40%, is a relative contraindication<br>Recent pulmonary embolism (within 6 weeks) is also a contraindication |
| Diabetes | Uncontrolled diabetes ($HbA_{1C}$ > 7.5% or 58 mmol/mol) or diabetes with significant end-organ damage is a relative contraindication |
| Renal dysfunction | eGFR < 30 is a relative contraindication |
| Hepatic dysfunction | Cirrhosis with portal hypertension is a relative contraindication |
| Peripheral vascular disease | Severe disease not amenable to revascularization is an absolute contraindication |
| Infection | Active infections except LVAD-related infections are contraindications; HIV, Hepatitis B and Hepatitis C are not contraindications if not active and well-controlled by treatment as defined by viral load/CD4 thresholds<br>Latent TB and Chagas are not contraindications |
| Substance use | 6 months of abstinence from smoking, alcohol and illicit drugs is required; in critically ill patients, consultation with psychiatry and social work is essential. Marijuana is a controversial topic |
| Psychosocial issues | Non-compliance, lack of caregiver/social support, and dementia are absolute contraindications; mental retardation may be a relative contraindication |

BMI: body mass index; DLCO: lung diffusion capacity; eGFR: estimated glomerular filtration rate; FEV: forced expiratory volume; FVC: forced vital capacity; HbA1C: glycosylated hemoglobin; HIV: human immunodeficiency virus; LVAD: left ventricular assist device; mg: milligrams; mmol: millimoles; mol: moles; PVR: pulmonary vascular resistance; TPG: transpulmonary gradient; TB: tuberculosis; dl: deciliters

presence of comorbidities that might impact survival, rehabilitation potential, and quality of life.

## Obesity

Increasing rates of obesity are observed in the HTx population, with a significant increase in body mass index (BMI) over time [8]. Obesity with BMI ≥ 35 kg/m$^2$ is associated with increased waitlist time, increased waitlist mortality, and increased post-mortality [9, 10]. There is a graded relationship between increased BMI and worse post-transplant survival in multiple registries and meta-analyses, with the best survival observed in those patients with normal BMI but acceptable survival in those patients with BMI 30–35 kg/m$^2$ [11–14]. Considering obesity is a potentially modifiable risk factor, achieving a BMI under 35 kg/m$^2$ is preferred to optimize post-transplant quality of life and survival. For some patients, options including bariatric surgery may be considered, depending on center expertise, resources, and patient stability [15–17].

## Malignancy

Malignancy after HTx remains a significant cause of morbidity and mortality. All HTx candidates should be screened for breast, prostate, and colon cancer as indicated and recommended for the general population, as there is little data to support malignancy screening recommendations specific to the HTx candidate [18]. Skin cancer screening by full-body skin examination completed by a dermatologist for all HTx candidates can be useful given the high prevalence of skin cancer after HTx. For those HTx candidates with pre-transplant malignancies, collaboration with an oncologist is essential for an individualized approach to risk stratification. While a period of observation prior to transplant listing may be recommended, this will be unique and specific to the given patient's cancer history. An individualized approach with multidisciplinary collaboration is essential, as arbitrary time intervals for observation may result in unnecessary delays in transplant listing. Those candidates with low-risk pre-transplant malignancy, including early-stage cancers with full resection and/or low-risk features, including prostate adenocarcinoma, renal cell carcinoma, cervical cancer, and bladder cancer, may undergo HTx with minimal or no pre-transplant observation and plans for post-transplant intervention [19]. On the other hand, active and/or metastatic neoplasms, with the exception of non-melanoma skin cancer, are absolute contraindications to HTx, as the course of the tumor may be accelerated by immunosuppression and the utility of the donor heart would not be maximized. Further guidance is available in consensus statements from the American Society of Transplantation with granular recommendations on transplant candidacy in transplant candidates with pre-transplant malignancies [19, 20].

## Pulmonary Hypertension

Pulmonary hypertension (mean pulmonary artery pressure > 20 mm Hg), most commonly Group 2 due to left heart disease (pulmonary capillary wedge pressure > 15 mm Hg) [21–23], is common in patients with HF [24, 25], and an elevated pulmonary vascular resistance (PVR) ≥ 2.5 Wood units is associated with increased early post-transplant mortality [26]. Although elevations in pulmonary artery systolic pressure (PASP), transpulmonary gradient (TPG), and pulmonary vascular resistance (PVR) above certain thresholds have been proposed as contraindications to HTx listing, the risk associated with each parameter is continuous from low to high values and absolute cutoffs do not exist [27, 28]. Even so, in patients with PASP ≥ 50 mm Hg and either TPG ≥ 15 or PVR ≥ 3 Wood units, a vasodilator (e.g., inhaled nitric oxide or nitroprusside if nitric oxide is not available) should be administered to document an acute reduction in PVR to acceptable levels [29]. An appropriate response to the vasodilator challenge would be if the TPG can be reduced to ≤ 12–15 mm Hg and the PVR to ≤ 2.5–3 WU.

If the PVR is reversible but systolic blood pressure falls to < 85 mm Hg with pharmacologic maneuvers, the risk of right HF remains high [29, 30]. When the response to the acute vasodilator challenge is not acceptable, hospitalization with continuous vasoactive therapies and hemodynamic monitoring would be the next step in management [31], followed by implantation of temporary mechanical circulatory support or a durable left ventricular assist device (LVAD) in eligible candidates [32–38].

## Primary Pulmonary Disease

Up to one-third of unselected patients with HF have concurrent chronic obstructive pulmonary disease (COPD), largely attributed to the shared risk factor of smoking [39]. HF also commonly co-exists with other lung diseases, including interstitial lung disease [40]. Patients with HF and lung disease have an increased risk of longer post-transplant hospital stays and increased mortality [41, 42]. Thus, it is essential to screen HTx candidates for pulmonary parenchymal disease with pulmonary function testing, including spirometry, volume assessment, and diffusion capacity, as well as chest imaging, most commonly non-contrast computed tomography, to assess for parenchymal disease. As pulmonary congestion may interfere with the interpretation of these tests [43, 44], optimization of volume status with diuretic therapy should occur prior to pulmonary evaluation. Further testing may be required as dictated by a pulmonary specialist. Patients with moderate or severe airway obstruction (forced expiratory volume in 1 s (FEV1) to forced vital capacity (FVC) ratio < 0.7 and FEV1 < 80% predicted) had higher operative mortality after cardiac surgery, with the highest operative mortality in those patients with diffusing capacity of the lung for carbon monoxide < 50% of predicted [45]. In HTx recipients in particular, FEV1 < 50% predicted and FVC < 50% predicted each was associated with significantly higher post-transplant mortality, and these should be considered contraindications to transplantation in conjunction with input from pulmonary consultants [41]. In addition, chronic hypoxia requiring supplemental oxygen, attributable to a pulmonary source, would contraindicate transplantation. A pulmonary embolism within the last 6 weeks also serves as a contraindication to transplantation because of the fear of recurrent emboli from the original source and the potential for abscess formation at the embolism site. Such patients should be treated with anticoagulation and then re-evaluated 4–6 weeks later with pulmonary imaging to assess candidacy for listing.

## Diabetes Mellitus

Approximately 30% of patients with advanced HF and 20% of HTx recipients have preexisting diabetes [46, 47]. The presence of uncomplicated post-transplant diabetes is not associated with worse post-transplant survival [47]. However, those HTx candidates with diabetes-related complications, including obesity, kidney dysfunction, cerebrovascular disease, or peripheral vascular disease, have worse post-transplant survival as well as an increased risk of post-transplant infections and kidney failure in one registry analysis [47] and additional risks of late graft failure and mortality in other cohorts [48–53]. Therefore, diabetes per se is not considered a contraindication for HTx, but careful assessment of diabetic control and end-organ damage (atherosclerotic vascular disease, nephropathy, proliferative retinopathy) is necessary. Posttransplant use of calcineurin inhibitors and corticosteroids will worsen glycemic control [54], so pretransplant optimal control to achieve glycosylated hemoglobin (Hgb A1c) 7–8% in collaboration with endocrinologists is highly encouraged [55]. On a program-specific basis, centers may identify a Hgb A1c level that is considered a relative contraindication to transplantation, especially in conjunction with diabetes-related complications, which portend worse post-transplant outcomes and because poorly controlled diabetes may also be an indicator of suboptimal medical adherence in some cases.

## Renal Dysfunction

The goal of the pretransplant evaluation of kidney function is to differentiate chronic kidney disease (CKD) that will not improve post-HTx from acute kidney injury (AKI) or CKD, which may reverse with the hemodynamic optimization afforded by HTx. This evaluation should take into account (1) historical trends in kidney function during the months to years prior to cardiac decompensation, (2) current trends in kidney function when the patient is hemodynamically optimized, ideally over a few weeks duration, (3) comorbidities (e.g., diabetes, lupus) known to be associated with irreversible kidney damage (4), and other findings like the presence of proteinuria [56]. Transplant candidates should have two independent measurements for GFR at least 2 weeks apart using serum creatinine measurements and race-free equations for eGFR [57–59]. The confirmatory GFR measurement should be a measured GFR, such as 24-h creatinine clearance [60]. The results of ancillary testing may be used to assess for the presence, severity, and chronicity of intrinsic renal disease, including the presence of cortical scarring on renal ultrasound or proteinuria. A kidney biopsy is rarely required. While worse renal function pre- and post-HTx portends worse outcomes post-HTx [2, 61, 62], data demonstrating improved survival with simultaneous heart-kidney transplant versus HTx when pretransplant GFR is below a specific threshold are limited [63–66]. A UNOS registry analysis of over 13,000 recipients transplanted 2005–2018 determined that transplant recipients derived increased survival for simultaneous heart-kidney transplant vs. HTx if they had eGFR < 45 ml/min/1.73 m$^2$ though kidney graft survival was lower in patients after simultaneous heart-kidney transplant than kidney transplant alone (1-year graft loss 14.7% vs 4.5%) [67]. Another challenge is marked changes in kidney function in HTx candidates while on the waiting list. In situations where there is inadequate time to assess for AKI recovery, both heart and kidney specialists should weigh all factors (i.e., perceived kidney reserve and recovery potential, risk or presence of CKD) in order to decide simultaneous kidney and HTx vs HTx candidacy. A caveat to qualify for simultaneous kidney with HTx is that the patient must have evidence for CKD (eGFR < 60 ml/min/m$^2$ at 90 days apart. This policy was initiated as patients with AKI without CKD are mostly able to have kidney recovery after HTx. If patients with eGFR < 30 ml/min/m$^2$ are deemed ineligible for kidney transplantation, HTx alone should generally not be pursued, given worse outcomes in recipients of HTx alone compared with simultaneous kidney and HTx when eGFR < 30 ml/min/m$^2$ [67]. Collaboration with nephrologists is essential for optimal donor stewardship. In the United States, a Safety Net approach has been proposed to theoretically allow better prioritization of donor organs. In this policy, HTx recipients would qualify for the Safety Net kidney donor if they were (1) registered on the kidney waiting list prior to the one-year anniversary of their HTx and (2) were on chronic dialysis or had a measured or estimated creatinine clearance or GFR ≤ 20 ml/min/1.73 m$^2$ between day 60 to day 365 posttransplant [68]. Some critically ill HTx recipients face a high rate of renal allograft dysfunction due to peri-operative hemodynamic instability and may benefit from this option, assuming a living donor is not available.

## Hepatic Dysfunction

Patients with severe heart disease may have co-existing liver disease from various causes. Patients with advanced HF and chronic liver disease who undergo HTx alone have reduced survival compared to those without liver disease [69]. Irreversible hepatic cirrhosis can significantly increase the risks of a HTx and is usually considered an absolute contraindication unless a combined heart and liver transplant (CHLT) can be performed [70].

CHLT is increasingly offered as an option for such patients. In recent years, approximately 40–50 CHLT surgeries have been performed annually in 25 centers in the United States. The most common indications for liver transplant in CHLT include non-congenital heart disease with non-cardiac cirrhosis (e.g., hepatitis C virus (HCV), alcohol-associated cirrhosis), congenital heart disease (CHD) with congestive hepatopathy and variant transthyretin cardiac amyloidosis (though less common in the current era due to the advent of effective disease-directed therapies).

A meta-analysis found that a CHLT is a safe and effective procedure for managing progressive heart and/or liver failure [71]. This meta-analysis included 16 studies with 860 patients. The mortality rate following CHLT was 14.1%. One and five-year survival rates were 85.3 and 71.4%, while the heart and liver rejection rates were 6.1 and 9.1%, respectively. The hospital stay was 25.8 days, and the intensive care unit stay was 9.9 days. These results are comparable to heart-alone transplantation. The authors note that CHLT is a complex procedure that requires expert surgeons, multidisciplinary consultation, and advanced immunology and critical care knowledge.

Liver cirrhosis is generally considered a contraindication to a HTx. However, some studies suggest that patients with end-stage HTx and liver cirrhosis may be eligible for a HTx if cases are carefully selected [72]. However, liver cirrhosis has been linked to poor outcomes after a HTx, and one study found that liver cirrhosis with moderate to severe ascites can lead to worse overall survival for up to two years after the transplant [73]. In that study, between 1994 and 2018, 170 patients with advanced HTx underwent HTx. Abdominal sonography or CT was performed to assess ascites in 163 patients preoperatively. Among them, 49 patients (30.0%) had visualized ascites and enrolled in this study. These patients were divided into two groups [group A; mild ascites (n = 35), B; moderate to massive ascites (n = 14)] and compared the clinical outcomes. The 1, 2, 5 and 10-year survival rates were 82.8 versus 74.3%, 78.4 versus 74.3%, 74.6 versus 74.3% and 74.6 versus 74.3%, respectively, and the survival rates were significantly lower until 2 years in group B than A ($p = 0.035$). However, there was no difference after 2 years ($p = 0.793$). Cox-regression analysis showed a moderate to massive ascites was associated with an increased risk of all-cause death after transplantation ($p < 0.001$).

The decision of when liver transplantation is warranted in a patient with advanced HF and compensated chronic liver disease is challenged by difficulties in differentiating those patients with moderate hepatic fibrosis (which may be reversible) from those with advanced fibrosis and/or cirrhosis who could benefit from this intervention. This can be particularly challenging given the overlap in clinical symptoms in advanced cardiac and liver disease and the lack of rigorous data for CHLT. Dedicated liver imaging should be performed for HTx candidates with the presence or prior history of liver disease or greater than 10 years of cardiac disease. If the liver appears potentially cirrhotic (nodular) on imaging, then liver transplant evaluation should be pursued. In this situation, participants in a consensus conference on heart-liver transplantation agreed that a liver biopsy should be performed when technically feasible and acceptably safe [74]. A liver biopsy may not be required if there are stigmata of portal hypertension (e.g., varices, *ascites)*. In the presence of ascites, it is important to perform diagnostic paracentesis to determine the cause of ascites (hepatic or cardiac). Isolated hepatic venous pressure gradient (HVPG) should not be used to rule in or rule out portal hypertension, especially in patients with Fontan-associated liver disease (FALD), as it may not be reliable. If cross-sectional imaging reveals portosystemic collaterals, upper endoscopy should be performed for variceal screening and the need for primary prophylaxis. In lower-risk patients (those with compensated HF), a normal elastography result (consistent with a liver biopsy of F0/F1) can be used to exclude advanced liver disease.

Biopsy-proven cirrhosis, regardless of the presence of portal hypertension, is generally considered a contraindication for HT alone. Biopsy-proven stage 3 fibrosis (F3) and/or clinical evidence of portal hypertension should be a barrier to HT alone. The CHLT rate for adult

CHD in the U.S. has increased dramatically as more patients with CHD survive into adulthood. Many of these CHD patients have undergone the Fontan procedure, with an estimated global population of 70,000 by 2025, which creates the potential for chronic congestive hepatopathy, known as FALD, warranting CHLT. Survival has been shown to be comparable between the CHD-HTx alone and CHD-CHLT groups [75]. Therefore, it is important that chronic CHD patients with a disease of several years undergo a liver assessment to exclude the need for CHLT [76].

## Cerebrovascular and Peripheral Vascular Disease

Post-operative stroke after HTx is associated with reduced functional capacity [77], and survival and HTx recipients with a history of transient ischemic attack (TIA) or stroke are at increased risk of stroke after transplantation [77–79]. Thus, efforts to reduce the risk of post-transplant strokes are paramount to the evaluation process, and screening for carotid artery stenosis is recommended for all HTx candidates with a history of stroke or neurologic signs or symptoms concerning for cerebrovascular disease, typically with carotid duplex ultrasonography (DUS). Further testing with imaging of the brain and cranial vessels may be required as dictated by neurologic consultation. For those HTx candidates with cerebrovascular disease, the presence of carotid disease warranting revascularization independent of transplant evaluation would be a contraindication until addressed. Consultation with a neurologist and/or vascular surgeon can be useful in this assessment. Another potential contraindication to transplant listing would be deficits from prior cerebrovascular accidents that impair rehabilitation efforts or increase the risk of aspiration and pulmonary infection. These decisions are necessarily individualized based on the patient's overall risk. Similarly, the presence of peripheral arterial disease portends worse survival in patients after HTx, and evaluation for peripheral arterial disease with ankle brachial indices is recommended for all candidates with claudication, diminished peripheral pulses, atherosclerotic disease, or the presence of risk factors associated with peripheral arterial disease. Further testing with arterial ultrasound, CT angiography, or invasive angiography may be required as dictated by the results of initial testing and vascular surgery consultation [80, 81]. There are certain characteristics of peripheral arterial disease that would impact post-transplant outcomes and quality of life and, therefore, could be considered contraindications. First, if a patient has disabling claudication not amenable to revascularization, transplantation would not offer an improvement in quality of life, and the claudication would impair rehabilitation efforts. Second, if a patient has non-healing ischemic ulcers, immunosuppression offers a prohibitive risk of infection and delayed wound healing.

## Frailty

Frailty is a syndrome of reduced physiological reserve resulting in a reduced capacity for an individual to tolerate minor or major stressors and can be observed in association with a variety of chronic disease states and at any age [82, 83]. There is no universally accepted definition of frailty, though the most commonly used frailty instrument in patients with HTx is the Physical Frailty Phenotype (FPF), composed of 5 physical domains—slowness, weakness, weight loss, reduced activity, and exhaustion [82, 84, 85]. Frailty, as measured by the FPF is common in HTx, occurring in up to 50% of patients [84, 86]. And is an independent predictor of mortality, including in those who were actively listed for HTx [86–88]. Frail HTx candidates are also at increased risk for post-transplant mortality [89]. Frailty can be at least partially reversible after LVAD implantation and HTx [90, 91]. However, whether those patients who reverse frailty while awaiting transplantation have better outcomes after transplantation remains unclear. An assessment of frailty can be useful as part of advanced care planning, incorporating both a patient's current functional status and future goal of care into the shared decision-making process [92]. Frailty needs to be re-assessed as time passes for patients with high urgency status awaiting HTx in hospital, especially if on temporary mechanical circulatory support. Those patients who had an acceptable level of frailty when listed as outpatients may no longer be suitable for transplantation after prolonged bed rest. However, the potential for successful post-transplant recovery should be considered when weighing the impact of a candidate's frailty; the ability to ambulate and quadriceps muscle strength may offer insight into recovery potential [93]. A frail candidate with a poor potential for recovery despite post-transplant rehabilitation should not be considered for transplantation, though the criteria for acceptability and prediction of post-transplant recovery is not well established and must be individualized based on the patient's specific clinical picture and center-specific thresholds of risk.

## Infections

In HTx candidates with certain infections, HTx is not recommended; these include (1) active infections requiring ongoing antibiotic treatment (with the possible exception of durable LVAD driveline infection) and (2) HIV with opportunistic infections or related malignancy, lack of stable antiretroviral regimen, detectable viral load, and/or low CD4 count. Other chronic infections such as Hepatitis B and C are no longer absolute contraindications, given advances in the treatment of these conditions. Vaccinations are part of health care maintenance, and as such, initiating or updating life-saving vaccines is the best practice in contemporary transplant medicine [94]. Detailed vaccination schedules are also publicly available and regularly updated by organizations such as the United States Advisory Committee on Immunization Practices [95]. Pre-transplant vaccination is essential, as the candidate is generally not immunosuppressed and thus expected to mount a more robust immune response than after transplantation; this has been observed most dramatically with vaccination against SARS-CoV-2 [96–99]. Ideally, vaccination should be completed at least 2 weeks prior to transplantation in order to optimize immune response. Refusal to accept guideline-recommended vaccinations may be considered a contraindication to transplantation. If live-attenuated vaccines are utilized, the transplant should be deferred for 4 weeks to reduce the risk of active viral replication at the time of transplant [94].

### HIV

Current guidelines currently suggest that selected HIV-positive patients may be considered for transplantation if they have had no active or prior opportunistic infections for 1 month and are clinically stable and adherent with antiretroviral therapy for at least 3 months. Laboratory thresholds of undetectable HIV RNA viral load, CD4 counts greater than 200 cells/microliter for at least 3 months must also be met [100]. Within the HIV-positive population, the guidelines regarding past neoplasms such as squamous cell carcinoma apply: if in remission and upon consultation with oncology, the patient may still be considered for transplantation. The management of HIV-positive transplant candidates requires a multidisciplinary approach to cope with the complex drug interactions during the perioperative period.

### Hepatitis B

While acute or fulminant Hepatitis B (HBV) infection is an absolute contraindication to transplant, patients with either chronic or previously resolved infections may still be considered for transplantation. All patients should undergo complete HBV viral evaluation at 3-month intervals while on the waitlist prior to transplantation, in order to distinguish active from chronic and previously resolved infections. This includes Hepatitis B core antigen (HBcAg), Hepatitis B surface antigen (HBsAg), Hepatitis B envelope antigen (HBeAg), and IgG/IgM antibodies against Hepatitis B core antigen (anti-HBc), antibody against Hepatitis B surface antigen (anti-HBs) and antibody against Hepatitis B envelope antigen (anti-HBe). Prior HBV infection is defined by positive anti-HBc or anti-HBs with negative HBsAg, while chronic infection is defined by HBsAg positivity or the presence of an antiviral drug regimen. It is also recommended that patients with chronic HBV infection undergo liver biopsy in order to exclude severe disease before listing for transplantation. Any clinical, radiologic, or biochemical (including alpha-fetoprotein levels) signs of cirrhosis, portal hypertension, or hepatocellular carcinoma are contraindications to transplantation.

### Hepatitis C

Treatment for Hepatitis C (HCV) with direct-acting antiviral agents can result in a sustained virologic response, and thus, HCV is no longer considered an absolute contraindication to transplant. HCV antibody testing and HCV ribonucleic acid polymerase chain reaction (RNA PCR) testing should be performed at 3-month intervals after initial screening until the time of transplantation to monitor viral loads and identify the status of infection. As with HBV, HCV patients require thorough liver evaluation, including biopsy; any clinical, radiologic, or biochemical (including alpha-fetoprotein levels) signs of cirrhosis, portal hypertension, or hepatocellular carcinoma are contraindications to transplantation [100].

### Tuberculosis

While active tuberculosis is a contraindication to transplant, latent TB should not be, as treatment is effective. All transplant candidates should be screened for latent tuberculosis infection (using a tuberculin skin test or interferon-gamma release assay), and if positive, undergo sputum or bronchoalveolar lavage testing to exclude active TB. Subsequent treatment should not interfere with the timing of transplantation; treatment can commence prior to and continue after transplantation.

### Chagas Disease

All patients born or who spent significant time in Latin America should undergo serologic testing for Trypanosoma cruzi, the parasite that leads to Chagas cardiomyopathy. If positive, treatment with benznidazole or nifurtimox should be administered. HTx is the treatment of choice for these candidates and is therefore not contraindicated in this population, although there is the risk of reactivation of disease. Collaboration with an infectious disease specialist in these cases is recommended.

## Substance Use

Illicit drug use, alcohol use, and tobacco smoking prior to HTx can increase the candidate's risk for poor post-surgical outcomes and mortality [101–104]. A thorough evaluation of the HTx candidate's substance use history should be performed and should include an assessment of any past or current illicit drug use, alcohol use, and tobacco use. Such an evaluation should examine frequency, amount, duration of use, and length of abstinence, as well as the level of impairment that affects the candidate's health, job, and relationships. Any current treatment for substance abuse and the patient's willingness to seek treatment should also be assessed. The presence of substance abuse should be assessed by patient reporting, questionnaires, and biochemical testing. Referrals to addiction services should be made for patients with active substance use disorders. In the critically ill patient who urgently needs transplantation, the assessment of illicit substance use may be difficult to make, and a period of abstinence may not be medically feasible. In this setting, consultation with social work and psychiatric specialists would be essential to gauge the HTx candidate's potential for abstinence and post-transplant adherence. Active tobacco smoking is a contraindication to HTx due to the significant increase in malignancy, cardiac allograft vasculopathy, renal dysfunction, and death associated with tobacco use in HTx recipients [105–107]. A patient can demonstrate candidacy for transplant by abstaining from tobacco use for at least six months. Abstinence from tobacco can be monitored using serum or urine cotinine levels [108]. Given the lack of information currently on e-cigarette use, avoidance of all nicotine products is preferred. Excessive alcohol use is associated with poor medication adherence and adverse outcomes post-transplant [101, 109], including increased mortality, and is an absolute contraindication for HTx. Large international variation exists on acceptable alcohol intake; hence, the national recommendations and standards may be useful in defining excessive alcohol use. Because of the association of shorter time periods of abstinence with relapse post-transplant, the recommended time period for abstinence from alcohol is at least six months [110]. Although marijuana is now legal in many regions for medical and recreational use, inhaled or vaporized cannabis use post-transplant has been linked to increased infection risks and fungal lung infections. In addition, cannabis may alter the metabolism of immunosuppressive medications [111]. Thus, programs will likely continue to make their own center-specific decisions regarding marijuana use and transplant candidacy [112], though it would be safest to emphasize avoidance of marijuana, regardless of legalization.

## Other Systemic Diseases

Active diseases that may or may not contribute to the etiology of HTx but have systemic involvement should be evaluated on a case-by-case basis with regard to potential impact on post-transplant survival and quality of life, preferably in collaboration with a specialist in the relevant field. Evaluation of the potential effects of immunosuppression on the disease itself, as well as potential interactions with existing medications, should also be considered.

## Psychosocial Evaluation

HTx requires significant engagement from patients and their caregivers, as the post-transplant care typically is complex and necessitates regular clinic visits and testing, strict adherence to medications, and adoption of healthy lifestyle measures. The psychosocial evaluation is a key component of the multifaceted pre-transplant screening process, aimed at identifying those candidates at increased risk of poor post-transplant outcomes due to inadequate support, adherence, or optimal mental health; deficits in these factors are associated with poor post-transplant outcomes [103].

Psychosocial assessment should be performed prior to listing for transplantation. This includes assessments to determine the patient's ability to comprehend and comply with care instructions, as well as the patient's ability to give informed consent. Neurocognitive testing may be considered as part of this process. Poor adherence to drug regimens is a risk factor for graft rejection and mortality. Patients who have demonstrated a consistent inability to comply with drug therapy on multiple occasions should not receive transplantation. The ability to demonstrate social support with a dedicated caregiver after transplantation is also extremely important: patients have been denied transplantation because of a lack of social support. A standardized assessment across transplant programs is ideal to minimize inequity in candidate selection. Options for validated standardized assessments include the Stanford Integrated Psychosocial Assessment for Transplant (SIPAT) [113].

Psychiatric evaluation should also be incorporated into the overall evaluation process for HTx listing. This includes a determination of any active psychiatric disease that may have a negative association with adherence to care regimens both pre-and post-HTx. Transplantation can be an emotionally and psychologically taxing experience for candidates and recipients, who may contend with significant challenges related to the evaluation, listing, and waiting period for a suitable donor, as well as adjustment to life with a transplanted organ.

## Financial Considerations

HTx requires a significant financial commitment. The costs for pre-transplant testing, transplant surgery, hospitalization during recovery, and follow-up care, including immunosuppressive medications and monitoring for graft rejection, can be substantial, even with insurance benefits. It is important that patients understand the terms and conditions of their insurance plans and other benefits and have the resources necessary to manage the financial aspects of transplantation without undue stress. HTx is a covered expense for most insurance companies, but coverage varies on a case-by-case basis. Accordingly, a financial coordinator or counselor should review all coverage benefits as part of the evaluation process. This review should include prescription drug coverage, co-pays and deductibles, and requirements for prior authorizations. This information should be reviewed with patients prior to listing, and an estimate of out-of-pocket costs for the surgery and post-transplant care should be included, as well as an overview of fees associated with transplantation. The financial commitment involved is important to consider when moving forward with HTx.

## References

1. Tsao CW, Aday AW, Almarzooq ZI, Alonso A, Beaton AZ, Bittencourt MS, et al. Heart disease and stroke statistics—2022 update: a report from the American Heart Association. Circulation. 2022;145(8):e153-639.
2. Khush KK, Cherikh WS, Chambers DC, Harhay MO, Hayes D, Hsich E, et al. The International Thoracic Organ Transplant Registry of the International Society for Heart and Lung Transplantation: thirty-sixth adult heart transplantation report—2019; focus theme: donor and recipient size match. J Heart Lung Transplant. 2019;38(10):1056–66.
3. Weiss ES, Nwakanma LU, Patel ND, Yuh DD. Outcomes in patients older than 60 years of age undergoing orthotopic heart transplantation: an analysis of the UNOS database. J Heart Lung Transplant. 2008;27(2):184–91.
4. Wever-Pinzon O, Edwards LB, Taylor DO, Kfoury AG, Drakos SG, Selzman CH, et al. Association of recipient age and causes of heart transplant mortality: implications for personalization of post-transplant management—an analysis of the International Society for Heart and Lung Transplantation Registry. J Heart Lung Transplant. 2017;36(4):407–17.
5. Laks H, Marelli D, Fonarow GC, Hamilton MA, Ardehali A, Moriguchi JD, et al. Use of two recipient lists for adults requiring heart transplantation. J Thorac Cardiovasc Surg. 2003;125(1):49–59.
6. Jawitz OK, Raman V, Klapper J, Hartwig M, Patel CB, Milano C. Donor and recipient age matching in heart transplantation: analysis of the UNOS registry. Transpl Int. 2019;32(11):1194–202.
7. Dalal AR. Philosophy of organ donation: review of ethical facets. World J Transplant. 2015;5(2):44.
8. Hsich E, Singh TP, Cherikh WS, Harhay MO, Hayes D, Perch M, et al. The International thoracic organ transplant registry of the international society for heart and lung transplantation: Thirty-ninth adult heart transplantation report—2022; focus on transplant for restrictive heart disease. J Heart Lung Transplant. 2022;41(10):1366–75.
9. Weiss ES, Allen JG, Russell SD, Shah AS, Conte JV. Impact of recipient body mass index on organ allocation and mortality in orthotopic heart transplantation. J Heart Lung Transplant. 2009;28(11):1150–7.
10. Chouairi F, Milner A, Sen S, Guha A, Stewart J, Jastreboff AM, et al. Impact of obesity on heart transplantation outcomes. J Am Heart Assoc. 2021;10(23):e021346.
11. Doumouras BS, Fan CS, Mueller B, Dipchand AI, Manlhiot C, Stehlik J, et al. The effect of pre–heart transplant body mass index on posttransplant outcomes: an analysis of the ISHLT registry data. Clin Transplant. 2019;33(7):e13621.
12. Liu Y, Padilla FA, Graviss EA, Nguyen DT, Lamba HK, Gnanashanmugam S, et al. Outcomes of heart transplant recipients with class II obesity: a United Network for Organ Sharing database analysis. J Surg Res. 2022;272:69–78.
13. Foroutan F, Doumouras BS, Ross H, Alba AC. Impact of pretransplant recipient body mass index on post heart transplant mortality: a systematic review and meta-analysis. Clin Transplant. 2018;32(8):e13348.
14. Russo MJ, Hong KN, Davies RR, Chen JM, Mancini DM, Oz MC, et al. The effect of body mass index on survival following heart transplantation: do outcomes support consensus guidelines? Ann Surg. 2010;251(1):144–52.
15. Okoh AK, Selevany M, Heaton J, Al-Obaidi N, Vucicevic D, Tayal R, et al. Outcomes of

obese patients bridged to heart transplantation with a left ventricular assist device. ASAIO J. 2021;67(2):137–43.
16. Challapalli J, Maynes EJ, O'Malley TJ, Cross DE, Weber MP, Choi JH, et al. Sleeve gastrectomy in patients with continuous-flow left ventricular assist devices: a systematic review and meta-analysis. Obes Surg. 2020;30:4437–45.
17. Choudhury RA, Foster M, Hoeltzel G, Moore HB, Yaffe H, Yoeli D, et al. Bariatric surgery for congestive heart failure patients improves access to transplantation and long-term survival. J Gastrointest Surg. 2021;25(4):926–31.
18. Smith RA, Andrews KS, Brooks D, Fedewa SA, Manassaram-Baptiste D, Saslow D, et al. Cancer screening in the United States, 2018: a review of current American Cancer Society guidelines and current issues in cancer screening. CA Cancer J Clin. 2018;68(4):297–316.
19. Al-Adra DP, Hammel L, Roberts J, Woodle ES, Levine D, Mandelbrot D, et al. Pretransplant solid organ malignancy and organ transplant candidacy: a consensus expert opinion statement. Am J Transplant. 2021;21(2):460–74.
20. Al-Adra DP, Hammel L, Roberts J, Woodle ES, Levine D, Mandelbrot D, et al. Preexisting melanoma and hematological malignancies, prognosis, and timing to solid organ transplantation: a consensus expert opinion statement. Am J Transplant. 2021;21(2):475–83.
21. Humbert M, Kovacs G, Hoeper MM, Badagliacca R, Berger RMF, Brida M, et al. 2022 ESC/ERS guidelines for the diagnosis and treatment of pulmonary hypertension. Eur Respir J. 2023;61(1).
22. Guazzi M, Borlaug BA. Pulmonary hypertension due to left heart disease. Circulation. 2012;126(8):975–90.
23. Simonneau G, Montani D, Celermajer DS, Denton CP, Gatzoulis MA, Krowka M, et al. Haemodynamic definitions and updated clinical classification of pulmonary hypertension. Eur Respir J. 2019;53(1).
24. Bursi F, McNallan SM, Redfield MM, Nkomo VT, Lam CSP, Weston SA, et al. Pulmonary pressures and death in heart failure: a community study. J Am Coll Cardiol. 2012;59(3):222–31.
25. Damy T, Goode KM, Kallvikbacka-Bennett A, Lewinter C, Hobkirk J, Nikitin NP, et al. Determinants and prognostic value of pulmonary arterial pressure in patients with chronic heart failure. Eur Heart J. 2010;31(18):2280–90.
26. Vakil K, Duval S, Sharma A, Adabag S, Abidi KS, Taimeh Z, et al. Impact of pre-transplant pulmonary hypertension on survival after heart transplantation: a UNOS registry analysis. Int J Cardiol. 2014;176(3):595–9.
27. Kirklin JK, Naftel DC, Kirklin JW, Blackstone EH, White-Williams C, Bourge RC. Pulmonary vascular resistance and the risk of heart transplantation. J Heart Transplant. 1988;7(5):331–6.
28. Matkovic M, Milicevic V, Bilbija I, Aleksic N, Cubrilo M, Nestorovic E, et al. Pulmonary artery hypertension as a risk factor for long-term survival after heart transplantation. In: The Heart Surgery Forum. 2021. p. E544–9.
29. Costard-Jäckle A, Fowler MB. Influence of preoperative pulmonary artery pressure on mortality after heart transplantation: testing of potential reversibility of pulmonary hypertension with nitroprusside is useful in defining a high risk group. J Am Coll Cardiol. 1992;19(1):48–54.
30. Butler J, Stankewicz MA, Wu J, Chomsky DB, Howser RL, Khadim G, et al. Pre-transplant reversible pulmonary hypertension predicts higher risk for mortality after cardiac transplantation. J Heart Lung Transplant. 2005;24(2):170–7.
31. Zern EK, Cheng S, Wolfson AM, Hamilton MA, Zile MR, Solomon SD, et al. Angiotensin receptor-neprilysin inhibitor therapy reverses pulmonary hypertension in end-stage heart failure patients awaiting transplantation. Circ Heart Fail. 2020;13(2):e006696.
32. Kutty RS, Parameshwar J, Lewis C, Catarino PA, Sudarshan CD, Jenkins DP, et al. Use of centrifugal left ventricular assist device as a bridge to candidacy in severe heart failure with secondary pulmonary hypertension. Eur J Cardiothorac Surg. 2013;43(6):1237–42.
33. Mikus E, Stepanenko A, Krabatsch T, Loforte A, Dandel M, Lehmkuhl HB, et al. Reversibility of fixed pulmonary hypertension in left ventricular assist device support recipients. Eur J Cardiothorac Surg. 2011;40(4):971–7.
34. Zimpfer D, Zrunek P, Roethy W, Czerny M, Schima H, Huber L, et al. Left ventricular assist devices decrease fixed pulmonary hypertension in cardiac transplant candidates. J Thorac Cardiovasc Surg. 2007;133(3):689–95.
35. John R, Liao K, Kamdar F, Eckman P, Boyle A, Colvin-Adams M. Effects on pre-and posttransplant pulmonary hemodynamics in patients with continuous-flow left ventricular assist devices. J Thorac Cardiovasc Surg. 2010;140(2):447–52.
36. Thangappan K, Morales DLS, Vu Q, Lehenbauer D, Villa C, Wittekind S, et al. Impact of mechanical circulatory support on pediatric heart transplant candidates with elevated pulmonary vascular resistance. Artif Organs. 2021;45(1):29–37.
37. Moayedifar R, Zuckermann A, Aliabadi-Zuckermann A, Riebandt J, Angleitner P, Dimitrov K, et al. Long-term heart transplant outcomes after lowering fixed pulmonary hypertension using left ventricular assist devices†. Eur J Cardio-Thorac Surg [Internet]. 2018;54(6):1116–21. https://doi.org/10.1093/ejcts/ezy214.
38. de Frutos F, Díez-López C, Sánchez-Salado JC, Miralles A, Manito N, González-Costello J.

Left ventricular assist devices in patients eligible for heart transplant with irreversible pulmonary hypertension. Rev Esp Cardiol (Engl Ed). 2020;73(7):583–6.
39. Hawkins NM, Petrie MC, Jhund PS, Chalmers GW, Dunn FG, McMurray JJV. Heart failure and chronic obstructive pulmonary disease: diagnostic pitfalls and epidemiology. Eur J Heart Fail. 2009;11(2):130–9.
40. Carter P, Lagan J, Fortune C, Bhatt DL, Vestbo J, Niven R, et al. Association of cardiovascular disease with respiratory disease. J Am Coll Cardiol. 2019;73(17):2166–77.
41. Lundgren SW, Lowes BD, Lyden E, Zolty R, Burdorf A, Hyden M, et al. Pulmonary function testing pre–heart transplant predicts posttransplant survival. Transplant Direct. 2021;7(10):e752.
42. Rivinius R, Helmschrott M, Ruhparwar A, Schmack B, Darche FF, Thomas D, et al. COPD in patients after heart transplantation is associated with a prolonged hospital stay, early posttransplant atrial fibrillation, and impaired posttransplant survival. Clin Epidemiol. 2018;1359–69.
43. Huang WM, Feng JY, Cheng HM, Chen SZ, Huang CJ, Guo CY, et al. The role of pulmonary function in patients with heart failure and preserved ejection fraction: looking beyond chronic obstructive pulmonary disease. PLoS ONE. 2020;15(7):e0235152.
44. Magnussen H, Canepa M, Zambito PE, Brusasco V, Meinertz T, Rosenkranz S. What can we learn from pulmonary function testing in heart failure? Eur J Heart Fail. 2017;19(10):1222–9.
45. Adabag AS, Wassif HS, Rice K, Mithani S, Johnson D, Bonawitz-Conlin J, et al. Preoperative pulmonary function and mortality after cardiac surgery. Am Heart J. 2010;159(4):691–7.
46. Dunlay SM, Killian JM, Mccoy RG, Redfield MM. Diabetes mellitus in advanced heart failure. J Card Fail. 2022;28(3):503–8.
47. Russo MJ, Chen JM, Hong KN, Stewart AS, Ascheim DD, Argenziano M, et al. Survival after heart transplantation is not diminished among recipients with uncomplicated diabetes mellitus: an analysis of the United Network of Organ Sharing database. Circulation. 2006;114(21):2280–7.
48. Saraiva J, Sola E, Prieto D, Antunes MJ. Diabetes as an outcome predictor after heart transplantation. Interact Cardiovasc Thorac Surg. 2011;13(5):499–504.
49. Rivinius R, Gralla C, Helmschrott M, Darche FF, Ehlermann P, Bruckner T, et al. Pre-transplant type 2 diabetes mellitus is associated with higher graft failure and increased 5-year mortality after heart transplantation. Front Cardiovasc Med. 2022;9:890359.
50. Foroutan F, Alba AC, Guyatt G, Posada JD, Hing NNF, Arseneau E, et al. Predictors of 1-year mortality in heart transplant recipients: a systematic review and meta-analysis. Heart. 2018;104(2):151–60.
51. López-Sainz Á, Barge-Caballero E, Barge-Caballero G, Couto-Mallón D, Paniagua-Martin MJ, Seoane-Quiroga L, et al. Late graft failure in heart transplant recipients: incidence, risk factors and clinical outcomes. Eur J Heart Fail. 2018;20(2):385–94.
52. Radovancevic B, Konuralp C, Vrtovec B, Radovancevic R, Thomas CD, Zaqqa M, et al. Factors predicting 10-year survival after heart transplantation. J Heart Lung Transplant. 2005;24(2):156–9.
53. Jalowiec A, Grady KL, White-Williams C. Heart transplant outcomes in patients with pretransplant diabetes mellitus. Am J Crit Care. 2017;26(6):482–90.
54. Newman JD, Schlendorf KH, Cox ZL, Zalawadiya SK, Powers AC, Niswender KD, et al. Post-transplant diabetes mellitus following heart transplantation. J Heart Lung Transplant. 2022;41(11):1537–46.
55. Qaseem A, Wilt TJ, Kansagara D, Horwitch C, Barry MJ, Forciea MA, et al. Hemoglobin A1c targets for glycemic control with pharmacologic therapy for nonpregnant adults with type 2 diabetes mellitus: a guidance statement update from the American College of Physicians. Ann Intern Med. 2018;168(8):569–76.
56. Kobashigawa J, Dadhania DM, Farr M, Tang WHW, Bhimaraj A, Czer L, et al. Consensus conference on heart-kidney transplantation. Am J Transplant. 2021;21(7):2459–67.
57. Delgado C, Baweja M, Crews DC, Eneanya ND, Gadegbeku CA, Inker LA, et al. A unifying approach for GFR estimation: recommendations of the NKF-ASN task force on reassessing the inclusion of race in diagnosing kidney disease. J Am Soc Nephrol. 2021;32(12):2994–3015.
58. Panchal S, Serper M, Bittermann T, Asrani SK, Goldberg DS, Mahmud N. Impact of race-adjusted glomerular filtration rate estimation on eligibility for simultaneous liver-kidney transplantation. Liver Transpl. 2022;28(6):959–68.
59. Dadhania DM, Doshi MD. Achieving equity for liver transplantation recipients with chronic kidney disease. Liver Transplant. 2022;28(6):920–2.
60. Kolsrud O, Ricksten SE, Holmberg E, Felldin M, Karason K, Hammarsten O, et al. Measured and not estimated glomerular filtration rate should be used to assess renal function in heart transplant recipients. Nephrol Dial Transplant. 2016;31(7):1182–9.
61. Habib PJ, Patel PC, Hodge D, Chimato N, Yip DS, Hosenpud JD, et al. Pre-orthotopic heart transplant estimated glomerular filtration rate predicts post-transplant mortality and renal outcomes: an analysis of the UNOS database. J Heart Lung Transplant. 2016;35(12):1471–9.

62. Kolsrud O, Karason K, Holmberg E, Ricksten SE, Felldin M, Samuelsson O, et al. Renal function and outcome after heart transplantation. J Thorac Cardiovasc Surg. 2018;155(4):1593–604.
63. Agarwal KA, Patel H, Agrawal N, Cardarelli F, Goyal N. Cardiac outcomes in isolated heart and simultaneous kidney and heart transplants in the United States. Kidney Int Rep. 2021;6(9):2348–57.
64. Karamlou T, Welke KF, McMullan DM, Cohen GA, Gelow J, Tibayan FA, et al. Combined heart-kidney transplant improves post-transplant survival compared with isolated heart transplant in recipients with reduced glomerular filtration rate: analysis of 593 combined heart-kidney transplants from the United Network Organ Sharing Database. J Thorac Cardiovasc Surg. 2014;147(1):456–61.
65. Russo MJ, Rana A, Chen JM, Hong KN, Gelijns A, Moskowitz A, et al. Pretransplantation patient characteristics and survival following combined heart and kidney transplantation: an analysis of the United Network for Organ Sharing Database. Arch Surg. 2009;144(3):241–6.
66. Kilic A, Grimm JC, Whitman GJR, Shah AS, Mandal K, Conte JV, et al. The survival benefit of simultaneous heart-kidney transplantation extends beyond dialysis-dependent patients. Ann Thorac Surg. 2015;99(4):1321–7.
67. Itagaki S, Toyoda N, Moss N, Mancini D, Egorova N, Mikami T, et al. Outcomes of simultaneous heart and kidney transplantation. J Am Coll Cardiol. 2023;81(8):729–40.
68. Establish Eligibility Criteria and Safety Net for Heart-Kidney and Lung-Kidney Allocation - OPTN [Internet]. https://optn.transplant.hrsa.gov/policies-bylaws/public-comment/establish-eligibility-criteria-and-safety-net-for-heart-kidney-and-lung-kidney-allocation/. Accessed 21 May 2024
69. Khush KK, Hsich E, Potena L, Cherikh WS, Chambers DC, Harhay MO, et al. The International Thoracic Organ Transplant Registry of the International Society for Heart and Lung Transplantation: thirty-eighth adult heart transplantation report—2021; focus on recipient characteristics. J Heart Lung Transplant. 2021;40(10):1035–49.
70. Sasevich MJ, Esmailian F, Rihbany K, Pouldar T, Yu Z, Liou F, et al. Is Pre-Existing Liver Cirrhosis and Fibrosis a Contraindication to Heart Transplantation? J Heart Lung Transplant. 2014;33(4):S157.
71. Frountzas M, Karampetsou N, Nikolaou C, Schizas D, Tsapralis D, Avgerinos D, et al. Combined heart and liver transplantation: an updated systematic review. Ann R Coll Surg Engl. 2022;104(2):88–94.
72. Hsu RB, Chang CI, Lin FY, Chou NK, Chi NH, Wang SS, et al. Heart transplantation in patients with liver cirrhosis. Eur J Cardiothorac Surg. 2008;34(2):307–12.
73. Kim H, Kim J, Lee S, Joo H, Yoo K, Youn Y. Heart transplantation outcomes in liver cirrhosis: influence of ascites on post-transplantation survival. J Heart Lung Transplant. 2019;38(4):S289-90.
74. Kobashigawa J, VanWagner LB, Hall S, Emamaullee J, Entwistle JW, Ganger D, et al. Summary of a consensus conference on heart-liver transplantation. Am J Transplant. 2024;24(3):380–90.
75. Bryant R 3rd, Rizwan R, Zafar F, Shah SA, Chin C, Tweddell JS, et al. Contemporary outcomes of combined heart-liver transplant in patients with congenital heart disease. Transplantation. 2018;102(2):e67-73.
76. Emamaullee J, Zaidi AN, Schiano T, Kahn J, Valentino PL, Hofer RE, et al. Fontan-associated liver disease: screening, management, and transplant considerations. Circulation. 2020;142(6):591–604.
77. Patlolla V, Mogulla V, DeNofrio D, Konstam MA, Krishnamani R. Outcomes in patients with symptomatic cerebrovascular disease undergoing heart transplantation. J Am Coll Cardiol. 2011;58(10):1036–41.
78. Alnsasra H, Asleh R, Kumar N, Lopez C, Toya T, Kremers WK, et al. Incidence, risk factors, and outcomes of stroke following cardiac transplantation. Am Heart Assoc. 2021.
79. Alvarez P, Kitai T, Okamoto T, Niikawa H, McCurry KR, Papamichail A, et al. Trends, risk factors, and outcomes of post-operative stroke after heart transplantation: an analysis of the UNOS database. ESC Heart Fail. 2021;8(5):4211–7.
80. Enciso JS, Kato TS, Jin Z, Chung C, Yang J, Takayama H, et al. Effect of peripheral vascular disease on mortality in cardiac transplant recipients (from the United Network of Organ Sharing Database). Am J Cardiol. 2014;114(7):1111–5.
81. Gerhard-Herman MD, Gornik HL, Barrett C, Barshes NR, Corriere MA, Drachman DE, et al. 2016 AHA/ACC guideline on the management of patients with lower extremity peripheral artery disease: executive summary: a report of the American College of Cardiology/American Heart Association Task Force on Clinical Practice Guidelines. Circulation. 2017;135(12):e686-725.
82. Fried LP, Tangen CM, Walston J, Newman AB, Hirsch C, Gottdiener J, et al. Frailty in older adults: evidence for a phenotype. J Gerontol A Biol Sci Med Sci. 2001;56(3):M146-57.
83. Clegg A, Young J, Iliffe S, Rikkert MO, Rockwood K. Frailty in elderly people. The Lancet. 2013;381(9868):752–62.
84. Denfeld QE, Winters-Stone K, Mudd JO, Gelow JM, Kurdi S, Lee CS. The prevalence of frailty in heart failure: a systematic review and meta-analysis. Int J Cardiol. 2017;236:283–9.
85. McDonagh J, Martin L, Ferguson C, Jha SR, Macdonald PS, Davidson PM, et al. Frailty

assessment instruments in heart failure: a systematic review. Eur J Cardiovasc Nurs. 2018;17(1):23–35.
86. Jha SR, Hannu MK, Chang S, Montgomery E, Harkess M, Wilhelm K, et al. The prevalence and prognostic significance of frailty in patients with advanced heart failure referred for heart transplantation. Transplantation. 2016;100(2):429–36.
87. Jha SR, Hannu MK, Gore K, Chang S, Newton P, Wilhelm K, et al. Cognitive impairment improves the predictive validity of physical frailty for mortality in patients with advanced heart failure referred for heart transplantation. J Heart Lung Transplant. 2016;35(9):1092–100.
88. Moayedi Y, Duero Posada JG, Foroutan F, Goldraich LA, Alba AC, MacIver J, et al. The prognostic significance of frailty compared to peak oxygen consumption and B-type natriuretic peptide in patients with advanced heart failure. Clin Transplant. 2018;32(1):e13158.
89. Kobashigawa J, Shah P, Joseph S, Olymbios M, Bhat G, Dhital K, et al. Frailty in heart transplantation: report from the heart workgroup of a consensus conference on frailty. Am J Transplant. 2021;21(2):636–44.
90. Maurer MS, Horn E, Reyentovich A, Dickson VV, Pinney S, Goldwater D, et al. Can a left ventricular assist device in individuals with advanced systolic heart failure improve or reverse frailty? J Am Geriatr Soc. 2017;65(11):2383–90.
91. Jha SR, Hannu MK, Newton PJ, Wilhelm K, Hayward CS, Jabbour A, et al. Reversibility of frailty after bridge-to-transplant ventricular assist device implantation or heart transplantation. Transplant Direct. 2017;3(7):e167.
92. Allen LA, Stevenson LW, Grady KL, Goldstein NE, Matlock DD, Arnold RM, et al. Decision making in advanced heart failure: a scientific statement from the American Heart Association. Circulation. 2012;125(15):1928–52.
93. Walsh JR, Chambers DC, Hopkins PMA. The emerging importance of skeletal muscle function in assessing candidates for transplantation. Transplantation. 2017;101(9):1967–8.
94. Danziger-Isakov L, Kumar D, practice ASTIDC of. Vaccination of solid organ transplant candidates and recipients: guidelines from the American society of transplantation infectious diseases community of practice. Clin Transplant. 2019;33(9):e13563.
95. Kroger A, Bahta L, Long S, Sanchez P. General best practice guidelines for immunization: best practices guidance of the Advisory Committee on Immunization Practices (ACIP). 2023.
96. Aslam S, Danziger-Isakov L, Mehra MR. COVID-19 vaccination immune paresis in heart and lung transplantation. J Heart Lung Transplant. 2021;40(8):763–6.
97. Peled Y, Ram E, Lavee J, Sternik L, Segev A, Wieder-Finesod A, et al. BNT162b2 vaccination in heart transplant recipients: clinical experience and antibody response. J Heart Lung Transplant. 2021;40(8):759–62.
98. Boyarsky BJ, Werbel WA, Avery RK, Tobian AAR, Massie AB, Segev DL, et al. Antibody response to 2-dose SARS-CoV-2 mRNA vaccine series in solid organ transplant recipients. JAMA. 2021;325(21):2204–6.
99. Wadei HM, Gonwa TA, Leoni JC, Shah SZ, Aslam N, Speicher LL. COVID-19 infection in solid organ transplant recipients after SARS-CoV-2 vaccination. Am J Transplant. 2021;21(10):3496.
100. Mehra MR, Canter CE, Hannan MM, Semigran MJ, Uber PA, Baran DA, et al. The 2016 International Society for Heart Lung Transplantation listing criteria for heart transplantation: a 10-year update. J Heart Lung Transplant. 2016;35(1):1–23.
101. Dew MA, DiMartini AF, Steel J, De Vito DA, Myaskovsky L, Unruh M, et al. Meta-analysis of risk for relapse to substance use after transplantation of the liver or other solid organs. Liver Transplant. 2008;14(2):159–72.
102. Bui QM, Allen LA, LeMond L, Brambatti M, Adler E. Psychosocial evaluation of candidates for heart transplant and ventricular assist devices: beyond the current consensus. Circ Heart Fail. 2019;12(7):e006058.
103. Dew MA, DiMartini AF, Dobbels F, Grady KL, Jowsey-Gregoire SG, Kaan A, et al. The 2018 ISHLT/APM/AST/ICCAC/STSW recommendations for the psychosocial evaluation of adult cardiothoracic transplant candidates and candidates for long-term mechanical circulatory support. Psychosomatics. 2018;59(5):415–40.
104. Owen JE, Bonds CL, Wellisch DK. Psychiatric evaluations of heart transplant candidates: predicting post-transplant hospitalizations, rejection episodes, and survival. Psychosomatics. 2006;47(3):213–22.
105. Duerinckx N, Burkhalter H, Engberg SJ, Kirsch M, Klem ML, Sereika SM, et al. Correlates and outcomes of posttransplant smoking in solid organ transplant recipients: a systematic literature review and meta-analysis. Transplantation. 2016;100(11):2252–63.
106. Roussel JC, Baron O, Périgaud C, Bizouarn P, Pattier S, Habash O, et al. Outcome of heart transplants 15 to 20 years ago: graft survival, post-transplant morbidity, and risk factors for mortality. J Heart Lung Transplant. 2008;27(5):486–93.
107. Botha P, Peaston R, White K, Forty J, Dark JH, Parry G. Smoking after cardiac transplantation. Am J Transplant. 2008;8(4):866–71.
108. Kim S. Overview of cotinine cutoff values for smoking status classification. Neurosci Nicotine. 2019;419–31.

109. Parker R, Armstrong MJ, Corbett C, Day EJ, Neuberger JM. Alcohol and substance abuse in solid-organ transplant recipients. Transplantation. 2013;96(12):1015–24.
110. Tome S, Said A, Lucey MR. Addictive behavior after solid organ transplantation: what do we know already and what do we need to know? Liver Transplant. 2008;14:127–9. Wiley Online Library.
111. Thompson GR, Tuscano JM, Dennis M, Singapuri A, Libertini S, Gaudino R, et al. A microbiome assessment of medical marijuana. Clin Microbiol Infect. 2017;23(4):269–70.
112. Neyer J, Uberoi A, Hamilton M, Kobashigawa JA. Marijuana and listing for heart transplant: a survey of transplant providers. Circ Heart Fail. 2016;9(7):e002851.
113. Maldonado JR, Sher Y, Lolak S, Swendsen H, Skibola D, Neri E, et al. The Stanford Integrated Psychosocial Assessment for Transplantation: a prospective study of medical and psychosocial outcomes. Psychosom Med. 2015;77(9):1018–30.

# Part II
# Pre-Heart Transplant Considerations

# 5 Listing Criteria and Optimization of the Pre-transplant Patient

Michelle M. Kittleson

**Abstract**

Once evaluation as a potential transplant candidate is complete, there are still many processes that a patient must undergo before receiving a donor heart. All transplant candidates spend time on the waitlist after listing; the current donor heart shortage means that, unfortunately, waitlist mortality remains a significant problem. This chapter aims to provide an overview of the listing process, the current US system of heart allocation, medical surveillance, immunological optimization, and other considerations of patients on the waiting list.

**Keywords**

Heart failure · Heart transplantation · Allocation · Policy · Donor heart

M. M. Kittleson (✉)
Cedars-Sinai Smidt Heart Institute, Los Angeles, CA, USA
e-mail: michelle.kittleson@cshs.org

## Clinical Pearls

- Heart Transplant Candidates undergo rigorous evaluation, culminating in multi-disciplinary selection meetings that include transplant and heart failure (HF) cardiologists, transplant surgeons, a psychiatrist, social workers, transplant coordinators, apharmacist, and a dietician, to determine suitability for transplant. If approved, the patient is then listed for transplant.
- Advantages of the new 2018 six-tiered heart allocation system include prioritization of more unstable inpatient candidates,such as those with ECMO support (Status 1), over those receiving inotropic support with hemodynamic monitoring (Status 3).
- Once listed, patients should be frequently clinically reevaluated and managed accordingly, taking into account HF symptoms,hemodynamic stability, and exercise capacity as priority status may change.
- Factors associated with increased HTx waitlist mortality include older age, lower BMI, male sex, diabetes, dialysis, poorfunctional status at listing, and higher urgency status.
- Patients on the heart transplant waitlist should be monitored at least annually for the detection of circulating anti-HLA antibodies, as these may decrease the donor pool while awaiting an immunologically compatible donor.



J. Kobashigawa (ed.), *Clinical Guide to Heart Transplantation*, https://doi.org/10.1007/978-3-031-88290-6_5

- Special considerations for patients on the waitlist include a switch from DOAC to Coumadin, discontinuation of antiplatelet-drugs to minimize perioperative bleeding.
- Monitoring of waitlist patients with pulmonary hypertension with regularly scheduled echocardiograms (at least q 6 months)and/or intra-pulmonary artery device may be helpful to avoid right ventricular failure of the donor heart at the time of implantation.

## Listing Process

Once evaluation as a potential transplant candidate is complete, there are still many processes that a patient must undergo before receiving a donor heart. All transplant candidates spend time on the waitlist after listing; the current donor heart shortage means that, unfortunately, waitlist mortality remains a significant problem [1]. As described in Chaps. 3 and 4, heart transplant (HTx) candidates undergo rigorous medical and psychosocial evaluation for transplant suitability. In most institutions, the culmination of this process is a final review of relevant information at regularly scheduled multi-disciplinary meetings, including the transplant and heart failure (HF) cardiologists, transplant surgeons, other physicians involved with the patient's care, psychiatrist, social workers, transplant coordinators, pharmacist, and dietician. At these meetings, a final decision regarding suitability for transplant is made, and the patient, if suitable, is listed for transplant. The HTx waiting list is a national, computerized list that is managed and maintained by the Organ Procurement and Transplantation Network (OPTN). Listing includes relevant recipient patient variables, including patient name, weight, weight range of acceptable donors, blood group, unacceptable antigens, immunological virtual crossmatch data, and whether a prospective crossmatch will be required (for highly sensitized patients) at the time of donor selection. Each patient is also assigned an urgency status code according to the priority level on the list (see below for more details). Within a status code level, candidates are ordered by time spent on the waiting list. As a donor becomes available, the donor's heart is offered to the highest recipient on the list that matches in terms of sizing, weight, blood group, and immunological criteria; if declined, the heart is offered to the next candidate on the list.

## Allocation Criteria

### A Brief History

The National Organ Transplant Act, which was enacted by Congress in 1984, was responsible for the formation of the OPTN, a unified transplant network that governs organ transplantation in the United States. Since the inception of the OPTN, allocation policy has undergone several iterations. A formal urgency-based system was first adopted in 1988 by the Department of Health and Human Services (DHHS). Initially, there were only two status levels: Status 1 and Status 2, with the sickest patients in Status 1, and others in Status 2 [2, 3]. Further major revisions occurred in 1999, with the introduction of a higher priority level for sicker Status 1 patients, dividing the Status 1 classification into Status 1A and 1B. The Final Rule, issued by the DHHS in 2000, dictated that policy must attempt to balance the difficult combination of equitable organ allocation (including across regions) while prioritizing according to severity of illness. Unfortunately, unlike kidneys, explanted hearts are currently only viable for a maximum of 4–6 h, so allocation needs to be delineated within geographic regions, further affecting distribution equity. In an update in 2005, patients listed for cardiac transplantation were stratified into a three-tiered system of escalating urgency for HTx to enhance broader access to donors. By 2015, the sickest patients in the Status 1A tier increased 5-fold and accounted for two-thirds of HTx recipients [4].

## The 2018 Allocation Revision

Despite good intentions to optimize organ allocation, there were critiques of the 2005 system [4] namely that the former Status 1A provided inadequate resolution among the sickest patients: a heterogenous group of unstable HTx candidates received the same prioritization despite different waitlist mortality [2]. The Thoracic Organ Transplantation Committee redesigned a six-tiered heart allocation system with a broader geographic sharing policy, implemented on October 18, 2018 (Table 5.1).

Advantages of the new system include prioritization of more unstable inpatient candidates, such as those with ECMO support (Status 1), over those receiving inotropic support with hemodynamic monitoring (Status 3), as well as prioritization of ambulatory HTx candidates with poorer prognosis, those with infiltrative or hypertrophic cardiomyopathy (Status 4), over those with nonischemic dilated cardiomyopathy (Status 6). There have been significant shifts in HTx practices and patient outcomes following the implementation of the new policy, including changes in listing practices, waitlist time and mortality, transplant donor characteristics, post-transplantation outcomes, and mechanical circulatory support use (Fig. 5.1) [5].

In a comparative analysis of the 2 eras, a larger proportion of transplantation procedures (78 vs. 68%) were performed in the highest-priority patients following the policy change [6]. Interestingly, an analysis that applied the new risk stratification rules to candidates from the pre-policy era demonstrated 17% more status 2 listings than anticipated, corresponding to the observed increase in the use of IABP, and the odds of high-priority listing were 5 times greater

**Table 5.1** Heart transplant allocation system as of October 2018

| Status | Status description |
|---|---|
| 1 | VA-ECMO |
| | Non-dischargeable surgically implanted Bi-VAD |
| | LVAD with life-threatening VT or VF |
| 2 | Non-dischargeable surgically implanted LVAD |
| | IABP |
| | Life-threatening VT or VF |
| | LVAD with mechanical failure, admitted to the hospital |
| | Percutaneous endovascular pump (e.g. Impella®) |
| | TAH, Bi-VAD, RVAD, or VAD for single ventricle patient |
| 3 | LVAD discharged with discretionary 30 days |
| | LVAD with device infection, hemolysis, pump thrombosis, right heart failure, mucosal bleeding or aortic regurgitation |
| | Multiple inotropes or single high dose inotrope with PA catheter |
| | VA-ECMO, IABP, or percutaneous endovascular pump that downgrades |
| 4 | Dischargeable LVAD without discretionary 30 days |
| | Multiple inotropes or single high dose inotrope without PA catheter |
| | Congenital heart disease, refractory angina, re-transplantation |
| | Amyloidosis, Hypertrophic or Restrictive cardiomyopathy |
| 5 | Listed for heart transplant and at least one other organ |
| 6 | All other adult heart candidates not meeting higher Status |
| 7 | Inactive |

*Source* Publicly available at: https://optn.transplant.hrsa.gov/media/km0bko0h/adult_heart_criteria.pdf
VA-ECMO, Veno-arterial extracorporeal membranous oxygenation; Bi-VAD, Biventricular assist device; LVAD, Left ventricular assist device; VT, Ventricular tachycardia; VF, Ventricular fibrillation; IABP, Intra-aortic balloon pump; Impella® (ABIOMED Inc., Danvers MA, USA); TAH, Total artificial heart; RVAD, Right ventricular assist device

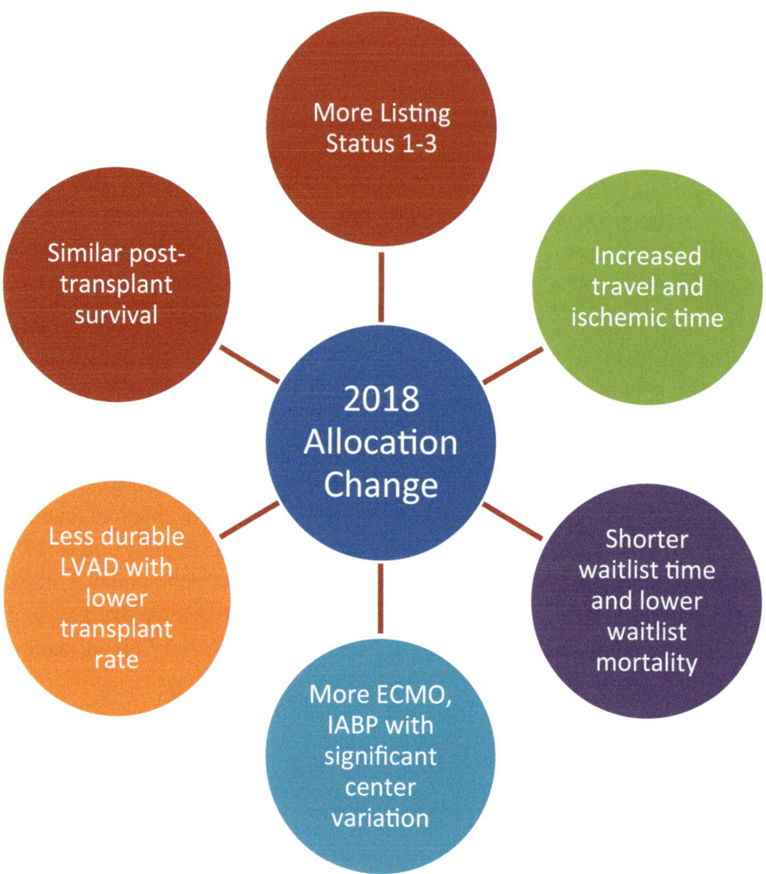


**Fig. 5.1** Summary of the impact of 2018 Allocation Change. ECMO = extracorporeal membrane oxygenation; IABP = intra-aortic balloon pump; ICU = intensive care unit; LVAD = left ventricular assist device

than expected following the policy change despite similar candidate characteristics [7]. On the other hand, the placement of durable mechanical circulatory support devices has decreased [8, 9]. Without a clear change in candidate characteristics nor overall number of listings, these phenomena may reflect a concerted change in clinical practice by transplant providers to meet the new high-priority criteria for patients that had lower urgency by previous era criteria. Despite a greater proportion of highest priority additions (statuses 1–3) to the waitlist in the new era, waitlist mortality is similar in some studies and even reduced in others, both at 90 days and 1 year [10, 11]. Despite the highest priority listings in the new era, the similar, if not improved, waitlist mortality is suggestive of the policy change functioning as intended, although further data will continue to assess waitlist outcomes.

## Optimization of the Pre-transplant Patient

### Medical Surveillance on the Waitlist

Medical treatment of HF and the evaluation criteria for HTx candidacy have already been covered in Chaps. 1–4. However, even once listed, patients should be frequently clinically reevaluated and managed accordingly, taking into account HF symptoms, hemodynamic stability (including blood pressure and EF

**Table 5.2** Guidelines for consideration of inactivation of heart transplant waitlist candidates due to clinical improvement

| Clinical criteria | Exercise criteria (assuming initial peak oxygen consumption of <14 ml/kg/min) |
|---|---|
| • Stable fluid balance without orthopnea, elevated jugular venous pressures or other evidence of congestion<br>• Stable blood pressure with systolic ≥ 80 mmHg<br>• Stable serum sodium (≥133 mEq/L)<br>• Stable renal function (BUN < 50 mg/dl, creatinine < 2 mg/dl)<br>• Absence of symptomatic ventricular arrhythmia<br>• Absence of frequent angina<br>• Absence of severe drug side effects<br>• Stable or improving activity level without dyspnea during self-care or 1-block exertion<br>• Increasing ejection fraction by echocardiogram | • Improvement in peak oxygen consumption of ≥2 mg/kg/min<br>• Peak oxygen consumption of ≥14 ml/kg/min |

Reused with permission: Michelle Kittleson, Jon Kobashigawa, Minh Luu, Listing, Donor Allocation and and Optimization of the Pre-transplant Patient, Clinical Guide to Heart Transplantation, 37–45, 2017, Springer Nature; https://doi.org/10.1007/978-3-319-43773-6_4

by echocardiography), and exercise capacity. Serum electrolytes and renal function should also be reviewed. The general aim is to maintain or even improve the level of function at listing until transplantation, essentially to make sure each patient remains an optimal candidate and is appropriately risk-stratified. A formal reevaluation on a yearly basis is required to reassess each patient's ongoing candidacy for transplant. A significant number of patients initially listed for transplantation may have clinical improvement, no longer requiring active transplant listing. In these cases, the patient should still undergo exercise testing, clinical evaluation, and hemodynamic assessment every few months. A detailed list of criteria for inactivation of HTx candidates due to clinical improvement is given in Table 5.2 Alternatively, some patients may have further clinical deterioration, requiring the difficult task of delisting them. Ideally, palliative care teams should be involved with all patients evaluated and undergoing HTx to assist with the complex issues involved. Pre-transplant outcomes indicate that 1-year survival on the HTx waiting list was 63.9% between 2007 and 2017 [12]. Thus, vigilance for indications of worsening HF or complications related to HF is crucial in both the inpatient and outpatient waitlist candidates.

In the outpatient waitlist candidate, such a scenario should necessitate immediate admission for evaluation and appropriate treatment. Likewise, inpatients should be monitored daily for the above. Ultimately, the goal is to prevent conditions that may subsequently negatively affect the perioperative outcomes, as well as death on the waitlist. A full list of indications for readmission is summarized in Table 5.3. Factors associated with increased HTx waitlist mortality include older age, lower BMI, male sex, diabetes, dialysis, poor functional status at listing, and higher urgency status [12]. These patients should, therefore, be monitored especially closely. Should a patient deteriorate and consequently display a relative contraindication to transplantation, the patient is placed on the inactive list (Status 7), and medical or device therapy is administered as appropriate. Once the patient has improved, the patient is reevaluated for transplanted suitability and is able to return to the transplant list without penalty (i.e., the time previously spent on the waitlist is counted).

## Immunological Optimization

While this topic will only be touched upon briefly here (it is covered in greater detail in Chap. 12), a notable proportion of waitlist patients display elevated levels of circulating anti-HLA antibodies as well as donor-specific

**Table 5.3** General indications for admission of waitlist candidates

| |
|---|
| • Unstable angina |
| • Syncope |
| • Frequent implantable cardioverter-defibrillator discharges |
| • Suspected embolic event |
| • Refractory congestive symptoms despite compliance with increased diuretics, which may: |
| – Render patients bedridden |
| – Cause increased hepatic congestion |
| – Worsen pre-existing pulmonary hypertension |
| • Persistently low blood pressure < 80 mmHg |
| • Pulse pressure < 12 mm Hg with cool extremities |
| • Chronic renal failure, creatinine > 2 mg/dl |
| • Clinical evidence of severe or progressive low cardiac output |
| • Clinical or catheterization evidence of severe pulmonary hypertension (systolic PA pressure > 60 mmHg) |

Reused with permission: Michelle Kittleson, Jon Kobashigawa, Minh Luu, Listing, Donor Allocation and and Optimization of the Pre-transplant Patient, Clinical Guide to Heart Transplantation, 37–45, 2017, Springer Nature; https://doi.org/10.1007/978-3-319-43773-6_4

anti-HLA antibodies. These anti-HLA antibodies may develop from events such as previous pregnancy, prior blood transfusions, or implantation of a mechanical circulatory support device. Patients with high levels of circulating anti-HLA antibodies are considered "sensitized" and, as a cohort, demonstrate poorer outcomes post-transplant [13], including increased rejection (acute and chronic) and increased mortality. Furthermore, the chances of an immunologically compatible donor are much lower. Therefore, any events such as blood transfusions need to be documented and preformed antibody levels rechecked, with leukocyte filtered blood administered whenever possible to reduce the risk of further sensitization. Desensitization therapy is an option for end-stage HF waitlist patients who are highly sensitized and would otherwise have a low chance of finding an acceptable donor organ [14, 15]. Desensitization may include intravenous immune globulin, rituximab, bortezomib, or tocilizumab [16]. In highly sensitized patients for whom a donor becomes available, a prospective crossmatch will also be performed shortly before transplant. The purpose is to definitively identify donor hearts that would be at risk of exposure to the specific circulating cytotoxic antibodies of the potential recipient. The need to physically transport the recipient's blood to the donor location reflects a geographical limitation of transplant in these highly sensitized patients.

## Other Considerations for Patients on the Waitlist

Patients on anticoagulation with one of the novel oral anticoagulants or on antiplatelet agents such as clopidogrel or prasugrel may be changed to more easily reversible options, since there may be little time from notification to the surgical procedure. Patients with histories of recent cigarette or other drug use should have periodic toxicology screening while waiting. All patients should be monitored for adherence to visits and the medical regimen and instructed to notify the team of any change in their medical condition or residence to reinforce the importance of these factors post-transplant. Once a donor heart is made available, the patient is typically contacted by the on-call transplant coordinator and if an outpatient, promptly admitted. The patient is told to refrain from eating or drinking. A brief re-evaluation of the potential recipient is performed to ensure that they have not developed any contraindications that may compromise the goals of early management post-transplant. The pre-transplant evaluation summaries should be reviewed for any additional comorbidities or conditions which may require specialized care during and after the transplant operation. For example, patients with pre-existing arrhythmias who are on amiodarone must be carefully watched, as this medication can slow the donor heart rate post-transplantation. A final compatibility check is run, including checking whether the blood type matches appropriately and whether the donor is of an appropriate size for the patient's height and weight. Pre-operative management includes special considerations for those with a history of pulmonary hypertension, as well as those with a predilection for increased bleeding. In those with pre-existing pulmonary hypertension, placement of a pulmonary artery catheter and measurement of pulmonary artery pressure is recommended prior to transplantation. If necessary, pharmacological adjustment through selective vasodilation to reduce pulmonary artery pressure should be performed, in order to prevent acute right HF of the donor heart. Information based on this may also be used to make a final decision regarding whether to accept the donor heart, especially where the donor heart is undersized. For those recipients at risk of increased intra-operative bleeding (usually due to previous sternotomy, mechanical circularity support device, long-term right HF, or chronic warfarin therapy), vitamin K (10 mg subcutaneously) and fresh frozen plasma may be administered prophylactically prior to the operation. Standard pre-operative measures also include immunosuppression, such as administration of pre-operative corticosteroids at some centers (500 mg IV 4 h before transplantation; 250 mg IV 1 h before), as they are thought to help reduce the damaging inflammatory processes that are the result of cardiopulmonary bypass. At some centers, pre-operative administration of anti-proliferative and calcineurin inhibitors occurs, whereas other centers prefer to initiate these agents' peri-operatively or shortly after transplant. Pre-operative broad-spectrum antibiotic prophylaxis is also administered to protect against gram-positive and gram-negative organisms.

## References

1. Colvin M, Smith JM, Ahn Y, Skeans MA, Messick E, Bradbrook K, et al. OPTN/SRTR 2020 annual data report: heart. Am J Transplant. 2022;22(Suppl 2):350–437.
2. Meyer DM, Rogers JG, Edwards LB, Callahan ER, Webber SA, Johnson MR, et al. The future direction of the adult heart allocation system in the United States. Am J Transplant. 2015;15(1):44–54.
3. Van Meter CH. The organ allocation controversy: how did we arrive here? Ochsner J. 1999;1(1):6–11.
4. Committee OUTOT. Proposal to modify the adult heart allocation system. 2016.
5. Maitra NS, Dugger SJ, Balachandran IC, Civitello AB, Khazanie P, Rogers JG. Impact of the 2018 UNOS heart transplant policy changes on patient outcomes. Heart Fail. 2023;11(5):491–503.
6. Goff RR, Uccellini K, Lindblad K, Hall S, Davies R, Farr M, et al. A change of heart: preliminary results of the US 2018 adult heart allocation revision. Am J Transplant. 2020;20(10):2781–90.
7. Ran G, Chung K, Anderson AS, Gibbons RD, Narang N, Churpek MM, et al. Between-center variation in high-priority listing status under the new heart allocation policy. Am J Transplant. 2021.
8. Jawitz OK, Fudim M, Raman V, Bryner BS, DeVore AD, Mentz RJ, et al. Reassessing recipient mortality under the new heart allocation system: an updated UNOS registry analysis. JACC Heart Fail. 2020;8(7):548–56.
9. Clerkin KJ, Salako O, Fried JA, Griffin JM, Raikhelkar J, Jain R, et al. Impact of temporary percutaneous mechanical circulatory support before transplantation in the 2018 heart allocation system. Heart Fail. 2022;10(1):12–23.
10. Stern LK, Velleca A, Nishihara K, Shen A, Zaliznyak M, Patel J, et al. Impact of the United Network for organ sharing 2018 donor heart allocation system on transplant morbidity and mortality. Clin Transplant. 2021;35(2):e14181.
11. Kilic A, Mathier MA, Hickey GW, Sultan I, Morell VO, Mulukutla SR, et al. Evolving trends in adult heart transplant with the 2018 heart allocation policy change. JAMA Cardiol. 2021;6(2):159–67.
12. Bakhtiyar SS, Godfrey EL, Ahmed S, Lamba H, Morgan J, Loor G, et al. Survival on the heart transplant waiting list. JAMA Cardiol. 2020;5(11):1227–35.
13. Kransdorf EP, Pando MJ, Gragert L, Kaplan B. HLA population genetics in solid organ transplantation. Transplantation. 2017;101(9):1971–6.
14. Kobashigawa J, Colvin M, Potena L, Dragun D, Crespo-Leiro MG, Delgado JF, et al. The management of antibodies in heart transplantation: an ISHLT consensus document. J Heart Lung Transplant. 2018;37(5):537–47.
15. Kobashigawa J, Mehra M, West L, Kerman R, George J, Rose M, et al. Report from a consensus conference on the sensitized patient awaiting heart transplantation. J Heart Lung Transplant. 2009;28(3):213–25.
16. DeFilippis EM, Kransdorf EP, Jaiswal A, Zhang X, Patel J, Kobashigawa JA, et al. Detection and management of HLA sensitization in candidates for adult heart transplantation. J Heart Lung Transplant. 2023;42(4):409–22.

# 6 Overview of Transplantation Immunobiology

Xiaohai Zhang

**Abstract**

Immunosuppression after heart transplantation has significantly reduced the incidence of rejection and improved patient outcomes. However, long-term graft outcome is challenged by multiple factors, including the effects of the immunosuppressive drugs used and the chronic rejection process. A better understanding of the multiple mechanistic processes involved may provide evidence of the feasibility of the best approach to achieve the ultimate goal of donor-specific tolerance. This chapter will summarize the role of the immune systems in transplantation, focusing on the interaction between innate and adaptive immunity, Human Leukocyte Antigens (HLA) polymorphism and nomenclature, and outlines the pathways of alloantigen presentation. The chapter also covers T cell-mediated rejection, antibody responses, and immunosuppressive strategies and explores the concept of tolerance.

X. Zhang (✉)
HLA and Immunogenetics Laboratory, Comprehensive Transplant Center, Cedars-Sinai Medical Center, Los Angeles, CA, USA
e-mail: xiaohai.zhang@cshs.org

**Keywords**

Heart failure · Heart transplantation · Human leukocyte antigen · Major histocompatibility complex · Rejection · Antibodies · Donor-specific antibodies · T-cells · B-cells · Tolerance

## Clinical Pearls

- Both the innate and adaptive immune systems normally collaborate to mount a response to external pathogens, but the same mechanisms also play a role in allograft rejection and injury.
- Mismatched HLA alloantigens on the donor graft are targeted by the recipient's immune system.
- Donor graft alloantigens are presented to the recipient's T-cells through the indirect, direct, or semi-direct pathway, ultimately leading to CD8+ T-cell-mediated cytotoxic response; various effector T-cell subsets are implicated in the cellular rejection process.
- Alloantibodies to the donor graft, originating from plasma cells, damage the graft through complement-dependent cytotoxicity, antibody-dependent cellular cytotoxicity through natural killer cell recruitment, and endothelial activation.


J. Kobashigawa (ed.), *Clinical Guide to Heart Transplantation*, https://doi.org/10.1007/978-3-031-88290-6_6

- CD-20 is expressed on surfaces of B-cells and can be targeted by anti-CD20 monoclonal antibodies such as rituximab to reduce alloantibody production and thus subsequent antibody-mediated rejection.
- Bortezomib is a proteasome inhibitor used to inhibit antibody production by plasma cells.
- Tolerance may theoretically be induced by induction of chimerism, depletion of specific lymphoid tissues, costimulatory blockade and regulation through B-cell mechanism.

## Innate Versus Adaptive Immunity

The immune system protects us from infection by recognizing and destroying or containing pathogens. The immune system can be categorized into two branches: the innate immune system and the adaptive immune system. The innate immune system and adaptive immune system are not completely independent systems. Instead, there is crosstalk at multiple levels and collaboration with each other to mount immune responses to pathogens. The processes that initiate transplant-directed alloimmune responses are not mediated by components related to organ transplantation, but rather are developed from a system that maintains the integrity against various pathogens. Exposure to pathogens such as viruses, bacteria, fungi, and protozoa is first countered by the innate immune system composed of inflammatory cells, usually granulocytes, which include neutrophils, eosinophils, basophils, and mast cells. A second important cellular component of the innate immune response includes monocytes, macrophages, and dendritic cells, which can take up and process exogenous materials. Also included in the cellular innate immune response are the γδ and natural killer (NK) cells, which can kill virally infected cells without prior sensitization [1]. These same cells survey the periphery, including transplanted organs, with usually a slower response than that observed in innate immune responses against pathogens. The cellular components of the adaptive immune response include T and B cells, which express unique and polymorphic antigen receptors, T cell receptor (TCR), and B cell receptor (BCR). The process that generates the antigen-detecting region of these receptors provides the ability to recognize and potentiate the response to specific antigens, which may include pathogens but also self-antigens. During this process, T and B cells undergo a selective maturation process, which removes strongly binding, autoreactive cells. When an organ transplant occurs between genetically disparate individuals, T cell-mediated adaptive immune response must be addressed with immune modulation. The cells of the innate immune component also play a role in presenting the alloantigen to these T cells. The activated T cells can also help B cells produce alloantibodies as part of the humoral response, thereby damaging the graft. Further details of these cells that participate in the transplant immune response are included later in this chapter.

## Human Leukocyte Antigens Polymorphism and Nomenclature

### Overview and Polymorphism of HLA

The difference between proteins expressed by the recipient and donor is actively surveyed by the recipient's immune system. The most polymorphic proteins in humans are the human leukocyte antigens (HLA). More than 30,000 HLA alleles have been identified by the year 2023. The high degree of polymorphism is necessary for HLA molecules to present various peptides during the adaptive immune response to pathogens; however, this degree of polymorphism creates a substantial barrier to allo-transplant between individuals. It is very common for the donor and recipient to not share exactly the same HLA molecules. The mismatched HLA molecules are recognized as foreign and often targeted by the recipient's immune system. In humans, HLA molecules are encoded by a cluster of genes localized on chromosome 6. The HLA genes are grouped into two categories based on the protein structure and function: HLA class I, which includes HLA-A, HLA-B, and HLA-C, and HLA class II, which includes HLA-DRB1, HLA-DRB3/4/5, HLA-DQB1, HLA-DQA1, HLA-DPB1, and HLA-DPA1. Other two genes, Major Histocompatibility Complex Class I Chain-Related Gene A (MICA) and Major Histocompatibility Complex Class I Chain-Related Gene B (MICB), which are often referred to as non-classical HLA genes, are also localized in this region (Fig. 6.1).

HLA class I polypeptides (HLA-A, HLA-B, or HLA-C), noncovalently bound to a non-polymorphic polypeptide β2 microglobulin, function as a dimer to present intracellular peptides or virus proteins synthesized inside the cell to T cell receptor (TCR) expressed on CD8+ T cells. The HLA class I polypeptide is organized as α1, α2, α3, transmembrane and cytoplasmic domains. The α1 and α2 domains of the HLA class I polypeptide, forming the binding site of presented peptides, are more polymorphic than other domains. Because the HLA class I is constitutively expressed on all cells but mature red blood cells, mismatched donor HLA class I are more likely targeted by preformed donor-specific antibodies (DSA) or T cells in the setting of acute rejection. The HLA class II polypeptides (HLA-DR, DQ, or DP) also form a dimer comprised of α chain and β chain. The α chains of HLA-DR, DQ, or DP are encoded by genes HLA-DRA, DQA1, and DPA1, respectively. The β chains are encoded by genes HLA-DRB1, DQB1, or DPB1. Both the α chain and β chain can be polymorphic for HLA-DQ and DP. For HLA-DR, only HLA-DRB1 is polymorphic.

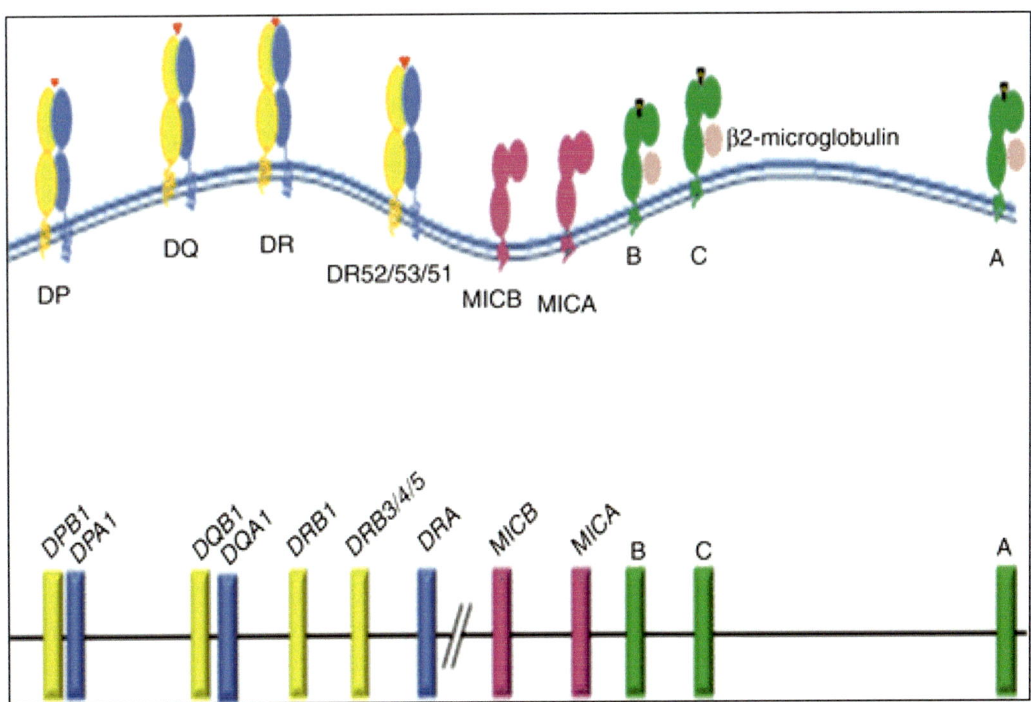


**Fig. 6.1** The HLA gene cluster is localized on chromosome 6. HLA class I genes (HLA-A, B, C) encode the HLA class I heavy chain, which pairs with non-polymorphic protein β2 -microglobulin on the cell membrane. HLA class II (HLA-DP, DQ, and DR) are also dimers, which are comprised of α chains and β chains. Some individuals may also express antigens DR52, DR53, and DR51, of which the β chain is encoded by genes DRB3, DRB4, and DRB5, respectively. MICA and MICB genes are also localized in this region. Reprinted with permission from Adapted with permission from Xiaohai Zhang, Nancy Reinsmoen, Jon Kobashigawa, Overview of Transplantation Immunobiology, Clinical Guide to Heart Transplantation, 47–56, 2017, Springer Nature. https://doi.org/10.1007/978-3-319-43773-6_5

The HLA class II polypeptide is organized as α1 and α2, transmembrane and cytoplasmic domains. The antigen recognition site of HLA class II peptides is contributed by α1 domains of both the α chain and β chain. HLA class II molecules present peptides derived from protein/pathogens from extracellular compartments to CD4+ T cells. HLA class II molecules are mainly expressed in antigen-presenting cells and B cells but not in other cells in the quiescent state. Expression of HLA class II can be stimulated in other cell types by cytokines, which usually exist in the inflammation environment. Levels of HLA class II expression can be different among different genes. HLA-DR is generally expressed higher than HLA-DQ, while HLA-DP expression is at the lowest among three HLA class II genes. The non-classic HLA gene, including MICA, is also localized in this region. MICA can be stress-induced and bind to and activate NK cells, which in turn can target stressed or damaged cells. MICA is not associated with β2 microglobulin and cannot present peptides to T cells. MICA has limited polymorphism, and mismatched MICA can be recognized by the recipient's adaptive immune system. The presence of MICA antibodies is suggested to be associated with transplant coronary artery disease in heart transplantation (HTx) [2].

## HLA Nomenclature

Each HLA allele has a unique number of up to four sets of digits, separated by colons. The name length depends on the allele's sequence and relation to similar alleles. The digits before the first colon represent the type, often corresponding to the antigen; the second set of digits represents subtypes, numbers being assigned in the order in which DNA sequences have been determined. The third set of digits is used to show synonymous DNA substitutions within the coding region. The fourth set of digits is used to show differences found in the non-coding regions. In addition, optional suffixes are added to indicate the allele's expression status, such as N (Null), L (Low expression on the cell surface), and S (Secreted protein), among others. A Convention for HLA allele naming is shown in Fig. 6.2 [3–5].

## Alloantigen Presentation

In order for the recipient's adaptive immune system to recognize mismatched alloantigens, they need to be presented as peptides by the HLA protein on antigen-presenting cells to the recipient's CD4+ T helper cells. Activation of the recipient's CD4+ T helper cells is a prerequisite to initiating CD8+ T cells mediated cytotoxic response and B cell-mediated humoral response against alloantigens. Alloantigens can be presented to the recipient's T cells through three pathways: the indirect, direct, and semi-direct pathways (Fig. 6.3). In the indirect pathway, alloantigens are presented in a similar way as antigens derived from pathogens. The recipient's antigen-presenting cells capture alloantigenes, which are shed from the graft, and present these antigens in the context of the recipient HLA class II to the recipient CD4+ T helper cells. Alloantigens targeted by de novo donor-specific antibodies are mainly presented through the indirect pathway [6]. Because in the indirect pathway, alloantigens have to be captured and processed first by the recipient's antigen-presenting cells before being presented to CD4+ T helper cells, it takes longer compared to the direct pathway of presentation of alloantigens. The recipient's immune system usually takes more than two weeks to develop de novo donor-specific antibodies. Different from the indirect pathway, alloantigens are presented directly by donor-derived antigen-presenting cells to the recipient's CD4+ T help cells in the direct pathway. These passenger donor-derived antigen-presenting cells in the allograft are transplanted into the recipient along with the graft. A special type of endothelial cells in allogeneic graft has also been identified to express MHC class II (equivalent to HLA class II in

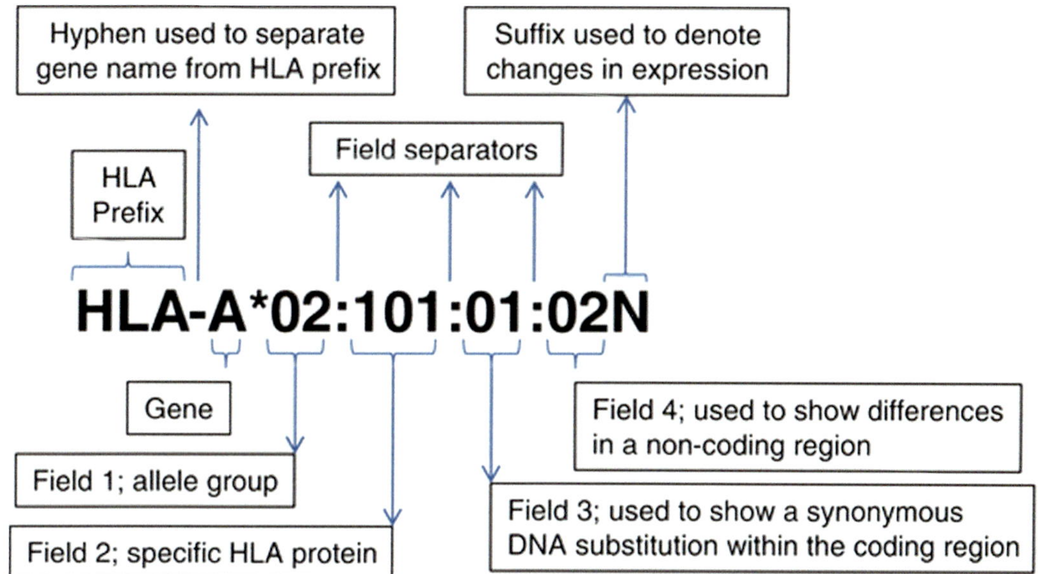


**Fig. 6.2** Convention for HLA allele naming. Reprinted with permission from Malek Kamoun, Jill A. Hollenbach, Steven J. Mack et al., Molecular HLA Typing, Molecular pathology in clinical practice, 867–885, 2016, Springer Nature. https://doi.org/10.1007/978-3-319-19674-9_58

humans) in a murine transplant model [7]. These endothelial cells and passenger antigen-presenting cells can interact with the recipient's CD4+ T helper cells directly and present alloantigens restricted by the donor HLA molecules to the CD4+ T helper cells to initiate adaptive immune response. In this pathway, antigen-presenting cells don't need to process new antigens, and an immune response is activated relatively fast. This pathway usually is responsible for the acute cellular-mediated immune response [8]. Immune response to alloantigens can also be initiated by the third pathway, the semi-direct pathway. In this pathway, the recipient antigen-presenting cells, mainly dendritic cells, obtain donor HLA peptide complexes by capturing the membrane from the donor passenger antigen-presenting cells or endothelial cells. These recipient dendritic cells then can present HLA alloantigens to both CD8+ cytotoxic T cells as an intact protein and to CD4+ T help cells as processed allopeptides simultaneously. This semi-direct pathway explains how CD8+ cytotoxic T cells can target HLA alloantigens expressed on the graft. This semi-direct pathway may be critical for CD8+ T cell-mediated cytotoxic response for mismatched HLA antigens between the donor and recipient [9].

## T Cell Mediated Response: Effector T Cells and the Memory Response

It has been shown that rejection of allografts may depend on certain T cell subsets. Single-cell sequencing of transplanted hearts has revealed that effector T cells and activated T cells are predominantly present in allogeneic grafts, while resting T cells mainly exist in syngeneic grafts in a murine model[7]. Blockade of T cell co-stimulation by CD154 antibody prolongs allograft survival in a nonhuman primate HTx model [10]. Studies in a HTx model have shown that rejection can occur in the absence of CD8+ T cells but not in the absence of CD4+ T cells[11]. Distinct effector phenotypes, Th1, Th2, and Th17, have been described; however, cytokines are pleiotropic and their role in the clinical rejection process remains somewhat controversial. Naïve T cells may

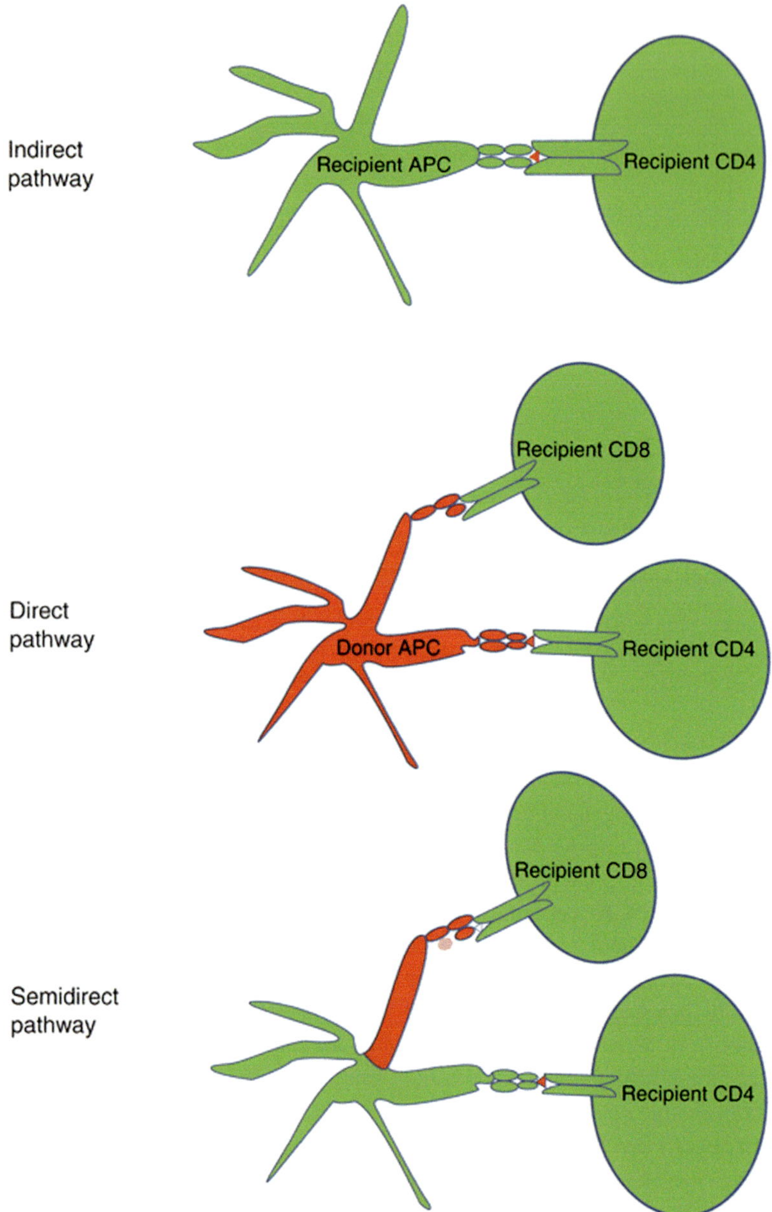


**Fig. 6.3** In the indirect pathway, recipient antigen-presenting cells (APC) present donor-derived peptides in the context of recipient HLA class II to recipient CD4+ T helper cells. This pathway is important for initiating antibody-mediated rejection. In the direct pathway, donor-derived APC present allopeptides restricted on donor HLA class II to recipient CD4+ T helper cells, and allopeptides restricted on donor HLA class I recipient CD8+ cytotoxicity cells. This pathway is usually responsible of acute cellular mediated immune response to intact donor HLA class I antigens. In the semidirect pathway, recipient APC capture membrane fragments bearing intact HLA class I antigens from donor cells, and present intact class I antigens to recipient CD8+ T cells. Allopeptide restricted on recipient HLA class II are also presented to recipient CD4+ T helper cells by the same APC. Reprinted with permission from Adapted with permission from Xiaohai Zhang, Nancy Reinsmoen, Jon Kobashigawa, Overview of Transplantation Immunobiology, Clinical Guide to Heart Transplantation, 47–56, 2017, Springer Nature. https://doi.org/10.1007/978-3-319-43773-6_5

differentiate into distinct helper T cell subsets based on cytokine signatures. Briefly, the Th1 cells secrete IL-2, IFN- γ, and TNF; Th2 cells secrete IL -4, IL-5, IL-10, and IL-13; Th17 cells secrete IL-17. Subsets of T cells, which can be either CD4+ or CD8+, can inhibit the immune response of other T cells and are termed regulatory T cells (Tregs). Although these various Th subsets were thought to be stable, more recent reports indicate these subsets may be flexible in their T cell phenotypes [12]. Naïve T cells proliferate through the autocrine growth factor IL-2 and can differentiate into various types based on their encounters with different cytokines. CD8+ T cells are usually termed as cytotoxic T cells. While CD4+ T cells can also be cytotoxic with the ability to secret granzyme B and perforin, CD4+ T cells are often termed T helper cells. When exposed to IL-12, activated CD4+ T cells can differentiate into a predominantly IFN- γ producing phenotype and are designated in the Th1 category. Activated T cells that are exposed to IL-4 predominantly differentiate into the Th2 cells that produce IL-4, IL-5, IL-10, and IL-13. Upon exposure to TGF-β and IL-6, they can differentiate into Th17 cells producing IL-17 (A and F) and IL-22 [13, 14]. The Th1 and Th17 cells have been associated with autoimmunity while the Th2 cells are often associated with asthma and allergies. The Th1 IFN- γ producing cells are often associated with acute allograft rejection along with the presence of IL-17. The Th2 cells have also been associated with the rejection process. After an initial antigenic challenge, a second stimulation by the same foreign antigen triggers a memory response characterized by a faster kinetics of lymphocyte activation for both the T and B cell compartments. In an initial response where the antigen is cleared, the number of effector cells peaks at about one week after which about 90% of the effector cells die. The remaining population is long-lived memory T cells with distinct phenotype and function. These memory T cells have a lower activation threshold allowing them to respond quickly upon restimulation. These effector memory T cells express homing receptors that allow for migration to non-lymphoid sites of inflammation [1]. Inhibition of T cell function is a routine strategy to treat and prevent transplant rejection. Depletion of T cells by photopheresis or antibodies, like anti-thymocyte globulin has been used for induction and treatment of acute cellular rejection [15]. In addition, blockade of T cell activation by antibodies against costimulatory ligand CD154 prolongs allograft survival and reduces DSA formation in a nonhuman primate HTx model [10].

## Antibody Production and Biology

Despite improvements to immune-suppressing regimens, antibody-mediated rejection (AMR) remains a major obstacle to long-term graft survival. With the help of CD4+ T helper cells, naïve B cells with an alloantigen bound on their B-cell antigen receptor (BCR) are primed. B cells go through the affinity maturation process, which requires interactions with both antigen-presenting cells (APC) and activated T helper cells, which facilitate the differentiation of activated B cells into memory B cells, plasmablasts, and plasma cells (Fig. 6.4) [16]. The later, secret antibodies against the antigen that can be originally recognized by the B cell, DSA, in case of organ transplantation, which, if not mitigated, may result in graft loss. Memory B cells, which can live for long periods of time, rapidly differentiate into plasma cells upon recurrent exposure to the initial antigens. The secondary response of the memory B cells is shorter (3–5 days) compared to the primary response (7–10 days). Antibodies produced by memory B cells have higher affinity and are usually characterized by isotype subgroups of IgG, IgA and IgE versus IgM in the primary response. Plasma cells can survive in niches, mainly in bone marrow, for long periods of time. Both memory B cells and long-lived plasma cells provide long-term humoral immunity [17]. Important to transplantation is that the long-term benefit of a therapy to treat AMR or to desensitize is mainly determined by its ability to remove antibody-producing cells, and attenuate antibody-rebound. CD20 protein is widely expressed on the surface of B cells during

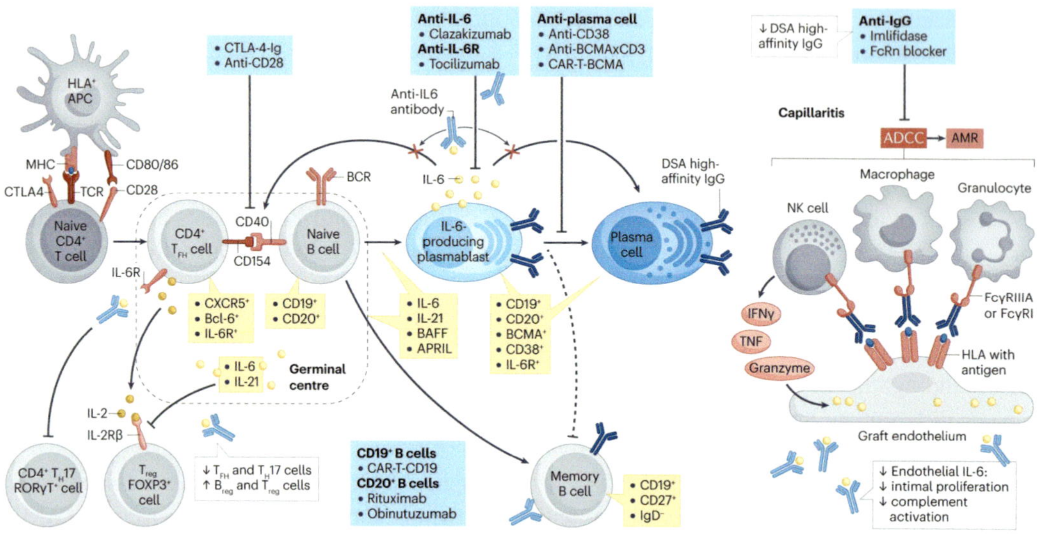


**Fig. 6.4** Alloimmune B cell differentiation pathways and their therapeutic targets

B-cell ontogeny and is necessary for B-cell activation. Anti-CD20 antibodies, like rituximab or obinutuzumab, are used to treat lymphoma and autoimmune disorders by depleting B cells through antibody-dependent or cell-dependent cytotoxicity. In the field of solid organ transplant, anti-CD20 antibodies are commonly used for desensitization and treatment of AMR. However, the expression of CD20 is lost after B cells differentiate into plasma cells. Therefore, the CD20 antibody therapy would be ineffective in removing antibodies after B cells differentiate into antibody-secreting plasma cells. This may be one of the reasons why CD20 antibody treatment is not always effective in desensitizing or treating AMR [16, 18]. CD38 is a type II transmembrane glycoprotein expressed throughout the immune system, especially NK and plasma cells [18]. Daratumumab, an anti-CD38 monoclonal antibody, has proven its efficacy in treating multiple myeloma and AL amyloidosis. Daratumumab depletes plasma and NK cells, which raised interest in its use for desensitization/AMR in organ transplant recipients [18]. Data in HTx patients remain limited, awaiting larger studies and outcomes of clinical trials to delineate its efficacy [19]. Another drug used for desensitization or treatment of AMR is bortezomib. Bortezomib is a proteasome inhibitor and originally is used to treat myeloma. Bortezomib is used to inhibit antibody production on the premise that plasma cells which synthesize a large amount of antibodies and need to degrade incorrectly folded proteins might be more sensitive to the inhibition of proteasome. It has been shown that proteasome inhibition in combination with T cells co-stimulation blockade can reduce HLA antibodies in HTx candidates [20]. However, the effectiveness of the current therapies is limited to certain patients. Developing novel therapies, such as chimeric antigen receptor T-cell (CAR T- cell) therapy targeting B-cell maturation antigen (BCMA), are needed [16]. In addition, the emergence of targeted bi-specific monoclonal antibodies that target plasma cells and CD3 T cells simultaneously has generated interest in its potential benefits for desensitization or treatment of AMR, and it's currently under investigation in highly sensitized patients awaiting kidney transplantation [16]. Relevant to AMR, targeting IL-6, with anti-IL-6 (clazakizumab) or anti-IL-6R monoclonal antibodies (tocilizumab), could disrupt plasma cell survival and differentiation. In addition, it can facilitate early termination of T follicular cell activity and enhance the generation of regulatory T cells. It can also limit graft damage by reducing endothelial injury and activation of pro-fibrotic genes [16, 21, 22]. In the HTx population, tocilizumab has only been explored as a pretransplant desensitization therapy, while very limited evidence is currently available on its safety and efficacy for the treatment of AMR [16, 23]. Another promising alternative agent is the immunoglobulin-depleting enzyme of Streptococcus pyogenes, IDES, or imlifidase. IDES neutralizes all serum IgG by separating the Fc and Fab fragments of the antibodies, thus reducing complement activation and any Fc-mediated antibody effect. Data from the use of IDES in renal transplant patients is encouraging [24, 25], but data in HTxs remains limited. Figure 6.4 illustrates Alloimmune B cell differentiation pathways and their therapeutic targets [16].

Antigen-presenting cells (APCs) display HLA antigens to naive CD4+ cells. Activated T and B cells migrate to germinal centers (GCs), and the former differentiate into T follicular (TFH) cells that facilitate the differentiation of activated B cells to memory B cells, plasmablasts, and antibody-secreting plasma cells that produce high-affinity donor-specific antibodies (DSAs), which, if unmitigated, mediate graft destruction. Several monoclonal antibodies have been developed that can target different B cell subsets for depletion, including plasmablasts (anti-CD20, anti-CD19) and plasma cells (anti-CD38, anti-B cell maturation antigen (BCMA)–CD3 and chimeric antigen receptor (CAR)-T-BCMA). Anti-IL-6 or anti-IL-6R monoclonal antibodies disrupt GC formation, memory B cell development, and differentiation of plasmablasts into antibody-secreting plasma cells; they can also reduce plasma cell survival. In addition, targeting the IL-6 axis can prevent IL-2 receptor-β (IL-2Rb) expression on TFH cells, which facilitates early termination of TFH cell activity and promotes the generation of regulatory T (Treg) cells, and can reduce endothelial injury and activation of pro-fibrotic genes, thus limiting damage to the allograft. Other important agents that inhibit T cell–B cell interactions and GC activity (CTLA4-Ig and anti-CD28), as well as monoclonals directed at natural killer (NK) cells, are highly likely to modulate antibody-mediated injury. DSAs can be targeted directly with IgG endopeptidase (imlifidase) and engineered IgG Fc fragments that block Fc receptor neonatal (FcRn) recycling of pathogenic IgGs and thus reduce their half-life. AMR, antibody-mediated rejection; ADCC, antibody-dependent cytotoxicity; BCR, B cell receptor; TCR, T cell receptor. Reprinted with permission form Peter S. Heeger et al., Translating B cell immunology to the treatment of antibody-mediated allograft rejection, Nature Reviews Nephrology, 20, 218–232, 2024, Springer Nature. https://doi.org/10.1038/s41581-023-00791-0.

Alloantibodies damage the graft mainly through three ways. The first is complement-dependent cytotoxicity. Upon binding to antigens on cells of the graft, alloantibodies recruit C1q, the first complement component activated in the classic complement pathway, through the Fc fraction of IgG [26]. There are 4 isotypes of IgG antibodies: IgG1, IgG2, IgG3 and IgG4. The affinity of these IgG to C1q is IgG3 > IgG1 > IgG2 > IgG4. IgG3 and IgG1 alloantibodies are more potent than IgG2 and IgG4 to activate the classic complement pathway. The presence of donor-specific IgG3 antibodies against HLA is associated with a high risk of AMR in renal transplant [27]. C1q binding to alloantibodies sequentially activates complement components C4, C3 and then C5, which in turn can lead to the formation of membrane attack complex. The membrane attack complex composes a pore in the cell membrane and causes cell death. As unintended activation of complement is detrimental to the tissue and organ, the activation of complement is tightly controlled by many negative regulators [28]. Even if alloantibodies are produced, complements may not necessarily be activated on the graft due to these negative regulations. C4d, a split product of complement C4 produced after the activation of the classic complement pathway, is covalently linked to the cell membrane. Its half-life is 12–31 days in vivo [29]. These characteristics make positive C4d staining on the biopsy as a useful marker for diagnosis of

AMR in kidney and heart transplantation. In the classic complement activation pathway, activation of complement C1 stimulates complement C4 to transform into active form C4b through proteolytic cleavage. The activity of C4b is negatively regulated by complement 4-bindig protein (C4BP). C4BP prevents C4b from activating the downstream complement cascade by degrading C4b through proteolytic cleavage. One of the cleavage products is C4d [28]. Thus, C4d deposition on the graft is dependent on both the activation of complement C1 and the presence of negative regulator of C4BP. When C4BP negative regulator is missing, or its activity is low, C4d will not be generated and detected even if the complement pathway is fully activated, which might be one of the reasons why a biopsy diagnosed with AMR can be negative for C4d staining. Activation of the complement pathway can also produce anaphylatoxin C3a and C5a which are cleavage products of the complement components C3 and C5. Due to the expression of multiple complement negative regulators on the cell surface of the graft, formation of membrane attack complexes and cell death do not always happen in AMR. Formation of C3a and C5a may be the major culprit for graft damage caused by complement activation. C5a is a pivotal chemoattractant for macrophages and neutrophils. Receptors for C3a and C5a are expressed on granulocytes and monocytes. Signaling activated by C3a and C5a triggers histamine release, oxidative burst and chemotaxis. Stimulation of C5a signaling can also upregulate the expression of activating Fc$\gamma$R receptor on macrophages, which further enhances antibody-dependent cell cytotoxicity. Eculizumab, a humanized monoclonal antibody against complement C5, is used to prevent/treat acute AMR in solid organ transplant [30]. Eculizumab binds to complement C5 can inhibit C5a production in addition to the blockade of membrane attack complex formation. In addition, antibodies against the allograft can cause graft damage through antibody-dependent cellular cytotoxicity by recruitment of NK cells. NK cell transcripts have been found enriched in kidney biopsies with AMR [31]. Most NK cells are activated in allogeneic heart allograft with acute rejection compared to syngeneic graft in a murine model [7]. Antibodies engage the innate immune system through the Fc fragment by interacting with the Fc receptors Fc$\gamma$RIIIa and/or Fc$\gamma$RIIc on NK cells. High affinity Fc$\gamma$RIIIa allele (FCGR3A-VV) in HTx recipients is associated with antibody-dependent NK cell cytotoxicity and cardiac allograft vasculopathy [32]. The signals activated through Fc receptors by antibodies cause NK cells to release cytokines, such as IFN -$\gamma$ which up-regulate HLA expression on the cell surface. Increased expression of allo-HLA molecules on the graft, in turn, enhances the potential for cytotoxic T cell recognition of allo-HLA antigens and thus promotes the induction of cell-mediated immunity to recruit adaptive immune cells. NK cells can also recognize antibody-coated cells through the Fc receptor and induce rapid apoptosis in target cells via the release of granzyme [33]. The requirement of NK cells in transplant vasculopathy has been demonstrated in a mouse model with cardiac allografts in which depletion of NK cells abolished donor MHC class I antibodies induced transplant vasculopathy [34].

## Endothelial Cell Activation by Antibodies

Transplant vasculopathy is characterized by concentric hyperplasia with intimal proliferation of the vessels of the allograft. Endothelial cells lining the blood vessels of allograft are directly targeted by the recipient's immune system. HLA antibodies can stimulate the proliferation and survival of endothelial cells and smooth muscle cells [35]. HLA molecules do not have intrinsic kinase activity. Instead, HLA class I molecules, upon ligation with antibodies, partner with integrin $\beta$4 to transduce intracellular signals [36]. Integrin $\beta$4 is a cell adhesion protein which regulates cell adhesion, migration, survival and proliferation. Depletion of integrin $\beta$4 dampens the proliferation of endothelial cells stimulated by HLA class I antibodies. HLA class II molecules can also transduce signals into the cell, but the protein that partners with HLA class II is not known yet. The mammalian target of rapamycin (mTOR) is at the center of the HLA signaling pathway. Ligation of HLA molecules with antibodies activates mTOR signaling through the SRC/FAK-PI3K-AKT pathway in endothelial cells. mTOR exists in two structurally and functionally distinct protein complexes: mTOR complex 1 (TORC1) and mTOR complex 2 (TORC2). TORC1 is pivotal in the regulation of mRNA translation, cell growth, and proliferation, while TORC2 stimulates actin cytoskeletal rearrangement and cell survival [37, 38]. Knockout of the PI3K gene in endothelial cells of allogeneic grafts prevents transplant vasculopathy in a murine HTx model [39]. The degree of HLA molecule crosslinking with antibodies may determine which mTOR complex is preferentially activated. Ligation of HLA class I with high titers of antibodies activates TORC1, which promotes endothelial cell proliferation. Activation of TORC1 stimulates phosphorylation of p70 ribosomal protein S6 kinase (S6K), which then phosphorylates S6 ribosomal protein (S6RP) and 4E-BP1 proteins. S6RP is essential for protein synthesis and cell growth and proliferation. Using a murine heart allograft model, increased phosphorylation of these proteins was observed in the endothelium after MHC-I (HLA class I in mouse) antibody injection. It is suggested that staining for phosphorylated S6K and phosphorylated S6RP can be useful markers for the diagnosis of AMR since expression of phosphorylated S6K and phosphorylated S6RP is significantly increased in capillary endothelial cells in endomyocardial biopsies with evidence of pathological AMR [40]. On the other hand, ligation of HLA class I with low titers of antibodies predominantly stimulates the TORC2 pathway with upregulation of cell survival proteins on the endothelium. Pretreatment with HLA class I antibodies at lower concentrations protects the endothelium from complement-mediated and cytotoxic T cell-mediated injury in a mouse model. However, extended exposure of the endothelium to HLA class I antibodies, even with low titers, may ultimately cause graft injury via activation of complement and recruitment of NK cells or monocytes. Rapamycin, used as an immunosuppressive agent for solid organ transplant, can block mTOR signaling. TORC1 is highly sensitive to rapamycin, whereas TORC2 is relatively insensitive. However, prolonged treatment or high concentrations of rapamycin can inhibit both TORC1 and TORC2 signaling. The core changes of endothelial cell activation include upregulation of leukocyte adhesion molecules and cytokine release. It is suggested that alloantibodies can contribute to the pathogenesis of AMR by activating human endothelial cell exocytosis and leukocyte trafficking. Treatment of endothelial cells with alloantibody promotes leukocyte recruitment [35]. Antibodies eluted from acutely rejected allografts can upregulate VCAM-1 and ICAM-1 expression on the surface of endothelial cells, which leads to an increase in leukocyte adhesion. Treatment of endothelial cells with HLA class I antibodies can also stimulate the release of P-selectin and von Willebrand Factor (vWF) by triggering calcium-mediated exocytosis. The release of P-selectin, in turn, enhances platelet and leukocyte adherence. Fc fragment of IgG is not required for alloantibodies to stimulate exocytosis because only the bivalent F (ab') 2 of HLA class I antibodies is effective in triggering exocytosis. Endothelial cells can also express HLA class II. Of note, a cluster of endothelial cells expressing MHC class II (HLA class II in mice) exclusively exists in allogeneic grafts but not in syngeneic grafts in a murine HTx model [7]. These endothelial cells may be targeted by HLA class II antibodies. Incubation of endothelial cells with HLA class II antibodies in vitro stimulates cell proliferation and migration [41].

## Tolerance

The seminal work of Billingham, Brent, and Medawar in 1953 established the groundwork for the discipline of transplant immunology and neonatal tolerance [42]. Since then, tolerance or operational tolerance has been a goal of transplantation. There have been sparse reports of allograft recipients with kidney or liver allograft who have achieved successful immunosuppression withdrawal [43]. However, the ability to predict the feasibility or signatures of tolerance is elusive. Tolerance appears to be achievable in experimental animal models but is rarely achieved in clinical transplantation. There are several mechanistic theories postulated for the development of tolerance including mixed chimerism: depletion of specific lymphoid tissues, costimulatory blockade, and regulation through B cell. Mixed chimerism can be achieved when bone marrow-derived cells of a recipient are replaced by donor cells after transfusion of donor cells. Depletion of recipient immune cells by total lymphoid irradiation or antibodies helps establish mixed chimerism [44]. The use of non-myeloablative conditioning using hematopoietic stem cells to establish chimerism has been reported to induce tolerance in renal transplant recipients [45]. In solid organ transplantation, however, this approach cannot be applied broadly since the donor needs to be HLA identical or genetically closely related to the recipient. In addition, with myeloablative condition requirements, there is a significant risk of infections and graft versus host disease-related morbidity. The feasibility of identifying a compatible donor for the marrow and concomitant solid organ transplant is slim for HTx. It is important to recognize that all transplant recipients are chimeric to a certain degree. Organs such as the liver, intestine, and lung contain massive amounts of donor cells capable of generating chimerism. The increased degree of chimerism has been shown to be associated with lower incidences of chronic rejection. This type of phenomenon is not uncommon and has been shown in the detection of cells from the offspring of women who have given birth decades before. On the other hand, offspring may also develop tolerance to non-inherited paternal antigens. This phenomenon has given rise to the theory of improved graft outcomes when non-inherited paternal antigens are expressed by the graft [46]. These studies enlighten us on the mechanisms necessary to achieve tolerance and the need to address a combination of multiple mechanisms to achieve tolerance. Co-stimulation blockade has also been proposed as a method to induce tolerance, but there have been discrepancies between results in animal models and humans [47]. There appear to be mechanistic barriers in humans complicating the development of tolerance by this approach. More recent studies using belatacept, a high-affinity CTLA4Ig, may prove to be a component of future therapeutic intervention [48]. Utilization of T regulatory cells is another potential approach to establish tolerance. Anti-HLA-A2-CAR regulatory T cells prolong graft survival in a murine model of heterotopic heart allotransplant [49]. The initial studies by Medawar conceptualized that tolerance was probably reversible due to continued pressures by inflammation and pathogen exposures. Regulation through various therapies, including T-regulatory cells, is a challenge due to the low frequency of these cells and the need for expansion. However, trials are underway to test the efficacy of expanding natural T regulatory cells in living donor kidney transplantation. B cell tolerance has been more difficult to achieve in human transplantation versus animal models. Various B cell targeted therapies have been used to treat AMR and to decrease antibody levels during desensitization but have failed to achieve tolerance. In conclusion, clinical transplantation requires chronic immunosuppression, with only anecdotal reports of patients weaned off all immunosuppression. Long-term graft outcome is challenged by multiple factors, including the effects of the immunosuppressive drugs used and the chronic rejection process. A better understanding of the multiple mechanistic processes involved may provide evidence of the feasibility of the best approach to achieve the ultimate goal of donor-specific tolerance.

## References

1. Turnquist HR, Giorgio; Metes, Diana; Angus, Thomson. An Overview of Physiologic Immunity. In: Kirk A, editor. Textbook of organ transplantation. Chichester, West Sussex: John Wiley & Sons, Inc.; 2014.

2. Zhang Q, Cecka JM, Gjertson DW, Ge P, Rose ML, Patel JK, et al. HLA and MICA: targets of antibody-mediated rejection in heart transplantation. Transplantation. 2011;91(10):1153–8.
3. Marsh SGE, Albert ED, Bodmer WF, Bontrop RE, Dupont B, Erlich HA, et al. Nomenclature for factors of the HLA system, 2010. Tissue Antigens. 2010;75(4):291.
4. Kamoun M, Hollenbach JA, Mack SJ, Williams TM. Molecular HLA typing. In: Molecular pathology in clinical practice; 2016. p. 867–85.
5. Nomenclature. Nomenclature for factors of the HLA system 2019. https://thehematologist.org/2020/02/16/nomenclature-for-hla-system/.
6. Colvin RB, Smith RN. Antibody-mediated organ-allograft rejection. Nat Rev Immunol. 2005;5(10):807–17.
7. Tang Y, Wang J, Zhang Y, Li J, Chen M, Gao Y, et al. Single-cell RNA sequencing identifies intra-graft population heterogeneity in acute heart allograft rejection in mouse. Front Immunol. 2022;13:832573.
8. Afzali B, Lombardi G, Lechler RI. Pathways of major histocompatibility complex allorecognition. Curr Opin Organ Transplant. 2008;13(4):438–44.
9. Harper SJF, Ali JM, Wlodek E, Negus MC, Harper IG, Chhabra M, et al. CD8 T-cell recognition of acquired alloantigen promotes acute allograft rejection. Proc Natl Acad Sci USA. 2015;112(41):12788–93.
10. Miura S, Habibabady ZA, Pollok F, Ma M, Rosales IA, Kinoshita K, et al. TNX-1500, a crystallizable fragment-modified anti-CD154 antibody, prolongs nonhuman primate cardiac allograft survival. Am J Transplant. 2023.
11. Szot GL, Zhou P, Rulifson I, Wang J, Guo Z, Kim O, et al. Different mechanisms of cardiac allograft rejection in wildtype and CD28-deficient mice. Am J Transplant. 2001;1(1):38–46.
12. Nakayamada S, Takahashi H, Kanno Y, O'Shea JJ. Helper T cell diversity and plasticity. Curr Opin Immunol. 2012;24(3):297–302.
13. Atalar K, Afzali B, Lord G, Lombardi G. Relative roles of Th1 and Th17 effector cells in allograft rejection. Curr Opin Organ Transplant. 2009;14(1):23–9.
14. Tay SS, Plain KM, Bishop GA. Role of IL-4 and Th2 responses in allograft rejection and tolerance. Curr Opin Organ Transplant. 2009;14(1):16–22.
15. Costanzo MR, Dipchand A, Starling R, Anderson A, Chan M, Desai S, et al. The International Society of Heart and Lung Transplantation Guidelines for the care of heart transplant recipients. J Heart Lung Transplant. 2010;29(8):914–56.
16. Heeger PS, Haro MC, Jordan S. Translating B cell immunology to the treatment of antibody-mediated allograft rejection. Nat Rev Nephrol. 2024:1–15.
17. Tangye SG. Staying alive: regulation of plasma cell survival. Trends Immunol. 2011;32(12):595–602.
18. Habal MV. Current desensitization strategies in heart transplantation. Front Immunol. 2021;12:702186.
19. Joher N, Matignon M, Grimbert P. HLA desensitization in solid organ transplantation: anti-CD38 to across the immunological barriers. Front Immunol. 2021;12:688301.
20. Alishetti S, Farr M, Jennings D, Serban G, Uriel N, Sayer G, et al. Desensitizing highly sensitized heart transplant candidates with the combination of belatacept and proteasome inhibition. Am J Transplant. 2020;20(12):3620–30.
21. Choi J, Aubert O, Vo A, Loupy A, Haas M, Puliyanda D, et al. Assessment of tocilizumab (anti–interleukin-6 receptor monoclonal) as a potential treatment for chronic antibody-mediated rejection and transplant glomerulopathy in HLA-sensitized renal allograft recipients. Am J Transplant. 2017;17(9):2381–9.
22. Miller CL, Madsen JC. IL-6 directed therapy in transplantation. Curr Transplant Rep. 2021;8(3):191–204.
23. Pottebaum AA, January SE, Liu C, Lavine S, Schilling JD, Lavine KJ. Feasibility of interleukin-6 receptor blockade in cardiac antibody-mediated rejection. Transplantation. 2024;108(2):539–44.
24. Jordan SC, Lorant T, Choi J, Kjellman C, Winstedt L, Bengtsson M, et al. IgG endopeptidase in highly sensitized patients undergoing transplantation. N Engl J Med. 2017;377(5):442–53.
25. Huang E, Jordan SC. Immunoglobulin G-Degrading Enzyme of Streptococcus pyogenes (IdeS), desensitization, and the kidney allocation system: complementary approaches to increase transplantation in highly HLA sensitized patients. Clin J Am Soc Nephrol. 2018;13(5):799–801.
26. Diebolder CA, Beurskens FJ, de Jong RN, Koning RI, Strumane K, Lindorfer MA, et al. Complement is activated by IgG hexamers assembled at the cell surface. Science. 2014;343(6176):1260–3.
27. Everly MJ, Rebellato LM, Haisch CE, Briley KP, Bolin P, Kendrick WT, et al. Impact of IgM and IgG3 anti-HLA alloantibodies in primary renal allograft recipients. Transplantation. 2014;97(5):494–501.
28. Bajic G, Degn SE, Thiel S, Andersen GR. Complement activation, regulation, and molecular basis for complement-related diseases. EMBO J. 2015;34(22):2735–57.
29. Nitsche JF, Tucker ES, 3rd, Sugimoto S, Vaughan JH, Curd JG. Rocket immunoelectrophoresis of C4 and C4d. A simple sensitive method for detecting complement activation in plasma. Am J Clin Pathol. 1981;76(5):679–84.
30. Coutance G, Kobashigawa JA, Kransdorf E, Loupy A, Desire E, Kittleson M, et al. Intermediate-term outcomes of complement inhibition for prevention of antibody-mediated rejection in immunologically high-risk heart allograft recipients. J Heart Lung Transplant. 2023.
31. Venner JM, Hidalgo LG, Famulski KS, Chang J, Halloran PF. The molecular landscape of antibody-mediated kidney transplant rejection: evidence for NK involvement through CD16a Fc receptors. Am J Transplant. 2015;15(5):1336–48.

32. Paul P, Picard C, Sampol E, Lyonnet L, Di Cristofaro J, Paul-Delvaux L, et al. Genetic and functional profiling of CD16-dependent natural killer activation identifies patients at higher risk of cardiac allograft vasculopathy. Circulation. 2018;137(10):1049–59.
33. Rocha PN, Plumb TJ, Crowley SD, Coffman TM. Effector mechanisms in transplant rejection. Immunol Rev. 2003;196:51–64.
34. Hirohashi T, Chase CM, Della Pelle P, Sebastian D, Alessandrini A, Madsen JC, et al. A novel pathway of chronic allograft rejection mediated by NK cells and alloantibody. Am J Transplant. 2012;12(2):313–21.
35. Zhang X, Valenzuela NM, Reed EF. HLA class I antibody-mediated endothelial and smooth muscle cell activation. Curr Opin Organ Transplant. 2012;17(4):446–51.
36. Zhang X, Rozengurt E, Reed EF. HLA class I molecules partner with integrin beta4 to stimulate endothelial cell proliferation and migration. Sci Signal. 2010;3(149):ra85.
37. Thoreen CC, Chantranupong L, Keys HR, Wang T, Gray NS, Sabatini DM. A unifying model for mTORC1-mediated regulation of mRNA translation. Nature. 2012;485(7396):109–13.
38. Jacinto E, Loewith R, Schmidt A, Lin S, Ruegg MA, Hall A, et al. Mammalian TOR complex 2 controls the actin cytoskeleton and is rapamycin insensitive. Nat Cell Biol. 2004;6(11):1122–8.
39. Masoud AG, Lin J, Zhu LF, Tao K, Ness NW, Kassiri Z, et al. Endothelial phosphoinositide 3-kinase-beta inactivation confers protection from immune-mediated vascular injury. Am J Transplant. 2023;23(2):202–13.
40. Li F, Wei J, Valenzuela NM, Lai C, Zhang Q, Gjertson D, et al. Phosphorylated S6 kinase and S6 ribosomal protein are diagnostic markers of antibody-mediated rejection in heart allografts. J Heart Lung Transplant. 2015;34(4):580–7.
41. Jin YP, Valenzuela NM, Zhang X, Rozengurt E, Reed EF. HLA class II-triggered signaling cascades cause endothelial cell proliferation and migration: relevance to antibody-mediated transplant rejection. J Immunol. 2018;200(7):2372–90.
42. Billingham RE, Brent L, Medawar PB. Actively acquired tolerance of foreign cells. Nature. 1953;172(4379):603–6.
43. Starzl TE, Murase N, Demetris AJ, Trucco M, Abu-Elmagd K, Gray EA, et al. Lessons of organ-induced tolerance learned from historical clinical experience. Transplantation. 2004;77(6):926–9.
44. Scandling JD, Busque S, Dejbakhsh-Jones S, Benike C, Millan MT, Shizuru JA, et al. Tolerance and chimerism after renal and hematopoietic-cell transplantation. N Engl J Med. 2008;358(4):362–8.
45. Leventhal J, Abecassis M, Miller J, Gallon L, Ravindra K, Tollerud DJ, et al. Chimerism and tolerance without GVHD or engraftment syndrome in HLA-mismatched combined kidney and hematopoietic stem cell transplantation. Sci Transl Med. 2012;4(124):124ra28.
46. Bracamonte-Baran W, Burlingham W. Non-inherited maternal antigens, pregnancy, and allotolerance. Biomed J. 2015;38(1):39–51.
47. Kirk AD. Crossing the bridge: large animal models in translational transplantation research. Immunol Rev. 2003;196:176–96.
48. Vincenti F, Larsen C, Durrbach A, Wekerle T, Nashan B, Blancho G, et al. Costimulation blockade with belatacept in renal transplantation. N Engl J Med. 2005;353(8):770–81.
49. Wagner JC, Ronin E, Ho P, Peng Y, Tang Q. Anti-HLA-A2-CAR Tregs prolong vascularized mouse heterotopic heart allograft survival. Am J Transplant. 2022;22(9):2237–45.

# The Sensitized Patient Awaiting Heart Transplantation

7

Jignesh Patel and Krishan Patel

**Abstract**

Pre-transplant sensitization is associated with an increased waiting time to transplant, increased wait-list mortality, and increased risk of rejection after transplant. In this chapter, we will focus on the role of antibodies in transplant patients, particularly donor-specific antibodies against human leukocyte antigens, and their clinical implications. In addition, we discuss risk factors for sensitization, antibody monitoring and detection methods, and desensitization strategies.

**Keywords**

Heart transplantation · HLA · Antibodies · Sensitized patients · Outcomes · Desensitization · Virtual crossmatch

J. Patel (✉) · K. Patel
Cedars-Sinai Smidt Heart Institute, Los Angeles, CA, USA
e-mail: jignesh.patel@cshs.org

K. Patel
e-mail: krishan.patel@cshs.org

## Clinical Pearls

- Sensitization of a pre-transplant patient is characterized by the development of alloreactive antibodies against HLA molecules and is associated with longer waitlist time and increased waitlist and post-transplant morbidity and mortality.
- Risk factors for sensitization include blood transfusions, prior pregnancy, prior transplantation, African American race, prior use of homografts, and the use of ventricular assist devices.
- Sensitization is measured by the calculated panel reactive antibody (cPRA) blood test, which defines the proportion of the donor population to whom the recipient has preformed potentially cytotoxic anti-HLA antibodies.
- High resolution solid phase immunoassays offer increased sensitivity and specificity for HLA antibody detection and allow determination of antibody specificity and binding strength; binding strength is measured by Mean Fluorescence Intensity.
- These immunoassays facilitate the use of the virtual crossmatch, in which potentially cytotoxic (based on binding strength) antibodies to donor HLA antigens are identified. The corresponding antigens to these antibodies are then avoided in any potential donor thus obviating the necessity of performing a



J. Kobashigawa (ed.), *Clinical Guide to Heart Transplantation*, https://doi.org/10.1007/978-3-031-88290-6_7

prospective donor-specific crossmatch, which expands the donor pool.

- Serum dilution assays, such as 1:8 dilutions, can provide advanced quantitative information regarding antibody levels. These assays also counter the prozone effect by diluting complement concentration which unshields antibodies allowing their detection.
- C1q binding assays are able to distinguish complement-fixing from non-complement-fixing antibodies. The ability of an antibody to bind C1q may be a better marker of potential cytotoxicity than antibody strength. Using a C1q threshold to determine incompatible donors instead of an MFI threshold would result in fewer antigen avoids and thus expand the donor pool. However, customized immune therapy may be needed if crossing high-level DSA.
- The cPRA defines the proportion of the donor population to whom the transplant candidate has preformed potentially cytotoxic anti-HLA antibodies and thus is a marker of the degree of sensitization and the wait time to transplant. In most programs, a threshold of cPRA>50% is used to consider desensitization.
- Therapeutic desensitization treatments may expand the donor pool and reduce waitlist time for sensitized patients: options include plasmapheresis and immunoadsorption, intravenous immunoglobulin, rituximab (anti-CD20), bortezomib (proteasome inhibitor), daratumumab (anti-CD38), and eculizumab (complement blockade affecting C5).
- Periodic monitoring of circulating antibodies in patients awaiting transplantation is warranted, especially after desensitization, as antibodies may potentially rebound.

## Introduction

The humoral theory of transplantation states that antibodies cause the rejection of allografts. This hypothesis was first proposed in the early twentieth century, when efforts were made to produce antibodies against tumors. However, it was soon realized that the antibodies were produced against antigens present on donor organs, not against the tumor-specific antigens. Development of inbred mice subsequently allowed identification of the transplant antigens determined by the H-2 locus of mice [1]. The analogous human leukocyte antigen (HLA) system was established by discovery of antibodies against leukocytes in multiple transfused patients [2] and analysis of lymphocytotoxic alloantibodies made by pregnant women, directed against mismatched paternal antigens of the fetus [3, 4]. In the field of transplantation, HLA antibodies were then found to cause rejection of kidneys [5]. Antibodies appeared in almost all patients after rejection of kidneys. Advances in antibody detection and understanding of humoral immunity would not have been possible without in vitro techniques developed initially by Pappenheimer and subsequently by Terasaki. The development of the dye exclusion test by Pappenheimer in 1917 [6] was a significant advance which allowed the in vitro assessment of the effect of antibodies on cells. Vital cells actively excluded the dye, while cells that were destroyed by antibodies and complement stained blue. This test still has important uses today.

A major advance in transplant immunobiology was made in 1964 with the development of the microlymphocytotoxic assay by Terasaki [7]. The test only requires 1 μl—one lambda—of serum and a similarly small amount of lymphocytes. The importance of this was that as little as 1 ml of serum facilitated up to 1000 tests. This allowed efficient sharing of serum between different laboratories. By 1967, The Third Histocompatibility Workshop determined that all observed reactions fit into a single genetic locus. This was subsequently named "HLA" in 1968 by the World Health Organization.

Elucidation of the molecular structure of HLA antigens allowed synthesis of single HLA lines using recombinant technology. In the early 2000s, Terasaki's group developed single antigen Luminex beads with a single HLA antigen on different colored beads, allowing accurate determination of antibody specificity and in particular, donor-specific antibodies (DSA) [8].

## Risk Factors for Sensitization

Risk factors for sensitization include race, blood transfusions, prior transplantation [9], use of homografts with prior cardiac surgeries [10], prior pregnancy [11] and the use of ventricular assist devices (VADs) prior to transplantation [12]. Registry data show that 31% of African-Americans awaiting transplant have Americans awaiting transplant have panel reactive antibody (PRA) > 10% compared to 23% of Caucasians [13]. In patients awaiting kidney transplantation, 20% percent of patients who received a transfusion exhibited an antibody response compared to 3% who did not [14]. Blood transfusion is likely to elicit an antibody response in women and African-Americans. Multiparous women are at risk of sensitization to paternal antigens [15]. VADs increase risk of sensitization due to the higher likelihood of needing blood transfusions, although biomaterials and textured surfaces have also been implicated in increasing immunologic risk through allosensitization. Sensitization after VAD implantation has been associated with an increased waiting time to transplant, increased risk of post-transplant acute rejection, and increased risk of primary graft dysfunction [16, 17]. More than half of all patients now undergoing heart transplant (HTx) are now bridged with mechanical circulatory support (MCS) [18]. In early cohorts, up to two-thirds of VAD patients were at risk of allosensitization [19, 20]. This risk has been particularly linked with older pulsatile devices, and the use of newer axial flow devices has been associated with a much lower risk of allosensitization [21, 22]. In one study, the risk of allosensitization within 3 months of implant was 28% with the HeartMate I device compared to only 8% with the HeartMate II or DeBakey devices ($p = 0.02$) [22]. The latest Heartmate 3 device has demonstrated an even lower risk of de novo HLA sensitization compared to Heartmate II [23]. Even the risk of allosensitization from transfusions in VAD patients may be further mitigated by the use of leukocyte-reduced, and ABO-identical blood products. In a study using this approach [24], de novo sensitization rates were maintained below 10%, with no patient developing broad sensitization (PRA > 50%) despite each patient receiving a mean of 90 blood components. In a recent large single-center study of sensitized MCS patients, significantly lower rates of antibody-mediated rejection (AMR) and an earlier decline in PRA levels following HTx were recorded compared to sensitized non-MCS patients, and it has been suggested that removal of MCS device at the time of transplantation may have contributed to these findings [25].

## Clinical Implication of HLA Antibodies

DSA present prior to HTx have been demonstrated to be a risk factor for poor patient and allograft survival [26, 27]. In an early study of over 600 HTx recipients [27], the presence of a positive lymphocytotoxic crossmatch at transplant was associated with a one-year survival of 56% compared to 73% for those with a negative crossmatch. In a study of 950 HTx recipients followed for 15 years after transplant, Ho et al. [28] demonstrated that 15-year graft survival was greatest in those patients who never developed HLA antibodies (70%) or only had antibodies prior to transplant (71%). In contrast, patients who demonstrated antibodies both before and after transplant had a graft survival of only 56%. Lowest survival was noted in patients who developed de novo antibodies after transplant (47%). The development of de novo antibodies was preceded in 76% of these patients by cellular rejection ISHLT grade 3, and the development of AMR had a significant negative impact on survival. In an analysis of 105 pediatric transplant recipients, 43% were noted to have developed de novo DSA. Patients with DSA had significantly higher rates of rejection, allograft vasculopathy and mortality at 5 years [29]. While a significant portion of HTx recipients appear to develop HLA antibodies, it appears that increased mortality is only noted in those patients with persistent DSA [30]. Non-DSA and transient DSA do not appear to be associated with poor outcomes. In this study of a pediatric population, persistent DSA was characterized by Class II antibodies in 88% of the cases, and the presence of antibodies to DQ was associated with the worst survival rate. In sensitized patients, the presence of alloantibodies limits the donor pool. This results in a prolonged time on the waitlist and a consequent increase in mortality while on the waitlist [31]. After transplant, the patient remains at risk of rejection, graft loss, development of allograft vasculopathy, and increased mortality.

## Methods of Assessment for HLA and Non-HLA Antibodies

### Panel Reactive Antibodies

PRA has been traditionally performed on patients waiting for solid organ transplants and measures circulating anti-HLA antibodies. The PRA score is given as a percentage and represents the portion of the sample population that the anti-HLA antibody in the recipient's blood reacts with.

Techniques for measuring HLA antibodies have evolved significantly over the last 20 years [32, 33] (Fig. 7.1). Traditionally, complement-dependent cytotoxicity (CDC) assays have been

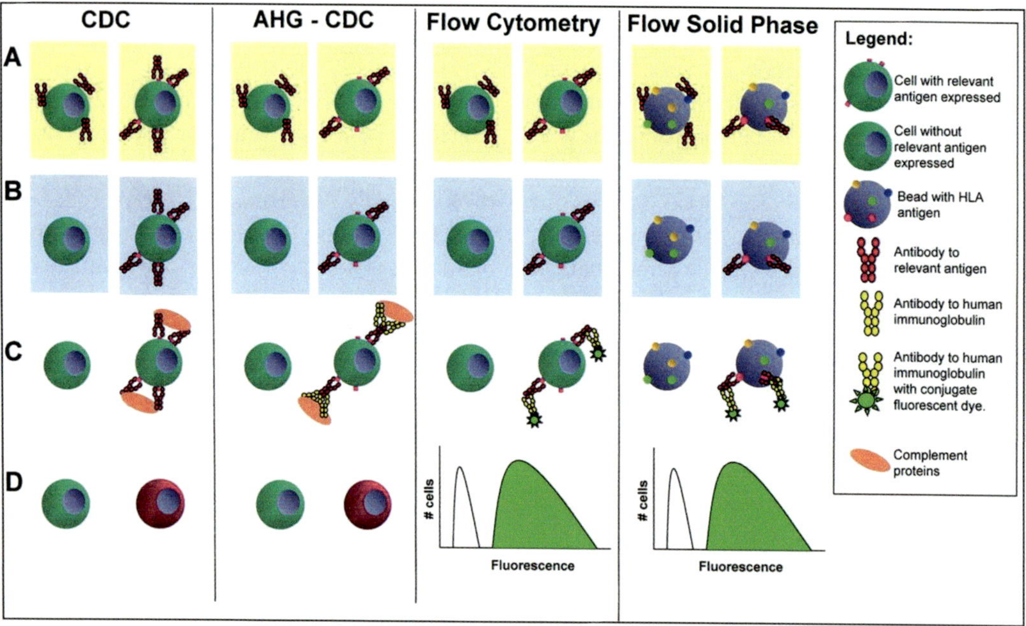


**Fig. 7.1** CDC and Flow Methods for Cross-Matching and Determination of Circulating HLA Alloantibodies. Abbreviations: CDC-Complement Dependent Cytotoxicity. AHG-Anti-human Globulin. Reused with permission from Kathryn Tinckam and Anil Chandraker, Mechanisms and Role of HLA and non-HLA Alloantibodies, Clinical Journal of the American Society of Nephrology, 1(3), 404–414 DOI: https://doi.org/10.2215/CJN.00270106; American Society of Nephrology

performed to assess the ability of recipient serum to lyse a panel of T or B cells obtained from a panel of volunteers, representative of the population. Addition of anti-human globulin (AHG) increased the sensitivity of CDC assays and allowed for detection of cytotoxic-negative, absorption-positive HLA alloantibodies. However, as both IgG and IgM can bind complement, neither test is able to distinguish between the immunoglobulin classes. The CDC tests also cannot distinguish between major histocompatibility (MHC) Class I or Class II antibodies. The CDC assay also requires a large number of cell panels from multiple donors to provide adequate sampling for detecting the most common HLA antigens, and rare or unusual antigens may be omitted [34]. More recent techniques using flow cytometry or enzyme-linked immunosorbent assay (ELISA) [33] are much more sensitive for the detection of antibodies and generally provide more reproducible results. The Luminex® test allows for simultaneous detection of multiple antibodies, as up to 100 color-coded antigen-coated microspheres can be detected in a single well [35]. The FlowPRA® test is a flow cytometry-based technique that consists of a pool of microparticle beads coated with full HLA Class I or Class II phenotype derived from purified HLA-bearing cell lines [36]. The percentage of PRAs can be determined by calculating the percentage of beads that react positively with patient sera. Due to variability in results between techniques, many laboratories will utilize multiple confirmatory tests.

While these assays are useful screening tools for the determination of PRA, further tests are required to determine the specificity and quantification of alloantibodies. The importance of the strength of circulating antibodies is increasingly recognized as an important factor determining the risk of a cytotoxic response. For determination of multiple antibody specificities and quantification of antibodies, single-antigen bead (SAB) assays are now commonly deployed [37]. These assays contain beads individually coated with a specific purified recombinant HLA molecule that identifies antibody specificity.

The ability to detect and quantify the strength of specific antibodies has allowed estimation of which recipient circulating antibodies are present at a strength that may prove to be cytotoxic for a potential donor organ. Laboratories will typically perform validation studies to determine the relationship between antibody levels determined by single antigen beads and flow crossmatch. For this purpose, the strength of antibody binding on single antigen beads, as represented by Mean Fluorescence Intensity (MFI), is compared to the degree of the flow crossmatch, which is reported as median channel shift (MCS). However, it is important to note that MFI is a measure of antibody-antigen binding or HLA molecule bead saturation rather than a direct measure of antibody titer.

MFI is also affected by several technical and biological factors. Antigen density on beads may vary depending on type of HLA molecule between different assay manufacturers' assay batches, and antigen density on beads may not reflect the natural expression of HLA molecules on cells in-vivo. Antibodies against public HLA epitopes (antigenic determinants produced by more than one gene) may be under-estimated and appear as weak antibodies due to a dilutional effect resulting from a single antibody being distributed across many beads. The presence of endogenous C1q inhibitors can also mask the detection of HLA antibodies. This is known as the "prozone effect." These C1q inhibitors may be diluted out through 1:8 dilution or eliminated by heat inactivation or denaturing with dithiothreitol (DTT) or ethylenediaminetetraacetic acid (EDTA) [38–40] in order to expose antibodies. The process of HLA molecule purification and coating onto the bead surface may also alter the natural conformation of antigens, leading to exposure or loss of antigenic epitopes. Therefore, HLA antibodies may remain undetected if they are unable to bind to the distorted HLA molecule. Conversely, clinically irrelevant antibodies may be detected that bind to the denatured but not intact antigen. In one study, a fifth of patients awaiting an HTx had at least one antibody to cryptic epitopes, which led to a false increase in calculated PRA (cPRA) by 5% [41].

Importantly, the technique allows the detection of low-level antibodies, which may trigger a strong amnestic immune response upon re-exposure to the antigen.

## Virtual Crossmatch

In the past, sensitized patients needed a prospective crossmatch to ensure allograft compatibility before transplantation. A prospective crossmatch identifies donor hearts that may be at risk of exposure to circulating cytotoxic antibodies. This method, however, can be logistically challenging as recipient blood has to be available close to the donor in order for the test to be performed in a timely manner. The test also requires local expertise, and samples also need to be kept updated as clinical conditions change for the recipient, who may be challenged with further potentially sensitizing events such as blood transfusions or VAD placement while awaiting transplantation. Recipient blood from sensitized patients has to be sent out to several locations where donors could potentially become available. The need for a prospective crossmatch inherently limits the geographical area from which sensitized patients may qualify for organ donors and, therefore, substantially increases the waiting time for transplants.

The ability to perform high-resolution antibody screening with solid phase assays has fortunately simplified appropriate donor selection by the use of a process termed "the virtual crossmatch." In a virtual crossmatch, the recipient antibody profile is determined at the time of listing, and potentially cytotoxic antibodies to HLA antigens are identified. Cytotoxicity is presumed from the strength of the antibody following correlation studies with flow cytometry crossmatch as described above [42]. The corresponding antigens are then documented as unacceptable on the transplant list. The principal advantage of his strategy is that it obviates the need to send out recipient blood and, therefore, substantially increases the geographical region from which a donor may be accepted. This approach has been shown to substantially decrease the waiting time to transplant [43]. The virtual crossmatch also helps identify patients who are potentially at elevated risk of rejection in whom immunosuppression may need to be augmented after transplantation. The use of the virtual crossmatch has been validated in several studies. In pediatric HTx recipients, the use of the virtual crossmatch was associated with a significantly decreased waiting time for transplant and improved survival compared to patients listed with a prospective crossmatch [44]. In another study, the accuracy of virtual crossmatch was compared to prospective AHG-CDC crossmatch [45]. Based on analysis of 257 T-cell AHG-CDC crossmatch tests, the positive predictive value of virtual crossmatch (the likelihood of an incompatible virtual crossmatch resulting in an incompatible T-cell CDC-AHG crossmatch) was 79%, and the negative predictive value of virtual crossmatch (the likelihood of a compatible virtual crossmatch resulting in a compatible T-cell CDC-AHG crossmatch) was 92%. When used prospectively in a cohort of 28 sensitized patients awaiting HTx, 14 received allografts based on a compatible virtual crossmatch alone from donors in geographically distant locations. Compared with the other 14 sensitized patients who underwent transplants after a compatible prospective serologic crossmatch, the rejection rates and survival were similar. More than 65% of HTx centers in the United States utilize the virtual crossmatch [46].

It is, however, unlikely that all classes and types of HLA antibodies have an equal impact on their ability to mount allograft rejection. The role of HLA-C and HLA-DP mismatches, for example, in allograft survival and their consideration in virtual crossmatch is still undetermined.

In contrast with CDC assays, conventional solid-phase assays do not discriminate between complement-fixing and non-complement-fixing antibodies. Avoidance of non-complement fixing and, therefore, non-cytotoxic antibodies in the virtual crossmatch may unnecessarily restrict the donor pool. A novel C1q assay developed to detect the sub-set of immunoglobulin G (IgG) antibodies capable of fixing complement may allow further expansion of the donor pool by allowing the exclusion of only complement-fixing antibodies in the virtual crossmatch [47]. In this study, the identification of complement-fixing antibodies in a standard virtual crossmatch correlated with a higher incidence of AMR compared to a virtual crossmatch with no complement-fixing antibodies. Another important observation is that the ability of an antibody to fix complement is independent of the strength of the antibody, and C1q fixation is independent of MFI values [48]. The C1q assay appears to be much more sensitive than the standard CDC at detecting complement-fixing antibodies.

Given the variety of testing now available to evaluate the sensitized HTx candidate, an algorithm for the assignment of unacceptable antigens for the virtual crossmatch has been used to allow transplantation of highly sensitized patients across the DSA barrier with survival rates comparable to DSA negative HTx recipients [49]. In this protocol, 4 antibody detection methods were used to prioritize unacceptable antigens- Luminex single antigen (LSA), LSA with 1:8 dilution, C1q LSA, and CDC panel.

## Non-HLA Antibodies

Antibody responses to non- HLA have been reported in solid organ transplantation and may occur as alloantibodies or autoantibodies. In thoracic organ transplantation, several have been implicated in acute and chronic allograft rejection. The antibodies identified include those against major histocompatibility class I chain-related gene A (MICA) [50, 51], angiotensin II type 1 receptor ($AT_1R$) [52], endothelin-1 type A receptor (ETAR) [53]endothelial cell antigens [54], vimentin [55], K-alpha-1-Tubulin (KA1T) [56], and collagen-V [57] and other non-HLA IgM antibodies. In cardiac transplantation, anti-MICA and anti-endothelial antibodies have been associated with increased AMR [58] and the development of cardiac allograft vasculopathy [50]. AT1R and ETAR have been implicated in the development of ACR, AMR, and early-onset microvasculopathy [53].

The detection of these antibodies in the setting of acute and chronic rejection, however, remains for investigational use, and none of the assays used to detect these antibodies have been routinely used for clinical evaluation. The clinical significance and the role of these antibodies in mediating thoracic allograft injury currently remains chiefly undetermined.

## Calculated PRA (cPRA)

Not all sensitized patients require treatment to decrease antibody burden. The need for therapy is dictated by cPRA. The cPRA value represents the percentage of donor hearts in a given population to which an HTx candidate will have cytotoxic anti-HLA antibodies. The cPRA is determined based on the antibody strength threshold (MFI) for cytotoxicity determined by the individual center's laboratory. For example, if the laboratory determines that antibodies with MFI>5000 correlate with cytotoxicity, only those corresponding antigens will be entered into the calculator available online at the Organ Procurement and Transplantation Network website from the US Department of Health and Human Services. The current cPRA data was updated in 2022, utilizing a larger data set than the original with expanded ethnic groups and a genotype-based algorithm rather than haplotype-based [59]. As the cPRA is an estimation of the proportion of the donors not suitable for the sensitized patients, generally, patients with a cPRA>50% may be considered for desensitization therapies as less than half the donor pool would be suitable for transplantation without treatment [60]. Patients awaiting HTx with cPRA>50% have a 49% lower likelihood of transplantation and a 70% higher risk of wait-list removal or death compared to those with cPRA<10% [61]. The aim of desensitization therapy is to reduce antibody burden, facilitate a reduction in the cPRA, and increase the chances of obtaining a suitable organ.

**Table 7.1** Strategies to prevent antibody-mediated rejection

| Approaches | Therapies |
|---|---|
| Antibody removal | Therapeutic plasma exchange, immunoadsorption |
| To alter antibody production<br>B-cell modulation<br>Plasma cell depletion | Rituximab, ATG, Bortezomib, Daratumumab, Tocilizumab |
| Immunomodulation (Ab inactivation) | IVIG |
| Suppression of the T-cell response | Steroids, ATG, MMF, CNI, PSI, Tocilizumab |
| Complement blockade | Eculizumab |

Abbreviations: Ab: antibody; ATG: anti-thymocyte globulin; IVIG: intravenous immunoglobulin; MMF: mycophenolate mofetil; CNI: calcineurin inhibitor; PSI: proliferation signal inhibitor

## Therapeutic Options for the Sensitized Patient

The humoral response involves B cells, plasma cells, antibodies, and complement. All of these have been commonly targeted as therapeutic options for desensitization (Table 7.1). Strategies for desensitization continue to evolve, but published clinical data remain sparse, and protocols in HTx have been adapted from experience in renal transplantation. The general approach is to use multiple complementary therapies, which are aimed at removing or neutralizing alloantibodies and suppressing further production.

### Plasmapheresis and Immunoadsorption

Plasmapheresis allows the physical removal of circulating antibodies. In one study, sensitized HTx candidates treated with pre-operative plasmapheresis and intravenous immunoglobulin (IVIG) had similar rates of rejection and allograft survival compared to non-sensitized controls [62]. Antibody rebound due to rapid diffusion from the extravascular space and reflex stimulation of plasma cells leading to increased production can occur, and multiple treatments are usually needed to achieve low circulating antibody levels. Large-bore intravenous access is required, and filtration of clotting factors with plasmapheresis may require replacement with fresh frozen plasma instead of albumin to correct coagulopathy. Immunoadsorption is an alternate form of plasmapheresis that uses IgG-specific columns to remove antibodies and then returns the patient's plasma, allowing targeted removal of alloantibodies, which may be more effective than untargeted plasmapheresis [63].

### Intravenous Immune Globulin (IVIg)

IVIG is a product of pooled IgG antibodies (immunoglobulin) extracted from the plasma of up to 100,000 blood donors. Originally developed for the treatment of primary immunodeficiency disorders, the product was found to have significant immunomodulatory effects. Its use was therefore expanded to treat autoimmune and inflammatory diseases and subsequently in organ transplantation. IVIg has multiple immune effects, including Fc receptor blockade, inhibition of complement deposition, enhancement of regulatory T cells, inhibition or neutralization of cytokines and B cell growth factors, accelerated clearance of autoantibodies, modulation of adhesion molecules and cell receptors, cross-linking B-cell receptor and FcγRIIB, which reduce APC activity and induce B-cell apoptosis and activation of regulatory macrophages [64, 65] (Fig. 7.2). A randomized placebo-controlled trial in sensitized patients awaiting renal transplantation revealed the efficacy of high-dose IVIg in reducing PRA, leading to improved transplant rates, but had no effect on rejection or graft loss

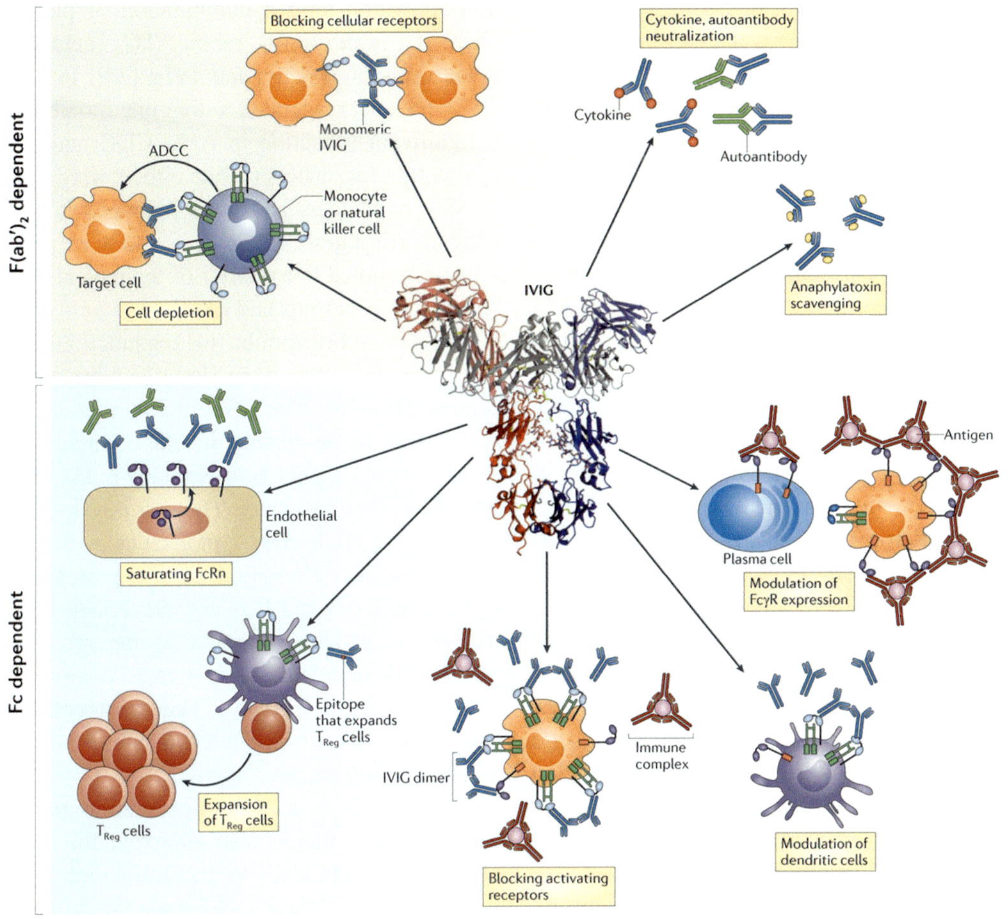


**Fig. 7.2** Mechanism of Intravenous Immunoglobulin (IVIg) activity. Reused with permission from Inessa Schwab et al., Intravenous immunoglobulin therapy: how does IgG modulate the immune system? Nature Reviews Immunology, 13(3), 176–189, 2013, Springer Nature. https://doi.org/10.1038/nri3401

[66]. In a study of sensitized LVAD recipients awaiting HTx [67], patients received monthly courses of either IVIg or plasmapheresis in conjunction with cyclophosphamide. Prolongation in transplant waiting time was related to the presence of Class I antibodies. Infusion of IVIg (2 g/kg) caused a mean reduction of 33% in anti-HLA class I alloreactivity within 1 week. Waiting time to transplantation was significantly reduced by IVIg therapy and subsequently matched non-sensitized patients. Although plasmapheresis caused a similar reduction in antibodies, this effect was achieved after longer treatment. Plasmapheresis was associated with an unacceptably high frequency of infectious complications. In this study, IVIg appeared to be more effective than plasmapheresis in reducing PRA with a superior safety profile.

## Rituximab

Rituximab is a chimeric monoclonal antibody against CD20 expressed on pre-B and mature B lymphocytes and was developed for the treatment of lymphoma. CD20 has an important role in B-cell maturation, regulating the early stages of cell cycle initiation and differentiation.

Rituximab causes B-cell depletion by complement and antibody-dependent cytotoxicity and apoptosis. In sensitized patients awaiting renal transplantation, rituximab in conjunction with IVIg has been shown to significantly reduce PRA, shorten time to transplant, and provide excellent 12-month graft and patient survival [68]. In HTx [69], 21 patients treated with a combination of plasmapheresis, IVIG, and rituximab had a mean reduction of PRA from 70.5 to 30.2%, resulting in a negative prospective donor-specific crossmatch and successful HTx. Compared with the control group (PRA < 10%), the treated sensitized group had similar 5-year survival and freedom from cardiac allograft vasculopathy. In a prospective study, 14 sensitized pediatric patients awaiting HTx underwent desensitization with high-dose IVIg and rituximab [70]. Eight patients had a significant decrease in cPRA, although 6 required multiple doses for a response. The total number of unacceptable antigens decreased for all 8 responders, leading to a median increase in the percentage of potential donors in the overall population from 10% pre-treatment to 85% post-treatment. Obinutuzumab is a second-generation fully humanized CD20 monoclonal antibody that may be more effective in depleting B cells, with published reports of use in desensitization limited to renal transplant candidates [71, 72].

## Proteasome Inhibitors

Although plasmapheresis, IVIg, and rituximab variably reduce antibody burden, these modalities have no suppressive effect on the cell responsible for antibody production, the mature plasma cell. Bortezomib is a selective, reversible 26S proteasome inhibitor used in the treatment of multiple myeloma, a plasma cell neoplasm. In vitro, bortezomib demonstrated plasma cell apoptosis and blocked anti-HLA antibody production [73]. In contrast, IVIG, rituximab, and anti-thymocyte globulin had no effect on suppressing antibody production by plasma cells. In one study, 34 highly sensitized patients awaiting living-related donor renal transplant underwent desensitization with a combination of plasmapheresis, bortezomib, rabbit-ATG, mycophenolate mofetil (MMF) and IVIg [74]. In total, 29/34 patients responded within one month with a significant reduction in AHG-CDC and flow cytometry crossmatches. Side effects were noted in 38% of patients and were manageable. Two patients lost a graft at one year, and acute rejections were noted in a quarter of the patients who responded to steroids and rATG.

In HTx, bortezomib, in conjunction with plasmapheresis, has been described by several centers [75, 76]. The response to this combination was noted mainly in class I antibodies (Class I cPRA 90–74% in Brinkley et al., 60.5–54.9% in Dhillon et al.). The primary route of synthesis of HLA class I molecules is dependent on peptide generation by the proteasome, whereas that of class II is not. Nevertheless, the majority of patients were able to undergo transplants with one-year survival rates comparable to non-sensitized patients. The most common side effects were thrombocytopenia, neutropenia, and peripheral neuropathy.

Carfilzomib is a second-generation proteasome inhibitor that is also approved for multiple myeloma and leads to irreversible inhibition of plasma cells. There has been a single center report describing the experience of 9 patients undergoing carfilzomib therapy combined with plasmapheresis and IVIg, demonstrating effectiveness in class I antibody reduction (total cPRA 76–40% and C1q-fixing antibodies 56–4%) and facilitation of transplant in 6 patients with acceptable outcomes [77]. It should be noted, though, that the majority of these patients had LVADs who may have a more benign phenotype of sensitization and that there has been significant cardiotoxicity associated with carfilzomib in patients with hematologic malignancies [78].

The combination of plasmapheresis with proteasome inhibitors may be more effective than plasmapheresis monotherapy because the removal of circulating antibodies by plasmapheresis results in increased metabolic demands on B-cells, memory B-cells, and plasma cells to produce more antibodies. This metabolic stress enhances the sensitivity of plasma cells to proteasome inhibition. Plasmapheresis during proteasome inhibitor therapy also provides the additional benefit of removing pre-existing circulating antibodies. This combination is primarily used in the inpatient setting.

## Emerging Desensitization Strategies

The CD38 monoclonal antibody daratumumab was similarly also originally developed for multiple myeloma but has shown utility in desensitization. CD38 is present on plasma cells and other immune cells. Experience in HTx candidates has been limited to case reports/series [79, 80].

Animal models have demonstrated the potential utility of antibodies against CTLA4 in inhibiting de novo DSA production [81]. Belatacept, which is a T-cell costimulation blocker that functions as an antibody against CD80/CD86 fused with CTLA4, has been trialed in conjunction with proteasome inhibitors in highly sensitized patients, demonstrating significant reductions in both HLA class I and II antibodies, including those that were previously C1q-binding [82].

Tocilizumab is an IL-6 inhibitor, which downregulates T and B cell differentiation and proliferation. In an early phase study of kidney transplant candidates who were unresponsive to desensitization with IVIg, rituximab, and/or plasma exchange, tocilizumab with IVIg led to a fall in class I/II cPRAs from $74 \pm 31\%$ and $93 \pm 5\%$ to $59 \pm 41\%$ and $89 \pm 9\%$, respectively, and 5/10 patients went onto successful transplant, all of which were free of AMR [83]. A humanized IL-6 inhibitor, clazakizumab, is also under investigation.

## Splenectomy

Splenectomy reduces plasma and precursor cells and impairs B-cell immune surveillance. It can be performed using minimally invasive techniques. It is, however, associated with a life-long risk of sepsis from encapsulated bacteria, and its effect on the immune system is permanent. This significantly limits its use in highly sensitized patients already at increased infection risk due to other desensitization therapies. Splenectomy has been shown to be effective in permitting ABO and HLA incompatible renal transplantation against a positive crossmatch when used in conjunction with plasmapheresis and immunoglobulin [84]. However, the use of this modality has waned due to potential complications and unintended consequences.

## Eculizumab

Antibody-mediated injury predominantly relies on the activation of complement. The complement system may be activated by 3 separate pathways that converge to C5, and the subsequent formation of the membrane attack complex (C5b-C9), which has proinflammatory and chemotactic properties and, importantly, promotes cell lysis. An approach preventing complement activation may, therefore, be effective in preventing AMR in sensitized patients after HTx. Eculizumab is a monoclonal antibody that specifically binds to the complement protein C5 with high affinity and inhibits its cleavage to C5a and C5b, thus preventing the generation of the terminal membrane attack complex C5b-9. C5a is also a potent immunomodulator involved in chemotaxis, macrophage cytokine production, and ischemia–reperfusion injury. One potential advantage of targeting the terminal components of the complement system is that the early components are preserved to remain active in immune defense. For example, C3b is an important opsonin against microbial infection. Eculizumab is approved for the treatment of paroxysmal nocturnal hemoglobinuria and atypical hemolytic uremic syndrome.

In renal transplantation, the incidence of biopsy-proven AMR in the first 3 months in 26 highly sensitized recipients treated with eculizumab was significantly reduced compared to a matched historical cohort (7.7 vs 41.2%; $p = 0.003$) [85]. A single-center pilot study of

**Table 7.2** Key takeaways from the 2023 Consensus Conference on Emerging Understanding of Antibodies and Antibody-Mediated Rejection in Heart Transplantation

| | |
|---|---|
| 1. | Stratify antibody risk by Mean Fluorescent Intensity (MFI) in the undiluted assay: |
| | • Low risk < 5,000 MFI |
| | • Moderate risk 5,000-8,000 MFI |
| | • High risk > 8,000 MFI. |
| 2. | Consider desensitizing if the calculated panel reactive antibody (cPRA) is >50%, depending on patient/antibody characteristics and center support/infrastructure. The goal of pre-transplant desensitization therapy is to lower the cPRA to broaden the donor pool and minimize the risk of post-transplant AMR. |
| 3. | There is a need for precision in defining ABO-related histocompatibility between donor and recipient to enable clinicians to carefully analyze risk and benefit while expanding this platform from infants to older children and select adults. |
| 4. | Induction therapy (antithymocyte globulin (ATG) or basiliximab) may be considered peri-transplant for sensitized patients. |
| 5. | Crossing donor-specific antibodies (DSA) in experienced centers may be considered for sensitized patients but should take into account patient characteristics, antibody attributes, and their biological significance. |
| 6. | If crossing DSA at the time of heart transplant, induction therapy (ATG) or IVIG/plasmapheresis are common therapies. |
| 7. | Several variables should be considered to treat patients with post-transplant DSA, including cardiac dysfunction by imaging, abnormal hemodynamics, an increasing MFI trend in DSA, the presence of early DSA, antibody attributes (C1q+ binding, detection of DSA in dilution assay), biopsy-proven pAMR ≥ 2, and abnormal molecular findings (dd-cfDNA and/or the MMDx) as available. However, the clinical utility of treating asymptomatic post-transplant DSA remains unclear. |
| 8. | Endomyocardial biopsy is not mandated in patients with asymptomatic post-transplant DSA but should be performed when DSA are associated with signs of clinical or subclinical graft dysfunction or graft injury. |
| 9. | Testing and treatment of non-HLA antibodies have not been recommended until a causal role in graft injury and defined thresholds are established. |
| 10. | Sensitization should be factored into donor heart allocation policy. |

the use of eculizumab at the time of transplantation and two months afterward in 20 highly sensitized patients demonstrated that despite positive B cell and T cell flow crossmatches in 14 and 11 patients, only 4 patients went onto have pAMR2 or greater and/or left ventricular dysfunction. Survival was 90% at 1 year [86].

## Monitoring of Sensitized Patients While Awaiting Transplantation

Antibodies may potentially rebound following the completion of desensitization therapy, and additional treatment may need to be considered. Further opportunities for sensitization may also present in patients receiving blood products, MCS, or developing infection. Circulating antibodies, therefore, need to be periodically monitored while awaiting HTx. For sensitized patients (PRA > 10%), circulating antibodies should be checked at 6–12 month intervals and/or if sensitizing events (blood transfusions) have occurred.

Consensus conferences took place in 2008 [46], 2016 [87], and 2023 [88, 89] to assess the prevalence of sensitization in patients awaiting HTx, the use and efficacy of desensitization therapies, and the outcomes of desensitized patients after HTx. Recently published key takeaways from the 2023 Consensus Conference on Emerging Understanding of Antibodies and Antibody-Mediated Rejection in Heart Transplantation are summarized in Table 7.2 [88, 89].

## Conclusions

HTx waitlists continue to grow as demand for organs has vastly out-stripped the donor pool despite expansion made possible by the use of Hepatitis C donors and donation after cardiac death. In this scenario, sensitized patients awaiting HTx represent a particular challenge. Due to a limited donor supply, an increasing number of patients awaiting HTx are on MCS, and these patients are at particular risk for sensitization. Pre-transplant sensitization is associated with an increased waiting time to transplant, increased wait-list mortality, and increased risk of rejection after transplant. Solid-phase immunoassays offer increased sensitivity and specificity for HLA antibody detection. These high-resolution tests allow patients to be listed for transplant by virtual cross-match, thereby increasing the donor pool. However, unlike the CDC assay, these assays do not distinguish complement fixing from non-complement fixing antibodies, and antibody strength and serial dilution serve as surrogates for cytotoxicity. The C1q binding assay further distinguishes HLA antibodies that can bind the first component of complement and may further help expand the donor pool by identifying the most pathogenic antibodies. Treatment options for sensitized patients remain an area of active investigation and focus on antibody removal (plasmapheresis and immunoadsorption), targeting B cells and immunomodulation (rituximab and IVIg), plasma cell depletion (proteasome inhibitors) and complement blockade (eculizumab). The most effective approach for reducing alloantibodies requires a combination of therapies.

## References


1. Gorer PA, Schutze H. Genetical studies on immunity in mice: II. Correlation between antibody formation and resistance. J Hyg (Lond). 1938;38(6):647–62.
2. Dausset J. Iso-leuko-antibodies. Acta Haematol. 1958;20(1–4):156–66.
3. Van Rood JJ, Eernisse JG, Van Leeuwen A. Leucocyte antibodies in sera from pregnant women. Nature. 1958;181(4625):1735–6.
4. Payne R, Rolfs MR. Fetomaternal leukocyte incompatibility. J Clin Investig. 1958;37(12):1756–63.
5. Terasaki PI, Kreisler M, Mickey RM. Presensitization and kidney transplant failures. Postgrad Med J. 1971;47(544):89–100.
6. Pappenheimer AM. Experimental studies upon lymphocytes: I. The reactions of lymphocytes under various experimental conditions. J Exp Med. 1917;25(5):633–50.
7. Terasaki PI, McClelland JD. Microdroplet assay of human serum cytotoxins. Nature. 1964;204:998–1000.
8. Pei R, Lee JH, Shih NJ, Chen M, Terasaki PI. Single human leukocyte antigen flow cytometry beads for accurate identification of human leukocyte antigen antibody specificities. Transplantation. 2003;75(1):43–9.
9. Karwande SV, Ensley RD, Renlund DG, Gay WA, Jr., Richenbacher WE, Doty DB, et al. Cardiac retransplantation: a viable option? The Registry of the International Society for Heart and Lung Transplantation. Ann Thorac Surg. 1992;54(5):840–4; discussion 5.
10. Hooper DK, Hawkins JA, Fuller TC, Profaizer T, Shaddy RE. Panel-reactive antibodies late after allograft implantation in children. Ann Thorac Surg. 2005;79(2):641–4; discussion 5.
11. Hyun J, Park KD, Yoo Y, Lee B, Han B, Song E, et al., editors. Effects of different sensitization events on HLA alloimmunization in solid organ transplantation patients. In: Transplantation proceedings. Elsevier; 2012.
12. John R, Boyle A, Pagani F, Miller L. Physiologic and pathologic changes in patients with continuous-flow ventricular assist devices. J Cardiovasc Transl Res. 2009;2(2):154–8.
13. OPTN/SRTR. Annual data report. http://www.srtr.org/annual_Reports/archives/2004/2004_Annual_Report/default.htm2004.
14. Leffell MS, Kim D, Vega RM, Zachary AA, Petersen J, Hart JM, et al. Red blood cell transfusions and the risk of allosensitization in patients awaiting primary kidney transplantation. Transplantation. 2014;97(5):525–33.
15. Reed E, Beer AE, Hutcherson H, King DW, Suciu-Foca N. The alloantibody response of pregnant women and its suppression by soluble HLA antigens and anti-idiotypic antibodies. J Reprod Immunol. 1991;20(2):115–28.
16. John R, Lietz K, Schuster M, Naka Y, Rao V, Mancini DM, et al. Immunologic sensitization in recipients of left ventricular assist devices. J Thorac Cardiovasc Surg. 2003;125(3):578–91.
17. Arnaoutakis GJ, George TJ, Kilic A, Weiss ES, Russell SD, Conte JV, et al. Effect of sensitization in

US heart transplant recipients bridged with a ventricular assist device: update in a modern cohort. J Thorac Cardiovasc Surg. 2011;142(5):1236–45, 45 e1.
18. Jawitz OK, Fudim M, Raman V, Bryner BS, DeVore AD, Mentz RJ, et al. Reassessing recipient mortality under the new heart allocation system: an updated UNOS registry analysis. Heart Fail. 2020;8(7):548–56.
19. John R, Rajasinghe H, Chen JM, Weinberg AD, Sinha P, Itescu S, et al. Impact of current management practices on early and late death in more than 500 consecutive cardiac transplant recipients. Ann Surg. 2000;232(3):302–11.
20. Massad MG, Cook DJ, Schmitt SK, Smedira NG, McCarthy JF, Vargo RL, et al. Factors influencing HLA sensitization in implantable LVAD recipients. Ann Thorac Surg. 1997;64(4):1120–5.
21. Drakos SG, Kfoury AG, Kotter JR, Reid BB, Clayson SE, Selzman CH, et al. Prior human leukocyte antigen-allosensitization and left ventricular assist device type affect degree of post-implantation human leukocyte antigen-allosensitization. J Heart Lung Transplant Off Publ Int Soc Heart Transplant. 2009;28(8):838–42.
22. George I, Colley P, Russo MJ, Martens TP, Burke E, Oz MC, et al. Association of device surface and biomaterials with immunologic sensitization after mechanical support. J Thorac Cardiovasc Surg. 2008;135(6):1372–9.
23. Jain R, Habal MV, Clerkin KJ, Latif F, Restaino SW, Zorn E, et al. De novo human leukocyte antigen allosensitization in Heartmate 3 versus Heartmate II left ventricular assist device recipients. ASAIO J. 2022;68(2):226–32.
24. Coppage M, Baker M, Fialkow L, Meehan D, Gettings K, Chen L, et al. Lack of significant de novo HLA allosensitization in ventricular assist device recipients transfused with leukoreduced, ABO identical blood products. Hum Immunol. 2009;70(6):413–6.
25. Youn J-C, Zhang X, Nishihara K, Kim I-C, Baek SH, Seguchi O, et al. Post-transplantation outcomes of sensitized patients receiving durable mechanical circulatory support. J Heart Lung Transplant. 2022;41(3):365–72.
26. Nwakanma LU, Williams JA, Weiss ES, Russell SD, Baumgartner WA, Conte JV. Influence of pretransplant panel-reactive antibody on outcomes in 8,160 heart transplant recipients in recent era. Ann Thorac Surg. 2007;84(5):1556–62; discussion 62–3.
27. Smith JD, Danskine AJ, Laylor RM, Rose ML, Yacoub MH. The effect of panel reactive antibodies and the donor specific crossmatch on graft survival after heart and heart-lung transplantation. Transpl Immunol. 1993;1(1):60–5.
28. Ho EK, Vlad G, Vasilescu ER, de la Torre L, Colovai AI, Burke E, et al. Pre- and posttransplantation allosensitization in heart allograft recipients: major impact of de novo alloantibody production on allograft survival. Hum Immunol. 2011;72(1):5–10.
29. Tran A, Fixler D, Huang R, Meza T, Lacelle C, Das BB. Donor-specific HLA alloantibodies: Impact on cardiac allograft vasculopathy, rejection, and survival after pediatric heart transplantation. J Heart Lung Transplant Off Publ Int Soc Heart Transplant. 2016;35(1):87–91.
30. Irving CA, Carter V, Gennery AR, Parry G, Griselli M, Hasan A, et al. Effect of persistent versus transient donor-specific HLA antibodies on graft outcomes in pediatric cardiac transplantation. J Heart Lung Transplant Off Publ Int Soc Heart Transplant. 2015;34(10):1310–7.
31. Lund LH, Edwards LB, Kucheryavaya AY, Dipchand AI, Benden C, Christie JD, et al. The Registry of the International Society for Heart and Lung Transplantation: thirtieth official adult heart transplant report–2013; focus theme: age. J Heart Lung Transplant Off Publ Int Soc Heart Transplant. 2013;32(10):951–64.
32. Tinckam KJ, Chandraker A. Mechanisms and role of HLA and non-HLA alloantibodies. Clin J Am Soc Nephrol. 2006;1(3):404–14.
33. Schlaf G, Pollok-Kopp B, Manzke T, Schurat O, Altermann W. Novel solid phase-based ELISA assays contribute to an improved detection of anti-HLA antibodies and to an increased reliability of pre- and post-transplant crossmatching. NDT Plus. 2010;3(6):527–38.
34. Altermann WW, Seliger B, Sel S, Wendt D, Schlaf G. Comparison of the established standard complement-dependent cytotoxicity and flow cytometric crossmatch assays with a novel ELISA-based HLA crossmatch procedure. Histol Histopathol. 2006;21(10):1115–24.
35. Smith JD, Hamour IM, Banner NR, Rose ML. C4d fixing, luminex binding antibodies - a new tool for prediction of graft failure after heart transplantation. Am J Transplant Off J Am Soc Transplant Am Soc Transplant Surg. 2007;7(12):2809–15.
36. Won DI, Jung HD, Jung OJ, Huh S, Suh JS. Flow cytometry PRA using lymphocyte pools from random donors. Cytom B Clin Cytom. 2007;72(4):256–64.
37. El-Awar N, Lee J, Terasaki PI. HLA antibody identification with single antigen beads compared to conventional methods. Hum Immunol. 2005;66(9):989–97.
38. Zachary AA, Lucas DP, Detrick B, Leffell MS. Naturally occurring interference in Luminex assays for HLA-specific antibodies: characteristics and resolution. Hum Immunol. 2009;70(7):496–501.
39. Schnaidt M, Weinstock C, Jurisic M, Schmid-Horch B, Ender A, Wernet D. HLA antibody specification using single-antigen beads–a technical solution for the prozone effect. Transplantation. 2011;92(5):510–5.

40. Zeevi A, Lunz J, Feingold B, Shullo M, Bermudez C, Teuteberg J, et al. Persistent strong anti-HLA antibody at high titer is complement binding and associated with increased risk of antibody-mediated rejection in heart transplant recipients. J Heart Lung Transplant Off Publ Int Soc Heart Transplant. 2013;32(1):98–105.
41. Oaks M, Michel K, Sulemanjee NZ, Thohan V, Downey FX. Practical value of identifying antibodies to cryptic HLA epitopes in cardiac transplantation. J Heart Lung Transplant. 2014;33(7):713–20.
42. Reinsmoen NL, Lai CH, Vo A, Cao K, Ong G, Naim M, et al. Acceptable donor-specific antibody levels allowing for successful deceased and living donor kidney transplantation after desensitization therapy. Transplantation. 2008;86(6):820–5.
43. Yanagida R, Czer LS, Reinsmoen NL, Cao K, Rafiei M, De Robertis MA, et al. Impact of virtual cross match on waiting times for heart transplantation. Ann Thorac Surg. 2011;92(6):2104–10; discussion 11.
44. Zangwill S, Ellis T, Stendahl G, Zahn A, Berger S, Tweddell J. Practical application of the virtual crossmatch. Pediatr Transplant. 2007;11(6):650–4.
45. Stehlik J, Islam N, Hurst D, Kfoury AG, Movsesian MA, Fuller A, et al. Utility of virtual crossmatch in sensitized patients awaiting heart transplantation. J Heart Lung Transplant Off Publ Int Soc Heart Transplant. 2009;28(11):1129–34.
46. Kobashigawa J, Mehra M, West L, Kerman R, George J, Rose M, et al. Report from a consensus conference on the sensitized patient awaiting heart transplantation. J Heart Lung Transplant Off Publ Int Soc Heart Transplant. 2009;28(3):213–25.
47. Chin C, Chen G, Sequeria F, Berry G, Siehr S, Bernstein D, et al. Clinical usefulness of a novel C1q assay to detect immunoglobulin G antibodies capable of fixing complement in sensitized pediatric heart transplant patients. J Heart Lung Transplant. 2010;30(2):158–63.
48. Chen G, Sequeira F, Tyan DB. Novel C1q assay reveals a clinically relevant subset of human leukocyte antigen antibodies independent of immunoglobulin G strength on single antigen beads. Hum Immunol. 2011;72(10):849–58.
49. Reinsmoen NL, Patel J, Mirocha J, Lai CH, Naim M, Ong G, et al. Optimizing transplantation of sensitized heart candidates using 4 antibody detection assays to prioritize the assignment of unacceptable antigens. J Heart Lung Transplant Off Publ Int Soc Heart Transplant. 2016;35(2):165–72.
50. Kauke T, Kaczmarek I, Dick A, Schmoeckel M, Deutsch MA, Beiras-Fernandez A, et al. Anti-MICA antibodies are related to adverse outcome in heart transplant recipients. J Heart Lung Transplant. 2009;28(4):305–11.
51. Angaswamy N, Saini D, Ramachandran S, Nath DS, Phelan D, Hachem R, et al. Development of antibodies to human leukocyte antigen precedes development of antibodies to major histocompatibility class I-related chain A and are significantly associated with development of chronic rejection after human lung transplantation. Hum Immunol. 2010;71(6):560–5.
52. Cao K, Lai C-H, Flores SV, Rafiei M, Mirocha J, Haas M, et al. Anti Angiotensin Type 1 Receptor (AT1R) antibodies together with anti-HLA Donor Specific Antibodies (HLA-DSA) identify patients at risk for immune complication in heart transplant. J Heart Lung Transplant. 2012.
53. Hiemann NE, Meyer R, Wellnhofer E, Schoenemann C, Heidecke H, Lachmann N, et al. Non-HLA antibodies targeting vascular receptors enhance alloimmune response and microvasculopathy after heart transplantation. Transplantation. 2012;94(9):919–24.
54. Faulk WP, Rose M, Meroni PL, Del Papa N, Torry RJ, Labarrere CA, et al. Antibodies to endothelial cells identify myocardial damage and predict development of coronary artery disease in patients with transplanted hearts. Hum Immunol. 1999;60(9):826–32.
55. Jurcevic S, Ainsworth ME, Pomerance A, Smith JD, Robinson DR, Dunn MJ, et al. Antivimentin antibodies are an independent predictor of transplant-associated coronary artery disease after cardiac transplantation. Transplantation. 2001;71(7):886–92.
56. Goers TA, Ramachandran S, Aloush A, Trulock E, Patterson GA, Mohanakumar T. De novo production of K-alpha1 tubulin-specific antibodies: role in chronic lung allograft rejection. J Immunol. 2008;180(7):4487–94.
57. Iwata T, Philipovskiy A, Fisher AJ, Presson RG Jr, Chiyo M, Lee J, et al. Anti-type V collagen humoral immunity in lung transplant primary graft dysfunction. J Immunol. 2008;181(8):5738–47.
58. Zhang Q, Cecka JM, Gjertson DW, Ge P, Rose ML, Patel JK, et al. HLA and MICA: targets of antibody-mediated rejection in heart transplantation. Transplantation. 2011;91(10):1153–8.
59. Kransdorf EP, Pando MJ, Stewart D, Lindblad K, Bray R, Murphey C, et al. Stem cell donor HLA typing improves CPRA in kidney allocation. Am J Transplant. 2021;21(1):138–47.
60. Colvin MM, Cook JL, Chang PP, Hsu DT, Kiernan MS, Kobashigawa JA, et al. Sensitization in heart transplantation: emerging knowledge: a scientific statement from the American Heart Association. Circulation. 2019;139(12):e553–78.
61. Kransdorf EP, Kittleson MM, Patel JK, Pando MJ, Steidley DE, Kobashigawa JA. Calculated panel-reactive antibody predicts outcomes on the heart transplant waiting list. J Heart Lung Transplant. 2017;36(7):787–96.
62. Pisani BA, Mullen GM, Malinowska K, Lawless CE, Mendez J, Silver MA, et al. Plasmapheresis with intravenous immunoglobulin G is effective in patients with elevated panel reactive antibody

prior to cardiac transplantation. J Heart Lung Transplant Off Publ Int Soc Heart Transplant. 1999;18(7):701–6.
63. Rummler S, Barz D. Plasma exchange and immunoadsorption of patients with thoracic organ transplantation. Transfus Med Hemotherapy: offizielles Organ der Deutschen Gesellschaft fur Transfusionsmedizin und Immunhamatologie. 2012;39(4):234–40.
64. Ballow M. The IgG molecule as a biological immune response modifier: mechanisms of action of intravenous immune serum globulin in autoimmune and inflammatory disorders. J Allergy Clin Immunol. 2011;127(2):315–23; quiz 24–5.
65. Schwab I, Nimmerjahn F. Intravenous immunoglobulin therapy: how does IgG modulate the immune system? Nat Rev Immunol. 2013;13(3):176–89.
66. Jordan SC, Tyan D, Stablein D, McIntosh M, Rose S, Vo A, et al. Evaluation of intravenous immunoglobulin as an agent to lower allosensitization and improve transplantation in highly sensitized adult patients with end-stage renal disease: report of the NIH IG02 trial. J Am Soc Nephrol. 2004;15(12):3256–62.
67. John R, Lietz K, Burke E, Ankersmit J, Mancini D, Suciu-Foca N, et al. Intravenous immunoglobulin reduces anti-HLA alloreactivity and shortens waiting time to cardiac transplantation in highly sensitized left ventricular assist device recipients. Circulation. 1999;100(19 Suppl):II229–35.
68. Vo AA, Lukovsky M, Toyoda M, Wang J, Reinsmoen NL, Lai CH, et al. Rituximab and intravenous immune globulin for desensitization during renal transplantation. N Engl J Med. 2008;359(3):242–51.
69. Kobashigawa JA, Patel JK, Kittleson MM, Kawano MA, Kiyosaki KK, Davis SN, et al. The long-term outcome of treated sensitized patients who undergo heart transplantation. Clin Transplant. 2011;25(1):E61-7.
70. Schumacher KR, Ramon DS, Kamoun M, Caruthers R, Gajarski RJ. HLA desensitization in pediatric heart transplant candidates: efficacy of rituximab and IVIg. J Heart Lung Transplant Off Publ Int Soc Heart Transplant. 2012;31(9):1041–2.
71. Redfield RR, Jordan SC, Busque S, Vincenti F, Woodle ES, Desai N, et al. Safety, pharmacokinetics, and pharmacodynamic activity of obinutuzumab, a type 2 anti-CD20 monoclonal antibody for the desensitization of candidates for renal transplant. Am J Transplant. 2019;19(11):3035–45.
72. NasrAllah MM, Elalfy M, El Ansary M, Elmeseery Y, Amer I, Malvezzi P, et al. Obinutuzumab in kidney transplantation: effect on B-cell counts and crossmatch tests. Transplantation. 2022;106(2):369–72.
73. Perry DK, Burns JM, Pollinger HS, Amiot BP, Gloor JM, Gores GJ, et al. Proteasome inhibition causes apoptosis of normal human plasma cells preventing alloantibody production. Am J Transplant Off J Am Soc Transplant Am Soc Transplant Surg. 2009;9(1):201–9.
74. Kute VB, Vanikar AV, Trivedi HL, Shah PR, Goplani KR, Patel HV, et al. Desensitization protocol for highly sensitized renal transplant patients: a single-center experience. Saudi J Kidney Dis Transplant Off Publ Saudi Center Organ Transplant Saudi Arabia. 2011;22(4):662–9.
75. Brinkley DM, Mangione M, Fossey SC, Harrison KM, Zalawadiya S, Rali AS, et al. Efficacy of bortezomib desensitization among heart transplant candidates. Clin Transplant. 2023;37(4):e14907.
76. Dhillon M, Kobashigawa JA, Kittleson M, Jain R, Patel N, Singer-Englar T, et al. Does bortezomib influence pre-transplant desensitization therapy or benefit post-heart transplant outcomes for highly sensitized patients? Clin Transplant. 2024;38(1):e15165.
77. Sriwattanakomen R, Xu Q, Demehin M, Shullo MA, Mangiola M, Hickey GW, et al. Impact of carfilzomib-based desensitization on heart transplantation of sensitized candidates. J Heart Lung Transplant. 2021;40(7):595–603.
78. Shah C, Bishnoi R, Jain A, Bejjanki H, Xiong S, Wang Y, et al. Cardiotoxicity associated with carfilzomib: systematic review and meta-analysis. Leuk Lymphoma. 2018;59(11):2557–69.
79. Curtis A, Guha A, Bhimaraj A, Kim J, Suarez E, Trachtenberg B, et al. Use of daratumumab for desensitization prior to cardiac transplantation: a case report. J Heart Lung Transplant. 2021;40(4):S493.
80. Atteneder C, Moayedifar R, Koren D, Fischer G, Nackenhorst M, Uyanik-Uenal K, et al. CD38-antibody daratumumab in allosensitized recipients for heart transplantation: outcomes and 3-years of single-centre experience. J Heart Lung Transplant. 2024;43(4):S103.
81. Kim I, Wu G, Chai N-N, Klein AS, Jordan S. Ibrutinib suppresses alloantibody responses in a mouse model of allosensitization. Transplant Immunol. 2017;45:59–64.
82. Alishetti S, Farr M, Jennings D, Serban G, Uriel N, Sayer G, et al. Desensitizing highly sensitized heart transplant candidates with the combination of belatacept and proteasome inhibition. Am J Transplant. 2020;20(12):3620–30.
83. Vo AA, Choi J, Kim I, Louie S, Cisneros K, Kahwaji J, et al. A phase I/II trial of the interleukin-6 receptor–specific humanized monoclonal (tocilizumab)+ intravenous immunoglobulin in difficult to desensitize patients. Transplantation. 2015;99(11):2356–63.
84. Warren DS, Zachary AA, Sonnenday CJ, King KE, Cooper M, Ratner LE, et al. Successful renal transplantation across simultaneous ABO incompatible and positive crossmatch barriers. Am J Transplant Off J Am Soc Transplant Am Soc Transplant Surg. 2004;4(4):561–8.

85. Stegall MD, Diwan T, Raghavaiah S, Cornell LD, Burns J, Dean PG, et al. Terminal complement inhibition decreases antibody-mediated rejection in sensitized renal transplant recipients. Am J Transplant Off J Am Soc Transplant Am Soc Transplant Surg. 2011;11(11):2405–13.
86. Patel JK, Coutance G, Loupy A, Dilibero D, Hamilton M, Kittleson M, et al. Complement inhibition for prevention of antibody-mediated rejection in immunologically high-risk heart allograft recipients. Am J Transplant. 2021;21(7):2479–88.
87. Kobashigawa J, Colvin M, Potena L, Dragun D, Crespo-Leiro MG, Delgado JF, et al. The management of antibodies in heart transplantation: An ISHLT consensus document. J Heart Lung Transplant. 2018;37(5):537–47.
88. Kobashigawa J, Zuckermann A, Zeevi A, Barten MJ, Chang PP, Colvin M, Coutance G, Dipchand A, Ensminger S, Farrero M,Habal M. Summary of the International Society for Heart and Lung Transplantation consensus conference on emergingunderstanding of antibodies and antibody-mediated rejection in heart transplantation. J Heart Lung Transplant. 2025 Jun 11.
89. Kobashigawa J, Zuckermann A, Zeevi A, Barten MJ, Chang PP, Colvin M, Coutance G, Dipchand A, Ensminger S, Farrero M, Habal M. The Authors' Perspective on' Summary of the International Society for Heart and Lung Transplantation ConsensusConference on Emerging Understanding of Antibodies and Antibody-mediated Rejection in Heart Transplantation'. J Heart Lung Transplant. 2025 Aug 1;44(8):1195-8.

# Donor Organ Procurement and Preservation

8

Pedro Catarino

**Abstract**

With the expanding burden of advanced heart failure and the scarcity of donor hearts, several innovations in organ procurement and preservation have emerged to help facilitate and improve the clinical outcomes of heart transplantation. This chapter explores donor referral and evaluation, focusing on both brain death and circulatory death donors. In addition, this chapter covers donor heart procurement and preservation techniques.

**Keywords**

Heart transplantation · Donor · Procurement · Brain death · Circulatory death · Organ preservation

## Clinical Pearls

- Intermediary organizations take responsibility for the process of consent, donor management and evaluation, and donor allocation, removing any conflict of interest from both those caring for potential donors and those providing transplants to potential recipients.
- For potential donors it is essential to obtain as complete a picture as possible regarding their social and medical history and any condition that might be a contra-indication to organ donation.
- Goal-directed intensive care management with attention to hemodynamics, fluid and electrolyte management, and ventilatory parameters are important to optimize the viability of all organs.
- The use of normothermic or hypothermic ex vivo machine perfusion has been shown to mitigate risk in extended criteria donors, more complex recipients, and predicted long ischemic times.
- The consideration of any donor's heart needs to be made in the context of the recipient's situation, with individual risk–benefit analyses carried out in each case. This requires an understanding of the overall availability and quality of donors.
- Donation after circulatory death (DCD) has significantly increased the donor pool by including patients who are not braindead but have a determination of futility of further active treatment. In these patients, there has been a planned withdrawal oflife-supporting therapies (WLST) resulting in irreversible cessation of circulatory function, at which time they are declared deadand can become organ donors (after a 5-minute standoff period).

P. Catarino (✉)
Cedars-Sinai Smidt Heart Institute, Los Angeles, CA, USA
e-mail: pedro.catarino@cshs.org





J. Kobashigawa (ed.), *Clinical Guide to Heart Transplantation*, https://doi.org/10.1007/978-3-031-88290-6_8

## Donation After Brain Death (DBD)

Death may be determined in the patient who has suffered a catastrophic brain injury on the basis of coma, brainstem areflexia, and apnea. Since brainstem function predicts the permanence of coma, most of the testing focuses on demonstrating loss of brainstem reflexes (absence of pupillary and corneal reflexes, absent response to pain above the neck, and absent caloric oculo-vestibular reflex). Apnea requires a setting of adequate stimulus for breathing, typically hypercarbia. All testing requires the absence of confounding factors such as hypotension, hypothermia, metabolic derangements, or drug effects. Diagnosis of brain death is primarily a clinical diagnosis, with ancillary imaging only performed as a backup measure. However, evidence of a brain injury compatible with brain death is essential to the diagnosis. There are specific guidelines with a standardized approach to testing applicable to particular jurisdictions [1, 2]. These patients are legally dead if confirmed by brain death testing. At this point, they may be referred for potential organ donation. The heart continues to beat, and organ viability is maintained by mechanical ventilation and intensive care measures.

## Donation After Circulatory Death (DCD)

DCD refers to organ donation, which takes place after a patient has been declared dead on the basis of irreversible cessation of respiratory and circulatory function [3]. For heart donation, this is currently only feasible in the setting where there has been a planned withdrawal of life-supporting therapies (WLST) following a determination of the futility of further active treatment. These are referred to as Maastricht category III donors to distinguish them from other potential DCDs that occur in uncontrolled settings.

Here, the WLST is coordinated with the organ procurement process. WLST is followed by a decline in the patient's vital signs, culminating in circulatory arrest. Death is determined on the basis of mechanical (not electrical) asystole—a flat arterial trace—and the absence of breathing. After a standoff period, which is usually 5 min, the absence of spontaneous autoresuscitation confirms permanence or irreversibility and allows confirmation of death. The donor is transferred to the operating theatre for organ procurement. There is no circulation, and the organs all suffer a warm ischemic injury during this period.

## Donor Referral and Evaluation

Organ donation represents a remarkable act of compassion and solidarity for our fellow man and maybe the final autonomous wish of patients. Healthcare providers who deliver end-of-life care have a duty to refer potential donors to fulfill this wish. Intermediary organizations take responsibility for the process of consent, donor management and evaluation, and donor allocation, removing any conflict of interest between those caring for potential donors and those providing transplants to potential recipients.

Potential donors require due diligence to obtain as complete a picture as possible regarding their social and medical history and any condition that might be a contraindication to organ donation. Standard laboratory tests, electrocardiograms, and chest X-rays are performed, as is serology for a range of blood-borne pathogens and human leukocyte antigen typing.

Specific testing for heart donors includes transthoracic echocardiography. Coronary angiography may be performed selectively, usually in donors with risk factors for coronary artery disease, including age over 45 years. This may be declined in the DCD setting, where invasive testing may not be felt to be in the best interests of the not-yet-deceased patient. In DCD, the management of the patient continues under their usual physicians, and the needs of the patient remain the priority of care. In DBD, management transfers to the organ procurement intermediary team and may last many hours or days. The period of donor evaluation is also one of goal-directed intensive care management, with attention to hemodynamics, fluid and electrolyte management, and ventilatory parameters with the aim of optimizing the viability of all organs. Adjuncts such as steroid or thyroxine supplementation have been used historically, but there is limited evidence of their effectiveness.

## Donor Acceptability and Recipient Matching

The consideration of any donor's heart needs to be made in the context of the recipient's situation, with individual risk–benefit analyses carried out in each case. This requires an understanding of the overall availability and quality of donors. Individual transplant centers' ability to absorb risk may also be a factor. Standard acceptable donors are of age 45 years or younger, with a normal echo [specifically EF > 50%, normal valves, and no left ventricular hypertrophy (wall thickness < 14 mm)], and normal hemodynamics [MAP > 60 mmHg, CVP ≤ 12 mmHg and cardiac index > 2.4 L/min/m$^2$]. In some situations, extended criteria donors would also be acceptable [4].

The up-to-date functional assessment of the heart by hemodynamics and echocardiography carries the most weight. This means that the circumstances of the death, for example, provoked cardiac arrest with a long downtime or cardiopulmonary resuscitation and raised biomarkers, would be mitigated by evidence of functional recovery after the event. Brainstem coning at the time of brain death results in a catecholamine storm, which can impair ventricular function, inducing a Takotsubo cardiomyopathy, which may take days to resolve. Repeated evaluations may be helpful.

ABO blood group matching to the recipient is essential, as is size-matching. Predicted heart mass provides the best metric for size-matching accounting for age, gender, height, and weight [5]. Online calculators are available. Generally, up to 10% under-sizing relative to the recipient's predicted heart mass would be acceptable, whereas more than 15% under-sizing would be too small. Increased risk factors such as high pulmonary vascular resistance in the recipient, the presence of a durable left ventricular assist device, and longer ischemic time would, however, influence this decision, as would other features of the donor.

Logistic factors will also come into play, particularly the predicted ischemic time. Ischemic time in DBD starts at the time of application of the aortic cross-clamp in the donor. It includes the time for cardioplegia flush and cardiac explant, travel time between donor and recipient centers, and time for implant in the recipient until the recipient's aortic cross-clamp is removed. Ischemic times over 4 h correlate with a higher incidence of primary graft dysfunction. The use of normothermic or hypothermic machine perfusion has been shown to mitigate risk in extended criteria donors, more challenging recipients, and long-predicted ischemic times [6, 7].

## DCD Heart Evaluation

The evaluation of DCD hearts follows similar principles to those outlined above for DBD hearts. Two main differences exist:

1. Only around 50% of patients suffer circulatory arrest following WLST within the time permitted, typically two hours. Therefore, the prediction of which donors will decline in a suitable time is part of their acceptability. Several scoring systems exist but have not proved clinically useful. Glasgow Coma Score (GCS) = 3 is associated with around a 2/3rds chance of rapid decline, but overbreathing on the ventilator reduces this probability. A low $PaO_2$:$FIO_2$ ratio is one of the strongest predictors.
2. There is an inevitable warm ischemic injury prior to procurement. Once the donor's systolic blood pressure drops below 50 mmHg, "functional warm ischemia" ensues, which continues until the donor's heart is perfused (either with blood or with cardioplegia). To maximize functional recovery, this period

should be kept below 30 min. This warm ischemic injury results in a substantial depletion of the metabolic substrate in the donor heart. The need to replenish these substrates prior to transport means that standard procurement strategies for DBD (i.e., cardioplegia followed by cold static storage) are poorly effective in DCD. Warm ischemic injury means that, until now, mainly standard criteria for hearts as defined for DBD have been accepted in the DCD setting. It remains to be seen what the results will be with extended criteria DCD hearts.

## Donor Heart Procurement

### DBD

Standard DBD heart procurement is performed by beating the heart and supporting the circulation in the setting of a multi-organ procurement [8]. It is essential that there is good communication between teams and that equipment is prepared, such as adequate field suction, to facilitate visualization during the period of organ flush. Sternotomy is followed by opening the pericardium and visualizing the heart, including right and left ventricular distension wall motion and coronary artery palpation. This visualization is usually sufficient to determine acceptability but may be augmented by direct pressure measurements, e.g., left atrial and even pulmonary artery catheter measurements. At this point, the recipient team can be given the go-ahead to start the recipient procedure.

The surgical technique of donor heart procurement will be detailed in Chap. 9. The explanted heart is moved to the back table to be prepared for transportation. In the great majority of cases, the heart is placed in a cold crystalloid solution surrounded by ice in a series of sterile containers, known as cold static storage. The goal of preservation in this setting is to minimize metabolic demand by producing a rapid mechanical and electrical arrest and inducing hypothermia. The actual cardioplegia solution would appear to be central to achieving these goals; however, limited evidence is available to support any particular solution.

### DCD

There are two distinct protocols that have been developed for the procurement of DCD heart.

#### Direct Procurement and Machine Perfusion (DP/MP)

This technique requires rapid explant of the heart and ex-situ warm blood re-perfusion. The TransMedics Organ Care System (OCS) Heart device is the only device currently available to achieve this. Donor blood is required to prime the device, and so the first step in surgery is to aspirate 1.2–1.5L of donor blood from the right atrium without any contamination from solutions used to flush the other organs, especially the liver. Once this is collected, the heart and other organs can be flushed, the heart with 500–1000 ml of cold crystalloid cardioplegia (Del Nido and St Thomas' solution are the most used, sometimes supplemented with GTN and erythropoietin). The heart is explanted as described above for DBD, with a longer main pulmonary artery preferred and high placement of the cardioplegia cannula so that this is excised when the aorta is transected. The explanted heart is moved to the back table, which is prepared for connection to the OCS heart device [9].

#### Normothermic Regional Perfusion (NRP)

This technique involves the rapid in-situ reperfusion of all the organs while excluding the cerebral circulation. The term TA-NRP is used to emphasize thoracic and abdominal organ perfusion. The donor is cannulated for cardiopulmonary bypass, usually draining the right atrium and re-infusing oxygenated blood into the ascending aorta. The aortic arch branches are clamped or ligated and may be vented, thereby preventing cerebral perfusion. A modified extracorporeal membrane oxygenation circuit with a hard-shell reservoir is used.

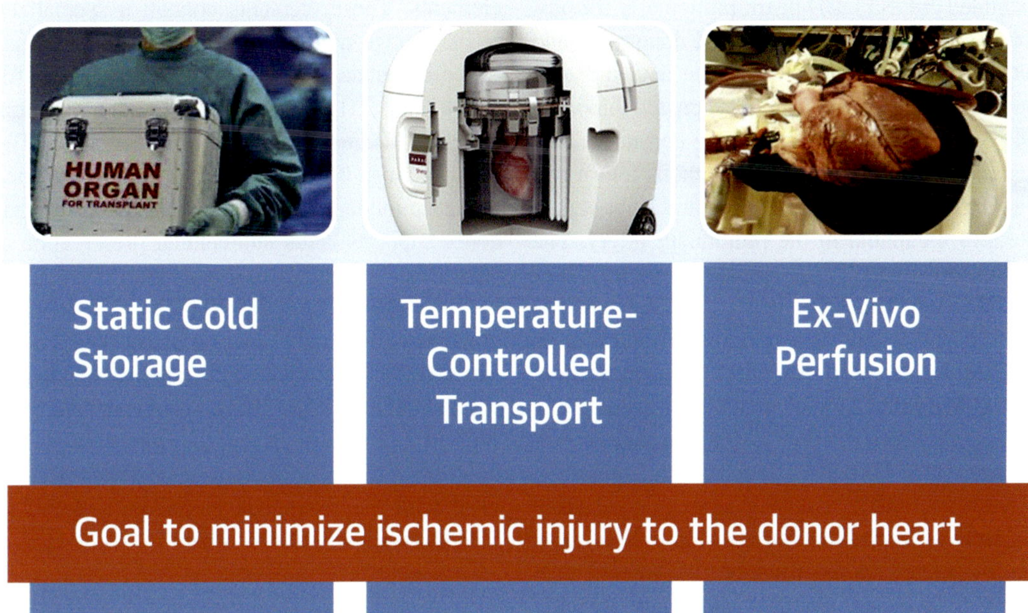


**Fig. 8.1** Advances in Donor Heart Preservation. Reprinted from Journal of the American College of Cardiology, 79(11), Ersilia M. DeFilippis, Kiran K. Khush, Maryjane A. Farr, Amy Fiedler, Arman Kilic, Michael M. Givertz, Evolving Characteristics of Heart Transplantation Donors and Recipients JACC Focus Seminar, 1108–1123., Copyright (2022), with permission from Elsevier

The DCD heart typically re-animates within one minute of NRP, which is then continued for around 40 min, with the aim of correcting the metabolic imbalance that has accumulated in the agonal and circulatory arrest periods. During this time, the lungs can be re-intubated and recruited, and a bronchoscopy can be performed. The abdominal surgical preparation can continue, and the external iliac arteries can be ligated to augment visceral perfusion. The NRP can then be weaned off, allowing the heart to support the thoraco-abdominal regional perfusion. Functional assessment of the heart can be carried out by visualization and basic hemodynamics, or more advanced measures applied like Swan-Ganz catheterization and/or transesophageal echocardiography. The donor has now become similar to a DBD donor, and further procurement proceeds as it would in that situation, including cardiac preservation with cold crystalloid cardioplegia and transportation in cold static storage [10].

## Donor Heart Preservation

Standard preservation is cold static storage, which involves placing the heart in a cold crystalloid solution surrounded by ice, which has generally been considered safe for 4 h of total ischemic time. Nevertheless, primary graft dysfunction may still occur even within this limit, especially if there are other adverse features of the donor organ. This has led to an increasing use of alternative approaches to preservation (Fig. 8.1). These include normothermic machine perfusion, controlled temperature static storage, and hypothermic machine perfusion.

## Normothermic Machine Perfusion

The TransMedics Organ Care System for Heart delivers normothermic blood perfusion to the ex-situ heart. It is essential to the strategy of DP/MP as described above [9] but is also useful in extended criteria DBD heart, particularly for prolonged ischemic times, increased donor age, and reduced ejection fraction [6]. The device uses a pulsatile pump to deliver oxygenated blood at 34 °C into the aorta and down the coronary arteries, recirculating the coronary venous return and passing through the right atrium and right ventricle into a cannula in the pulmonary artery. The left atrium is open and vented, so the left heart is unloaded. The heart beats typically in sinus rhythm, but it can also be paced. Adenosine is infused to prevent coronary vasoconstriction, and epinephrine is used to control aortic pressure. A wireless monitor displays real-time aortic pressure, coronary flow rate, temperature, oxygen saturation, and hematocrit. Visualization of wall motion is possible, although it must be interpreted in the light of the left side not being loaded and the right side only partially so. Trends in the aortic pressure (65–90 mmHg) required to achieve a given coronary blood flow (650–850 ml/min), as well as the venous versus arterial blood lactate levels, provide some functional assessment as surrogates for microvascular function and cardiac metabolism. Preservation times of 4–8 h are common. Once the recipient is ready for the implant, the heart can be cooled and re-arrested with cold crystalloid cardioplegia prior to separation from the device.

The key studies that underpin the use of the OCS Heart are the EXPAND trial and its continued access protocol, which showed that a high proportion (87%) of extended criteria hearts could be used with an acceptable safety profile, with comparable outcomes to general HTx [5]; and the US DCD Heart study which showed early outcomes for DCD HTx with a DP/MP strategy to be comparable to those of general DBD HTx [9].

## Controlled Temperature Static Storage

The Paragonix SherpaPak is designed to keep the donor heart at 4–8 °C. The donor's heart is suspended by the aorta in a cold preservation solution container, which is placed in a sterile canister around temperature-controlled packaging elements. These elements contain a specialized phase-change material that can absorb or release heat and sustain the desired temperature range for many hours. The transport device also monitors and logs the temperature in the container. The main premise of the technology is the avoidance of freeze-induced injury, although increasing evidence supports better sub-cellular preservation at temperatures higher than 0 °C [11].

The GUARDIAN-Heart registry is a manufacturer-supported international multicenter database that allows for propensity-matched cohort comparisons. These types of analyses support a reduction in severe primary graft dysfunction and an improvement in one-year survival with the SherpaPak compared to standard cold storage, particularly where ischemic time is increased [12].

## Hypothermic Machine Perfusion

The XVIVO hypothermic perfusion apparatus consists of a reservoir from which a blood-based perfusate is pumped with a roller pump through an oxygenator, leucocyte filter, and heater-cooler unit into the aorta of the donor heart. The perfusate is at eight °C and has a hematocrit of 15%. The aortic pressure is controlled at 20 mmHg, producing a coronary flow rate of 150–250 ml/min. The device has been used in several clinical studies in DBD transplants [7], in a small number of clinically directly procured DCD transplants, and in the first clinical xenotransplants.

## References

1. Greer DM, Kirschen MP, Lewis A, Gronseth GS, Rae-Grant A, Ashwal S, et al. Pediatric and adult brain death/death by neurologic criteria consensus guideline: report of the AAN guidelines subcommittee, AAP, CNS, and SCCM. Neurology. 2023;101(24):1112–32.
2. Shemie SD, Wilson LC, Hornby L, Basmaji J, Baker AJ, Bensimon CM, et al. A brain-based definition of death and criteria for its determination after arrest of circulation or neurologic function in Canada: a 2023 clinical practice guideline. Can J Anesthesia/Journal canadien d'anesthésie. 2023;70(4):483–557.

3. Statement on Controlled Organ Donation After Circulatory Death [Internet]. https://www.asahq.org/standards-and-practice-parameters/statement-on-controlled-organ-donation-after-circulatory-death. Accessed 13 Oct 2024
4. Copeland H, Knezevic I, Baran DA, Rao V, Pham M, Gustafsson F, et al. Donor heart selection: evidence-based guidelines for providers. J Heart Lung Transplant. 2023;42(1):7–29.
5. Kransdorf EP, Kittleson MM, Benck LR, Patel JK, Chung JS, Esmailian F, et al. Predicted heart mass is the optimal metric for size match in heart transplantation. J Heart Lung Transplant. 2019;38(2):156–65.
6. Schroder JN, Patel CB, DeVore AD, Casalinova S, Koomalsingh KJ, Shah AS, et al. Increasing utilization of extended criteria donor hearts for transplantation: the OCS Heart EXPAND trial. Heart Fail. 2024;12(3):438–47.
7. Rega F, Lebreton G, Para M, Michel S, Schramm R, Begot E, et al. Hypothermic oxygenated perfusion of the donor heart in heart transplantation: the short-term outcome from a randomised, controlled, open-label, multicentre clinical trial. The Lancet. 2024;404(10453):670–82.
8. Copeland H, Hayanga JWA, Neyrinck A, MacDonald P, Dellgren G, Bertolotti A, et al. Donor heart and lung procurement: a consensus statement. J Heart Lung Transplant. 2020;39(6):501–17.
9. Schroder JN, Patel CB, Devore AD, Bryner BS, Casalinova S, Shah A, et al. Transplantation outcomes with donor hearts after circulatory death. N Engl J Med. 2023;388(23):2121–31.
10. Hoffman JRH, Hartwig MG, Cain MT, Rove JY, Siddique A, Urban M, et al. Consensus statement: technical standards for thoracoabdominal normothermic regional perfusion. Ann Thorac Surg. 2024.
11. Radakovic D, Karimli S, Penov K, Schade I, Hamouda K, Bening C, et al. First clinical experience with the novel cold storage SherpaPak™ system for donor heart transportation. J Thorac Dis. 2020;12(12):7227.
12. D'Alessandro D, Schroder J, Meyer DM, Vidic A, Shudo Y, Silvestry S, et al. Impact of controlled hypothermic preservation on outcomes following heart transplantation. J Heart Lung Transplant. 2024;43(7):1153–61.

# Surgical Considerations in Heart Transplantation

9

Fardad Esmailian and Andrew Lin

**Abstract**

Heart transplantation (HTx) represents one of the seminal accomplishments of cardiac surgery. This chapter reviews the evolution of surgical techniques for donor heart recovery and HTx. We also shed light on surgical strategies to optimize outcomes of complex cases.

**Keywords**

Heart transplantation · Donor · Procurement · Brain death · Donor selection · Organ preservation · Bicaval · Biatrial · Cardiothoracic surgery

## Clinical Pearls

- Various surgical techniques for organ procurement exist, but key universal principles include occluding or venting systemic and pulmonary venous return, ensuring excellent delivery of cardioplegia with rapid and effective arrest, prevention of ventricular distention, and avoiding injury to any structure that is utilized in donor implant.
- The bicaval technique is the most common operative technique for heart transplant in the modern era, but the biatrial technique is useful where dissection of the vena cavae is hazardous.
- Transplant candidates with existing mechanical circulatory support devices or previous sternotomies usually have significant mediastinal adhesions; in these situations, the operating team should be given sufficient time to prepare the recipient to minimize ischemic time.
- Any patient being considered for heart transplantation via redo sternotomy should have a preoperative computed tomography scan of the chest performed as part of the preoperative workup in order to better evaluate the intrathoracic anatomy

## Introduction

Heart transplantation (HTx) represents one of the seminal accomplishments in the field of cardiac surgery. The first successful human heart implant was performed on December 3, 1967, by Dr. Christiaan Barnard in Cape Town, South Africa. Several weeks later, Dr. Norman E.

F. Esmailian (✉)
Cedars-Sinai Smidt Heart Institute, Los Angeles, CA, USA
e-mail: fardad.esmailian@cshs.org

A. Lin
Aurora St. Luke's Medical Center, Milwaukee, WI, USA



J. Kobashigawa (ed.), *Clinical Guide to Heart Transplantation*, https://doi.org/10.1007/978-3-031-88290-6_9

Shumway of Stanford University performed the first adult HTx in the United States [1]. Since the era of these early pioneers, nearly all elements of the procedure have undergone significant modification and refinement. In 1983, the use of cyclosporine and subsequent improvement in the medical management of organ rejection allowed HTx outcomes to improve as well as the therapy to be widespread [2]. Currently, over 4000 transplants are performed in the United States annually. While organ procurement and preservation are discussed in Chap. 8, we review surgical techniques for donor heart recovery and HTx in this chapter.

## Surgical Technique of Donor Heart Recovery

The donor is transported to the operating room from the Intensive Care Unit with a secure airway and continuous monitoring. They are supine with tucked arms and a slight pad under the scapulae. Skin is cleansed, and sterile draping is undertaken. A sternotomy is performed, taking care to avoid injury to the underlying heart and lungs. The pericardium is divided and retracted. The heart may then be assessed for donor suitability, with special attention given to the size of the organ, ventricular function, and evidence of gross abnormalities such as trauma or coronary artery disease. Various surgical techniques for organ procurement exist, but key universal principles include (i) occluding or venting systemic and pulmonary venous return, (ii) ensuring excellent delivery of cardioplegia with rapid and effective arrest, (iii) prevention of ventricular distention, and (iv) avoiding injury to any structure that is utilized in donor implant. It is also important to be conscientious of the needs of the other organs undergoing procurement, such as the length of the Inferior Vena Cava (IVC) for the liver and lengths of the atrial cuff and pulmonary arteries (PA) for the lungs.

A typical operative sequence for procurement in a brain-dead donor may proceed as follows:

(i) Mobilize the ascending aorta and encircling with an umbilical tape to allow separation from the underlying right pulmonary artery
(ii) Mobilize the superior vena cava (SVC) and place a snare around it superior to the azygos vein; dissect the azygos and ligate with free tie
(iii) In conjunction with other organ procurement teams, administer heparin and place antegrade cardioplegia/pressure monitoring catheter in the ascending aorta and connect arterial pressure monitoring line
(iv) When all teams ready, the SVC can be snared with a Rummel tourniquet to limit upper body venous return
(v) Pulmonary venous return is drained by venting of the left atrium by rapidly transecting the pulmonary vein (our preference is the right superior or left inferior when no lung team is present); in the presence of a lung team, the left atrial appendage or incision of the left atrium between the orifice of the right pulmonary veins and Sondegaard's groove
(vi) Incise the anterior IVC just above the diaphragm
(vii) With the heart empty, cross-clamp aorta and begin antegrade cardioplegia with a goal aortic root pressure tracing of 60–80 mmHg (we believe it is important to measure the aortic root pressure to ensure adequate delivery of cardioplegia since finger palpation will not be accurate; one must be extremely cautious in accepting the organ if the preservation solution cannot be delivered with adequate aortic root pressure); place ice slush around heart and complete the cardioplegia infusion ( approximately 15 cc/kg) while checking for left ventricular distention

(viii) Divide IVC at junction with right atrium; divide left and right pulmonary veins or left atrium if lungs are being procured; divide ascending aorta distally, divide pulmonary arteries, divide SVC distal to the azygos vein; we recommend taking an extended length of SVC for complex redo cases

(ix) Inspect the heart on the back table for any abnormality (e.g., patent foramen ovale, valvular pathology), (xv) place the heart in cold preservation.

In cases of procuring the heart and lungs, care must be taken to avoid delivery of the pulmonary preservation solution into the coronary circulation. This can be achieved by dividing the ascending aorta as soon as cardioplegia delivery is completed and ensuring a very large incision in the left atrial appendage and/or opening the interatrial groove to aspirate the return from the pulmonary veins.

## Biatrial Orthotopic Cardiac Transplantation

### Indications

The biatrial method represents the original operative technique for HTx and was widely utilized in the 1980's. This operation has essentially been replaced by the bicaval method, but it remains useful in certain surgical circumstances. A review of the UNOS database by Davies et al. revealed that the biatrial technique was associated with increased need for permanent pacemaker (OR 2.6, CI 2.2–3.1) and that the bicaval technique was associated with improved 30-day survival (OR 0.83, CI 0.75–0.93) [3]. The major advantage of the biatrial technique in the modern era is for circumstances in which dissecting out the SVC and IVC represent severe hazards, such as in redo operations with dense adhesions.

### Technique

The recipient is brought to the operating room, and appropriate monitoring lines are inserted, including arterial line and central venous line. Once the donor's heart is confirmed to be appropriate for procurement, the implanting team can begin preparing for the implant operation. The sternal incision is made 60–90 min prior to the anticipated time of organ arrival, and preferably earlier in the setting of redo sternotomy. The ascending aorta is typically cannulated just proximal to the aortic arch, but the axillary or femoral arteries may prove useful in special circumstances such as a heavily calcified ascending aorta or a difficult preoperative mediastinum. The SVC and IVC are then snared and cannulated distally to allow room for anastomoses. A left ventricular vent may be placed at the discretion of the implanting surgeon to avoid rewarming of the heart by the blood returning from the pulmonary veins from collateral flow during the implantation. Once the donor's heart is confirmed to have arrived safely, cardiopulmonary bypass is initiated, and the aorta is cross-clamped. The native heart is then excised, taking care to leave an appropriate cuff of tissue along the aorta, PA, right atrium, and left atrium. Any defibrillator leads are excised as proximal as possible at this time without a forceful pull to avoid tearing the SVC or innominate vein. The donor's heart is inspected on the back table and assessed for any potential valvular abnormalities, a patent foramen ovale requiring closure, or structural injury requiring repair. Once the back-table preparation is complete, the organ is removed from the ice bath and brought into the surgical field. The left atrial anastomosis is performed first. This suture line must be performed with meticulous attention to hemostasis, as accessibility is difficult upon completion of the implantation. The donor's right atrium is then opened from the right atrial appendage to the IVC, taking care not to injure the sinoatrial node. The donor SVC is oversewn. The donor's right atrial cuff is anastomosed to the recipient's right atrium, starting directly over the left atrial suture line and continuing circumferentially along the atrial free wall. Next, one-half of the PA anastomosis is performed, followed by the aortic anastomosis. Several minutes prior to the release of the cross clamp, systemic glucocorticoids (e.g., solumedrol) are administered. An aortic root vent is placed, and the aortic cross-clamp is then removed by venting the aortic root to prevent the introduction of air into the coronary circulation. After reperfusion of the donor graft, the remaining half of the PA anastomosis is completed if not previously performed in its entirety. The patient is then weaned off cardiopulmonary bypass after initiation of the inotropic support and de-airing of the left ventricle. Protamine is administrated, and decannulation is performed in the standard fashion. A partial left pericardectomy can be performed to decrease the chance of significant pericardial effusion in the postoperative period, especially in cases where there is a very large pericardial space in comparison to the size of the donor organ. The defibrillator generator and the remnant of the pacing leads, if present, are then removed with the chest still open. Chest tubes and pacing wires are placed. Hemostasis is optimized, and the wound is closed. An illustrative comparison between the biatrial and bicaval techniques is demonstrated in Fig. 9.1 [4].

## Bicaval Technique

### Operative Technique

Preparation of the recipient mediastinum is largely similar to the biatrial technique, with the major alteration being the isolation of the SVC and IVC. The SVC is divided at the cavoatrial junction, and the free wall of the right atrium is trimmed to allow for a sewing cuff just above the true IVC. The left atrial anastomosis is performed first, followed by the IVC and PA anastomoses. The posterior portions of the IVC and PA anastomoses can be performed prior to reperfusion to reduce warm ischemic time. The aortic anastomosis is completed, and the cross-clamp is released. The remaining PA anastomosis is completed. The donor SVC is then opened into the azygos vein to allow a large anastomosis and prevent postoperative stenosis. Care must be taken to keep the orientation of the SVC and avoid any kinking. The anterior anastomosis of the IVC is then completed. Weaning from cardiopulmonary bypass is initiated, and the operation is completed, as discussed previously.

## Heterotopic Heart Transplantation

### Indications

Heterotopic HTx is not widely utilized and is useful only for select circumstances. Accepted indications include (1) irreversible high pulmonary vascular resistance (PVR) in the recipient and (2) severe donor-recipient size mismatch. A potential third indication in the future may include xenotransplant bridging, as immunomodulation advances may eventually make this a feasible option. As the donor graft serves to augment the native heart, it functions as a de facto bi-ventricular assist device. One advantage of the heterotopic technique is preservation of the native heart as a safety margin in case of graft dysfunction. Recognized complications include a high incidence of ventricular dysrhythmias, anatomic compression by the graft (e.g., right lung), and a high incidence of premature structural deterioration of the donor organ [5–7].

### Operative Technique

Cardiopulmonary bypass is established, and the right pleura is incised. An opening is made on the donor's left atrium just below the interatrial groove, and this is anastomosed to a cuff of the recipient's right pulmonary vein. A longitudinal incision is then made on the recipient's right atrium and extended to the SVC. The donor right atrium and SVC are similarly incised, and a running anastomosis is performed. The donor

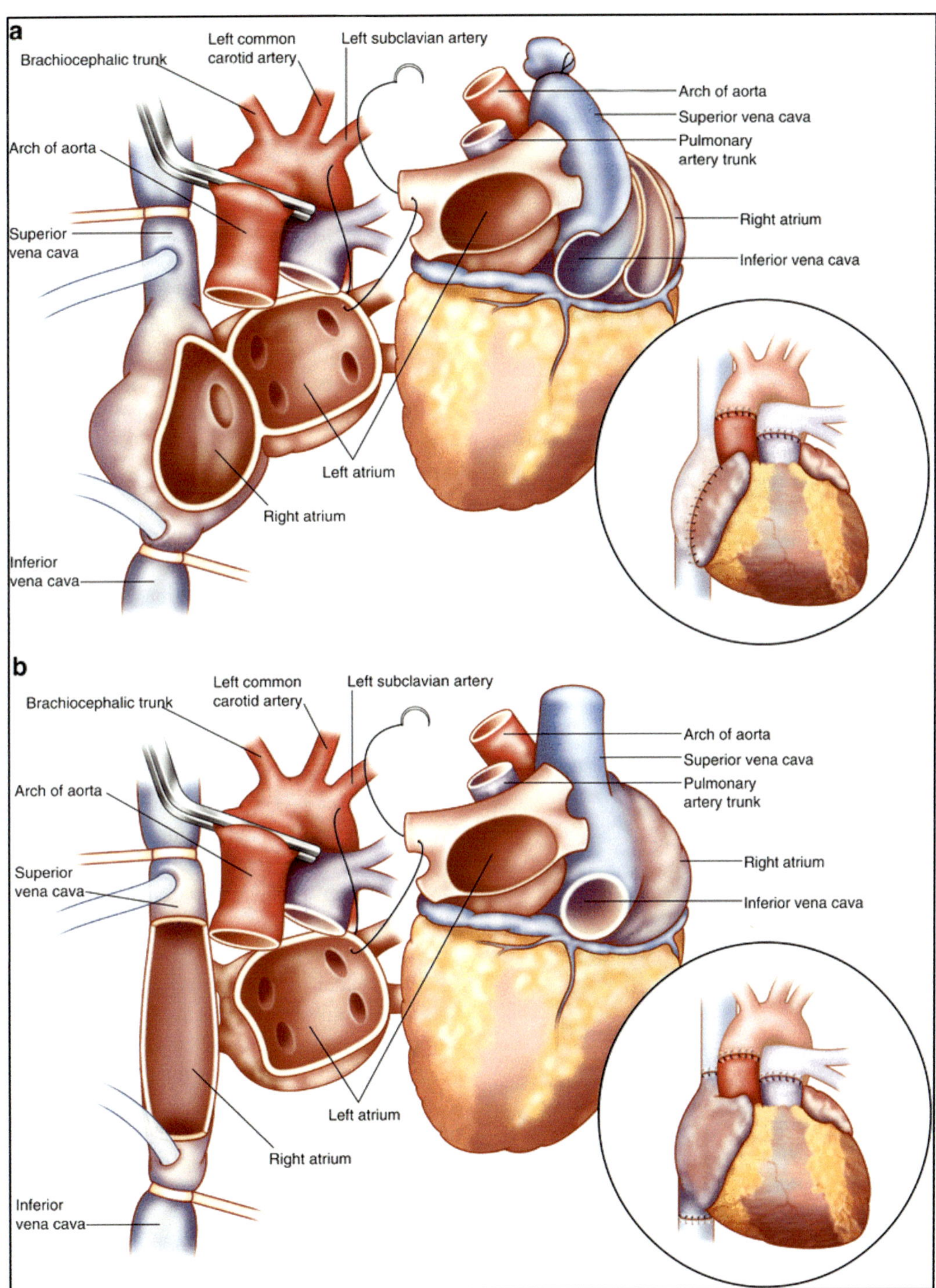


**Fig. 9.1** Different techniques of implantation. **a** The heart implantation was performed using a biatrial approach. The inset shows the completed implantation. **b** The heart implantation is performed using a bicameral approach. Reused with permission from Arie Blitz, Surgical Techniques of Heart Transplantation and Heart–Lung Transplantation, Anesthesia and Perioperative Care for Organ Transplantation, 137–161, 2016, Springer Nature. https://doi.org/https://doi.org/10.1007/978-1-4939-6377-5_12

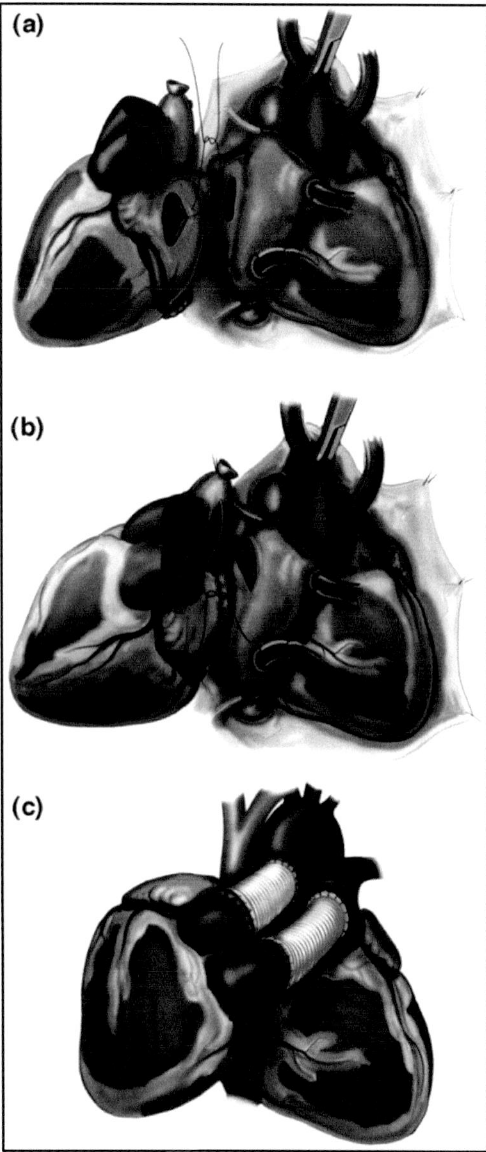


**Fig. 9.2** Heterotopic heart transplantation. Reused with permission from Kadner, Alexander; Chen, Raymond H, Heterotopic heart transplantation: experimental development and clinical experience, European Journal of Cardio-Thoracic Surgery, 2000, 17(4), 474–481, by permission of Oxford University Press, European Association for Cardio-Thoracic Surgery

pulmonary artery and aorta are then anastomosed to their respective structures on the recipient in an end-to-side fashion; these connections often require prosthetic graft augmentation to provide adequate length [6]. An illustration of the technique is provided in Fig. 9.2.

## Special Considerations

It is quite common for HTx recipients to require redo sternotomy, as many heart failure patients have previously undergone operations such as coronary artery bypass, valve replacement, correction of congenital abnormality, mechanical circulatory support device implantation, or prior HTx. Previous thoracic operations can significantly elevate the complexity and hazard of the surgical dissection and may result in increased use of blood products and operative time. Any patient being considered for HTx via redo sternotomy should have a preoperative CT scan of the chest performed as part of the preoperative workup in order to better evaluate the intrathoracic anatomy (e.g., course of the inominate vein and proximity of the aorta and/or right ventricle to the sternum). At the time of implant surgery, the operative team must have a clearly defined strategy that should include strong consideration of alternative cannulation options, such as femoral or axillary artery cannulation. The IVC may be cannulated percutaneously via the femoral vein using a guide wire and serial dilators. Utilizing peripheral vascular access can allow for initiation of cardiopulmonary bypass prior to sternotomy. Both short-term and durable mechanical circulatory support devices have been commonly utilized for bridge-to-transplantation. Centrally implanted devices, such as left ventricular assist devices or total artificial heart, in particular, are associated with a high degree of mediastinal adhesions and increased risk and difficulty at the time of redo sternotomy. In these instances, the operating team must be given sufficient time to prepare the recipient for implant prior to the arrival of the donor organ to minimize ischemic time injury. When prolonged donor organ ischemic time is encountered, the operative sequence may be altered by performing the aortic anastomosis immediately after the left atrial. This allows for early removal of the aortic cross-clamp and organ perfusion. The remaining anastomoses may then be performed with the donor's heart beating. When implanting durable mechanical circulatory support devices in potential transplant recipients, it is often referred to 'protect' the mediastinum with adhesion-resistant prostheses (e.g., polytetrafluoroethylene membrane) to facilitate safe and efficient re-entry at the time of transplantation [8].

## References


1. Silbergleit A, Norman E. Shumway and the early heart transplants. Tex Heart Inst J. 2006;33(2):274.
2. Dandel M, Lehmkuhl HB, Knosalla C, Hetzer R. Impact of different long-term maintenance immunosuppressive therapy strategies on patients' outcome after heart transplantation. Transpl Immunol. 2010;23(3):93–103.
3. Davies RR, Russo MJ, Morgan JA, Sorabella RA, Naka Y, Chen JM. Standard versus bicaval techniques for orthotopic heart transplantation: an analysis of the United Network for Organ Sharing database. J Thorac Cardiovasc Surg. 2010;140(3):700–8.
4. Blitz A. Surgical techniques of heart transplantation and heart–lung transplantation. In: Anesthesia and perioperative care for organ transplantation; 2017. p. 137–61.
5. Akasaka T, Lythall D, Cheng A, Yoshida K, Yoshikawa J, Mitchell A, et al. Continuous aortic regurgitation in severely dysfunctional native hearts after heterotopic cardiac transplantation. Am J Cardiol. 1989;63(20):1483–8.
6. Kadner A, Chen RH, Adams DH. Heterotopic heart transplantation: experimental development and clinical experience. Eur J Cardiothorac Surg. 2000;17(4):474–81.
7. Reichenspurner H, Hildebrandt A, Boehm D, Kaulbach HG, Willems S, Odell JA, et al. Heterotopic heart transplantation in 1988–recent selective indications and outcome. J Heart Transplant. 1989;8(5):381–6.
8. Ihnken KA, Ramzy D, Esmailian F, Trento A, Arabía FA. Surgical technique to facilitate explantation of mechanical circulatory support devices: LVADs, BiVADs, and TAHs before heart transplantation. ASAIO J. 2016;62(2):211–3.

# Part III
# Post-Heart Transplant Patient Management

# Physiology of the Transplanted Heart

# 10

Andriana P. Nikolova

**Abstract**

Surgical excision of the heart from the donor results in the immediate denervation of both the sympathetic and parasympathetic nervous fibers. This chapter will provide a comprehensive overview of the denervation and electrophysiology of the transplanted heart and the resulting changes in heart rate regulation and exercise capacity. The chapter also covers the reinnervation process and explores differences in the response to medications in the transplanted heart.

**Keywords**

Denervated heart · Physiology · Exercise · Autonomic nervous system · Sympathetic nervous system · Parasympathetic nervous system · Drugs and the denervated heart · Reinnervation

A. P. Nikolova (✉)
Cedars-Sinai Smidt Heart Institute, Los Angeles, CA, USA
e-mail: andriana.nikolova@csmc.edu

## Clinical Pearls

- Surgical excision of the heart from the donor results in the immediate denervation of both the sympathetic and parasympathetic nervous fibers.
- The reliance on circulating catecholamines means that the denervated heart shows a much slower increase in heart rate and a lower peak heart rate in response to exercise.
- Heart transplant recipients have a much lower $VO_2$ max when compared with age-adjusted, non-transplant cardiac patients.
- Exercise regimens help improve the exercise capacity of heart transplant recipients by improving peripheral factors and improving the chronotropic response.
- The loss of sensory fibers from the transplanted heart means that ischemia is often silent.
- Atropine and digoxin do not have any effect on the denervated heart and should not be used to treat arrhythmias in heart transplant patients.

## Introduction

The normal heart is innervated by sympathetic and parasympathetic fibers of the autonomic nervous system (ANS). The ANS exerts chronotropic and inotropic control over the heart and



J. Kobashigawa (ed.), *Clinical Guide to Heart Transplantation*, https://doi.org/10.1007/978-3-031-88290-6_10

supplies visceral sensory fibers to the pericardium. Heart transplantation (HTx) results in the denervation of the donor's heart by surgical dissection of postganglionic neurons. Within days, cardiac stores of norepinephrine become depleted, and autonomic influence over the heart is lost.

The lack of parasympathetic tone means that HTx recipients have a higher average resting heart rate (HR) of 95 beats per minute (bpm) compared with 66 bpm for non-transplant cardiac patients [1]. Despite significant improvements in exercise tolerance compared with the end stages of heart failure (HF), patients still show a reduction in maximum achievable exertion when compared with normal individuals of the same age [2]. This is accounted for by the chronotropic incompetence of the denervated heart as well as peripheral factors that will be discussed later. The normal heart will show a rapid acceleration in HR in response to exercise that peaks during exercise and rapidly recover. The transplanted heart shows a delayed chronotropic response to exercise due to a reliance on circulating catecholamines. Norepinephrine and epinephrine levels are either normal or elevated in the transplant recipient [3]. The lack of nervous supply and reliance on humoral mechanisms causes a shift from predominately type-1 to type-2 beta-adrenergic receptors on cardiac myocytes [4].

## The Autonomic Nervous System

### Functional Anatomy

Cardiovascular regulation by the autonomic nervous system has its origins in the medulla oblongata. The medulla contains two regions, the cardioaccelerator and cardioinhibitory centers, that regulate the HR. The heart is able to contract independently of extrinsic innervation due to the specialized pacemaker cells found in the sinus node. Sympathetic innervation to the heart is from the cervical ganglia and T1-T4 of the thoracic ganglia of the sympathetic chain. Parasympathetic innervation comes from branches of the vagus nerve [5]. At the base of the heart, autonomic nerves form the cardiac plexus. This plexus contains the postganglionic sympathetic fibers and the preganglionic parasympathetic fibers. The cardiac plexus is found within the adventitia of the great vessels, the aortic arch, anterior to the right pulmonary artery, and anterior to the bifurcation of the trachea.

Visceral sensory fibers arise from the phrenic and vagus nerves. The phrenic nerve innervates the fibrous pericardium and the parietal layer of the serous pericardium. The vagus nerve innervates the visceral layer of the serous pericardium.

### Parasympathetic Fibers

The vagus nerve (cranial nerve X) contains both motor and sensory fibers. The preganglionic fibers of the parasympathetic nervous system supplying the heart are found within 3 nuclei (the nucleus ambiguus, the dorsal nucleus, and the solitary nucleus). The right and left vagus nerves are contained within the carotid sheath, lateral to the carotid artery. The nerve travels through the lower brain stem and leaves the skull at its base. It follows the path of the carotid in the neck, penetrates the chest, and supplies the heart and lungs. The vagus nerve then branches to supply the sinus node and the atrioventricular (AV) node, as well as the atria and ventricles directly [5]. As with the majority of the parasympathetic nervous system, the presynaptic neurons synapse at ganglia within the target organ, leaving short postsynaptic neurons to supply the organ itself.

Most parasympathetic innervation to the heart is directed at the sinus and AV nodes. Normally, the right vagus supplies the sinus node, and the left supplies the AV node. However, a normal anatomical variant exists where fibers from the right and left vagus cross over.

## Sympathetic Fibers

The preganglionic sympathetic nervous supply to the heart arises in the lateral column of the spinal cord. The cervical ganglia and first four thoracic ganglia of the sympathetic chain supply the postganglionic fibers [5]. Sympathetic stimulation results in an increase in HR, contractility, and faster conduction (positive dromotropy).

## Cardiac Pacemaker

The cells of the sinus node have no resting membrane potential but instead have what is known as a pacemaker potential [6]. Other cells maintain a resting potential as a result of potassium ions continuously flowing out of the cell through potassium channels. Pacemaker cells differ by having a membrane that decreases its permeability for potassium ions over time. Additionally, there is a slow influx of sodium ions through specialized channels, forming what is known as the "funny" current [6]. These two currents cause the membrane potential to slowly increase until reaching a threshold potential of −40 mV when an action potential is initiated (see Fig. 10.1 for a comparison between the ordinary action potential and the pacemaker potential). Even without nervous stimulation, the sinus node will depolarize at a rate of 100 per minute.

## Autonomic Physiology

At rest, the heart receives autonomic tone from both the sympathetic and parasympathetic nervous systems. However, the vagal tone predominates in suppressing the resting HR. The preganglionic neurons of both the sympathetic and parasympathetic nervous systems release acetylcholine that binds to nicotinic receptors on the cell bodies of the postganglionic neurons. Postganglionic sympathetic fibers synapsing at the heart release norepinephrine, which binds to type-1 beta-adrenergic receptors. Postganglionic parasympathetic fibers of the vagus nerve release acetylcholine to stimulate type-2 muscarinic receptors ($M_2$) on the heart. Both receptors are G-protein coupled receptors. The type-1 beta receptor is a stimulatory G-protein-linked receptor, and the type-2 muscarinic receptor is inhibitory. G-protein dissociates upon ligand binding and either stimulates or inhibits adenylyl cyclase. This results in either increased or decreased cAMP production, respectively. Increasing cAMP leads to an increase in HR and contractility and vice-versa [7]. Additionally, acetylcholine release from the parasympathetic fibers bind to ligand-gated potassium channels to decrease the rate of depolarization and slow the HR.

Both muscarinic and beta-adrenergic receptors are found on the sinus node, AV node, and atria; however, only beta receptors are present on the ventricles. Thus, the parasympathetic nervous system has no influence on ventricular contractility.

## Homeostasis of the Cardiovascular System

Homeostasis of the cardiovascular system is controlled primarily by the baroreceptor and chemoreceptor pathways. Changes in arterial pressure, $O_2$ concentration, and, to a lesser extent, $CO_2$ concentration are detected and result in appropriate autonomic responses to sustain the blood pressure in the short term [8].

### Baroreceptor Reflex

A decrease in arterial pressure is detected by baroreceptors in the carotid sinus and aortic arch. They are stretch receptors that inhibit sympathetic stimulation to the heart. Signals are sent via afferent fibers of the vagus and glossopharyngeal nerves to the solitary nucleus in the medulla. When blood pressure falls, the baroreceptors detect a decrease in wall tension. The receptors, in turn, decrease their rate of

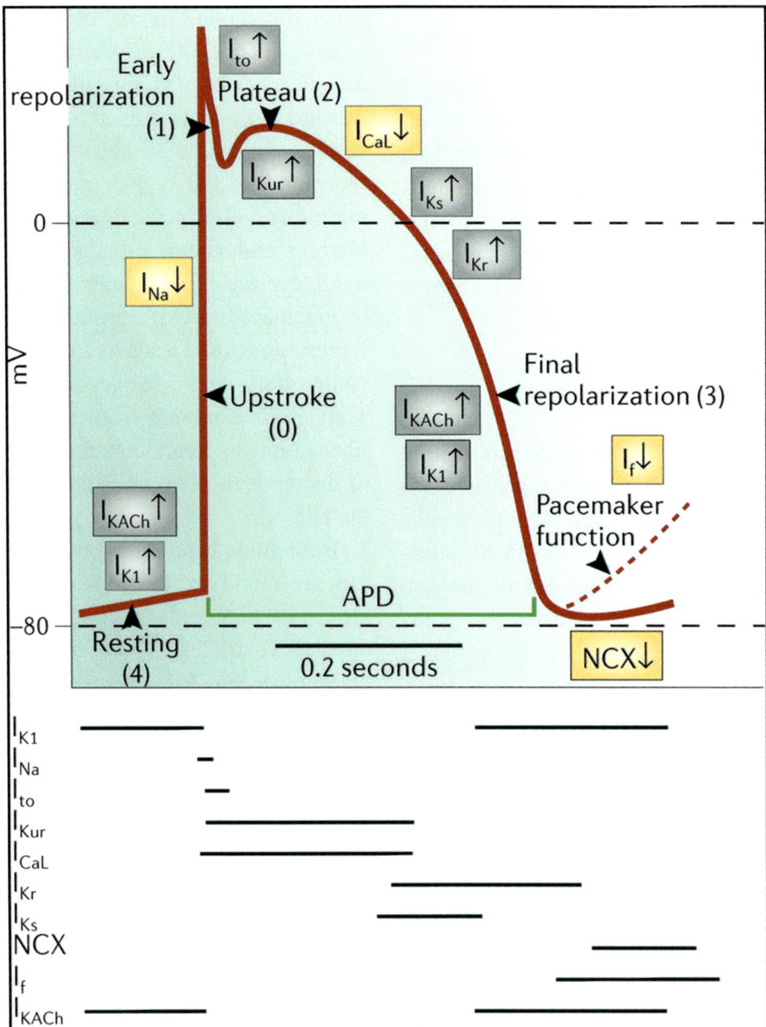


**Fig. 10.1** Membrane currents that generate the normal action potential. Resting (4), upstroke (0), early repolarization (1), plateau (2), and final repolarization are the 5 phases of the action potential. A decline of potential at the end of phase 3 in pacemaker cells, such as the sinus node, is shown as a broken line. The inward currents, INa, ICa, and If, are shown in yellow boxes; the sodium-calcium exchanger (NCX) is also shown in yellow. It is electrogenic and may generate inward or outward current. IKAch, IK1, Ito, IKur, IKr, and IKs are shown in gray boxes. The action potential duration (APD) is approximately 200 ms. Reused with permission from Augustus O. Grant, Cardiac Ion Channels, Circulation: Arrhythmia and Electrophysiology, 2(2), 185–194 and https://doi.org/10.1161/CIRCEP.108.789081; American Heart Association

firing, which disinhibits the sympathetic nervous system and results in an increase in total vascular resistance HR and contractility [8]. Similar to the baroreceptor reflex is the atrial reflex (also known as the Bainbridge reflex), which is when stretch receptors of the atria detect changes in venous return to the heart. An increase in venous return causes an increase in HR through the efferent limb of the reflex to the sinus node. The opposite is also true.

## Chemoreceptor Reflex

Chemoreceptors located in the carotid and aortic bodies respond primarily to changes in the partial pressure of oxygen but also monitor the partial pressure of carbon dioxide and pH. Hypoxia, hypercapnia, or acidosis will increase the firing rate of chemoreceptors and result in an increase in both the rate and depth of respiration. The sympathetic tone of the heart is then increased through both direct and indirect mechanisms [8]. Chemoreceptors have a direct effect on medullary vasomotor neurons supplying the heart. Indirectly, by increasing the depth of breathing, stretch receptors in the lung result in increased sympathetic stimulation to the heart [8].

## Exercise and the Denervated Heart

Exercise tolerance post-transplantation is greatly improved compared with end-stage HF but peak oxygen uptake ($VO_2$ max) in recipients is reported at only 50–70% of age-adjusted expected values [2]. A lower $VO_2$ max correlates strongly with morbidity and mortality [9]. One of the goals in the long-term management of the HTx patient, therefore, is to optimize exercise capacity. This lower observed exercise capacity is not only the result of the denervated heart but also due to peripheral factors. Examples include impairments to vasodilation and a decline in skeletal muscle function. These changes occur during HF pre-transplantation and are reversible through exercise, although not entirely [10]. At levels of exercise below the maximum, appropriate cardiac outputs are observed in the HTx recipient [9]. Ejection fraction and systolic function are normal during exercise. There is diastolic dysfunction that must be compensated for with higher filling pressures. Pulmonary artery wedge pressures of twice the resting value have been demonstrated during maximal exercise in HTx patients [11].

## Allograft Response to Exercise

Dynamic exercise requires an increase in CO to meet the increased metabolic demands of skeletal muscle and maintain aerobic respiration. The two components of CO are HR and stroke volume (SV). The normal heart responds to exercise predominantly by increasing its HR in response to the neural and hormonal effects on the sinus and AV nodes. A decrease in vagal tone allows the HR to rise to the intrinsic rate of depolarization of the sinus node. A further increase in HR occurs due to sympathetic stimulation. This is augmented by circulating catecholamines. HR promptly drops after the cessation of exercise. During strenuous exercise, SV will also increase in the normal heart. Skeletal muscle vasodilation causes a decrease in peripheral vascular resistance, an increase in venous return and therefore an increase in SV.

In contrast, the denervated heart does increase its HR in response to exercise but more slowly and achieves a lower maximum HR. The increase in HR is in response to circulating catecholamines rather than from the effects of the autonomic nervous system [12]. HR is slower to normalize and actually peaks after exercise stops. The transplanted heart is said to be "preload dependent" since SV relies on venous return [13]. During mild exercise, left ventricular end-diastolic volume and pressure increase. This increase in venous return will further stretch the myocardial fibers, leading to greater contractility (Frank-Starling's mechanism). Over time, the donor heart becomes increasingly sensitive to catecholamines [12].

In the normal patient isometric exercise causes muscles to produce metabolites such as lactate that stimulate the autonomic nervous system to increase the HR and constrict peripheral arterioles. The arterial blood pressure elevates, and CO increases slightly [14]. The transplant patient shows a similar response to isometric exercise with a slight increase in CO and increases in systolic and diastolic arterial pressures [15]. Mechanisms controlling changes to peripheral vascular resistance remain intact. The significant difference is the lack of HR acceleration seen in normal patients performing isometric exercise [16]. The transplanted heart is unable to reach the CO of the normal heart at rest and during exercise. Transplant patients cannot sustain exercise for as long as control individuals. Oxygen extraction is heightened and reflected in an increased arterio-venous (AV) oxygen gradient. Transplant recipients also undergo more anaerobic respiration when exercising, as demonstrated by an increase in lactate concentration [17].

## Peripheral Factors Affecting Exercise

HF patients, especially those who ultimately undergo HTx, spend prolonged periods of time in a state of deconditioning due to a decline in exercise capacity, decompensations, hospitalizations, and being in a bed-ridden state. The peripheral skeletal muscles decrease in mass and, on a microscopic level, show fewer mitochondria and a shift towards a predominance of fast-twitch fibers, an increase in glycolytic enzymes, and a decrease in oxidative enzymes and creatine kinase. As such, these muscles are preferentially glycolytic and produce more lactate [18]. Although the oxidative capacity of skeletal muscle normalizes after transplantation, the capillary beds do not regrow entirely. These persisting vascular abnormalities contribute to decreased exercise capacity post-transplantation [19].

Pulmonary function declines in severe HF. Although there is a marked improvement in pulmonary function tests after transplantation, the lung diffusion of carbon monoxide (DLCO) remains below the predicted value even when there is no underlying lung disease. This is because the pulmonary capillary wedge pressure is elevated in HF, leading to the capillary endothelium becoming irreversibly damaged; in HTx patients who have a DLCO of <50% of predicted, exercise results in respiratory acidosis and hypoxemia [20].

## Exercise Protocols for the Heart Transplant Recipient

The chronotropic incompetence seen in HTx patients improves after the first year post-transplantation, with resting HR decreasing, maximum HR increasing, and peak $VO_2$ increasing even without a prescribed regimen of exercise [21]. However, the benefits of exercise were demonstrated by Kobashigawa et al. in a randomized control trial [22] which has been affirmed by numerous studies since then. Increases in $VO_2$ max after exercise regimens ranged from 13 to 28 mL/kg/min [23–29]. Patients who are motivated and follow a supervised training program show a 50% improvement in $VO_2$ max compared with recipients who remain sedentary [19]. Previously, it was thought that the loss of chronotropy due to denervation meant that exercise regimens needed to be limited to moderate training protocols. It was also thought that central factors influenced exercise capacity more than others. Evidence now suggests that peripheral factors have a larger impact on the decreased exercise capacity post-transplantation [30]. It has also been demonstrated that chronotropy can normalize both early and late post-transplantation [31, 32].

## High-Intensity Interval Training

With an improved understanding of the physiology of the transplanted heart and the impact of peripheral factors on exercise tolerance in the heart transplant recipient, the effectiveness of high-intensity interval training (HIIT) has been demonstrated [27–29, 32, 33]. HIIT has long been a therapeutic tool in the long-term management of cardiovascular disease and HF. These patients have shown a marked improvement in exercise tolerance with an increase in $VO_2$ max of 46% and even a reversal of ventricular structural changes after 12 weeks [34].

HIIT requires the patient to engage in aerobic exercise until a $VO_2$ of 85–95% of max or an HR of 90%-95% of the predicted max is achieved (see Fig. 10.2 for a comparison

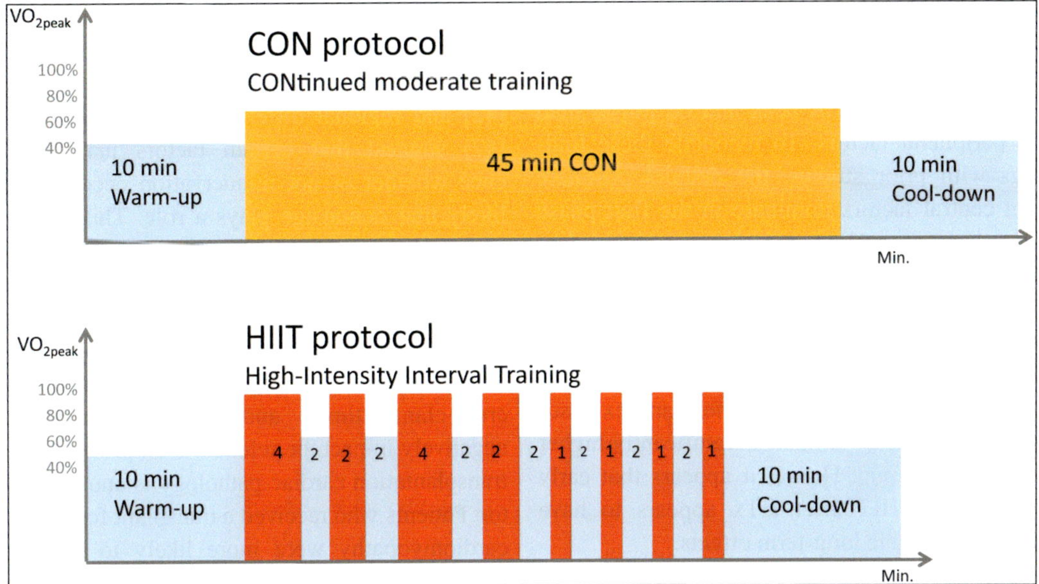


**Fig. 10.2** The HIIT training protocol (10-min warm-up, 16 min of HIIT training [>80% of $VO_2$peak] + 14 min of recovery and 10-min cool-down) and the CON training protocol (10-min warm-up, 45 min of CON training [~60–70% of $VO_2$peak] and 10-min cool-down). Reprinted from The Journal of Heart and Lung Transplantation, 34(8), Christian H. Dall, Finn Gustafsson, Stefan B. Christensen, Flemming Dela, Henning Langberg, Eva Prescott, Effect of moderate- versus high-intensity exercise on vascular function, biomarkers and quality of life in heart transplant recipients: A randomized, crossover trial, 1033–1041, Copyright (2015), with permission from Elsevier

between HIIT and continued moderate training). This is followed by a period of rest until HR falls to 60–70% of max. The cycle is then repeated four times [35]. The transplant patient must augment this regimen with both a cool-down and a warm-up period due to chronotropic incompetence and a reliance on circulating catecholamines to increase CO, as discussed earlier. Compliance is an issue when prescribing exercise protocols to patients, especially when psychological co-morbidities such as depression and anxiety exist.

With HIIT training, some patients are able to attain a $VO_2$ max of 80–89% of predicted [29]. Systolic systemic blood pressure falls by an average of 3 mmHg. Resting HR decreases slightly with HIIT, but no change is seen in patients on protocols of moderate exercise [32]. HR recovery time improves after both moderate exercise protocols and HIIT, with HIIT proving slightly more beneficial. This is important because HR recovery time strongly correlates with mortality [36]. Peripheral factors also show an improvement with skeletal muscle mass increasing and an increase in mitochondrial density [29].

HIIT improves $VO_2$ max more so than moderate training programs. This has been demonstrated in one of the largest multicenter clinical trials where 81 patients were randomized at a mean of 11 weeks post-heart transplant to 9 months of either HIIT or moderate-intensity continuous training [33]. At 1-year follow-up, the HIT group demonstrated greater improvements in the $VO_2$ peak (mean difference between groups, 1.8 mL·kg$^{-1}$·min$^{-1}$ corresponding to approximately 0.5 metabolic equivalents), the anaerobic threshold (0.28 L/min), the peak expiratory flow (11%), and the extensor muscle exercise capacity (464 J). In

sympathetic nervous system. HTx patients who undergo sympathetic reinnervation are able to experience during ischemic episodes. Those who remain denervated suffer silent ischemia [45].

Another role of the sympathetic nervous system is to regulate coronary blood flow. Even within the same patient, there are prominent differences in myocardial blood flow depending on the extent of reinnervation. Areas with sympathetic reinnervation had increased blood flow [46].

## Parasympathetic Reinnervation

The functional significance of parasympathetic reinnervation is unknown. The extent to which it occurs is contentious and not well defined due to difficulties in measuring parasympathetic activity in the heart. Early studies found that histological evidence of parasympathetic reinnervation only appeared 10 years after transplantation [58]. Physiological studies similarly only demonstrated parasympathetic tone after 8 years [59, 60]. These findings may be the result of surgical techniques. The biatrial method was the standard until the mid-to-late 1990s, until the bicaval method predominated. Parasympathetic reinnervation has been demonstrated in patients who underwent bicaval anastomosis within a year of transplantation. This could be because the bicaval technique results in both the parasympathetic and sympathetic fibers of the recipient being dissected, whereas in the bilateral technique, approximately half of the sympathetic fibers are cut, and the parasympathetic fibers of the recipient are left intact. Surgical dissection of nerves may stimulate axonal regrowth [61].

HTx patients have markedly delayed HR recovery times. In healthy subjects, HR recovery is associated with parasympathetic tone [62]. In addition to being lower than predicted, peak HR is achieved after the cessation of exercise, a feature unique to HTx patients. This is due to a lack of vagal innervation required to decelerate the HR and the time taken to metabolize circulating catecholamines [43]. Parasympathetic reinnervation might occur as early as 6 months post-transplantation [43] and may result in improved HR recovery times and a lower resting HR [29].

## Electrophysiology of the Transplanted Heart

The transplanted heart invariably has a different electrophysiology from the normal heart. Surgical technique, denervation, ischemia, fibrosis, CAV, and reinnervation all play a role in altering the conduction system, sometimes leading to clinically significant arrhythmias [63].

There is a wide range for the incidence of atrial arrhythmias post-transplantation in the literature. Atrial fibrillation (AF) is reported at 0.3–24% after HTx [64–67]. Larger studies tend to report lower numbers [64, 65, 67]. Early AF is rarer after HTx than after other forms of cardiac surgery, such as coronary artery bypass grafting or valve replacement. This may be because the donor's heart is usually healthier than the hearts of other cardiac patients.

Whether rejection causes AF or atrial flutter is equivocal. There may be an association between sustained AF or atrial flutter and episodes of rejection [64, 66–68]. Therefore, a finding of AF or atrial flutter should be investigated to exclude rejection [68]. Repeated episodes of rejection scar the atria, which can lead to atrial flutter [64]. Atrial flutter is more common than AF in HTx patients and usually occurs later after transplantation [66, 68]. Donor age and use of the biatrial method are risk factors [69]. Patients who develop atrial flutter are at increased risk of developing LV dysfunction and early death [64]. Once primary etiologies have been excluded, sustained atrial flutter can be treated with radiofrequency ablation.

Denervation and reinnervation impact the electrophysiology of the transplanted heart. As mentioned earlier, denervation results in a decrease in HR variability and an increase in resting HR. The corrected QT interval correlates with sympathetic reinnervation. Heterogeneous reinnervation increases the risk of ventricular arrhythmias [70].

After transplantation, it is common for patients to become bradycardic as a result of sinus node ischemia [71]. A subset of these patients develops a form of sick sinus syndrome known as bradycardia-tachycardia syndrome [71]. Caution should be exercised in these patients if treating AF, as some therapeutic agents can worsen bradycardia. Complete AV block manifests later on after transplantation and is probably due to progressive ischemic injury to the conduction system from CAV [72]. Approximately 10% of HTx patients with bradycardia will need a permanent pacemaker [73]. This number may decline in the future because biatrial anastomosis is a major risk factor for needing a permanent pacemaker. Interestingly, needing a permanent pacemaker does not impact survival [74].

Ventricular arrhythmias are relatively common immediately following transplantation. Later on, ventricular tachycardia (VT) could be the result of CAV and should be followed up with coronary angiography and an endomyocardial biopsy [75]. The placement of an implantable cardioverter defibrillator may be required [76].

Improvements in the survival of HTx recipients mean that the electrophysiology of the transplanted heart and resultant arrhythmias are important causes of morbidity and mortality.

## Pharmacology of the Transplanted Heart

The donor heart is distinct from the normal heart in its response to certain drugs. As discussed earlier, denervation means that normal autonomic regulation during exertion can be diminished or absent. This creates a dependence on circulating catecholamines to increase CO even with minimal stress. Cardiac myocytes shift from a predominance of type-1 to type-2 beta-adrenergic receptors. The most profound differences in the pharmacokinetics of the transplanted heart are unsurprisingly found with beta-blockers and drugs targeting the autonomic nervous system.

### Beta-Blockers

Beta-blockers are sometimes used post-transplantation to treat hypertension that is refractory to other agents [77]. The innervated heart can respond to mild and moderate exertion with little or no increase in SV. The denervated heart, however, increases CO principally via the Frank-Starling mechanism, increasing SV as a result of increased venous return, even with mild exercise. Beta blockade in HTx patients has the unsurprising effect of reducing exercise capacity by 34% [78]. When compared with a control group, ejection fraction and cardiac index were significantly lower in HTx patients, highlighting the detrimental impact of beta-blockers on ventricular function [79]. However, the use of beta blockers later after transplantation (more than 6 months) appears to be tolerated. In addition, using beta blockers for atrial arrhythmias is acceptable. The reduction in CO is not too profound in most patients.

### Beta-Adrenergic Receptor Agonists

Beta receptor agonists are positive inotropes used to treat ventricular dysfunction. They have a positive chronotropic effect by directly stimulating type-1 beta receptors on the heart and indirectly by inducing a reflex tachycardia in response to vasodilation from type-2 beta receptor stimulation [80]. The donor's heart shows increased sensitivity to beta-agonists, with HR increasing more than those of controls [81]. Despite this increase in responsiveness, there is no upregulation or increased sensitivity of beta receptors on the donor heart [82]. The supersensitivity is because of presynaptic nerve terminals at the sinus node not clearing beta-agonists [83].

### Atropine

Atropine is an anticholinergic drug normally used to treat bradyarrhythmias. The mechanism of action is via the parasympathetic nervous

variability and positron emission tomography. J Heart Lung Transplant. 2000;19(4):317–23.
42. Bengel FM, Ueberfuhr P, Ziegler SI, Nekolla S, Reichart B, Schwaiger M. Serial assessment of sympathetic reinnervation after orthotopic heart transplantation: a longitudinal study using PET and C-11 hydroxyephedrine. Circulation. 1999;99(14):1866–71.
43. Imamura T, Kinugawa K, Fujino T, Inaba T, Maki H, Hatano M, et al. Recipients with shorter cardiopulmonary bypass time achieve improvement of parasympathetic reinnervation within 6 months after heart transplantation. Int Heart J. 2014;55(5):440–4.
44. Schwaiblmair M, von Scheidt W, Überfuhr P, Ziegler S, Schwaiger M, Reichart B, et al. Functional significance of cardiac reinnervation in heart transplant recipients. J Heart Lung Transplant. 1999;18(9):838–45.
45. Stark RP, McGinn AL, Wilson RF. Chest pain in cardiac-transplant recipients: evidence of sensory reinnervation after cardiac transplantation. N Engl J Med. 1991;324(25):1791–4.
46. Di Carli MF, Tobes MC, Mangner T, Levine AB, Muzik O, Chakroborty P, et al. Effects of cardiac sympathetic innervation on coronary blood flow. N Engl J Med. 1997;336(17):1208–16.
47. Wilson RF, Laxson DD, Christensen BV, McGinn AL, Kubo SH. Regional differences in sympathetic reinnervation after human orthotopic cardiac transplantation. Circulation. 1993;88(1):165–71.
48. Terenghi G. Peripheral nerve regeneration and neurotrophic factors. J Anat. 1999;194(1):1–14.
49. Dickason A, Isaacson L. Plasticity of aged perivascular axons following exogenous NGF: analysis of catecholamines. Neurobiol Aging. 2002;23(1):125–34.
50. Bengel FM, Ueberfuhr P, Hesse T, Schiepel N, Ziegler SI, Scholz S, et al. Clinical determinants of ventricular sympathetic reinnervation after orthotopic heart transplantation. Circulation. 2002;106(7):831–5.
51. Stein PK, Bosner MS, Kleiger RE, Conger BM. Heart rate variability: a measure of cardiac autonomic tone. Am Heart J. 1994;127(5):1376–81.
52. Estorch M, Campreciós M, Flotats A, Marí C, Bernà L, Catafau AM, et al. Sympathetic reinnervation of cardiac allografts evaluated by 123I-MIBG imaging. J Nucl Med. 1999;40(6):911–6.
53. Wilson RF, Christensen BV, Olivari MT, Simon A, White CW, Laxson DD. Evidence for structural sympathetic reinnervation after orthotopic cardiac transplantation in humans. Circulation. 1991;83(4):1210–20.
54. Schuurman H-J, Plomp S, Wijngaard PL, Slootweg PJ, De Jonge N. Innervation of the endomyocardium in the first period after heart transplantation. Transplantation. 1993;56(1):85–7.
55. Buendia-Fuentes F, Almenar L, Ruiz C, Vercher J, Sánchez-Lázaro I, Martínez-Dolz L, et al., editors. Sympathetic reinnervation 1 year after heart transplantation, assessed using iodine-123 metaiodobenzylguanidine imaging. In: Transplantation proceedings. Elsevier; 2011.
56. Cooper T, Willman VL, Jellinek M, Hanlon CR. Heart autotransplantation: effect on myocardial catecholamine and histamine. Science. 1962;138(3536):40–1.
57. Koglin J, Gross T, Uberfuhr P, Von Scheidt W. Time-dependent decrease of presynaptic inotropic supersensitivity: physiological evidence of sympathetic reinnervation after heart transplantation. J Heart Lung Transplant. 1997;16(6):621–8.
58. Rowan R, Billingham M. Myocardial innervation in long-term heart transplant survivors: a quantitative ultrastructural survey. J Heart Transplant. 1988;7(6):448–52.
59. Halpert I, Goldberg AD, Levine AB, Levine TB, Kornberg R, Kelly C, et al. Reinnervation of the transplanted human heart as evidenced from heart rate variability studies. Am J Cardiol. 1996;77(2):180–3.
60. Keeley EC, Toth ZK, Goldberg AD. Long-term assessment of heart rate variability in cardiac transplant recipients. J Heart Lung Transplant. 2000;19(3):310–2.
61. Bernardi L, Valenti C, Wdowczyck-Szulc J, Frey AW, Rinaldi M, Spadacini G, et al. Influence of type of surgery on the occurrence of parasympathetic reinnervation after cardiac transplantation. Circulation. 1998;97(14):1368–74.
62. Imai K, Sato H, Hori M, Kusuoka H, Ozaki H, Yokoyama H, et al. Vagally mediated heart rate recovery after exercise is accelerated in athletes but blunted in patients with chronic heart failure. J Am Coll Cardiol. 1994;24(6):1529–35.
63. Thajudeen A, Stecker EC, Shehata M, Patel J, Wang X, McAnulty JH Jr, et al. Arrhythmias after heart transplantation: mechanisms and management. J Am Heart Assoc. 2012;1(2):e001461.
64. Ahmari SA, Bunch TJ, Chandra A, Chandra V, Ujino K, Daly RC, et al. Prevalence, pathophysiology, and clinical significance of post-heart transplant atrial fibrillation and atrial flutter. J Heart Lung Transplant. 2006;25(1):53–60.
65. Cohn WE, Gregoric ID, Radovancevic B, Wolf RK, Frazier O. Atrial fibrillation after cardiac transplantation: experience in 498 consecutive cases. Ann Thorac Surg. 2008;85(1):56–8.
66. Dizon J, Chen K, Bacchetta M, Argenziano M, Mancini D, Biviano A, et al. A comparison of atrial arrhythmias after heart or double-lung transplantation at a single center: insights into the mechanism of post-operative atrial fibrillation. J Am Coll Cardiol. 2009;54(22):2043–8.
67. Khan M, Kalahasti V, Rajagopal V, Khaykin Y, Wazni O, Almahameed S, et al. Incidence of atrial fibrillation in heart transplant patients: long-term follow-up. J Cardiovasc Electrophysiol. 2006;17(8):827–31.

68. Vaseghi M, Boyle NG, Kedia R, Patel JK, Cesario DA, Wiener I, et al. Supraventricular tachycardia after orthotopic cardiac transplantation. J Am Coll Cardiol. 2008;51(23):2241–9.
69. Dasari TW, Pavlovic-Surjancev B, Patel N, Williams AA, Ezidinma P, Rupani A, et al. Incidence, risk factors, and clinical outcomes of atrial fibrillation and atrial flutter after heart transplantation. Am J Cardiol. 2010;106(5):737–41.
70. Vrtovec B, Radovancevic R, Thomas CD, Yazdabakhsh AP, Smart FW, Radovancevic B. Prognostic value of the QTc interval after cardiac transplantation. J Heart Lung Transplant. 2006;25(1):29–35.
71. DiBiase A, Tse T-M, Schnittger I, Wexler L, Stinson EB, Valantine HA. Frequency and mechanism of bradycardia in cardiac transplant recipients and need for pacemakers. Am J Cardiol. 1991;67(16):1385–9.
72. Leonelli FM, Dunn JK, Young JB, Pacifico A. Natural history, determinants, and clinical relevance of conduction abnormalities following orthotopic heart transplantation. Am J Cardiol. 1996;77(1):47–51.
73. Cooper MM, Smith CR, Rose EA, Schneller SJ, Spotnitz HM. Permanent pacing following cardiac transplantation. J Thorac Cardiovasc Surg. 1992;104(3):812–6.
74. Cantillon DJ, Gorodeski EZ, Caccamo M, Smedira NG, Wilkoff BL, Starling RC, et al. Long-term outcomes and clinical predictors for pacing after cardiac transplantation. J Heart Lung Transplant. 2009;28(8):791–8.
75. Costanzo MR, Dipchand A, Starling R, Anderson A, Chan M, Desai S, et al. The International Society of Heart and Lung Transplantation guidelines for the care of heart transplant recipients. Elsevier; 2010. p. 914–56.
76. Ptaszek LM, Wang PJ, Hunt SA, Valantine H, Perlroth M, Al-Ahmad A. Use of the implantable cardioverter-defibrillator in long-term survivors of orthotopic heart transplantation. Heart Rhythm. 2005;2(9):931–3.
77. Ghotra AS, Angus C, Price J, Hussain Z, McCants K, Slaughter MS, et al. Safety and long term outcomes of using beta blockers after heart transplantation. J Cardiac Fail. 2015;8(21):S37–8.
78. Bexton RS, Milne JR, Cory-Pearce R, English T, Camm A. Effect of beta blockade on exercise response after cardiac transplantation. Heart. 1983;49(6):584–8.
79. Verani MS, Nishimura S, Mahmarian JJ, Hays JT, Young JB. Cardiac function after orthotopic heart transplantation: response to postural changes, exercise, and beta-adrenergic blockade. J Heart Lung Transplant. 1994;13(2):181–93.
80. Arnold J, McDevitt D. Contribution of the vagus to the haemodynamic responses following intravenous boluses of isoprenaline. Br J Clin Pharmacol. 1983;15(4):423–9.
81. Yusuf S, Theodoropoulos S, Mathias C, Dhalla N, Wittes J, Mitchell A, et al. Increased sensitivity of the denervated transplanted human heart to isoprenaline both before and after beta-adrenergic blockade. Circulation. 1987;75(4):696–704.
82. Denniss AR, Marsh JD, Quigg RJ, Gordon JB, Colucci WS. Beta-adrenergic receptor number and adenylate cyclase function in denervated transplanted and cardiomyopathic human hearts. Circulation. 1989;79(5):1028–34.
83. Gilbert EM, Eiswirth CC, Mealey PC, Larrabee P, Herrick CM, Bristow MR. Beta-adrenergic supersensitivity of the transplanted human heart is presynaptic in origin. Circulation. 1989;79(2):344–9.
84. Ellenbogen KA, Thames MD, DiMarco JP, Sheehan H, Lerman BB. Electrophysiological effects of adenosine in the transplanted human heart. Evidence of supersensitivity. Circulation. 1990;81(3):821–8.

# Immediate Post-operative Management After Heart Transplantation

11

Evan Kransdorf, Lily Stern, and Yosef Manla

**Abstract**

The optimal immediate postoperative management in patients undergoing heart transplantation is a crucial determinant of clinical outcomes. This chapter provides an overview of the management in the immediate post-transplant period, encompassing monitoring and management of hemodynamics and arrhythmias, along with addressing non-cardiac complications such as renal, neurological, and gastrointestinal dysfunctions. It also covers infection prophylaxis, nutrition, and debility considerations for the early post-transplant period.

**Keywords**

Heart failure · Heart transplantation · Inotropes · Perioperative management · Mechanical circulatory support · Pulmonary hypertension · Primary graft dysfunction · Renal dysfunction

E. Kransdorf (✉) · L. Stern · Y. Manla
Cedars-Sinai Smidt Heart Institute, Los Angeles, CA, USA
e-mail: evan.kransdorf@cshs.org

L. Stern
e-mail: Lily.stern@cshs.org

Y. Manla
e-mail: Yosef.manla1@gmail.com

## Clinical Pearls

- For optimal hemodynamic monitoring, invasive monitoring of arterial pressure, central venous pressure, pulmonary artery pressure, wedge pressure, cardiac output, continuous measurement of arterial oxygen saturation, intermittent measurement of mixed venous saturation, and systemic vascular resistance should be performed immediately following transplantation.
- Continuous infusion of an inotropic agent or a combination of agents should be used to maintain hemodynamic stability post-operatively and be weaned as tolerated over the first three to five days.
- Post-operatively, mechanical circulatory support with an intra-aortic balloon pump or temporary assist device such as VA-ECMO should be considered if there is a failure to wean from cardiopulmonary bypass or if there is persistent hemodynamic instability resistant to treatment with upward titration of vasoactive agents.
- Causes of early hemodynamic instability include hyperacute rejection, intrathoracic hemorrhage, cardiac tamponade, elevated pulmonary vascular resistance (causing right ventricular dysfunction), and primary graft dysfunction.



J. Kobashigawa (ed.), *Clinical Guide to Heart Transplantation*, https://doi.org/10.1007/978-3-031-88290-6_11

- Norepinephrine is considered the first-line agent for the treatment of vasoplegia, followed by vasopressin.
- Pulmonary vasodilators with minimal effect on systemic arterial pressure, such as inhaled nitric oxide or prostacyclin analogs, should be considered in the management of right ventricular dysfunction ± pulmonary hypertension.
- Sinus node dysfunction is common post-transplant (especially in patients on amiodarone pre-transplant), resulting in post-transplantation relative bradycardia that resolves over 4 weeks; rarely, permanent pacing may be required.
- Renal dysfunction is common 24–48 h post-transplant; therefore, continuous assessment of urine output in the early post-operative period is important.
- Early mobilization of heart transplant recipients and involvement of physical therapy with subsequent cardiac rehabilitation demonstrated to be beneficial.

## Introduction

The purpose of heart transplantation (HTx) is to provide long-term survival and improve the quality of life for patients with end-stage heart disease [1]. The immediate post-operative period is crucial in achieving this outcome. HTx clinicians should be familiar and comfortable with treating multiple transplant-specific and medical issues in HTx recipients. This chapter aims to provide an overview of the management in the immediate post-transplant period, including perioperative management strategies, frequently encountered early morbidities, and short-term complications. Although both induction and maintenance immunosuppression are initiated in the early post-transplant period, these regimens will be discussed in depth in Chaps. 12 and 13, respectively.

## Monitoring and Management of Hemodynamics in the Early Post-transplant Period

### Recommended Hemodynamic Monitoring

As cardiac allograft dysfunction is common in the early post-transplant period [2], adequate hemodynamic monitoring of the post-transplant patient is crucial. The 2023 International Society for Heart and Lung Transplantation (ISHLT) guidelines for the care of HTx recipients advised that monitoring should include (a) invasive arterial pressure monitoring, (b) direct measurement of right atrial pressure/central venous pressure (CVP), (c) measurement of left atrial or pulmonary capillary wedge pressure, (d) intermittent measurement of cardiac output, (e) intermittent measurement of systemic vascular resistance, (f) continuous measurement of arterial oxygen saturation, (g) intermittent measurement of mixed venous saturation, (h) intraoperative transesophageal echocardiogram (TEE), and (i) continuous assessment of urinary output [1].

### Causes of Cardiac Allograft Dysfunction

Numerous pre- and peri-transplant factors can contribute to the development of cardiac allograft dysfunction early (days 0–7) after HTx. These factors will be discussed here. Causes of cardiac allograft dysfunction are generally classified as primary, where the dysfunction is intrinsic to the allograft, or due to a secondary cause, including rejection, intrathoracic hemorrhage, cardiac tamponade, or pulmonary hypertension [2]. The presence of early cardiac allograft dysfunction is typically marked by systemic arterial hypotension, abnormally low cardiac output/index despite inotropic support and/or abnormally high filling pressures. These abnormally high filling pressures include CVP on the right ventricular (RV) side and left atrial/pulmonary capillary wedge pressure on the left ventricular side. In some cases, systemic arterial pressure will be preserved, and disproportionately elevated pulmonary artery pressures will be present. In either situation, hemodynamic instability can contribute to the development of renal dysfunction as marked by decreased urine output and elevated laboratory makers such as blood urea nitrogen/creatinine and/or hepatic dysfunction as marked by coagulopathy and elevated laboratory markers such as total bilirubin. When assessing a patient with cardiac allograft dysfunction, the first step is to rule out secondary causes of cardiac allograft dysfunction. Hyperacute rejection can manifest immediately after allograft reperfusion and can be difficult to identify since specific immunologic markers like a crossmatch or donor-specific antibody testing can take several days to return. Nevertheless, hyperacute rejection should remain on the list of possible causes of cardiac allograft dysfunction, especially in recipients with a history of pre-transplant allosensitization [3]. The presence of intrathoracic hemorrhage can be identified based on high chest tube output. Tamponade should be suspected when refractory hypotension is present and can be confirmed with bedside echocardiography. Pulmonary hypertension often leads to predominantly RV dysfunction and should be suspected with pulmonary artery systolic pressures $\geq 50$ mmHg.

## Primary Graft Dysfunction

If cardiac allograft dysfunction is present but there is no apparent secondary cause of cardiac allograft dysfunction present, primary graft dysfunction (PGD) should be suspected. PGD is defined as allograft dysfunction within 24 h of HTx unrelated to a secondary cause [2]. The ISHLT has developed a classification system for PGD based on the degree of ventricular dysfunction (i.e., mild, moderate, or severe) and the ventricular function affected (i.e., RV versus LV versus both) [2] (Table 11.1). According to a recent meta-analysis by Buchan et al., pooled incidences of mild, moderate, severe, and isolated RV-PGD were 3.5, 6.6, 7.7, and 1.6%, with a 1-year mortality rate of 15, 21, 41, and 35%, respectively [4]. The pathophysiology of PGD is not fully understood, but numerous risk factors have been identified (Table 11.2). These risk factors can be divided into donor, transplant, and recipient factors and vary between studies [2, 4]. In terms of donor factors, increasing donor age has been associated with an increased risk of PGD in numerous studies. In terms of transplant factors, increased allograft ischemic time [4] and use of a donor undersized by donor-recipient predicted heart mass ratio have been associated with an increased risk of PGD [5]. In terms of recipient factors, recipient mechanical circulatory support (MCS) [4], and treatment with amiodarone plus beta-blocker have been associated with an increased risk of PGD [6]. Recently, insights on the utility of recipients' pre-transplant-microvesicle proteomics have expanded our understanding of molecular pathways and inflammatory biomarkers implied in the PGD disease process and identified novel biomarkers of PGD that can improve PGD prediction accuracy. Giangreco et al. studied 88 HTx recipients who developed severe PGD post-HTx, incorporating pre-transplant data on 37 clinical characteristics and 181 protein markers; the authors identified 16 proteins predictive of severe PGD occurrence [7] and seven proteins predictive of survival post-HTx in these patients [8]. Plasma kallikrein, peroxiredoxin, tropomyosin alpha-4, and myeloperoxidase were among the proteins predictive of severe PGD occurrence [7].

## Management of Cardiac Allograft Dysfunction

Inotropic and vasoactive pharmacologic support is necessary to augment cardiac allograft function in the immediate post-cardiopulmonary bypass period. Furthermore, the catecholamine stores of the newly transplanted heart are often

**Table 11.1** Definition of severity scale for primary graft dysfunction (PGD)

| Category | Severity/Grade | Criteria |
|---|---|---|
| Left ventricle (LV) | Mild PGD–LV: One of the following criteria must be met | LVEF ≤ 40% by echo<br>-OR-<br>Hemodynamics with RAP > 15 mmHg, PCWP > 20 mmHg, CI < 2.0 L/min/m² (lasting > 1 h) requiring low-dose inotropes |
| | Moderate PGD-LV: Must meet one criterion from I and another criterion from II | I. One criteria from the following:<br>i. LVEF ≤ 40% by echo<br>-OR-<br>ii. Hemodynamics with RAP > 15 mmHg, PCWP > 20 mmHg, CI < 2.0 L/min/m², hypotension with MAP < 70 mmHg (lasting > 1 h)<br>II. One criteria from the following:<br>i. High-dose inotropes – inotrope score > 10<br>-OR-<br>ii. Newly placed IABP (regardless of inotropes) |
| | Severe PGD-LV | Dependence on left or biventricular mechanical support including ECMO, LVAD, BiVAD, or percutaneous LVAD. Excludes requirement for IABP |
| Right ventricle (RV) | Diagnosis requires either both i and ii, or iii alone | i. Hemodynamics with RAP > 15 mm Hg, PCWP < 15 mm Hg, CI < 2.0 L/min/m²<br>ii. TPG < 15 mm Hg and/or pulmonary artery systolic pressure < 50 mm Hg,<br>or<br>iii. Need for RVAD |

*Abbreviations* BiVAD = biventricular assist device; CI = cardiac index; ECMO = extracorporeal membrane oxygenation; IABP = intra-aortic balloon pump; LVAD = left ventricular assist device; LVEF = left ventricular ejection fraction; PCWP = pulmonary capillary wedge pressure; RAP = right atrial pressure; RVAD = right ventricular assist device; TPG = transpulmonary pressure gradient. Reprinted from The Journal of Heart and Lung Transplantation, 33(4), Jon Kobashigawa, Andreas Zuckermann, Peter Macdonald, Pascal Leprince, Fardad Esmailian, Minh Luu, Donna Mancini, Jignesh Patel, Rabia Razi, Hermann Reichenspurner, Stuart Russell, Javier Segovia, Nicolas Smedira, Josef Stehlik, Florian Wagner, Report from a consensus conference on primary graft dysfunction after cardiac transplantation, 327–340, Copyright (2014), with permission from Elsevier

depleted, requiring exogenous supplementation [9]. The 2023 ISHLT guidelines for the care of HTx recipients recommend that continuous infusion of an inotropic agent or a combination of agents should be used to maintain hemodynamic stability post-operatively and be weaned as tolerated over the first three to five days. As far as agent choice, the guidelines recommend the following agents: (a) isoproterenol, 1–10 μg/min, or (b) dobutamine, 1–10 μg/kg/min ± dopamine 1–10 μg/kg/min, or (c) isoproterenol, 1–10 μg/min ± dopamine 1–10 μg/kg/min, or (d) milrinone, 0.375–0.75 μg/kg/min, or (e) milrinone, 0.375–0.75 μg/kg/min ± epinephrine 0.01–0.1 μg/kg/min [1]. If pharmacologic treatment alone is insufficient to support allograft function, MCS is required. According to the ISHLT guidelines [1], MCS should be considered as

**Table 11.2** Risk factors for primary graft dysfunction

| Donor risk factors | Recipient risk factors | Surgical procedural risk factors |
|---|---|---|
| Age | Age | Ischemic time |
| Cause of death | Weight | Donor-recipient size mismatch |
| Trauma | Mechanical support | Weight mismatch |
| Cardiac dysfunction | Congenital heart disease as etiology of heart failure | Non-cardiac organ donation |
| Inotropic support | Multiple reoperations | Experience of procurement team and center volume |
| Comorbidities: diabetes, hypertension | LVAD explant | Cardioplegia solution |
| Downtime of cardiac arrest | Comorbidities: renal dysfunction, liver dysfunction (high MELD), DM | Increased blood transfusions |
| Drug abuse: alcohol, cocaine, amphetamines | Ventilator dependent | Elective versus emergency transplant |
| Left ventricular hypertrophy | Multiorgan transplant | |
| Valvular disease | Elevated PVR | |
| Hormone treatment | Allosensitization | |
| CAD/wall motion abnormalities on TTE | Infection | |
| Sepsis | Retransplant | |
| Alternate list/marginal donor allocation—not increased risk | | |
| Troponin trend | | |
| Hypernatremia | | |

CAD, coronary artery disease; DM, diabetes mellitus; LVAD, left ventricular assist device; MELD, Model for End-stage Liver Disease; PGD, primary graft dysfunction; PVR, peripheral vascular resistance; TTE, transthoracic echocardiogram; UNOS, United Network for Organ Sharing. Reprinted from The Journal of Heart and Lung Transplantation, 33(4), Jon Kobashigawa, Andreas Zuckermann, Peter Macdonald, Pascal Leprince, Fardad Esmailian, Minh Luu, Donna Mancini, Jignesh Patel, Rabia Razi, Hermann Reichenspurner, Stuart Russell, Javier Segovia, Nicolas Smedira, Josef Stehlik, Florian Wagner, Report from a consensus conference on primary graft dysfunction after cardiac transplantation, 327–340, Copyright (2014), with permission from Elsevier

early as during the operation if there is a failure to wean from cardiopulmonary bypass (CPB). Post-operatively, MCS should be considered if there is persistent hemodynamic instability due to cardiac allograft dysfunction that is resistant to treatment with upward titration of vasoactive agents. A variety of MCS devices may be used. The ISHLT guidelines recommend that an intra-aortic balloon pump (IABP) is attempted prior to other forms of MCS. The IABP is often effective in establishing sufficient pulsatility to improve coronary perfusion and cardiac performance to separate from cardiopulmonary bypass. Extracorporeal membrane oxygenation (ECMO) is a frequently used short-term MCS device for recipients with cardiac allograft dysfunction unresponsive to vasoactive agents and/or IABP. Patients with severe PGD requiring VA-ECMO appear to benefit from plasmapheresis in the immediate post-transplant period, potentially by alleviating the inflammatory milieu contributing to its development [10]. Approximately 50% of patients with severe PGD requiring ECMO will have normalization of allograft function and consequently will be able to be weaned off of ECMO [6]. Patients who are placed on ECMO post-transplant and are subsequently able to be weaned off ECMO have a similar survival to those who did not require ECMO at 1-year post-transplant but have a lower number of days alive out of the hospital [11].

## Management of Vasoplegia

Vasoplegia is a hemodynamic complication that can occur post-transplant that can overlap in presentation with cardiac allograft dysfunction in that severe systemic arterial hypotension is present but distinct in that cardiac allograft function is preserved. Vasoplegia is more common after HTx in recipients with older age, longer cardiopulmonary bypass time, higher pre-transplant creatinine, chronic liver disease and pre-transplant durable MCS [12]. However, unlike recipients with severe PGD, patients with vasoplegia did not exhibit a higher risk of mortality 1-year post-transplant. The 2023 ISHLT guidelines for the care of HTx recipients recommend that norepinephrine is considered the first-line agent for the treatment of vasoplegia, followed by vasopressin [1]. Additional vasoactive agents that can be utilized include epinephrine, norepinephrine, dopamine, and angiotensin II. Adjunctive medications, including methylene blue, ascorbic acid, and hydrocortisone, may also play a supportive role [13].

## Management of Specific Causes of Cardiac Allograft Dysfunction

### Hyperacute Rejection

Hyperacute rejection is a very rare complication that occurs early post-transplant when pre-formed anti-ABO or anti-HLA antibodies bind to the cardiac allograft and fix complement, resulting in severe allograft dysfunction. It typically presents immediately following reperfusion of the allograft. This phenomenon is covered in more detail in Chap. 19. The development and use of the prospective cytotoxic crossmatch, and subsequently the virtual crossmatch, has greatly reduced the frequency of this complication [14]. Treatment for hyperacute rejection should be initiated as soon as the diagnosis is suspected. In addition to standard management for cardiac allograft dysfunction, aggressive immunosuppression consisting of high-dose intravenous corticosteroids, plasmapheresis, intravenous immunoglobulin, anti-thymocyte globulin cytolytic agents, and eculizumab, as well as immediate initiation of intensified maintenance immunosuppression including a calcineurin inhibitor and metabolic cycle inhibitors or mammalian target of rapamycin (mTOR) inhibitors [1].

### Intrathoracic Hemorrhage and Cardiac Tamponade

In the immediate post-operative period in the intensive care unit, output from chest tubes is to be expected. However, output of 1500 mL within an hour or 200 mL/h over four hours suggests active intrathoracic bleeding and may be accompanied by hemodynamic compromise. Likewise, the sudden appearance of systemic arterial hypotension accompanied by cardiac allograft dysfunction may indicate the accumulation of blood in the pericardium. Cardiac tamponade should be excluded as a possible cause by bedside echocardiography. If intrathoracic hemorrhage or cardiac tamponade is present, direct surgical exploration is indicated to prevent further hemodynamic decompensation.

### Pulmonary Hypertension

Elevated recipient pre-transplant pulmonary vascular resistance (PVR) is known to be a significant risk factor for early post-transplant RV dysfunction and subsequent mortality [1, 15, 16]. The risk of RV failure is as high as 75%, with a 15% mortality risk among patients with pre-transplant PVRi (indexed to body surface area)>6 Wood units x $m^2$. In contrast, patients without increased pre-transplant PVR only demonstrate a 20% risk of RV failure [17, 18]. The mechanism of RV failure in the immediate post-transplant period is thought to be multifactorial. The donor's RV is particularly vulnerable to peri-procedural myocardial strain, ischemia, cardioplegia, and surgical trauma. When exposed to elevated recipient PVR, factoring in complications from transitional pulmonary vascular hyper-reactivity resulting from cardiopulmonary bypass [19], the sudden and dramatic increase in PVR can cause RV failure. This situation is exacerbated by a donor heart that is too small for a larger recipient [20]. Thus, in all patients, particular attention should be given to continuous monitoring of the post-operative pulmonary artery pressures. An invasive pulmonary arterial line, as per ISHLT recommendations [1], permits continuous post-operative pulmonary arterial pressure monitoring and facilitates treatment when elevated to prevent subsequent RV failure. Broadly speaking, management of pulmonary hypertension-induced RV dysfunction can be approached on four fronts: (a) preload optimization with CVP maintained at 5–12 mmHg, (b) maintenance of sinus rhythm and atrioventricular synchrony, (c) ventilatory support, and (d) appropriate pharmacologic and/or mechanical support to stabilize hemodynamic function. For preload optimization, diuretics should be utilized to achieve CVP goals. If diuretics are not able to achieve CVP goals, then ultrafiltration/renal replacement therapy may be needed. Ventilatory parameters that may help improve pulmonary hypertension include avoiding hypercapnia or hypoxia. Pharmacologic support for RV dysfunction is the same as that for left ventricular dysfunction: inotropic agents such as isoproterenol, milrinone, dobutamine, and epinephrine [1]. However, to specifically target pulmonary arterial hypertension (high pulmonary artery pressure and normal pulmonary capillary wedge pressure), as compared to pulmonary venous hypertension (high pulmonary artery pressure and high pulmonary capillary wedge pressure), selective pulmonary vasodilating agents may be beneficial. Examples of selective vasodilators include epoprostenol (inhaled), iloprost (inhaled), nitric oxide (inhaled), and sildenafil (oral). All of the aforementioned agents have proven effective at decreasing PVR and improving pulmonary artery pressures in a small series of adult post-transplant recipients [21–24].

## Monitoring and Management of Arrhythmias in the Early Post-Transplant Period

### Electrical Monitoring

In the immediate postoperative period, the ISHLT guidelines recommend the use of both continuous electrocardiographic monitoring and post-operative 12-lead electrocardiography [1]. Furthermore, it is recommended that both atrial and ventricular temporary epicardial pacing wires be placed at the time of the HTx surgery, even if the initial rhythm is sinus.

### Sinus Node Dysfunction

While most cardiac allografts return to sinus rhythm after reperfusion in the operating room, dysfunction of the sinus node is very common, with prevalence as high as 50% [25]. The electrophysiologic parameters affected may include prolonged sinus node recovery time, prolonged corrected sinus node recovery time, and abnormal sinoatrial conduction time. Post-transplant sinus node dysfunction is believed to be multifactorial in origin, including surgical trauma, cardiac denervation, and ischemia–reperfusion injury [26]. Sinus bradycardia is also common for recipients who received amiodarone prior to transplant, as amiodarone has a very long half-life (average 60 days), and so will remain in the recipient's system for a prolonged period after HTx. Recipients who receive amiodarone prior to a HTx are at an increased risk of needing a pacemaker after HTx [27]. In the immediate postoperative period, the cardiac allograft exhibits a restrictive hemodynamics [28], and consequently, a high heart rate needs to be maintained to support adequate cardiac output (due to smaller stroke volume). The 2023 ISHLT guidelines for the care of HTx recipients recommend pharmacologic treatment or temporary pacing to maintain a minimum heart rate of at least 90 bpm [1]. Such pharmacologic agents may include isoproterenol while awaiting the return of normal sinus node function. Although sinus node dysfunction is typically transient [29], a few patients display permanent sinus node dysfunction and require permanent pacing. Recommendations suggest delaying pacemaker implantation until at least three weeks after HTx. A 2–10% prevalence of pacemaker placement during the transplant hospitalization has been reported [30, 31].

### Atrial Fibrillation

Atrial fibrillation is common in the early postoperative period after a HTx, affecting approximately 14% of patients in one cohort study [32]. Its frequency is not surprising, given that atrial fibrillation is a common complication of cardiac surgery. However, in HTx recipients, older studies suggest that atrial fibrillation can be a sign of rejection, and as such, it is also prudent to rule out rejection in HTx patients presenting with atrial fibrillation [33]. The use of vasoactive agents, as well as the lack of cardiac innervation, lead to high ventricular rates when HTx patients have atrial fibrillation early after HTx. Thus, hemodynamic instability may develop, and emergent restoration of sinus rhythm via synchronized cardioversion may be needed. In the absence of hemodynamic instability, amiodarone can be used to control ventricular rate urgently and potentially restore sinus rhythm. Beta-blockers or calcium channel blockers can be used if the patient has sufficient systemic blood pressure for the addition of these agents. Digoxin is not recommended as it is not effective in HTx recipients, given the lack of parasympathetic innervation [34]. If atrial fibrillation is recurrent, anticoagulation may be needed to reduce the risk of stroke. Given the need for procedures such as endomyocardial biopsy early after HTx, direct oral anticoagulants have been used successfully [35].

### Ventricular Tachycardia

Non-sustained ventricular tachycardia is very common in the early postoperative period due to the use of vasoactive agents and electrolyte abnormalities. In contrast, sustained ventricular tachycardia is rare and should prompt consideration for causes of allograft dysfunction, such as hyperacute rejection or PGD.

## Non-cardiac Medical Issues After Heart Transplant

### Renal Dysfunction

Renal reserves are often impaired prior to HTx due to the prolonged low cardiac output and chronic administration of diuretics that occurs in end-stage heart failure. This vulnerability combines with the renal effects of cardiopulmonary bypass, post-transplant hemodynamic complications, and initiation of calcineurin inhibitor immunosuppression to cause acute kidney injury (AKI) in about 40% of HTx recipients [36]. Specific complications associated with an increased risk of AKI include tamponade, hemorrhage, and RV failure. In patients with AKI and oliguria (urine output < 0.5 mL/kg/h), high-dose diuretics, potentially including the use of both loop and thiazide diuretics, should be undertaken. If the patient fails to respond and CVP continues to increase, the ISHLT guidelines recommend renal replacement therapy [1]. For patients with pre-existing renal insufficiency, the use of induction immunosuppression with delayed initiation of calcineurin inhibitor may be helpful to mitigate worsening kidney function [37]. Thus, early involvement and consultation of Nephrology is essential. Subsequent to the changes to the heart allocation system in the United States in 2018, about 13% of post-transplant patients required de novo hemodialysis [38]. Patients who required hemodialysis had decreased survival at 1- and 2 years post-transplant. Pre-transplant renal function (as measured by the glomerular filtration rate) and pre-transplant ECMO were strong predictors of the need for post-transplant hemodialysis.

## Neurological Dysfunction

Neurological dysfunction in the early post-transplant period may present in several forms: focal neurological deficit (e.g., unilateral upper and/or lower extremity motor deficits), seizures, or encephalopathy. These differing presentations may arise from several causes: hypotension associated with cardiac allograft dysfunction, stroke from systemic embolus, metabolic derangements, or side effects of calcineurin inhibitors [1]. With regards to the latter, tacrolimus in the presence of low lipid levels has been associated with an increased risk of encephalopathy, as low lipids result in higher amounts of free tacrolimus, which can more easily translocate across the blood–brain barrier [39]. In this situation, switching from tacrolimus to cyclosporine has been helpful. Both stroke and seizures require the involvement of neurology care, and thus, early consultation is imperative.

## Gastrointestinal Dysfunction

HTx recipients are at increased risk of intraabdominal complications in the early postoperative period, affecting 20% or more of HTx recipients in older cohort series [40, 41]. The most common events include ischemic bowel, viscus perforation, cholecystitis, and gastrointestinal hemorrhage. These complications can be difficult to identify in the setting of HTx recipients with multiple ongoing medical issues, and thus, clinicians should maintain a high index of suspicion.

## Antibiotic Use for Prophylaxis of Infection

In the first month post-transplant, infections are most commonly bacterial and typically related to indwelling catheters and wound infections. Coagulase-negative Staphylococci and S. aureus (MRSA and MSSA) are the most common pathogens causing surgical site infections in HTx recipients; other encountered pathogens include gram negatives and Candida spp. For prophylactic purposes, broad-spectrum antibiotics such as first/third-generation cephalosporin with/without vancomycin are commonly used [1]. For prophylaxis against Pneumocystis jiroveci, the preferred agent is trimethoprim-sulfamethoxazole. For cytomegalovirus (CMV) prevention, the ISHLT recommended that the CMV serologic status of the donor and recipient should be used to risk stratify patients for post-transplant CMV infection. Acyclovir (if low risk) or valganciclovir (if high risk) are being used. For prophylaxis against mucocutaneous candidiasis, nystatin or clotrimazole are used.

## Nutritional Insufficiency

Nutritional insufficiency and cachexia are common in patients with end-stage heart failure [42], and thus, returning to an adequate nutritional state is an important endpoint for HTx recipients. For transplant recipients with a delay in extubation or inability to swallow safely, enteral nutritional supplementation should be initiated. Once the recipient has been extubated or can swallow safely, enteral nutritional supplementation can be discontinued. However, clinicians should continue to monitor the patient's oral intake to ensure that caloric needs are being met.

## Debility

Patients with end-stage heart failure who undergo HTx are likely to have been ill for a prolonged period of time. As a result of this, as well as immobility related to the HTx surgery, HTx recipients are likely to have debility that varies in severity from mild to severe. Early involvement of physical, occupational, and speech therapy (when needed) is important. For patients with severe debility, transfer to inpatient rehabilitation has been shown to improve functional status [43]. For patients with more mild debility, discharge with home therapy is appropriate. When the patient is ready (6–12 weeks post-procedure), completion of cardiac rehabilitation has been shown to improve functional status [44].

## Conclusions

Mortality in the first year after a HTx remains significant, ranging between 6% and 10% in most HTx programs in the United States. Thus, the events that occur immediately after surgery are critically important for the long-term survival of HTx recipients. Each HTx center uses its own set of protocols with regard to early post-transplant care in the intensive care unit and hospital, but here, we have outlined general principles and highlighted complications clinicians should be aware of to ensure optimal outcomes for HTx recipients.

## References


1. Velleca A, Shullo MA, Dhital K, Azeka E, Colvin M, DePasquale E, et al. The International Society for Heart and Lung Transplantation (ISHLT) guidelines for the care of heart transplant recipients. J Heart Lung Transplant. 2023;42(5):e1–141.
2. Kobashigawa J, Zuckermann A, Macdonald P, Leprince P, Esmailian F, Luu M, et al. Report from a consensus conference on primary graft dysfunction after cardiac transplantation. J Heart Lung Transplant. 2014;33(4):327–40.
3. Kobashigawa J, Mehra M, West L, Kerman R, George J, Rose M, et al. Report from a consensus conference on the sensitized patient awaiting heart transplantation. J Heart Lung Transplant. 2009;28(3):213–25.
4. Buchan TA, Moayedi Y, Truby LK, Guyatt G, Posada JD, Ross HJ, et al. Incidence and impact of primary graft dysfunction in adult heart transplant recipients: a systematic review and meta-analysis. J Heart Lung Transplant. 2021;40(7):642–51.
5. Gong TA, Joseph SM, Lima B, Gonzalez-Stawinski GV, Jamil AK, Felius J, et al. Donor predicted heart mass as predictor of primary graft dysfunction. J Heart Lung Transplant. 2018;37(7):826–35.
6. Benck L, Kransdorf EP, Emerson DA, Rushakoff J, Kittleson MM, Klapper EB, et al. Recipient and surgical factors trigger severe primary graft dysfunction after heart transplant. J Heart Lung Transplant. 2021;40(9):970–80.
7. Giangreco NP, Lebreton G, Restaino S, Farr MJ, Zorn E, Colombo PC, et al. Plasma kallikrein predicts primary graft dysfunction after heart transplant. J Heart Lung Transplant. 2021;40(10):1199–211.
8. Giangreco NP, Lebreton G, Restaino S, Farr M, Zorn E, Colombo PC, et al. Alterations in the kallikrein-kinin system predict death after heart transplant. Sci Rep. 2022;12(1):14167.
9. Mohanty PK, Sowers JR, Thames MD, Beck FW, Kawaguchi A, Lower RR. Myocardial norepinephrine, epinephrine and dopamine concentrations after cardiac autotransplantation in dogs. J Am Coll Cardiol. 1986;7(2):419–24.
10. Manla Y, Chang D, Patel J, Kanungo A, Nikolova A, Kransdorf E, et al. Therapeutic plasma exchange is associated with increased survival in heart transplant recipients experiencing severe primary graft dysfunction. J Heart Lung Transplant. 2025;44(4):627–633.
11. M'Pembele R, Roth S, Stroda A, Buse GL, Sixt SU, Westenfeld R, et al. Life impact of VA-ECMO due to primary graft dysfunction in patients after orthotopic heart transplantation. ESC Heart Fail. 2022;9(1):695–703.
12. Chan JL, Kobashigawa JA, Aintablian TL, Dimbil SJ, Perry PA, Patel JK, et al. Characterizing predictors and severity of vasoplegia syndrome after heart transplantation. Ann Thorac Surg. 2018;105(3):770–7.
13. Datt V, Wadhhwa R, Sharma V, Virmani S, Minhas HS, Malik S. Vasoplegic syndrome after cardiovascular surgery: a review of pathophysiology and outcome-oriented therapeutic management. J Card Surg. 2021;36(10):3749–60.
14. Morris AB, Sullivan H, Krummey SM, Gebel HM, Bray RA. Out with the old, in with the new: virtual versus physical crossmatching in the modern era. Hla. 2019;94(6):471–81.
15. Costard-Jackle A, Fowler MB. Influence of preoperative pulmonary artery pressure on mortality after heart transplantation: testing of potential reversibility of pulmonary hypertension with nitroprusside is useful in defining a high risk group. J Am Coll Cardiol. 1992;19(1):48–54.
16. Murali S, Kormos RL, Uretsky BF, Schechter D, Reddy PS, Denys BG, et al. Preoperative pulmonary hemodynamics and early mortality after orthotopic

cardiac transplantation: the Pittsburgh experience. Am Heart J. 1993;126(4):896–904.
17. Daftari B, Alejos JC, Perens G. Initial experience with sildenafil, bosentan, and nitric oxide for pediatric cardiomyopathy patients with elevated pulmonary vascular resistance before and after orthotopic heart transplantation. J Transplant. 2010;2010:656984.
18. Addonizio LJ, Gersony WM, Robbins RC, Drusin RE, Smith CR, Reison DS, et al. Elevated pulmonary vascular resistance and cardiac transplantation. Circulation. 1987;76(5 Pt 2):V52-5.
19. Kant S, Banerjee D, Sabe SA, Sellke F, Feng J. Microvascular dysfunction following cardiopulmonary bypass plays a central role in postoperative organ dysfunction. Front Med (Lausanne). 2023;10:1110532.
20. Shah M, Saeed O, Shin J, Murthy S, Sims DB, Vukelic S, et al. Predicted heart mass-based size matching among recipients with moderate pulmonary hypertension: outcomes and sex effect. J Heart Lung Transplant. 2020;39(7):648–56.
21. Rajek A, Pernerstorfer T, Kastner J, Mares P, Grabenwoger M, Sessler DI, et al. Inhaled nitric oxide reduces pulmonary vascular resistance more than prostaglandin E(1) during heart transplantation. Anesth Analg. 2000;90(3):523–30.
22. Ardehali A, Hughes K, Sadeghi A, Esmailian F, Marelli D, Moriguchi J, et al. Inhaled nitric oxide for pulmonary hypertension after heart transplantation. Transplantation. 2001;72(4):638–41.
23. Theodoraki K, Tsiapras D, Tsourelis L, Zarkalis D, Sfirakis P, Kapetanakis E, et al. Inhaled iloprost in eight heart transplant recipients presenting with post-bypass acute right ventricular dysfunction. Acta Anaesthesiol Scand. 2006;50(10):1213–7.
24. Kulkarni A, Singh TP, Sarnaik A, Walters HL, Delius R. Sildenafil for pulmonary hypertension after heart transplantation. J Heart Lung Transplant. 2004;23(12):1441–4.
25. McGiffin DC, Kirklin JK, Naftel DC, Bourge RC. Competing outcomes after heart transplantation: a comparison of eras and outcomes. J Heart Lung Transplant. 1997;16(2):190–8.
26. Bexton RS, Nathan AW, Hellestrand KJ, Cory-Pearce R, Spurrell RA, English TA, et al. Electrophysiological abnormalities in the transplanted human heart. Br Heart J. 1983;50(6):555–63.
27. Cooper LB, Mentz RJ, Edwards LB, Wilk AR, Rogers JG, Patel CB, et al. Amiodarone use in patients listed for heart transplant is associated with increased 1-year post-transplant mortality. J Heart Lung Transplant. 2017;36(2):202–10.
28. Young JB, Leon CA, Short HD, Noon GP, Lawrence EC, Whisennand HH, et al. Evolution of hemodynamics after orthotopic heart and heart-lung transplantation: early restrictive patterns persisting in occult fashion. J Heart Transplant. 1987;6(1):34–43.
29. Heinz G, Hirschl M, Buxbaum P, Laufer G, Gasic S, Laczkovics A. Sinus node dysfunction after orthotopic cardiac transplantation: postoperative incidence and long-term implications. Pacing Clin Electrophysiol. 1992;15(5):731–7.
30. Cantillon DJ, Tarakji KG, Hu T, Hsu A, Smedira NG, Starling RC, et al. Long-term outcomes and clinical predictors for pacemaker-requiring bradyarrhythmias after cardiac transplantation: analysis of the UNOS/OPTN cardiac transplant database. Heart Rhythm. 2010;7(11):1567–71.
31. Jones DG, Mortsell DH, Rajaruthnam D, Hamour I, Hussain W, Markides V, et al. Permanent pacemaker implantation early and late after heart transplantation: clinical indication, risk factors and prognostic implications. J Heart Lung Transplant. 2011;30(11):1257–65.
32. Darche FF, Helmschrott M, Rahm AK, Thomas D, Schweizer PA, Bruckner T, et al. Atrial fibrillation before heart transplantation is a risk factor for post-transplant atrial fibrillation and mortality. ESC Heart Fail. 2021;8(5):4265–77.
33. Cui G, Tung T, Kobashigawa J, Laks H, Sen L. Increased incidence of atrial flutter associated with the rejection of heart transplantation. Am J Cardiol. 2001;88(3):280–4.
34. Joglar JA, Wan EY, Chung MK, Gutierrez A, Slaughter MS, Bateson BP, et al. Management of arrhythmias after heart transplant: current state and considerations for future research. Circ Arrhythm Electrophysiol. 2021;14(3):e007954.
35. Henricksen EJ, Tremblay-Gravel M, Moayedi Y, Yang W, Lee R, Ross HJ, et al. Use of direct oral anticoagulants after heart transplantation. J Heart Lung Transplant. 2020;39(4):399–401.
36. Garcia-Gigorro R, Renes-Carreno E, Corres Peiretti MA, Arribas Lopez P, Perez Vela JL, Gutierrez Rodriguez J, et al. Incidence, risk factors and outcomes of early acute kidney injury after heart transplantation: an 18-year experience. Transplantation. 2018;102(11):1901–8.
37. Chang DH, Youn J-C, Dilibero D, Patel JK, Kobashigawa JA. Heart transplant immunosuppression strategies at cedars-sinai medical center. Int J Heart Fail. 2021;3(1):15.
38. Hong Y, Hess NR, Ziegler LA, Hickey GW, Huston JH, Mathier MA, et al. Clinical trends, risk factors, and temporal effects of post-transplant dialysis on outcomes following orthotopic heart transplantation in the 2018 United States heart allocation system. J Heart Lung Transplant. 2023;42(6):795–806.
39. Anghel D, Tanasescu R, Campeanu A, Lupescu I, Podda G, Bajenaru O. Neurotoxicity of immunosuppressive therapies in organ transplantation. Maedica (Bucur). 2013;8(2):170–5.
40. Watson CJ, Jamieson NV, Johnston PS, Wreghitt T, Large S, Wallwork J, et al. Early abdominal complications following heart and heart-lung transplantation. Br J Surg. 1991;78(6):699–704.

41. Augustine SM, Yeo CJ, Buchman TG, Achuff SC, Baumgartner WA. Gastrointestinal complications in heart and in heart-lung transplant patients. J Heart Lung Transplant. 1991;10(4):547–55; discussion 55–6.
42. Lv S, Ru S. The prevalence of malnutrition and its effects on the all-cause mortality among patients with heart failure: a systematic review and meta-analysis. PLoS ONE. 2021;16(10):e0259300.
43. Shiner CT, Woodbridge G, Skalicky DA, Faux SG. Multidisciplinary inpatient rehabilitation following heart and/or lung transplantation-examining cohort characteristics and clinical outcomes. PMR. 2019;11(8):849–57.
44. Kobashigawa JA, Leaf DA, Lee N, Gleeson MP, Liu H, Hamilton MA, et al. A controlled trial of exercise rehabilitation after heart transplantation. N Engl J Med. 1999;340(4):272–7.

# 12 Maintenance Immunosuppression Strategies in Heart Transplantation

Jignesh Patel and Krishan Patel

**Abstract**

Advancements in immunosuppression therapies have transformed the landscape of heart transplantation and significantly improved outcomes for transplant recipients. Modern immunosuppression strategy hinges on deploying a combination of immunosuppressive agents; this chapter will cover the different categories of maintenance immunosuppressive agents used in heart transplant patients, their clinical utility, and strategies involving different combinations of these agents to adjust to various clinical phenotypes.

**Keywords**

Heart failure · Heart transplantation · Immunosuppression · Rejection · Induction · Cardiac allograft vasculopathy · Outcomes

J. Patel (✉) · K. Patel
Cedars-Sinai Smidt Heart Institute, Los Angeles, CA, USA
e-mail: jignesh.patel@cshs.org

K. Patel
e-mail: krishan.patel@cshs.org

## Clinical Pearls

- While there is no accepted universal protocol for immunosuppression, common standard practice consists of "triple" therapy consisting of a calcineurin inhibitor, an anti-proliferative agent, and corticosteroids.
- Corticosteroid wean-to-off protocols are successful in a majority of patients at low risk for rejection with best results occurring when initiated within the first year post-transplant.
- Tacrolimus is generally preferred to cyclosporine due to reduced rejection and a more tolerable adverse effect profile.
- Common side effects of calcineurin inhibitors include hypertension, nephrotoxicity, hyperglycemia, hyperlipidemia, and neurotoxicity.
- Calcineurin inhibitors are metabolized by the cytochrome P-450 liver enzyme pathway and thus are susceptible to interactions, most notably with cytochrome P-450 inhibitors such as the –azole antifungals and grapefruit juice.
- Within the antiproliferatives, mycophenolate mofetil (MMF) is superior to azathioprine with improved survival, decreased incidence of rejection and a reduced adverse effect profile.
- Common side effects of the antiproliferatives include myelosuppression, fluid retention and nausea/vomiting.



J. Kobashigawa (ed.), *Clinical Guide to Heart Transplantation*, https://doi.org/10.1007/978-3-031-88290-6_12

- The proliferation signal inhibitors everolimus/sirolimus are superior to MMF in retarding cardiac allograft vasculopathy and may also enable early weaning of calcineurin inhibitors; however, they have also been associated with impaired wound healing and renal insufficiency as they potentiate calcineurin inhibitor nephrotoxicity.
- Immunosuppression regimens should be individualized to each patient's risk profile and medical history.

## Introduction to Transplant Immunosuppression

Initial immunosuppressive efforts in human cardiac transplantation were hindered by poor outcomes that resulted from suboptimal regimens, with the result frequently being overwhelming infection or allograft rejection. Initially, at the advent of modern cardiac transplantation, 1-year survival in the 1970s hovered around 50% [1]. At this stage, the only viable immunosuppressive techniques were the use of azathioprine, a purine analogue, and total body irradiation, both with many adverse effects. In the subsequent 30 years, improved donor heart management, refinement of donor and recipient selection methods, and the introduction of the calcineurin-inhibiting agent cyclosporine, followed by even more successful immunosuppressive agents and regimens, has improved survival considerably. With 1-year survival at 90%, a 5-year survival rate of approximately 70%, and a median survival in excess of 11 years, developments in immunosuppression have enabled heart transplantation (HTx) to become a definitive option for selected patients with end-stage heart failure [2]. There are three possible outcomes in the use of immunosuppressive drugs, some or all of which may overlap: the desired immunosuppressive effects, adverse effects of immunodeficiency such as infection and malignancy, and non-immune toxicities such as diabetes, hypertension, and renal insufficiency. In particular, malignancy is one of the most common causes of death post-cardiac transplant, accounting for 24% of deaths after 5 years [2]. The impaired immunoregulation that results from immunosuppression is synergistic with carcinogens such as nicotine or ultraviolet light exposure and oncogenic viruses such as the Epstein–Barr virus (EBV) and the papillomavirus (HPV) [3]. Lymphoproliferative diseases, skin cancers, and Kaposi sarcoma have a particularly high incidence relative to the general population.

In this field, it has always been crucial to maintain a delicate balance between the risk of rejection and the risk of immunosuppression-related adverse effects. Minimizing immunosuppression and immunosuppression-associated complications without sacrificing efficacy are the goals of post-transplantation management. Modern immunosuppression strategy hinges on the deployment of a combination of immunosuppressive agents, with each affecting a different pathway of T-cell activation (Fig. 12.1). This chapter will cover the different categories of maintenance immunosuppressive agents used in HTx patients, their clinical utility, and strategies involving different combinations of these agents.

Immunosuppressive agents commonly used in HTx patients and their mechanisms of action and common side effects are listed in Table 12.1, which gives trade names, pharmacology, necessary adjustments for renal or hepatic dysfunction, and dosing and general monitoring guidelines for each of the drugs. Table 12.2 lists the major adverse effects of immunosuppressive drugs.

## Immunosuppressive Agents for Maintenance Regimens

Immunosuppression regimens can be generally defined as induction, maintenance, or rejection regimens. Whereas "rejection" regimens refer to agents specifically used to treat rejection episodes (covered in Chap. 19), and "induction" refers to a brief period of intense perioperative immunosuppression, and will be covered later in Chap. 13, maintenance therapy refers to the ongoing immunosuppressive regimen that a

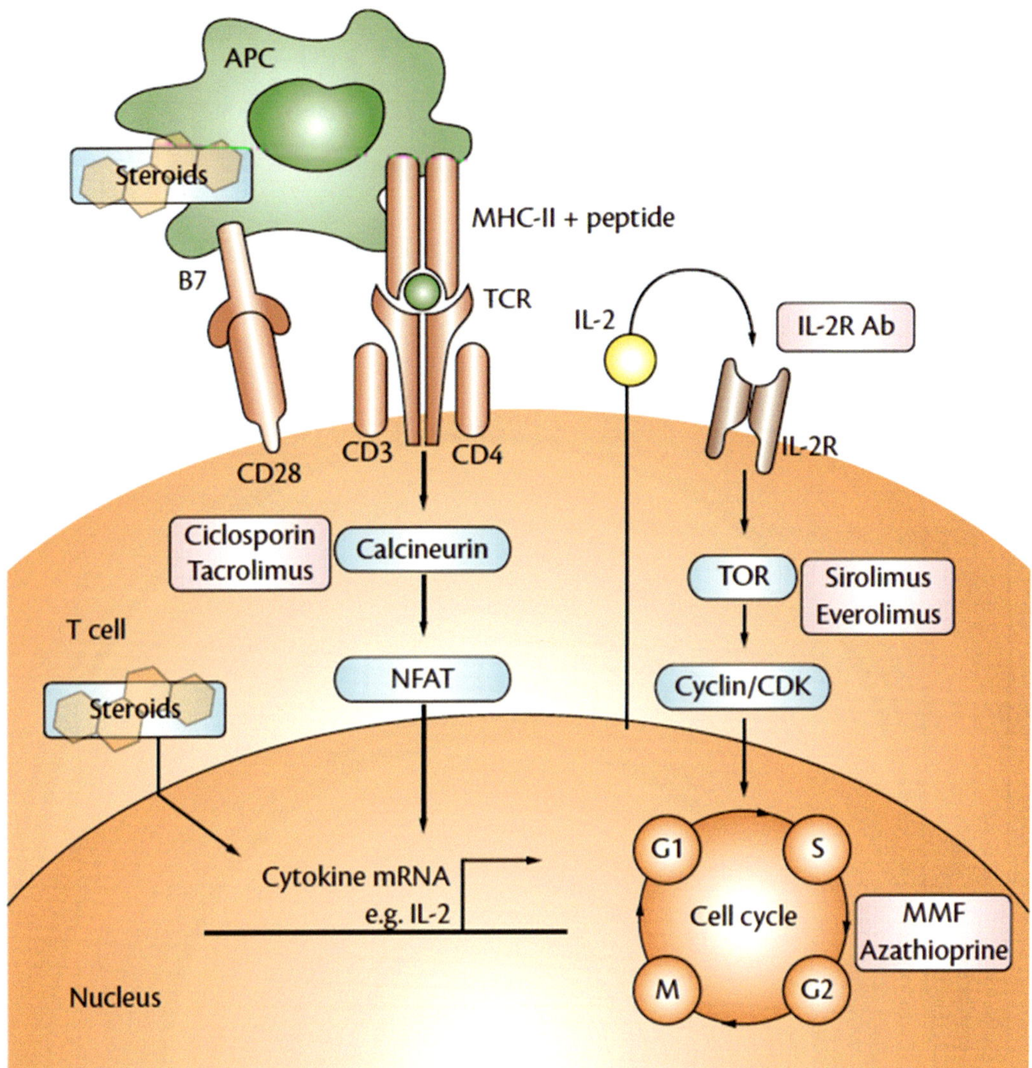


**Fig. 12.1** Diagram of mechanisms of action of common immunosuppressants in heart transplant. Through various pathways, the drugs inhibit T-cell proliferation. *Abbreviations* G1 (first growth phase), S (synthesis of DNA), G2 (second growth phase), and M (cell division) represent the phases of the cell cycle. APC, antigen-presenting cell; CDK, cyclin-dependent kinase; IL-2, interleukin-2; IL-2R, interleukin-2 receptor; IL-2R Ab, interleukin-2-receptor antibody; MHC, major histocompatibility complex; MMF, mycophenolate mofetil; mRNA, messenger RNA; NF-AT, nuclear factor of activated T cells; TCR, T-cell receptor; TOR, target of rapamycin protein. Reused with own rights according to Springer Nature Policy, Kobashigawa JA, Patel JK. Immunosuppression for heart transplantation: where are we now? Nature Clinical Practice Cardiovascular Medicine. 2006; 3(4): 203–12

cardiac transplant patient must undergo for the rest of their lives, to prevent rejection.

Remarkably, there remains no accepted uniform protocol for maintenance immunosuppression in cardiac transplant patients. The most common long-term regimen consists of a triple therapy regimen, consisting of a corticosteroid, calcineurin inhibitor, and antiproliferative. However, there remains controversy over which specific agents and combinations of agents are

**Table 12.1** Overview of commonly used immunosuppressive drugs in cardiac transplantation, including both maintenance and induction agents

| Drug | Trade name(s) | Pharmacology | Adjustment for renal/hepatic dysfunction | Dosing | | | Monitoring |
|---|---|---|---|---|---|---|---|
| | | | | Oral | Intravenous | Comments | |
| Prednisone | Deltasone<br>Generic | Processed in the liver and metabolites excreted in the urine | Consider prednisolone if hepatic dysfunction | × | | Intra and post: Solumedrol 5–10 mg/kg pre- or intraoperatively and 5–7 mg/kg in 3 divided doses over next 24 h; then rapidly tapered from 1 to 0.3 mg/kg/day at 3–6 mo to 0.1 mg/kg/day at 6 mo<br>For rejection: prednisone 1–3 mg/kg/day PO for 3–7 day or solumedrol 3–10 mg/kg/day IV; Lower doses have been used successfully | No currently available monitoring tool except clinical response |
| Prednisolone | Generic | Prednisone is converted to Prednisolone in liver | No | × | | | |
| Methylprednisolone | Medrol | Prednisone and Prednisolone have 4–5 times potency of hydrocortisone | No | × | | | |
| | Solumedrol | | | × | | | |
| Azathioprine | Imuran | Converted in liver to 6-mercaptopurine, which is inactivated by xanthine oxidase or TMPT predominantly in the liver | Decrease doses for renal dysfunction and lower dose range for hepatic dysfunction | × | × | 1–2 mg/kg per day PO or IV<br>Rarely used > 3 mg/kg<br>IV and oral the same dose | Monitoring of levels not clinically available<br>Dose is decreased if white blood cells < 3000–4000<br>Major drug interaction with allopurinol<br>Polymorphisms in *TMPT* may increase effect |

(continued)

**Table 12.1** (continued)

| Drug | Trade name(s) | Pharmacology | Adjustment for renal/hepatic dysfunction | Dosing | | | Monitoring |
|---|---|---|---|---|---|---|---|
| | | | | Oral | Intravenous | Comments | |
| MMF | Cellcept<br>Generic | Rapidly hydrolyzed to mycophenolic acid (MPA) and MPA to its gluronide, which is excreted in urine and bile | ≤1000 mg BID | × | × | 500–1500 mg BID<br>Higher doses have been used when monitoring trough MPA levels<br>IV and oral the same dose | Monitoring of MPA levels is controversial, but trough levels of 2.5–5.0 μg/mL have been suggested<br>CSA inhibits enterohepatic circulation of MPA, decreasing exposure and levels |
| Calcineurin inhibitors | | | | | | | |
| Cyclosporine | | | | | | | |
| Oil-based | Sandimmune<br>Generic | Oil-based formulation has unpredictable absorption secondary to need for emulsification by bile salts | Hepatic dysfunction:<br>Decrease dose by half and follow levers | 4–8 mg/kg per day in 2 divided doses | 1–2 mg/kg per day in 2 divided doses or as continuous infusion | Dosing is high early after transplantation and gradually decreases over time<br>Drugs that inhibit CYP-3A4 and p-GP may result in significantly higher levels<br>IV dose is 1/3–1/4 of oral dose<br>IV may be best administered in 2–6 h infusions | Abbott TDX assay most commonly used<br>CSA trough levels have been routinely used with levels of 300–350 ng/ml early postoperatively decreasing to 100–200 by 1 year<br>Levels at 2 h postdose appear to more accurately estimate area under the curve and may result in lower doses |
| Modified (oil-based formulation is not bioequivalent to modified preparation) | Neoral<br>Gengraf<br>Other generics | Modified for more predictable absorption<br>Both forms extensively metabolized by CYP-3A4 and are substrates and inhibitors of p-GP | | | | | |

(continued)

**Table 12.1** (continued)

| Drug | Trade name(s) | Pharmacology | Adjustment for renal/hepatic dysfunction | Dosing | | | Monitoring |
|---|---|---|---|---|---|---|---|
| | | | | Oral | Intravenous | Comments | |
| Tacrolimus | Prograf<br>Generic | Metabolized by CYP-3A4 and are substrates and inhibitors of p-GP | Follow levels for hepatic dysfun-ction | 0.05–0.1 mg/kg per day in 2 divided doses | 0.01–0.02 mg/kg per day in 2 divided doses or as continuous infusion | Doses are high early after transplantation and decrease over time<br>Drugs that inhibit CYP3A4 or p-GP may result in higher levels | Whole-blood levels of 10–15 ng/ml early after transplantation and 5–10 ng/ml by 1 year are targets |
| mTOR inhibitors | | | | | | | |
| Sirolimus | Rapamune | CYP-3A4 and p-GP substrate | ≤33% ↓ if hepatic dysfunction | × | | 2 mg/day in 1 dose (may be preceded by a single 6-mg loading dose) | Whole-blood trough levels of 4–15 ng/ml<br>Coadministration with CSA may increase CSA levels as much as 100%<br>Dose 4 h apart with CSA or tacrolimus |
| Everolimus | Zotress (US)<br>Certican (EU) | CYP-3A4 and p-GP substrate | ≤33% ↓ if hepatic dysfunction | × | | 0.75 mg BID | Therapeutic drug monitor is 3–8 ng/ml<br>Early renal insuf-ficiency seen when used with sd-CSA. rd-CSA recommended |

CNI, calcineurin inhibitor; CSA, cyclosporine; CYP, cytochrome P450; MMF, mycophenolate mofetil; p-GP, p-glycoprotein; rd-CSA, reduced-dose cyclosporine; sd-CSA, standardized-dose cyclosporine; TOR, target of rapamycin; TMPT, thiopurine methyltransferase. Reused with permission from JoAnn Lindenfeld, Geraldine G. Miller, Simon F. Shakar, Ronald Zolty, et al., Drug Therapy in the Heart Transplant Recipient: Part II: Immunosuppressive Drugs, Circulation, 110 (25), 3858–3865, https://doi.org/10.1161/01.CIR.0000150332.42276.69; American Heart Association.

**Table 12.2** Overview of major adverse effects of immunosuppressive drugs used in cardiac transplantation—listed by frequency scoring

| | Steroid | AZA | MMF | CSA | TAC | SIR | EVR |
|---|---|---|---|---|---|---|---|
| Potential for drug–drug interactions | 1 | 1 | 1 | 4 | 4 | 4 | 4 |
| Hypertension | 2 | | | 4 | 3 | 2 | |
| Diabetes | 3 | | | 1–2 | 2–3 | | |
| Obesity | 2 | | | | | | |
| Hyperlipidemia[a] | 2 | | | 3 | 3 | 3–4 | 3–4 |
| Renal insufficiency | | | | 3 | 3 | | 4[b] |
| Osteoporosis | 3 | | | 1–2 | 1–2 | | 1–2 |
| Avascular necrosis | 1 | | | | | | |
| Poor wound healing | 2 | | | | | 2[c] | 1–2 |
| Neurological minor tremors, paresthesias | | | | 3 | 3 | | |
| Neurological major seizures, cerebritis | | | | 1 | 1 | | |
| Hirsutism | 2 | | | 3 | | | |
| Alopecia | | 1 | | | 2 | | |
| Gingival hyperplasia | | | | 3 | | | |
| GI[d] | | 2 | 3 | 2 | 3 | 3 | 3 |
| Hepatic toxicity | | 2 | | 1 | 2 | 1 | 1 |
| Hypomagnesmia | | | | 3 | 3 | | |
| Hyperkalemia | | | | 2 | 2 | 2 | |
| Hyperuricemia | | | | 3 | 3 | 3 | |
| Anemia | | 2 | 3 | | | 3 | 3 |
| Thrombocytopenia | | 1 | 2 | | 3 | 3 | 3 |
| Neutropenia | | 3 | 3 | | | 3 | 3 |
| Cushingoid features | 3 | | | | | | |
| Cytokine release syndrome—mild | | | | | | | |
| Cytokine release syndrome—severe | | | | | | | |
| Serum sickness | | | | | | | |

AZA, azithoprine; CSA, cyclosporine; EVR, everolimus; GI, gastrointestinal; MMF, mycophenolate mofetil; SIR, sirolimus; TAC, tacrolimus

1, rare (<5%); 2, common (5–15%); 3, very common; 4, most patients

a. Hyperlipidemia defined as: (↑ total cholesterol, ↑↑LDL cholesterol, ↑ triglycerides) (16–50%)

b. When used concomitantly with cyclosporine

c. Wound healing (especially early after operation), >50%

d. GI problems: diarrhea, nausea, vomiting

Reused with permission from JoAnn Lindenfeld, Geraldine G. Miller, Simon F. Shakar, Ronald Zolty, et al., Drug Therapy in the Heart Transplant Recipient: Part II: Immunosuppressive Drugs, Circulation, 110 (25), 3858–3865, https://doi.org/10.1161/01.CIR.0000150332.42276.69; American Heart Association

most effective. This section will cover the most commonly used immunosuppressive agents in maintenance regimens.

## Corticosteroids

Corticosteroids, or simply steroids, are among the first immunosuppressive agents ever used in clinical transplantation, and, to this day, remain a cornerstone of post-transplant management. They exert potent immunosuppressive and anti-inflammatory effects. Uniquely, they play a major role in the induction phase immediately post-transplant, during maintenance, and as part of anti-rejection regimens. While highly effective for the prevention and treatment of acute rejection, their long-term use is associated with a number of adverse effects. For this reason, many centers attempt to wean prednisone, the most commonly used maintenance steroid, by 12 months post-transplant except for multi-organ transplant recipients or those with certain etiologies of their original cardiomyopathy, like sarcoidosis or giant cell myocarditis [4].

### Mechanism of Action

Corticosteroids act by altering the transcriptional regulation of multiple genes that affect leukocytes (T and B lymphocytes, granulocytes, macrophages, and monocytes) as well as endothelial cell function [5]. The major effect on lymphocytes is mediated by inhibition of the transcription factor activator protein 1 and nuclear factor kappa B (NF-kB), which negatively affect the expression of several genes, including those controlling cytokine production, growth factors, and adhesion molecules. Furthermore, steroids cause a decrease in the production of vasoactive/chemoattractant factors and lipolytic/proteolytic enzymes in non-lymphoid cells. Downstream, this results in inhibition of neutrophil adhesion to endothelial cells, prevention of macrophage differentiation, and down-regulation of endothelial function. Glucocorticoids also exert their anti-inflammatory effects through inducing the release of lipocortin, which acts by inhibiting phospholipase A2, in turn suppressing the production of prostaglandins and leukotrienes [6, 7].

### Adverse Effects

While effective at preventing rejection, steroids are associated with a significant number of long-term adverse effects. Hypertension, poor wound healing, gastric ulcers, emotional lability, cataracts, and proximal myopathy are all associated with corticosteroid therapy. Furthermore, cosmetic side effects such as hirsutism, acne, moon facies, easy bruising, skin fragility, "buffalo hump," and truncal obesity may also occur. From a metabolic point of view, hyperlipidemia, salt and water retention, diabetes mellitus, osteopenia, and growth retardation in children may result [6, 8]. If high-dose steroids are administered long-term, chronic adrenal suppression may result (via negative feedback mechanisms). Adrenal insufficiency may also follow a steroid taper or physiologic "stress" (illness, surgical procedures, infections).

## Calcineurin Inhibitors: Cyclosporine and Tacrolimus

The calcineurin inhibitors (CNIs), which include cyclosporine and tacrolimus, have become cornerstones of maintenance immunosuppressive therapy for transplant patients. Cyclosporine is a lipophilic undecapeptide which was initially isolated from the fungus Tolypocladium inflatum. The discovery of cyclosporine and subsequent use in HTx in the late 1970s enabled survival rates to drastically improve. Tacrolimus, in contrast, was more recently discovered in 1987 and only since the late 2000s has it become widely used in HTx patients. Tacrolimus is a macrolide and is produced by the fungus Streptomyces usukubaensis; it has a very similar mode of action to cyclosporine and is frequently used as an alternative to it.

### Mechanism of Action

Cyclosporine and tacrolimus both function by blocking calcium-activated calcineurin (Fig. 12.1) [9, 10]. The agents are able to enter cells through diffusion and bind to different immunophilins: cyclosporine binds to cyclophilin and tacrolimus to FK binding protein-12 (FKBP-12). This drug-immunophilin complex proceeds to bind to calcineurin, a phosphatase that dephosphorylates multiple molecules, including nuclear factor of activated T cells (NF-AT). In turn, dephosphorylated NF-AT translocates to the nucleus, where it binds to specific DNA sites in the promoter regions of several cytokine genes, including interleukin (IL)-2. Through this series of actions, cyclosporine and tacrolimus inhibit transcription of IL-2 and other cytokines, tumor necrosis factor alpha (TNF-a), granulocyte–macrophage colony-stimulating factor, and interferon-gamma [11]. In a mechanism specific to cyclosporine, transforming growth factor-ß (TGF-ß) production is also stimulated, augmenting its immunosuppressive activity [12]. Furthermore, cyclosporine has been found to suppress delayed-type hypersensitivity skin reactions to tuberculin in guinea-pigs but appeared have no effects on antibody synthesis, suggesting a mechanism of immunosuppression specific to T cells.

## Notes

Cyclosporine is available as oil-based or microemulsion formulations, as well as intravenous solution (for post-operative administration). Due to an improved pharmacokinetic profile and clinical data, microemulsion preparations are generally preferred over the older oil-based formulations [13]. Indeed, randomized studies comparing the two demonstrated similar survival at 2 years, but lower rates of treated rejection in the microemulsion group [14–16]. Furthermore, the microemulsion formulation exhibited better tolerance and fewer discontinuations, and allowed lower average doses of corticosteroids compared to the oil-based formulation.

Tacrolimus has become the most widely used CNI in recent years, preferred over cyclosporine. There is evidence from uncontrolled studies that tacrolimus results in lower rates of rejection and fewer adverse effects as compared to cyclosporine [17–19]. While there is no demonstrated difference in post-transplant survival between tacrolimus and oil-based cyclosporine [20, 21], randomized controlled trials show patients on tacrolimus display lower moderate-severe cellular rejection rates at 6 months compared to those on microemulsion cyclosporine [22]. Despite this, tacrolimus patients have been noted to display a higher incidence of de novo diabetes mellitus compared to microemulsion cyclosporine.

## Adverse Effects

While not an adverse effect per se, cyclosporine treatment has been previously noted to mask the clinical signs and symptoms of acute allograft rejection, making endomyocardial biopsy essential for rejection surveillance.

Cyclosporine is also noted to cause acute or chronic dose-related nephrotoxicity, with the possible sequelae of arteriolar sclerosis and tubulo-interstitial fibrosis (see Table 12.2). In most patients, hypertension and hyperlipidemia tend to occur [23] and the development of de novo diabetes mellitus is fairly common. Electrolyte abnormalities are common, especially hyperkalemia, but are rarely life-threatening if renal function remains intact. Hypertrichosis, which occurs in at least 50% of patients, and gingival hyperplasia are side effects seen with cyclosporine. Neurotoxic symptoms may also occur; such manifestations include tremor, paresthesias, headache, seizures, mental status changes, visual symptoms, and insomnia. Other possible side effects include nausea, vomiting, cholestasis/cholelithiasis, and long-term, may accelerate the development of osteoporosis (especially in combination with corticosteroids).

Tacrolimus has been noted to exhibit a similar side effect profile to cyclosporine, although the incidence of hyperlipidemia and hypertension are reduced (see Table 12.2) [20], while the incidence of hyperglycemia and neurotoxicity is relatively increased. There is some evidence to suggest that the onset of diabetes may be more common when tacrolimus is given with azathioprine compared to mycophenolate mofetil [24].

**Table 12.3** Overview of common calcineurin inhibitor drug interactions in cardiac transplantation

| Drugs that increase cyclosporine/tacrolimus levels | Drugs that decrease cyclosporine/tacrolimus Levels | Drugs that enhance nephrotoxicity |
|---|---|---|
| Calcium channel blockers: diltiazem, verapamil, nifedipine, nicardipine | Antibiotics: nafcillin and rifampin | Antibiotics: aminoglycosides, vancomycin, trimethoprim-sulfamethoxazole |
| Antibiotics: erythromycin, clarithromycin, doxycycline (cyclosporine only) | Anticonvulsants: phenytoin, phenobarbital, carbamazepine | NSAIDs: all formulations, colchicine |
| Antifungal: ketoconazole, voriconazole, fluconazole | Miscellaneous: *hypericum perforatum*, ticlopidine (cyclosporine only), cholestyramine | Antifungals: amphotericin B |
| GI agents: metoclopramide, cimetidine, omeprazole | | GI agents: cimetidine, ranitidine |
| HIV protease inhibitors | | Antivirals: aciclovir |
| Miscellaneous: amiodarone, allopurinol, grapefruit, grapefruit juice, methylprednisolone | | Antineoplastics: cisplatin |

*Abbreviations* GI: gastrointestinal; HIV: human immunodeficiency virus; NSAIDs: non-steroidal anti-inflammatory drugs



Care must be taken in specific demographic groups, such as African-Americans and females, with regard to high tacrolimus doses and hyperglycemia [25]. In contrast to the side effect profile seen with cyclosporine, hirsutism, and gingival hypertrophy do not occur with tacrolimus. But, alopecia may be a side effect of tacrolimus. Tacrolimus is frequently used as a substitute for cyclosporine when cyclosporine-related toxic effects occur; the converse is also applicable to tacrolimus-related toxic effects [25].

### Drug Interactions

The calcineurin inhibitors and proliferation signal inhibitors are extensively metabolized by the cytochrome P-450 3A4 enzyme pathway in the liver; as a result, their blood levels are affected by drugs that induce or inhibit this pathway. As a result, the nephrotoxic effects of CNIs may be enhanced. The interactions may occur with very commonly used drugs; as such, constant attention is required and vigilance as to potential interactions, and utmost care should be taken when introducing new drugs. Table 12.3 summarizes the potential interactions of CNIs with common, everyday medications. It should also be noted that cyclosporine, but not tacrolimus, inhibits P-glycoprotein membrane transporters that affect the metabolism of certain statins [26, 27].

## Antiproliferative

An antiproliferative agent is usually used in current immunosuppressive regimens; azathioprine and mycophenolate mofetil (MMF) are the most commonly used. Early immunosuppressive protocols in the 1970s used azathioprine with prednisone, with relatively poor 1-year survival of 60–65% and 5-year actuarial survival of 35–40% [28, 29]. The introduction of cyclosporine significantly improved survival and somewhat relegated the role of azathioprine to that of an adjunctive agent; with the introduction of MMF in the 1990s, azathioprine has further fallen out of favor.

## Azathioprine

### Mechanism of Action

Azathioprine is a prodrug that is hydrolyzed rapidly in the blood to 6-mercaptopurine, which is subsequently converted to thioinosine monophosphate, a purine analog that is its active metabolite (Fig. 12.1). This purine analog is incorporated into DNA, thereby inhibiting its synthesis and the consequent proliferation of both T and B lymphocytes.

### Adverse Effects

The major side effects of azathioprine are hematologic, and hence, complete blood counts should be regularly monitored. Myelosuppressive adverse effects, including leukopenia, anemia, and thrombocytopenia (see Table 12.2), may occur. Generally dose-dependent, these events typically resolve after 7–10 days with dose reduction. More rarely, pancreatitis, hepatitis, and hepatic veno-occlusive disease may also occur.

## Mycophenolate Mofetil (MMF)

### Mechanism of Action

MMF is a reversible inhibitor of inosine monophosphate dehydrogenase, a crucial enzyme in the de novo synthesis of guanine nucleotides. Proliferating lymphocytes are dependent on this pathway because it is their only pathway for purine synthesis and DNA replication. In contrast, other cells use both de novo and salvage pathways for purine synthesis. Therefore, MMF is a more selective inhibitor of lymphocyte proliferation than azathioprine. In vivo and in vitro, mycophenolic acid blocks the proliferation of T and B cells, inhibits antibody formation, and inhibits the generation of cytotoxic T cells [30]. Furthermore, MMF down-regulates the expression of adhesion molecules on lymphocytes.

### Notes

MMF is largely preferred over azathioprine due to its reduced adverse effect profile combined with superior efficacy in maintaining survival and preventing rejection. In a multi-center, active-controlled, randomized trial [31], MMF was compared with azathioprine when used in conjunction with cyclosporine and corticosteroids in 650 de novo HTx recipients. Because an intravenous form of the study drug was not available at the time of the trial, 11% of the patients withdrew before receiving the drug. Survival and rejection were similar in both groups when analyzed in an intention-to-treatment manner. However, among treated patients, MMF was associated with a significant reduction in both mortality (6 vs. 11%, $p=0.031$) and in the incidence of treatable rejection (66 vs. 74%, $p=0.026$) at one year. These findings are supported by retrospective data from the International Society for Heart and Lung Transplantation (ISHLT) Thoracic Registry [32], which find significantly superior actuarial 1 and 3-year survival in MMF patients compared to azathioprine patients. (1 year, 96 vs. 93%; 3 year, 91 vs. 86%; $p=0.0012$). MMF has also been demonstrated to be effective in reversing recurrent rejection when used in place of azathioprine [33, 34]. In patients with chronic renal dysfunction, switching from azathioprine to MMF in combination with cyclosporine reduction or withdrawal to improve renal function has also been employed as an effective strategy [33].

### Adverse Effects

MMF is considerably less myelosuppressive than azathioprine and is usually well tolerated (see Table 12.2). The most common side effects include nausea, vomiting, and diarrhea, which usually respond to dose adjustment. Mychophenolate sodium is an alternate formulation of mycophenolate that is enteric coated and delayed release, thus improving the upper gastroenintestinal tolerability [19]. There is some data to suggest that the risk of opportunistic infections may be higher in patients on MMF compared with azathioprine [31].

## Proliferation Signal Inhibitors (PSIs): Sirolimus and Everolimus

The proliferation signal inhibitors include sirolimus and everolimus. Sirolimus is a natural product of the actinomycete Streptomyces hygroscopicus [35, 36]. Like tacrolimus, sirolimus is a macrolide antibiotic and is structurally related. Everolimus is an analog of sirolimus, with a shorter half-life and identical mechanism of action to sirolimus. The proliferation signal inhibitors may be considered in select patients with cardiac allograft vasculopathy, malignancy, or renal dysfunction.

### Mechanism of Action

Sirolimus and everolimus bind to the same family of immunophilins as tacrolimus, the FKBPs, but instead of blocking calcineurin-dependent T-cell activation, the resultant complex inhibits a key regulatory kinase; mammalian target of rapamycin (mTOR) (Fig. 12.1). mTOR phosphorylates proteins that play a vital role in cell cycle regulation. In turn, connecting signals from the growth factor receptors to the cell nucleus stimulate growth and proliferation of T and B lymphocytes [37, 38]. In this way, sirolimus/everolimus is able to specifically inhibit cell division. Notably, sirolimus has also been noted to inhibit arterial smooth muscle and endothelial cell growth via inhibition of mTOR; this has translated to reduced allograft atherosclerosis in animal models [39, 40].

### Notes

Sirolimus, which was discovered before everolimus, has been shown to effectively inhibit acute graft rejection and treat refractory acute graft rejection in HTx recipients [39]. In randomized, open-label clinical trials, sirolimus has demonstrated reduced rejection compared to azathioprine, though with similar mortality [41]. Furthermore, sirolimus has been shown to decrease the development of cardiac allograft vasculopathy (CAV), as assessed by intravascular ultrasound (IVUS) at 6 months; the benefit was maintained at 2 years [41]. In existing patients with CAV, sirolimus was also demonstrated to slow the progression of CAV as per angiography [42]. Interestingly, sirolimus has also been noted for its antitumor effects; a useful quality in a field where a major cause of death after transplant is malignancy. In a recent study, the switch from cyclosporine to sirolimus in renal transplant recipients who subsequently developed Kaposi's sarcoma was shown to reduce tumor burden significantly [43].

Clinical trials involving everolimus have also demonstrated largely positive results. In a randomized double-blind prospective 634 patient three-arm trial that compared everolimus (1.5 or 3 mg) to azathioprine [44], significantly less patients on everolimus reached the 6-month composite endpoint of death, graft loss or retransplantation, loss to follow-up, biopsy-proven severe acute rejection, or rejection with hemodynamic compromise (36.4 and 27.0%, compared to 46.0%). Furthermore, a decrease in the development of CAV, as assessed by IVUS at 12 months, was observed in the everolimus groups compared to those on azathioprine. These study results are further supported by a clinical trial of 721 patients [45] which found no difference between everolimus and MMF in 2-year survival and rejection, and actually found a favorable effect of everolimus in reducing CAV compared to MMF [46]. Interestingly, the rates of cytomegalovirus (CMV) infection have been noted to be significantly lower in everolimus patients compared to azathioprine.

### Adverse Effects

When administered alone, sirolimus/everolimus are not noted to adversely affect renal function. Data from clinical trials shows that everolimus with low-dose cyclosporine has been shown not to worsen [47] and may even improve renal function when compared to standard-dose cyclosporine with MMF—a finding supported in multiple prospective studies [45, 47–50], including the NOCTET study by Gullestad et al. and the SCHEDULE trial, which showed regular everolimus with no cyclosporine (with MMF) to be superior to cyclosporine with MMF for renal function. In the MANDELA study, both everolimus with reduced CNI and everolimus as part of a CNI-free regimen improved and stabilized renal function by estimated GFR (moreso in the CNI-free group) [51]. However, in both the SCHEDULE and MANDELA studies (both CNI-free studies), there were more asymptomatic rejection episodes but no impact on survival. While potent effective immunosuppressive drugs, use of proliferation signal inhibitors following HTx has remained limited because of evidence from clinical trials regarding worsening CNI nephrotoxicity, delayed wound healing and dehiscence, and increased infection [52, 53]. Furthermore, data from the everolimus versus MMF trial showed an increased mortality from infection in the patient group with high-dose everolimus (3.0 mg) [45]. Other major adverse effects of the proliferation signal inhibitors include hyperlipidemia, hypertriglyceridemia with increased LDL cholesterol, mouth ulceration, deep venous thrombosis, proteinuria, and more rarely, thrombocytopenia, neutropenia, and anemia (see Table 12.2) [54–58]. Rarely, cases of noninfectious pneumonitis have been reported with sirolimus [54].

Hypercholesterolemia, hypertriglyceridemia, thrombocytopenia and mouth ulcers are generally at least partially responsive to dose reduction [54]. PSI-induced hyperlipidemia also responds to conventional treatment with HMG-CoA reductase inhibitors (statins) and fibric acid derivatives (fibrates) [59].

### Drug Interactions

It must be noted that interactions with sirolimus/everolimus and statins or fibrates may occur as a result of competitive metabolism via CYP3A [60]. Thus, heightened awareness is necessary for potential hepatic and muscular toxicity when combining statins or fibrates with sirolimus/everolimus. In a microcosm of immunosuppression, the risk of hyperlipidemia must be balanced against the powerful anti-atherogenic effects.

### Statins

The use of statins post-cardiac transplant is now widespread and will be discussed in Chap. 13. They are typically initiated a week or two after transplant.

## Major Clinical Trials of Maintenance Immunosuppression Regimens—Which Agent to Use?

Part of the reason that there remains no standardized protocol for immunosuppression is a lack of available evidence. Indeed, relatively few HTx procedures occur per year, thus limiting the number of randomized clinical trials available to inform treatment decisions. Consequently, the majority of ISHLT guideline recommendations are class IIa or IIb and based on level B or C evidence [61]. The most commonly used regimen consists of a triple therapy regimen, consisting of a corticosteroid, calcineurin inhibitor, and antiproliferative agent.

Typical major study endpoints of clinical trials of immunosuppression in HTx have included the following, either alone or in combination: survival, rejection, CAV, and adverse events. While survival is the most important endpoint, the low population typical of HTx studies means that most studies are not powered to demonstrate a mortality benefit. However, the clinical endpoints of rejection, CAV, and adverse events, which studies are often powered to detect differences in, are noted to either indirectly or directly affect mortality, morbidity, and quality of life and thus are considered clinically reasonable endpoints for the purposes of comparison.

Survival appears to be largely comparable in all the randomized clinical trials of immunosuppressants in HTx, and in any case, these studies were not powered to demonstrate survival difference. The other clinical endpoints of rejection, CAV, and adverse events have revealed differences between immunosuppressive regimens across several trials. The major randomized clinical trials of immunosuppressive therapy in HTx are summarized in Table 12.4 [19–22, 31, 41, 44, 45, 47, 50, 62–65].

## Comparison by Survival

Clinical trials have not demonstrated differences in survival among the various immunosuppressive regimens, primarily due to inadequate statistical power. There is, however, one notable exception; in a multicenter clinical trial of MMF compared to azathioprine, a treated-patient analysis demonstrated significant 1-year survival benefit for patients on MMF [31]. In this case, the intent-to-treat analysis was severely skewed by unusually high rates of perioperative mortality in the MMF group that occurred by chance, with patients having been randomized before transplant. Since this trial, and other subsequent trials confirming a benefit to MMF in not just survival but also CAV [66], MMF has become the antiproliferative of choice over azathioprine. Nevertheless, the randomized clinical trials comparing cyclosporine to tacrolimus [17, 18, 22], everolimus to MMF [45], sirolimus to MMF, sirolimus to azathioprine [41], and everolimus to azathioprine [44] have not shown a survival benefit.

## Comparison by Incidence of Rejection

Several immunosuppressive agents have been shown to decrease the incidence of rejection (Table 12.4). However, it must be noted that many of these trials assessing the efficacy of MMF [31], everolimus [44] and sirolimus [41] used azathioprine as the comparator, which itself has fallen out of favor—thus making the comparison less clinically useful. Nevertheless, more recent clinical trials for everolimus have used MMF as a comparator, including the large multicenter everolimus versus MMF trial [45].

A large 2006 European multicenter trial comparing tacrolimus to cyclosporine reported by Grimm et al. [22] revealed a significantly lower rejection rate at 6 months for tacrolimus compared to cyclosporine (both in combination with azathioprine). More recently, a three-arm trial compared regimens of tacrolimus/MMF, tacrolimus/sirolimus, and cyclosporine/MMF [19] (all in combination with corticosteroids) and found that both the tacrolimus regimens had significantly less treated rejection at 6 months than the regimen with cyclosporine/MMF. Furthermore, tacrolimus/MMF when compared only to cyclosporine/MMF had significantly lower incidences of cellular rejection (ISHLT grade > 3A/2R) and any treated rejections.

Therefore, the overall rejection data from the clinical trials suggest that tacrolimus-based regimens may have benefit over cyclosporine-based regimens (class IIb/level B of evidence) [19, 21]. Regarding specific combinations, comparisons of the contemporary immunosuppressive combination regimens of tacrolimus/MMF and cyclosporine/MMF suggest that tacrolimus/MMF may have benefit over cyclosporine/MMF for preventing rejection (class IIb/level B of evidence). Everolimus with reduced-dose cyclosporine has not been compared to tacrolimus/MMF in a randomized trial.

However, the relative advantage of tacrolimus-based therapy for rejection is balanced by an increased incidence of diabetes. Furthermore, the tacrolimus/sirolimus-treated patients in this three-arm trial had lower rejection but increased nephrotoxic events and impaired wound healing, rendering this regimen less desirable compared with tacrolimus/MMF [19].

A 721-patient multicenter clinical trial in 2013 compared everolimus to MMF; specifically, reduced dose everolimus 1.5 mg with reduced-dose cyclosporine was found to be no different to MMF with standard-dose cyclosporine in terms of 1 and 2-year biopsy-proven acute rejection, although 3-month mortality was found to be higher in everolimus patients who had undergone induction [45]. Other studies comparing everolimus with low-dose cyclosporine to MMF (with or without low-dose cyclosporine) also demonstrated no difference in rates of rejection compared to MMF [48, 49]. However, a Scandinavian trial investigating

**Table 12.4** Overview of results from major randomized multicenter clinical trials comparing efficacy of immunosuppressive drugs in cardiac transplantation [19–22, 31, 41, 44, 45, 47, 50, 62–65]

| Study | *n* | Follow-up | Survival | Rejection | CAV by IVUS | Renal function | Infections | Cholesterol and triglycerides | Hypertension | Hematologic | GI disorders | Other |
|---|---|---|---|---|---|---|---|---|---|---|---|---|
| Kobashigawa et al. 1998 MMF versus AZA [31] | 650 | 3 yrs | *MMF = higher survival | MMF = less rejection | NS; **MMF = less CAV at 1 year | | MMF = more any opportunistic infection | | | AZA = more leukopenia | MMF = more diarrhea and esophagitis | NS for hyperglycemia treatment |
| Reichart et al. 1998 TAC versus CSA [21] | 82 | 1 yr | NS | NS | | NS | NS | | CSA = more hypertension | | | NS for glucose intolerance |
| Taylor et al. 1999 TAC versus CSA [20] | 85 | 1 yr | NS | NS | | NS | NS | CSA = higher chol and tri | CSA = more hypertension | NS | | |
| Eisen et al. 2003 EVR versus AZA [44] | 634 | 1 yr | NS | EVR groups = less rejection | EVR groups = less CAV | EVR groups = worse renal function | EVR groups = lower viral/CMV but more bacterial infections | EVR groups = higher chol and tri | NS | NS | NS | NS for wound infection |
| Keogh et al. 2004 SIR versus AZA [41] | 136 | 2 yrs | NS | SIR groups = less rejection at 6 months | SIR groups = less CAV | SIR groups = worse renal function | SIR groups = lower CMV but more pneumonia | NS for chol; SIR groups = higher trig | NS | SIR groups = more anemia and thrombocytopenia | AZA = more nausea SIR groups = more diarrhea | AZA = more arrhythmia and atrial fibrillation; SIR groups = more mouth ulcers and abnormal healing |
| Grimm et al. (2006) TAC versus CSA [22] | 314 | 1.5 yr | NS | TAC = less rejection at 6 months | | NS | NS | CSA = higher chol and triglycerides | CSA = more hypertension | TAC = more anemia | CYA = more cholelithiasis | TAC = more diabetes mellitus and tremor; CSA = more gum hyperplasia and hirsutism |

(continued)

**Table 12.4** (continued)

| Study | *n* | Follow-up | Survival | Rejection | CAV by IVUS | Renal function | Infections | Cholesterol and triglycerides | Hypertension | Hematologic | GI disorders | Other |
|---|---|---|---|---|---|---|---|---|---|---|---|---|
| Kobashigawa et al. (2006) TAC/MMF versus TAC/SIR versus CSA/MMF [19] | 343 | 1 yr | NS | NS; TAC groups = lower any treated rejection | | TAC/MMF = best renal function | TAC/SIR = lower viral but more fungal infections | NS for chol TAC/MMF = lower trig | NS | NS | | TAC/SIR = more insulin therapy and impaired wound healing; NS for diabetes mellitus |
| Baran et al. 2007 TAC/MMF versus TAC [63] | 58 | 1 yr | NS | NS | NS | NS | TAC/MMF = more hospitalized infections | | | NS | | NS for malignancy |
| Lehmkuhl et al. 2008 EVR/rd-CSA versus MMFsd-CSA [47] | 176 | 1 yr | NS | NS | | NS | EVR = Less CMV infections | | | MMF = more leukopenia | | |
| Baran et al. 2011 TAC/MMF versus TAC alone [64] | 150 | 5 yrs | NS | NS | NS | NS; TAC alone group = numerically better renal function | TAC/MMF = more hospitalized infections | | | TAC alone = higher mean white blood cell count, but not clinically meaningful | | |
| Eisen et al. 2013 EVR-CSA versus MMF-CSA [45] | 721 | 2yrs | NS | EVR groups = numerically more rejection | EVR groups = less CAV | EVR groups = worse renal function | EVR = Less CMV infections | EVR groups = higher chol and triglycerides | NS | NS | NS | EVR 3.0mg high dose = higher overall rate of discontinuation due to increased mortality |

(continued)

**Table 12.4** (continued)

| Study | $n$ | Follow-up | Survival | Rejection | CAV by IVUS | Renal function | Infections | Cholesterol and triglycerides | Hypertension | Hematologic | GI disorders | Other |
|---|---|---|---|---|---|---|---|---|---|---|---|---|
| Andreassen et al. 2014 EVR-rd-CSA followed by EVR only (early CSA withdrawal) versus MMF-CSA [50, 65] | 115 | 3yrs*** | NS | More mild rejection in EVR only group, but no difference after 1 year | EVR group-less CAV | EVR group-better renal function | EVR-numerically more infections | EVR groups = higher chol and trigly-cerides | NS | NS | | |
| Barten et al. 2019 EVR-MMF-steroids (CNI-free) versus EVR-rd-CNI-MMF-ste-roids [51] | 162 | 1 yr | NS | EVR-rd-CNI-MMF-ste-roids = less rejection | | CNI-free—better renal function | CNI-free—less infections, inclu-ding CMV | NS | EVR-rd-CNI-MMF-ste-roids—more hypertension | NS | EVR-rd-CNI-MMF-ste-roids = more diarrhea | |

* Treated-patient population (see text)

** Reanalysis of MMF IVUS data

*** Subsequent 3-year follow up study, published 2016

CAV, cardiac allograft vasculopathy; CYA, cyclosporine; EVL, everolimus; EVL/rd, everolimus/reduced exposure; IVUS, intravascular ultrasound; MMF, mycophenolate mofetil; MMFsd, mycophenolate mofetil/standard exposure; NS, not statistically significant; SRL, sirolimus; TAC, tacrolimus.

low-dose everolimus with early cyclosporine withdrawal followed by regular everolimus dosing compared to standard cyclosporine therapy (both groups with MMF and steroids) showed higher asymptomatic rejection in the everolimus group, further supporting the notion that caution is required in the early initiation of everolimus [50]. The EVERHEART study demonstrated that delayed everolimus initiation avoided adverse events (via a primary composite safety endpoint) without compromising efficacy [67].

## Comparison by Effect on Cardiac Allograft Vasculopathy (CAV)

In many of the randomized trials of immunosuppression, CAV as an endpoint has been assessed through the use of IVUS assessment at 1-year post-transplant compared to baseline. Prior studies have established that an increase of 0.5 mm or more in maximal intimal thickness on coronary IVUS within the first year after HTx, is associated with a significantly increased risk of 5-year all-cause death, myocardial infarction, and the subsequent development of angiographic severe CAV. Thus, IVUS has served as a surrogate endpoint for CAV in subsequent immunosuppression trials. Furthermore, IVUS is increasingly used to identify patients at high risk for future cardiovascular events, and may aid in allowing therapeutic adjustment of immunosuppression [68]. Several of the recent randomized immunosuppressive trials including the MMF versus azathioprine [31], everolimus versus azathioprine [44] and sirolimus versus azathioprine [41] trials demonstrated benefit compared to azathioprine in the first-year IVUS results, with a lower incidence of patients developing CAV as defined by an increase of 0.5 mm or more in maximal intimal thickness on coronary IVUS within the first year after HTx.

The MMF versus azathioprine study showed benefit in CAV retardation using a threshold for first-year change in maximum intimal thickness greater than 0.3 mm, but at 0.5 mm significant benefit was no longer seen. The sirolimus versus azathioprine study [41] showed benefit for sirolimus therapy using the usual 0.5 mm threshold; however, patients were studied at baseline and at 6 months, not 12, after HTx, making IVUS less useful for predictions of subsequent CAV. Nevertheless, in a randomized study of cardiac transplant patients with established CAV, sirolimus has been demonstrated to slow disease progression as determined by angiography (not IVUS) [42].

In particular, the everolimus studies have been the clearest in demonstrating a benefit in CAV retardation over azathioprine and MMF. In the everolimus versus azathioprine trial, this was demonstrated using several IVUS parameters (intimal volume, intimal area, intimal index in addition to maximal intimal thickness > 0.5 mm) [44]. Additionally, in the multicenter trial comparing 1.5 mg everolimus as compared to standard MMF, there was significantly reduced proportion of patients on everolimus with CAV as defined by IVUS [45]. Furthermore, while not a direct comparison against MMF, the CAV benefits of everolimus are further supported by IVUS data from a Scandinavian trial investigating low-dose everolimus with early cyclosporine withdrawal followed by regular everolimus dosing compared to standard cyclosporine therapy (both groups with MMF and steroids), which show a lower incidence of 12-month > 0.5 mm increase in maximal intimal thickness in the everolimus group [65].

Thus, there is considerable evidence for CAV benefit with MMF, everolimus and sirolimus over azathioprine, and thus these drugs should be considered for inclusion (class IIb, level B) [41, 44, 66]. There is also strong evidence to suggest that everolimus is superior to MMF for CAV retardation [45]. However, there remain concerns with safety, regarding renal dysfunction for everolimus/sirolimus when combined with standard-dose cyclosporine, and thus caution should be exercised; with low-dose cyclosporine, everolimus appears safer in this regard [48–50]. Furthermore, the use of 0.5 mm change in maximal intimal thickness on 12-month IVUS as a surrogate for subsequent CAV and poor outcomes is only strictly applicable to the everolimus versus azathioprine and everolimus versus

MMF studies. Overall, the value of everolimus in retarding allograft vasculopathy appears superior to the competition, but this must be balanced against its negative aspects.

## Comparison by Adverse Effect Profile

While survival, rejection data and CAV data are comparable amongst the newer agents of MMF, everolimus and sirolimus, adverse events are often the deciding factor regarding the choice to use a specific drug regimen for a certain patient.

Regarding everolimus/sirolimus, the inferior renal function seen when in combination with standard-dose cyclosporine, along with other side effects of hyperlipidemia, edema and impaired wound healing and greater risk of infection, must be considered when seeking to use this combination. Sirolimus is also noted to cause significantly higher rates of anemia, thrombocytopenia, diarrhea and mouth ulceration. There appears to be a general trend for significantly increased serious adverse events in trials comparing everolimus, without affecting the primary endpoint [49, 50, 65]. Nevertheless, from a renal standpoint, the use of everolimus in more recent trials with reduced or even withdrawn cyclosporine has demonstrated either comparable or improved renal function, compared to MMF with standard-dose cyclosporine [45, 49, 50, 69].

Evidence from other, nonrandomized studies has also demonstrated that conversion from CNI-based immunosuppression to sirolimus-based immunosuppression results in improved renal function [70, 71]. A recent multicenter randomized trial demonstrated that conversion to CNI-free immunosuppression (MMF, sirolimus) was superior to CNI-reduced immunosuppression in improving renal failure in late HTx recipients (average 5 years post-transplant) with renal insufficiency [72].

Other side effects must also be considered: Patients on cyclosporine had higher cholesterol and triglyceride levels, and more hypertension, cholelithiasis, hirsutism, and gum hyperplasia than tacrolimus-treated patients [19–21]. However, tacrolimus-treated patients had more diabetes mellitus, tremor, and anemia than cyclosporine-treated patients. When comparing the regimen of tacrolimus/MMF compared to tacrolimus/sirolimus and cyclosporine/MMF had the best renal function and lowest triglyceride levels [19]. However, the tacrolimus/sirolimus group had a higher incidence of poor wound healing and the most patients on insulin therapy.

Overall, sirolimus/everolimus is often preferred in patients with CAV, but are generally not used in the first few months due to the drug leading to poor wound healing, increased infection risk, potentiating the calcineurin inhibitor nephrotoxic effects, and propensity for other adverse events and side effects.

## Individualizing Immunosuppression

Caution should be exercised in the interpretation of the aforementioned trials. The most appropriate dose of the medications is unknown, so outcomes in clinical trials may be affected by different doses. Adverse effects may result from a drug interaction within a combination (e.g. tacrolimus with sirolimus) rather than a drug by itself. Additionally, randomized clinical trials tend to include a lower risk population with many exclusion criteria (to exclude high risk patients) including renal dysfunction, older age, and pre-sensitized patients. Nevertheless, even taking these concerns into account, there are important findings that can be taken from the results of the randomized clinical trials and applied to our practice.

The adverse events observed for specific drugs and combinations in the randomized clinical trials further support need for individualization of immunosuppression. For example, patients with high risk for CMV infection might benefit from everolimus- or sirolimus-based immunosuppression; patients with gingival hyperplasia from a tacrolimus-based regimen; patients with pre-existing diabetes or excess tremors/peripheral neuropathy from a cyclosporine-based regimen. The adverse events listed in Table 12.4 (along with the results of the clinical trials) can be used to determine what immunosuppressive drugs would best serve patients with specific characteristics in the selection of a particular immunosuppression regimen.

Immunosuppression protocols vary by program, and selection of specific agents and combinations is generally based on that center's experience and their interpretation of randomized clinical trials in the literature. As immunosuppressive regimens continue to evolve with newer drugs becoming available, the choice of immunosuppression in HTx will change, depending on the results of future immunosuppressive randomized clinical trials.

## Conclusions

Advancements in immunosuppression have allowed HTx to become the gold standard therapy for end-stage heart failure. Comparisons of specific immunosuppression regimens have been limited by selection bias in retrospective analyses given distinct adverse event profiles of the different drugs and low statistical power in randomized clinical trials. Understanding the immune system and how to precisely manipulate the immune response is critical to allow for further breakthroughs in the field of transplantation.

## References


1. Caves PK, Stinson EB, Griepp RB, Rider AK, Dong E, Shumway NE. Results of 54 cardiac transplants. Surgery. 1973;74(2):307–14.
2. Stehlik J, Edwards LB, Kucheryavaya AY, Benden C, Christie JD, Dobbels F, et al. The registry of the International Society for Heart and Lung Transplantation: twenty-eighth adult heart transplant report—2011. J Heart Lung Transplant. 2011;30(10):1078–94.
3. Penn I. Post-transplant malignancy: the role of immunosuppression. Drug Saf. 2000;23(2):101–13.
4. Chang DH, Youn JC, Dilibero D, Patel JK, Kobashigawa JA. Heart transplant immunosuppression strategies at cedars-sinai medical center. Int J Heart Fail. 2021;3(1):15.
5. Cohen DJ. Action, efficacy and toxicities: corticosteroids. In: Primer on Transplantation. Mt Laurel, NJ: American Society of Transplantation; 2001. p. 146–51.
6. Kirklin JK. Immunosuppressive modalities. Heart Transplant. 2002.
7. Halloran PF, Gourishankar S. Principles and overview of immunosuppression. In: Primer on transplantation. Mt Laurel, NJ: American Society of Transplantation; 2001. p. 87–98.
8. Hardman JG. Adrenocortical steroids and their synthetic analogs. In: Goodman & Gilman's the pharmacological basis of therapeutics; 1996. p. 1481.
9. Clipstone NA, Crabtree GR. Identification of calcineurin as a key signalling enzyme in T-lymphocyte activation. Nature. 1992;357(6380):695–7.
10. Kahn BD. Cyclosporin. N Eng J Med. 1989;321:1725–38.
11. Reem GH. Molecular mode of action of cyclosporin and FK506in human thymocytes. J Autoimmun. 1992;5:159–65.
12. Shin GT, Khanna A, Ding R, Sharma VK, Lagman M, Li B, et al. In vivo expression of transforming growth factor-β1 in humans: stimulation by cyclosporine: 1. Transplantation. 1998;65(3):313–8.
13. Cooney GF, Jeevanandam V, Choudhury S, Feutren G, Mueller EA, Eisen HJ. Comparative bioavailability of Neoral and Sandimmune in cardiac transplant recipients over 1 year. In: Transplantation proceedings. 1998. p. 1892–4.
14. Yonan NA, Aziz T, El-Gamel A, Campbell CS, Rahman AN, Deiraniya AK. Long-term safety and efficacy of Neoral in heart transplantation. In: Transplantation proceedings. 1998. p. 1906–9.
15. Maccherini M, Bernazzali S, Diciolla F, Giunti G, Bizzarri F, Lisi GF, et al. Neoral versus Sandimmun: clinical impact and modification of immunosuppressive therapy in cardiac transplantation. In: Transplantation proceedings. 1998. p. 1904–5.
16. Carrier M, White M, Pellerin M, Pelletier GB, Pelletier LC. Comparison of Neoral and Sandimmune cyclosporine for induction of immunosuppression after heart transplantation. Can J Cardiol. 1997;13(5):469–73.
17. Pham SM, Kormos RL, Hattler BG, Kawai A, Tsamandas AC, Demetris AJ, et al. A prospective trial of tacrolimus (FK 506) in clinical heart transplantation: intermediate-term results. J Thorac Cardiovasc Surg. 1996;111(4):764–72.
18. Armitage JM, Kormos RL, Morita S, Fung J, Marrone GC, Hardesty RL, et al. Clinical trial of FK 506 immunosuppression in adult cardiac transplantation. Ann Thorac Surg. 1992;54(2):205–11.
19. Kobashigawa JA, Miller LW, Russell SD, Ewald GA, Zucker MJ, Goldberg LR, et al. Tacrolimus with mycophenolate mofetil (MMF) or sirolimus vs. cyclosporine with MMF in cardiac transplant patients: 1-year report. Am J Transplant. 2006;6(6):1377–86.

20. Taylor DO, Barr ML, Radovancevic B, Renlund DG, Mentzer RM Jr, Smart FW, et al. A randomized, multicenter comparison of tacrolimus and cyclosporine immunosuppressive regimens in cardiac transplantation: decreased hyperlipidemia and hypertension with tacrolimus. J Heart Lung Transplant. 1999;18(4):336–45.
21. Reichart B, Meiser B, Vigano M, Rinaldi M, Yacoub M, Banner NR, et al. European multicenter tacrolimus heart pilot study: three year follow-up. J Heart Lung Transplant. 2001;20(2):249–50.
22. Grimm M, Rinaldi M, Yonan NA, Arpesella G, Del Prado JMA, Pulpón LA, et al. Superior prevention of acute rejection by tacrolimus vs. cyclosporine in heart transplant recipients—a large European trial. Am J Transplant. 2006;6(6):1387–97.
23. Valantine H. Neoral use in the cardiac transplant recipient. In: Transplantation proceedings. 2000. p. 27S-44S.
24. Montori VM, Basu A, Erwin PJ, Velosa JA, Gabriel SE, Kudva YC. Posttransplantation diabetes: a systematic review of the literature. Diab Care. 2002;25(3):583–92.
25. Taylor DO, Barr ML, Meiser BM, Pham SM, Mentzer RM, Gass AL. Suggested guidelines for the use of tacrolimus in cardiac transplant recipients. J Heart Lung Transplant. 2001;20(7):734–8.
26. Migliozzi DR, Asal NJ. Clinical controversy in transplantation: tacrolimus versus cyclosporine in statin drug interactions. Ann Pharmacother. 2020;54(2):171–7.
27. Lemahieu W, Maes B, Pierik M, Verbeke K, Vanrenterghem Y. Combination of cyp3a4 measurement in vivo and genetic stratification for p-glycoprotein explains 71% of the variability of dose and weight normalized tacrolimus trough levels in stable renal transplant recipients. Transplantation. 2004;78(2):262.
28. Lu CY, Sicher SC, Vazquez MA. Prevention and treatment of renal allograft rejection: new therapeutic approaches and new insights into established therapies. J Am Soc Nephrol. 1993;4(6):1239–56.
29. Copeland JG, Mammana RB, Fuller JK, Campbell DW, McAleer MJ, Sailer JA. Heart transplantation: four years' experience with conventional immunosuppression. JAMA. 1984;251(12):1563–6.
30. Ensley RD, Bristow MR, Olsen SL, Taylor DO, Hammond EH, O'Connell JB, et al. The use of mycophenolate mofetil (RS-61443) in human heart transplant recipients. Transplantation. 1993;56(1):75–81.
31. Kobashigawa J, Miller L, Renlund D, Mentzer R, Alderman E, Bourge R, et al. A randomized active-controlled trial of mycophenolate mofetil in heart transplant recipients1. Transplantation. 1998;66(4):507–15.
32. Hosenpud JD, Bennett LE. Mycophenolate mofetil versus azathioprine in patients surviving the initial cardiac transplant hospitalization: an analysis of the Joint UNOS/ISHLT Thoracic Registry. Transplantation. 2001;72(10):1662–5.
33. Kirklin JK, Bourge RC, Naftel DC, Morrow WR, Deierhoi MH, Kauffman RS, et al. Treatment of recurrent heart rejection with mycophenolate mofetil (RS-61443): initial clinical experience. J Heart Lung Transplant. 1994;13(3):444–50.
34. Taylor DO, Ensley RD, Olsen SL, Dunn D, Renlund DG. Mycophenolate mofetil (RS-61443): preclinical, clinical, and three-year experience in heart transplantation. J Heart Lung Transplant. 1994;13(4):571–82.
35. Sehgal SN, Baker H, Vézina C. Rapamycin (AY-22, 989), a new antifungal antibiotic II. Fermentation, isolation and characterization. J Antibiot (Tokyo). 1975;28(10):727–32.
36. Vézina C, Kudelski A, Sehgal SN. Rapamycin (AY-22, 989), a new antifungal antibiotic I. taxonomy of the producing streptomycete and isolation of the active principle. J Antibiot (Tokyo). 1975;28(10):721–6.
37. Guba M, Von Breitenbuch P, Steinbauer M, Koehl G, Flegel S, Hornung M, et al. Rapamycin inhibits primary and metastatic tumor growth by antiangiogenesis: involvement of vascular endothelial growth factor. Nat Med. 2002;8(2):128–35.
38. Heitman J, Movva NR, Hall MN. Targets for cell cycle arrest by the immunosuppressant rapamycin in yeast. Science (1979). 1991;253(5022):905–9.
39. Degertekin M, Serruys PW, Foley DP, Tanabe K, Regar E, Vos J, et al. Persistent inhibition of neointimal hyperplasia after sirolimus-eluting stent implantation: long-term (up to 2 years) clinical, angiographic, and intravascular ultrasound follow-up. Circulation. 2002;106(13):1610–3.
40. Poston RS, Billingham M, Hoyt EG, Pollard J, Shorthouse R, Morris RE, et al. Rapamycin reverses chronic graft vascular disease in a novel cardiac allograft model. Circulation. 1999;100(1):67–74.
41. Keogh A, Richardson M, Ruygrok P, Spratt P, Galbraith A, O'Driscoll G, et al. Sirolimus in de novo heart transplant recipients reduces acute rejection and prevents coronary artery disease at 2 years: a randomized clinical trial. Circulation. 2004;110(17):2694–700.
42. Mancini D, Pinney S, Burkhoff D, LaManca J, Itescu S, Burke E, et al. Use of rapamycin slows progression of cardiac transplantation vasculopathy. Circulation. 2003;108(1):48–53.
43. Stallone G, Schena A, Infante B, Di Paolo S, Loverre A, Maggio G, et al. Sirolimus for Kaposi's sarcoma in renal-transplant recipients. N Engl J Med. 2005;352(13):1317–23.
44. Eisen HJ, Tuzcu EM, Dorent R, Kobashigawa J, Mancini D, Valantine-von Kaeppler HA, et al. Everolimus for the prevention of allograft rejection and vasculopathy in cardiac-transplant recipients. N Engl J Med. 2003;349(9):847–58.

45. Eisen HJ, Kobashigawa J, Starling RC, Pauly DF, Kfoury A, Ross H, et al. Everolimus versus mycophenolate mofetil in heart transplantation: a randomized, multicenter trial. Am J Transplant. 2013;13(5):1203–16.
46. Kobashigawa JA, Pauly DF, Starling RC, Eisen H, Ross H, Wang SS, et al. Cardiac allograft vasculopathy by intravascular ultrasound in heart transplant patients: substudy from the Everolimus versus mycophenolate mofetil randomized, multicenter trial. JACC Heart Fail. 2013;1(5):389–99.
47. Lehmkuhl HB, Arizon J, Viganò M, Almenar L, Gerosa G, Maccherini M, et al. Everolimus with reduced cyclosporine versus MMF with standard cyclosporine in de novo heart transplant recipients. Transplantation. 2009;88(1):115–22.
48. Potena L, Prestinenzi P, Bianchi IG, Masetti M, Romani P, Magnani G, et al. Cyclosporine lowering with everolimus versus mycophenolate mofetil in heart transplant recipients: long-term follow-up of the SHIRAKISS randomized, prospective study. J Heart Lung Transplant. 2012;31(6):565–70.
49. Gullestad L, Iversen M, Mortensen SA, Eiskjær H, Riise GC, Mared L, et al. Everolimus with reduced calcineurin inhibitor in thoracic transplant recipients with renal dysfunction: a multicenter, randomized trial. Transplantation. 2010;89(7):864–72.
50. Andreassen AK, Andersson B, Gustafsson F, Eiskjaer H, Rådegran G, Gude E, et al. Everolimus initiation and early calcineurin inhibitor withdrawal in heart transplant recipients: a randomized trial. Am J Transplant. 2014;14(8):1828–38.
51. Barten MJ, Hirt SW, Garbade J, Bara C, Doesch AO, Knosalla C, et al. Comparing everolimus-based immunosuppression with reduction or withdrawal of calcineurin inhibitor reduction from 6 months after heart transplantation: the randomized MANDELA study. Am J Transplant. 2019;19(11):3006–17.
52. Dean PG, Lund WJ, Larson TS, Prieto M, Nyberg SL, Ishitani MB, et al. Wound-healing complications after kidney transplantation: a prospective, randomized comparison of Sirolimus and Tacrolimus1. Transplantation. 2004;77(10):1555–61.
53. King-Biggs MB, Dunitz JM, Park SJ, Savik SK, Hertz MI. Airway anastomotic dehiscence associated with use of sirolimus immediately after lung transplantation. Transplantation. 2003;75(9):1437–43.
54. Kahan BD, Camardo JS. Rapamycin: clinical results and future opportunities1. Transplantation. 2001;72(7):1181–93.
55. Ponticelli C, MacDonald AS, Rajagopalan P, Sindhi R, Mathew T, Group RGS. Phase III trial of Rapamune versus placebo in primary renal allograft recipients. In: Transplantation proceedings. Elsevier; 2001. p. 2271–2.
56. Kreis H, Cisterne JM, Land W, Wramner L, Squifflet JP, Abramowicz D, et al. Sirolimus in association with mycophenolate mofetil induction for the prevention of acute graft rejection in renal allograft Recipients12. Transplantation. 2000;69(7):1252–60.
57. Groth CG, Bäckman L, Morales JM, Calne R, Kreis H, Lang P, et al. Sirolimus (RAPAMYCIN)-based therapy in human renal transplantation: similar efficacy and different toxicity compared with cyclosporine: 1, 2. Transplantation. 1999;67(7):1036–42.
58. Kahan BD. Efficacy of sirolimus compared with azathioprine for reduction of acute renal allograft rejection: a randomised multicentre study. The Lancet. 2000;356(9225):194–202.
59. Blum CB. Effects of sirolimus on lipids in renal allograft recipients: an analysis using the Framingham risk model. Am J Transplant. 2002;2(6):551–9.
60. Barshes NR, Goodpastor SE, Goss JA. Sirolimus-atorvastatin drug interaction in the pancreatic islet transplant recipient. Transplantation. 2003;76(11):1649–50.
61. Velleca A, Shullo MA, Dhital K, Azeka E, Colvin M, DePasquale E, et al. The International Society for Heart and Lung Transplantation (ISHLT) guidelines for the care of heart transplant recipients. J Heart Lung Transplant. 2023;42(5):e1-141.
62. Costanzo MR, Dipchand A, Starling R, Anderson A, Chan M, Desai S, et al. The International Society of Heart and Lung Transplantation Guidelines for the care of heart transplant recipients. J Heart Lung Transplant. Elsevier. 2010; 29:914–56.
63. Baran DA, Zucker MJ, Arroyo LH, Alwarshetty MM, Ramirez MR, Prendergast TW, et al. Randomized trial of tacrolimus monotherapy: tacrolimus in combination, tacrolimus alone compared (the TICTAC trial). J Heart Lung Transplant. 2007;26(10):992–7.
64. Baran DA, Zucker MJ, Arroyo LH, Camacho M, Goldschmidt ME, Nicholls SJ, et al. A prospective, randomized trial of single-drug versus dual-drug immunosuppression in heart transplantation: the tacrolimus in combination, tacrolimus alone compared (TICTAC) trial. Circ Heart Fail. 2011;4(2):129–37.
65. Andreassen AK, Andersson B, Gustafsson F, Eiskjaer H, Rådegran G, Gude E, et al. Everolimus initiation with early calcineurin inhibitor withdrawal in de novo heart transplant recipients: three-year results from the randomized SCHEDULE study. Am J Transplant. 2016;16(4):1238–47.
66. Kobashigawa JA, Tobis JM, Mentzer RM, Valantine HA, Bourge RC, Mehra MR, et al. Mycophenolate mofetil reduces intimal thickness by intravascular ultrasound after heart transplant: reanalysis of the multicenter trial. Am J Transplant. 2006;6(5):993–7.
67. Potena L, Pellegrini C, Grigioni F, Amarelli C, Livi U, Maccherini M, et al. Optimizing the safety profile of everolimus by delayed initiation in de novo heart transplant recipients: results of the prospective randomized study EVERHEART. Transplantation. 2018;102(3):493–501.

68. Kobashigawa JA, Tobis JM, Starling RC, Tuzcu EM, Smith AL, Valantine HA, et al. Multicenter intravascular ultrasound validation study among heart transplant recipients: outcomes after five years. J Am Coll Cardiol. 2005;45(9):1532–7.
69. Lebmkuhl H, Livi U, Arizon J, Vigano M, Magelli C, Boissonnat P, et al. Results of a 12 month, multicenter, randomized trial of everolimus with reduced-exposure cyclosporine versus MMF and standard-exposure cyclosporine in De Novo cardiac transplant recipients. J Heart Lung Transplant. 2008;27(2).
70. Raichlin E, Khalpey Z, Kremers W, Frantz RP, Rodeheffer RJ, Clavell AL, et al. Replacement of calcineurin-inhibitors with sirolimus as primary immunosuppression in stable cardiac transplant recipients. Transplantation. 2007;84(4):467–74.
71. Groetzner J, Meiser B, Landwehr P, Buehse L, Mueller M, Kaczmarek I, et al. Mycophenolate mofetil and sirolimus as calcineurin inhibitor-free immunosuppression for late cardiac-transplant recipients with chronic renal failure. Transplantation. 2004;77(4):568–74.
72. Groetzner J, Kaczmarek I, Schulz U, Stegemann E, Kaiser K, Wittwer T, et al. Mycophenolate and sirolimus as calcineurin inhibitor-free immunosuppression improves renal function better than calcineurin inhibitor-reduction in late cardiac transplant recipients with chronic renal failure. Transplantation. 2009;87(5):726–33.

# 13 Induction Strategies in Heart Transplantation

Lily Stern, Evan Kransdorf, and Yosef Manla

**Abstract**

Induction therapy refers to a brief period of intense immunosuppression administered pre-transplant with the intent to decrease rejection episodes and/or to delay the start of nephrotoxic immunosuppressive drugs for patients with renal insufficiency. The benefit of routine induction therapy has not been established. This chapter will summarize induction therapies commonly used in patients undergoing heart transplantation, including depleting and non-depleting antibodies, their efficacy, and adverse effects. Until further data is available, the risks and benefits of induction therapy following heart transplantation need to be carefully weighed.

**Keywords**

Induction · Heart failure · Heart transplantation · Immunosuppression · Sensitization · Renal dysfunction · Rejection · Outcome

L. Stern · E. Kransdorf (✉) · Y. Manla
Cedars-Sinai Smidt Heart Institute, Los Angeles, CA, USA
e-mail: evan.kransdorf@cshs.org

L. Stern
e-mail: Lily.stern@cshs.org

Y. Manla
e-mail: Yosef.manla@cshs.org; Yosef.Manla1@gmail.com

## Clinical Pearls

- Induction therapy refers to an intense period of perioperative immunosuppression in patients undergoing transplantation but its benefit for routine therapy has not been established.
- In patients with pre-transplant sensitization or those with renal dysfunction undergoing heart transplantation, induction therapy with anti-thymocyte globulin or basiliximab may be warranted.
- Anti-thymocyte globulin can cause cytokine release syndrome, prompting slow administration over 6–8 h with pre-medication with antipyretics, antihistamines, and corticosteroids.
- Basiliximab is notable for a significantly lower incidence of drug-related adverse events but less efficacy compared to anti-thymocyte globulin.
- The use of complement blockade given perioperatively could be considered in highly sensitized patients if crossing high donor-specific antibodies at the time of transplant.

## Introduction

"Induction therapy" refers to a brief period of intense immunosuppression administered pre-transplant and is generally indicated in cases of pre-transplant sensitization, given the


J. Kobashigawa (ed.), *Clinical Guide to Heart Transplantation*, https://doi.org/10.1007/978-3-031-88290-6_13

risk of hyperacute rejection in the immediate post-transplant period. Other indications for induction therapy encompass multi-organ transplantation and renal-sparing protocols to delay calcineurin inhibitor (CNI) therapy [1–3]. Currently, induction therapy is used in approximately 50% of heart transplant (HTx) patients [4, 5]. Induction therapy strategies include the use of antibodies that are primarily directed against T-cell activation and assist with the suppression of potentially harmful circulating alloantibodies as well as against pathways for formation of new alloantibodies in the perioperative period. Induction therapy can largely be divided into two categories: depleting antibodies and non-depleting antibodies [6]. Depleting antibodies include both monoclonal and polyclonal antibodies. Depleting antibodies reduce alloreactive T cells at the time of transplantation, in turn suppressing host response to the allograft. In contrast, nondepleting antibodies (such as basiliximab) inhibit critical T-cell activities, including IL-2-driven cell proliferation. Induction therapies have more potent immunomodulatory effects than maintenance immunosuppression, which can last for months. Recent evidence also suggested that the complement system could be a potential therapeutic target, which will also be discussed in this chapter [7]. Table 13.1 summarizes induction agents' trade names, pharmacology, necessary adjustments for renal or hepatic dysfunction, and dosing and general monitoring guidelines for commonly used intravenous induction immunosuppressive drugs [8]. Until further data is available, the disadvantages and benefits of induction therapy following HTx need to be carefully weighed.

## Depleting Antibodies

### Polyclonal Antibodies

Polyclonal anti-lymphocyte antibodies are available in two ATG formulations: ATGAM (equine ATG) and Thymoglobulin (rabbit ATG [rATG]) polyclonal antibodies. ATG is a polyclonal antibody derived from the immunization of rabbits or horses with human thymocytes. The final product includes antibodies against CD2, CD3, CD4, CD8, CD11a, CD18, CD25, CD44, CD45, HLA-DR, and HLA class I heavy chains and is effective in preventing cellular immune responses against a variety of antigenic stimuli through substantial lymphocyte depletion [9, 10]. Administration of ATG results in complement-dependent opsonization, eventual cell lysis, and apoptosis of these cells, thus preventing rejection. ATG predominantly affects naïve T cells and spares memory and regulatory T cells [11] which assists in the prevention of acute rejection in the perioperative period (induction therapy) or as part of acute allograft rejection treatment post-transplant (see Chap. 19). The effects of ATG usually last up to 3 months, but in some patients, it can last up to 1 year. ATG is generally given for 3–7 days postoperatively. According to the Registry of the International Society for Heart and Lung Transplantation., around 20% of HTx recipients received ATG as induction therapy [4]. With regard to the two formulations, Thymoglobulin is superior to ATGAM in that it has been associated with less serious adverse side effects, fewer opportunistic infections, and better efficacy. However, compared to ATGAM, leukopenia is more frequently observed with Thymoglobulin [12–14]. ATG induction is often reserved for sensitized patients (panel reactive antibody > 10%) and those with baseline serum creatinine > 2.0 mg/dL [3]. African American patients with a propensity for CYP3A single nucleotide polymorphisms that contribute to rapid metabolism and subtherapeutic levels of CNIs [15] and patients supported with ventricular assist devices with high levels of preformed antibodies may be the best candidates to undergo induction. In many programs, sensitized patients are administered ATG induction, commonly administered at 1.5 mg/kg for five days.

Retrospective analyses have investigated the utility of ATG induction. A national retrospective study in the United Kingdom [16], included over 2000 patients between 1995 and 2008, 1000 of whom had been inducted with

**Table 13.1** Overview of commonly used induction agents in cardiac transplantation

| Induction agent drug | Trade name(s) | Pharmacology | Adjustment for renal/ hepatic dysfunction | Dosing | Monitoring |
|---|---|---|---|---|---|
| **Polyclonal anti-lymphocyte preparations** | | | | | ATGAM requires skin test before first dose<br>Premedication to prevent cytokine release syndrome is required: anti-pyretics, IV steroids, antihistamines, H2 blockers<br>Monitoring is done by following CD3 counts<br>Various targets include CD3 at 5–10% baseline, <50 CD3+ cells/ml, 50–100 CD3+ cells/ml<br>Repeating daily dose when CD3+ cells increase may decrease number of daily doses, especially with Thymoglobulin<br>Dose reduction or discontinuation is required for thrombocytopenia |
| Anti-Thymocyte Globulin | ATGAM | Elimination by protein degradation and antibody formation to equine (ATGAM) or rabbit (Thymoglobulin) protein | No | 10–15 mg/kg/day IV over 6–8 h for 5–14 days | |
| | Thymoglobulin | | | 1.5 mg/kg/day IV over 6–8 h for 3–7 days | |
| **Monoclonal preparations** | | | | | |
| Alemtuzumab | Campath | CD52 antibody, depleting T cells as well as B cells and other lymphoid subsets | No | 30 mg IV over 2 h once intraoperatively | Premedication is required. Total lymphocyte counts should also be monitored |
| Basiliximab | Simulect | Elimination via protein degradation similar to IgG | No | 20 mg IV within 2 h of surgery and day 4 postoperatively | CD3 counts do not change. IL-2R+ lymphocytes may be measured but are generally followed clinically. Hypersensitivity may occur rarely |

Used with permission from For journal content: JoAnn Lindenfeld, Geraldine G. Miller, Simon F. Shakar, Ronald Zolty, et al., Drug Therapy in the Heart Transplant Recipient: Part I: Cardiac Rejection and Immunosuppressive Drugs, Circulation,110 (24), 3858–3865, https://doi.org/10.1161/01.CIR.0000149745.83186.89; American Heart Association.

ATG. The study found no significant difference in survival at 10 years between the two groups, but investigators did note lower rates of rejection over the first year. However, this potential benefit was accompanied by increased rates of infection. A single-center retrospective study of 103 patients who were transplanted between 2010 and 2012 and underwent baseline and 1-year IVUS demonstrated a decrease in CAV plaque progression at 1 year in the ATG arm (N = 46) despite having a higher rate of sensitization at the time of HTx compared to those who received standard triple therapy. There was no difference in survival or rates of rejection but with higher rates of infection by one-year post-HTx [17]. To date, no randomized prospective trial has been published that assesses the benefit of ATG induction in terms of survival, rejection, or cardiac allograft vasculopathy (CAV). The xenogeneic (horse/rabbit) origin of ATG may induce a host antibody response leading to acute hypersensitivity response or, rarely, serum sickness on subsequent exposure, which is characterized by fevers, chills, tachycardia, hypertension or hypotension, myalgias, and rash, and may occur after the first dose. Flow cytometry to monitor T cells is helpful in assessing effectiveness and adjusting dosing. Rarely, cytokine release syndrome can occur due to brief, initial T cell activation with surface receptor binding. To prevent this reaction, ATG infusions are given over 6–8 h with pre-dosing with acetaminophen, antihistamines, and corticosteroids. Hypertension, diarrhea, and headache are common. Furthermore, leukopenia and thrombocytopenia frequently occur (14–30% of patients [18]), sometimes necessitating either a reduction in dose or termination of therapy. There is an increased incidence of either primary or reactivated CMV infections with ATG use; therefore, prophylactic doses of ganciclovir are given during and for at least 3 months after commencing ATG [19]. A major risk of ATG over IL-2 receptor antagonists (discussed below) is malignancy, mainly consisting of virally induced cancers. The cumulative load of immunosuppression has been shown to be a primary determinant of post-transplant lymphoproliferative disorder (PTLD), including non-Hodgkin's lymphoma incidence early after transplantation [20] but these occurrences are rare.

## Monoclonal Antibodies

Alemtuzumab is a humanized rat monoclonal antibody that targets the CD52 antigen expressed on both T and B cells and is thus lymphocyte-depleting. It is used in less than 2% of heart transplants [4]. In kidney transplant recipients, the use of alemtuzumab has permitted the use of lower-intensity maintenance immunosuppression with reduced rates of biopsy-proven rejection in multiple randomized controlled trials when compared to basiliximab [21] or Thymoglobulin [21, 22] and without an appreciable increase in infection or mortality but a decrease in creatinine clearance in a meta-analysis of 6 trials when compared to Thymoglobulin induction [23]. Early experience in observational studies suggests that Alemtuzumab induction may decrease the incidence of early (<12 months) acute cellular rejection while allowing the use of lower intensity, steroid-free [24] or steroid minimized [25] maintenance immunosuppression. The reported effect on renal function has been variable. The most common adverse reaction to alemtuzumab is lymphopenia, which lasts for approximately six months and may persist for up to three years in some individuals. It sometimes requires a granulocyte colony-stimulating factor. Nevertheless, recent observational studies have not demonstrated an increase in infection [24, 25]. In a study by LaMattina et al. of 1687 renal transplant recipients, Alemtuzumab was found to be an independent risk factor for antibody-mediated rejection and, therefore, decreased graft survival compared to patients receiving either basiliximab or Thymoglobulin [26]. Other adverse reactions include anemia, thrombocytopenia, and infusion-related reactions.

The CTOT-11 (Prevention of Cardiac Allograft Vasculopathy Using Rituximab Therapy in Cardiac Transplantation [Clinical Trials in Organ Transplantation-11]) study was a randomized, placebo-controlled, multicenter, double-blinded clinical trial in non-sensitized primary HTx recipients. The study sought to determine whether B cell depletion therapy would attenuate the development of cardiac allograft vasculopathy with the primary outcome being the change in first-year IVUS parameter of percent atheroma volume (PAV). The study found a marked, unexpected increase in coronary artery PAV with rituximab compared to control during the first year in HTx recipients ($+6.8 \pm 8.2\%$ rituximab vs. $+1.9 \pm 4.4\%$ placebo, $p = 0.0019$). One-year survival was not impacted. This study suggests that abrogation of intact B cell function immediately after transplant by a CD20 receptor antagonist is deleterious. It is speculated that elimination of B cell regulatory properties may have precipitated the results of this study [27].

## Non-depleting Antibodies

### Basiliximab

Basiliximab is a monoclonal antibody that selectively binds to the IL-2 receptor of T-lymphocytes, blocks the binding of IL-2 to the receptor complex, and inhibits IL-2-mediated T-lymphocyte proliferation [28, 29]. Basiliximab was historically the most frequently used induction agent, with 30% of transplant patients undergoing induction (2). In renal transplantation, basiliximab is FDA-approved for the prophylaxis of acute organ rejection in patients as part of a regimen that also includes cyclosporine and corticosteroids. In HTx, it is generally used in high-risk patients, similar to how ATG is used, specifically, for those at the highest risk of rejection or renal failure. A 2018 Cochrane meta-analysis of randomized control trials and observational case–control studies [30] showed that patients receiving any induction therapy had a similar risk of moderate-to-severe rejection, all-cause death, infection, and cancer compared to those who did not receive any induction therapy. However, the use of IL-2 induction was associated with a higher risk of moderate-severe rejection than ATG but a similar risk of death, infections, and cancer. Analysis of data from the ISHLT registry of 9,324 patients who received induction therapy prior to HTx between the years 2000 and 2011 demonstrated that basiliximab was associated with increased mortality over 3-year follow-up compared to ATG use (hazard ratio 1.22); however, patients were not matched for sensitization or illness severity prior to transplant [31]. Basiliximab is notable for a significantly lower incidence of drug-related adverse events compared to ATG [32]. Unlike ATG, cytokine release syndrome has not been reported after administration of this type of drug, and there has been no established increased risk of malignancy [28, 29, 33, 34]. However, hypersensitivity has been reported with initial exposure and subsequent re-exposure to basiliximab. In such scenarios, the second dose should be withheld [35].

### Eculizumab

Eculizumab is a humanized monoclonal antibody that binds to the complement component (C5) and prevents its conversion to anaphylatoxin (C5a). Therefore, it blocks the constitution of the cell membrane attack complex (C5b-9), resulting in a powerful inhibition of the complement cascade [36]. Based on prior experience in highly sensitized kidney transplant patients [37, 38]. Patel et al. completed a trial on the perioperative use of eculizumab in patients with persistently elevated PRA and high-preformed ($MFI > 10{,}000$) DSA. The study included 20 patients with a median calculated panel reactive antibody of 95% (90–97%) and pre-formed donor-specific antibodies; patients were administered nine infusions of eculizumab during the first two months post-transplant. Survival at one year was 90%, with no deaths resulting from AMR. Comparing treated patients to matched control patients, there was a significant reduction in the risk of biopsy-proven AMR in patients treated with eculizumab (HR = 0.36, 95% CI [0.14–0.95], p = 0.032) [7]. The authors concluded that eculizumab may serve as a potential therapy with favorable outcomes at one year. Regarding adverse events, in the study by Patel et al., no side effects occurred at the time of eculizumab infusion. During the follow-up period, seven patients had bacterial infections, while six and two cases were diagnosed with viral and fungal infections, respectively. In one patient, a septic complication was thought to have contributed to the mortality.

## References


1. Cantarovich M, Metrakos P, Giannetti N, Cecere R, Barkun J, Tchervenkov J. Anti-CD25 monoclonal antibody coverage allows for calcineurin inhibitor "holiday" in solid organ transplant patients with acute renal dysfunction. Transplantation. 2002;73(7):1169–72.
2. Delgado DH, Miriuka SG, Cusimano RJ, Feindel C, Rao V, Ross HJ. Use of basiliximab and cyclosporine in heart transplant patients with pre-operative renal dysfunction. J Heart Lung Transplant. 2005;24(2):166–9.
3. Chang DH, Youn J-C, Dilibero D, Patel JK, Kobashigawa JA. Heart transplant immunosuppression strategies at cedars-sinai medical center. Int J Heart Fail. 2021;3(1):15.
4. Khush KK, Cherikh WS, Chambers DC, Harhay MO, Hayes D, Jr., Hsich E, et al. The International Thoracic Organ Transplant Registry of the International Society for Heart and Lung Transplantation: thirty-sixth adult heart transplantation report - 2019; focus theme: donor and recipient size match. J Heart Lung Transplant. 2019;38(10):1056–66.
5. Colvin M, Smith JM, Ahn Y, Skeans MA, Messick E, Goff R, et al. OPTN/SRTR 2019 annual data report: heart. Am J Transplant. 2021;21(Suppl 2):356–440.
6. Baran DA. Induction therapy in cardiac transplantation: when and why? Heart Fail Clin. 2007;3(1):31–41.
7. Patel JK, Coutance G, Loupy A, Dilibero D, Hamilton M, Kittleson M, et al. Complement inhibition for prevention of antibody-mediated rejection in immunologically high-risk heart allograft recipients. Am J Transplant. 2021;21(7):2479–88.
8. Lindenfeld J, Miller GG, Shakar SF, Zolty R, Lowes BD, Wolfel EE, et al. Drug therapy in the heart transplant recipient: part II: immunosuppressive drugs. Circulation. 2004;110(25):3858–65.
9. Bourdage JS, Hamlin DM. Comparative polyclonal antithymocyte globulin and antilymphocyte/antilymphoblast globulin anti-CD antigen analysis by flow cytometry. Transplantation. 1995;59(8):1194–200.
10. Padiyar A, Augustine JJ, Hricik DE. Induction antibody therapy in kidney transplantation. Am J Kidney Dis. 2009;54(5):935–44.
11. Ruzek MC, Neff KS, Luong M, Smith KA, Culm-Merdek K, Richards SM, et al. In vivo characterization of rabbit anti-mouse thymocyte globulin: a surrogate for rabbit anti-human thymocyte globulin. Transplantation. 2009;88(2):170–9.
12. Panackel C, Mathew JF, Jacob M. Immunosuppressive drugs in liver transplant: an insight. J Clin Exp Hepatol. 2022;12(6):1557–71.
13. Brennan DC, Flavin K, Lowell JA, Howard TK, Shenoy S, Burgess S, et al. A randomized, double-blinded comparison of thymoglobulin versus Atgam for induction immunosuppressive therapy in adult renal transplant Recipients 1, 2. Transplantation. 1999;67(7):1011–8.
14. Langrehr JM, Nüssler NC, Neumann U, Guckelberger O, Lohmann R, Radtke A, et al. A prospective randomized trial comparing interleukin-2 receptor antibody versus antithymocyte globulin as part of a quadruple immunosuppressive induction therapy following orthotopic liver transplantation. Transplantation. 1997;63(12):1772–81.
15. Kuehl P, Zhang J, Lin Y, Lamba J, Assem M, Schuetz J, et al. Sequence diversity in CYP3A promoters and characterization of the genetic basis of polymorphic CYP3A5 expression. Nat Genet. 2001;27(4):383–91.
16. Emin A, Rogers CA, Thekkudan J, Bonser RS, Banner NR. Antithymocyte globulin induction therapy for adult heart transplantation: a UK national study. J Heart Lung Transplant. 2011;30(7):770–7.
17. Azarbal B, Cheng R, Vanichsarn C, Patel JK, Czer LS, Chang DH, et al. Induction therapy with antithymocyte globulin in patients undergoing cardiac transplantation is associated with decreased coronary plaque progression as assessed by intravascular ultrasound. Circul Heart Fail. 2016;9(1):e002252.
18. Enderby C, Keller CA. An overview of immunosuppression in solid organ transplantation. Am J Manag Care. 2015;21(1 Suppl):s12-23.
19. Costanzo MR, Dipchand A, Starling R, Anderson A, Chan M, Desai S, et al. The International Society of Heart and Lung Transplantation guidelines for the care of heart transplant recipients. J Heart Lung Transplant. 2010;29(8):914–56.
20. Opelz G, Döhler B. Lymphomas after solid organ transplantation: a collaborative transplant study report. Am J Transplant. 2004;4(2):222–30.
21. Haynes R, Harden P, Judge P, Blackwell L, Emberson J, Landray MJ, et al. Alemtuzumab-based induction treatment versus basiliximab-based induction treatment in kidney transplantation

(the 3C Study): a randomised trial. Lancet. 2014;384(9955):1684–90.
22. Hanaway MJ, Woodle ES, Mulgaonkar S, Peddi VR, Kaufman DB, First MR, et al. Alemtuzumab induction in renal transplantation. N Engl J Med. 2011;364(20):1909–19.
23. Hill P, Cross NB, Barnett AN, Palmer SC, Webster AC. Polyclonal and monoclonal antibodies for induction therapy in kidney transplant recipients. Cochrane Datab Syst Rev. 2017;1(1):Cd004759.
24. Teuteberg JJ, Shullo MA, Zomak R, Toyoda Y, McNamara DM, Bermudez C, et al. Alemtuzumab induction prior to cardiac transplantation with lower intensity maintenance immunosuppression: one-year outcomes. Am J Transplant. 2010;10(2):382–8.
25. Gale SE, Ravichandran B, Ton VK, Pham S, Reed BN. Alemtuzumab induction versus conventional immunosuppression in heart transplant recipients. J Cardiovasc Pharmacol Ther. 2019;24(5):435–41.
26. LaMattina JC, Mezrich JD, Michael Hofmann R, Foley DP, D'Alessandro AM, Sollinger HW, et al. Alemtuzumab as compared to alternative contemporary induction regimens. Transpl Int. 2012;25(5):518–26.
27. Starling RC, Armstrong B, Bridges ND, Eisen H, Givertz MM, Kfoury AG, et al. Accelerated allograft vasculopathy with rituximab after cardiac transplantation. J Am Coll Cardiol. 2019;74(1):36–51.
28. Beniaminovitz A, Itescu S, Lietz K, Donovan M, Burke EM, Groff BD, et al. Prevention of rejection in cardiac transplantation by blockade of the interleukin-2 receptor with a monoclonal antibody. N Engl J Med. 2000;342(9):613–9.
29. Kahan BD, Rajagopalan PR, Hall M. Reduction of the occurrence of acute cellular rejection among renal allograft recipients treated with basiliximab, a chimeric anti-interleukin-2-receptor monoclonal antibody. United States Simulect Renal Study Group. Transplantation. 1999;67(2):276–84.
30. Briasoulis A, Inampudi C, Pala M, Asleh R, Alvarez P, Bhama J. Induction immunosuppressive therapy in cardiac transplantation: a systematic review and meta-analysis. Heart Fail Rev. 2018;23(5):641–9.
31. Ansari D, Lund LH, Stehlik J, Andersson B, Höglund P, Edwards L, et al. Induction with anti-thymocyte globulin in heart transplantation is associated with better long-term survival compared with basiliximab. J Heart Lung Transplant. 2015;34(10):1283–91.
32. Mattei MF, Redonnet M, Gandjbakhch I, Bandini AM, Billes A, Epailly E, et al. Lower risk of infectious deaths in cardiac transplant patients receiving basiliximab versus anti-thymocyte globulin as induction therapy. J Heart Lung Transplant. 2007;26(7):693–9.
33. Hershberger RE, Starling RC, Eisen HJ, Bergh CH, Kormos RL, Love RB, et al. Daclizumab to prevent rejection after cardiac transplantation. N Engl J Med. 2005;352(26):2705–13.
34. Nashan B, Moore R, Amlot P, Schmidt AG, Abeywickrama K, Soulillou JP. Randomised trial of basiliximab versus placebo for control of acute cellular rejection in renal allograft recipients. CHIB 201 International Study Group. Lancet. 1997;350(9086):1193–8.
35. Leonard PA, Woodside KJ, Gugliuzza KK, Sur S, Daller JA. Safe administration of a humanized murine antibody after anaphylaxis to a chimeric murine antibody. Transplantation. 2002;74(12):1697–700.
36. Yerly P, Rotman S, Regamey J, Aubert V, Aur S, Kirsch M, et al. Complement blockade with eculizumab to treat acute symptomatic humoral rejection after heart transplantation. Xenotransplantation. 2022;29(1):e12726.
37. Cornell L, Schinstock C, Gandhi M, Kremers W, Stegall M. Positive crossmatch kidney transplant recipients treated with eculizumab: outcomes beyond 1 year. Am J Transplant. 2015;15(5):1293–302.
38. Stegall M, Diwan T, Raghavaiah S, Cornell L, Burns J, Dean P, et al. Terminal complement inhibition decreases antibody-mediated rejection in sensitized renal transplant recipients. Am J Transplant. 2011;11(11):2405–13.

# Minimization of Immunosuppression in Heart Transplantation

14

David H. Chang and Yosef Manla

**Abstract**

The sequelae of rejection post-heart transplant (HTx) impact the quality of life as well as short- and long-term survival. The goal of optimal immunosuppression therapy after HTx is to achieve a state of immune quiescence, preventing rejection of the donor heart graft while minimizing immunosuppression complications. Despite advancements in the field of immunosuppression, a regimen that leads to prolonged survival and yet is void of associated morbidity, including infection, malignancy, and drug-related toxicities, has not been identified. Patients without elevated immunologic risk features may benefit from minimization of immunosuppression after HTx. In this chapter, we discuss various management approaches to minimize immunosuppression for HTx recipients, including prednisone weaning, calcineurin inhibitors (CNI) minimization, use of proliferation signal inhibitors (PSI) to reduce or replace CNI, tacrolimus monotherapy, in addition to leveraging novel assays (e.g., T cell immune function assay), artificial intelligence, and precision medicine to personalize immunosuppression therapy.

**Keywords**

Calcineurin inhibition · Anti-metabolite · Corticosteroid · Prednisone wean · Proliferation signal inhibitor · Precision medicine · Co-stimulation blockade

## Clinical Pearls

- The goal of maintenance immunosuppression is immune system quiescence and prevention of allograft rejection and dysfunction.
- Three major adverse clinical outcome sequelae of calcineurin inhibitor (CNI) based immunosuppression are infection, nephrotoxicity, and malignancy.
- Due to the long-term side effects of CNIs, CNI-reduced and CNI-free maintenance immunosuppression regimens are used in low-risk patients.
- Corticosteroid weaning is a common strategy of immunosuppression minimization.
- The proliferation signal inhibitors (PSI) everolimus and sirolimus can be effectively

D. H. Chang (✉) · Y. Manla
Cedars-Sinai Smidt Heart Institute, Los Angeles, CA, USA
e-mail: David.chang2@cshs.org

Y. Manla
e-mail: Yosef.manla@cshs.org



J. Kobashigawa (ed.), *Clinical Guide to Heart Transplantation*, https://doi.org/10.1007/978-3-031-88290-6_14

used to lower maintenance immunosuppression in select patients.
- Tacrolimus monotherapy can be used with acceptable outcomes in low-risk heart transplant recipients with severe infection or significant medication intolerance.

## Introduction

The sequelae of rejection post-heart transplant (HTx) impact the quality of life as well as short- and long-term survival [1, 2]. The goal of optimal immunosuppression therapy after HTx is to achieve a state of immune quiescence, preventing rejection of the donor heart graft while minimizing immunosuppression complications [1]. Despite advancements in the field of immunosuppression, a regimen that leads to prolonged survival and yet is void of associated morbidity, including infection, malignancy, and drug-related toxicities, has not been identified. Additionally, there is no standard combination of medications for maintenance immunosuppression after HTx, and each patient's immunosuppression is individualized. For maintenance immunosuppression, most patients are prescribed a combination of calcineurin inhibitor (tacrolimus), anti-metabolite (mycophenolate mofetil, MMF), and corticosteroid [3–8]. Similarly, there is no set standard of care with respect to induction therapy at the time of HTx. Approximately 50% of patients are treated with induction therapy at the time of HTx [9]. Induction therapy is generally applied to patients at higher risk of graft rejection and patients with renal insufficiency [10]. Patients at elevated immunologic risk who need heightened surveillance and more intense immunosuppression include patients who are sensitized pre-transplant, developed post-transplant cardiac dysfunction, developed de novo donor-specific antibodies (dn-DSA), and patients with rejection. Patients without these features are considered immunologically low risk and may benefit from minimization of immunosuppression after HTx.

## Sequelae of Immunosuppression

Immunosuppression side effects and complications can impact morbidity and mortality after solid organ transplantation. Drug-specific side effects and morbidity lead clinicians to minimize, as permitted, maintenance immunosuppression to improve patient symptoms and reduce the impact of maintenance immunosuppression. Three major adverse clinical outcome sequelae of immunosuppression include infection, renal insufficiency, and malignancy [9, 11, 12]. Infection is the cause of death in ~30% of HTx recipients from 1 month to 1-year post-transplant and the cause of death in ~10% of patients from 10 to 15 years post-transplant [9, 11, 12]. Renal insufficiency defined as creatinine > 2.5 mg/dL, dialysis or renal transplant was recorded in 8.6, 18.4, and 29.2% in survivors within 1-, 5-, and 10-years post-transplant [9, 11, 12]. Malignancy is the long-term leading cause of death after HTx, accounting for ~20% of deaths 3 years and afterward post-transplant [9, 11, 12]. Additionally, immunosuppression, including corticosteroids, contributes to hypertension and hyperlipidemia. Additional corticosteroid complications include glucose intolerance/diabetes, obesity, osteoporosis, avascular necrosis, cataracts, glaucoma, myopathy, Cushingoid features, and neuropsychiatric issues [13, 14].

## Minimization of Immunosuppression Strategies

### Standard Maintenance Immunosuppression

Calcineurin inhibitors (CNI) remain foundational to the maintenance of immunosuppression to prevent allograft rejection, particularly in the earliest phase after HTx. Trough levels are assessed and maintained in pre-specified target levels that are highest in the first month after transplant and tapered to steady-state levels 3 months after HTx. In our clinical practice, tacrolimus trough levels can be targeted to 10–15 ng/dL in the first month, 8–12 ng/dL in the second and third months, and 5–10 ng/dL after month 3. Mycophenolic acid (active metabolite of MMF) trough levels are not commonly tested as the dose of this medication is based on tolerance. Common side effects include nausea and/or diarrhea, leukopenia, anemia, and thrombocytopenia. Optimal target dose (based on clinical trial data) for MMF is 1500 mg twice daily [15].

In this chapter, we discuss various management approaches to minimize immunosuppression for HTx recipients, including prednisone weaning, CNI minimization, use of proliferation signal inhibitors (PSI) to reduce or replace CNI, tacrolimus monotherapy, in addition to leveraging novel assays (e.g., T Cell Immune function assay), artificial intelligence, and precision medicine to personalize immunosuppression therapy (Fig. 14.1).

## Prednisone Weaning

A commonly used strategy for minimization of immunosuppression is corticosteroid weaning. After HTx, high-dose IV steroids, including solumedrol, are routinely administered and transitioned to oral steroids. Per the most recent ISHLT guidelines for the care of HTx patients, corticosteroid withdrawal protocols can be used 3–12 months after HTx in low-risk patients to minimize steroid side effects [2]. An example of corticosteroid withdrawal is what follows. After an oral steroid taper, prednisone 10 mg twice daily is given for up to 1 month post-HTx. This dose is slowly weaned such that by 3 months post-transplant, prednisone is weaned to 10 mg daily, and by 6 months post-transplant, prednisone is weaned to 5 mg daily. Patients at low immunologic risk may then reduce prednisone slowly to off by weaning prednisone by 1 mg monthly until prednisone is stopped close to a year after HTx [10]. Asymptomatic rejection is

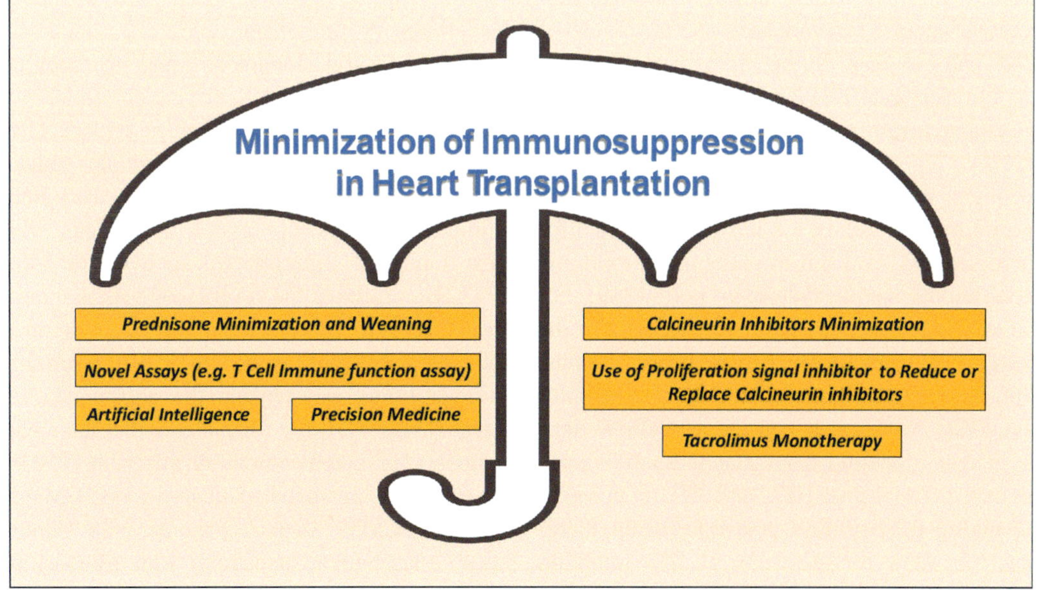


**Fig. 14.1** Management approaches to minimize immunosuppression for heart transplant recipients

possible during a prednisone weaning period, so routine surveillance is recommended either by endomyocardial biopsy or by non-invasive diagnostic tests (e.g., genome expression profiling donor-derived cell-free DNA). Patients often experience symptoms of fatigue, myalgias, and arthralgias during the process of a prednisone wean to off protocol. Some studies have effectively directed a more rapid prednisone wean. In the Tacrolimus In Combination, Tacrolimus Alone Compared (TICTAC) trial, patients were weaned off steroids approximately 8–9 weeks post-HTx with acceptable outcomes [16]. Patients with cardiac sarcoidosis, for example, who require HTx, should be maintained on low-dose corticosteroids to prevent recurrent disease [17, 18].

## Calcineurin Minimization

Due to the dose and time-dependent deterioration of renal function with CNI and the long-term risk of malignancy, efforts have been made to reduce calcineurin exposure or withdraw and replace the CNI with a different immunosuppressant agent. Predominantly due to the use of CNI, chronic renal failure [defined as glomerular filtration rate (GFR) < 30 ml/minute or the development of end end-stage disease (ESRD)] has been reported in approximately 10% of HTx recipients over 5 years after transplant [19]. The overall hazard ratio of 4.5 has been reported for increased risk of death in patients with chronic renal failure over the follow-up period [19]. For patients who undergo induction therapy at the time of HTx, there are two medications most commonly used, which include the IL2 receptor antagonist basiliximab and the polyclonal anti-thymocyte globulin (ATG). Basiliximab is given on days 0 and 4 post-HTx, and ATG is dosed at 1.5 mg/kg for 3–7 days post-HTx. Both therapies can allow for the delay of CNI initiation [20, 21]. ATG may be more potent than basiliximab, but it may carry a higher risk of infection [22]. Clinical trials have shown that in patients who receive ATG induction with maintenance immunosuppression, including cyclosporine and MMF, lower target cyclosporine levels can be maintained, resulting in improved renal function without increased risk of rejection [23, 24].

## Use of Proliferation Signal Inhibitors to Reduce or Replace Calcineurin Inhibitors

PSI including sirolimus and everolimus, can be used as maintenance immunosuppression with CNI to allow lower target doses of CNI or as an alternative medication in place of CNI. Clinical trials of PSI show improvements in cardiac allograft vasculopathy and renal function (in the absence of CNI). PSI intolerances overlap with MMF intolerance and include GI disturbance (nausea and/or diarrhea). Additional PSI intolerances include fluid retention, abdominal bloating, lower extremity edema, and oral aphthous ulcers. Approximately 10–35% of patients who trial PSI do not tolerate these medications due to medication side effects and need to revert back to prior immunosuppression medical treatments [25, 26]. Risks of PSI treatment include a higher risk of fungal infection, deep vein thrombosis/pulmonary embolism (DVT/PE), nephrotic range proteinuria, pneumonia, and pneumonitis [25, 26].

PSIs can be used to reduce or replace CNI in a CNI-free regimen to potentially reduce long-term nephrotoxicity. PSI may also help minimize immunosuppression in patients with post-transplant lymphoproliferative disorder (PTLD), minimize the severity of malignancies, including skin cancer, and theoretically reduce the long-term risk of malignancy [10]. Sirolimus or everolimus can replace the anti-metabolite agent (usually MMF) for patients that have had a history of cytomegalovirus infection (CMV) or are CMV mismatch patients (donor CMV+/recipient CMV- status), patients with donor-specific antibodies, or patients with a history of recurrent treated rejection post HTx [10]. Initial efforts to replace CNI with the PSI sirolimus after one year post-HTx showed that in patients with moderate renal impairment, there was an improvement in renal dysfunction without increased rates of rejection with PSI compared to patients continued on CNI [27–29]. In the Nordic Certican (Everolimus) Trial in heart and lung Transplantation (NOCTET) trial, standard CNI-based immunosuppression was compared to everolimus with reduced dose CNI in thoracic transplant patients more than one year after transplant [30]. 282 patients were randomized in this multi-center trial. The primary endpoint of change in mean GFR was met in the everolimus group without a significant increase in rejection compared to the control CNI-based group. Infections, including pneumonia, were significantly higher in the PSI group.

Initial efforts to replace CNI with PSI early post-HTx were not successful and were terminated. The Heart Save the Nephron multicenter randomized trial examined CNI withdrawal and replacement with sirolimus at 12 weeks. MMF and steroids were also used in maintenance of immunosuppression. The trial was terminated early as more than half of the seven patients randomized to PSI experienced significant cellular rejection, including one patient with hemodynamic compromise [31]. The Scandinavian HTx everolimus de novo study with early calcineurin inhibitor avoidance (SCHEDULE) trial included 115 patients and was a subsequent attempt at early conversion to a PSI-based regimen in patients after HTx [32]. In this randomized, open-label trial, ATG induction was used in all patients. Patients were randomized to low-dose everolimus (3–6 ng/ml) with low-dose cyclosporine in addition to MMF and corticosteroids or to a control group of standard-dose cyclosporine, MMF and corticosteroids. Between 7 and 11 weeks, cyclosporine was withdrawn, and everolimus was adjusted to target a trough level of 6–10 mg/ml in the everolimus group. The primary endpoint of GFR at 1-year post-transplant was significantly increased in the everolimus group. Intravascular ultrasound (IVUS) data at 1-year cardiac catheterization showed a significantly lower incidence of cardiac allograft vasculopathy (CAV) in the everolimus group. However, biopsy-proven rejection was higher in the everolimus arm at 1-year post-HTx but left ventricular function was similar between the two groups. There were higher rates of cellular rejection in the everolimus group but similar left ventricular ejection fraction between the two groups. The frequency of adverse and serious adverse events was higher in the everolimus group. There were more deaths in the CNI group compared to the PSI group. The SCHEDULE trial demonstrated that early CNI withdrawal is possible with everolimus with favorable effects on GFR and CAV, but rejection rates were higher in the PSI arm but did not lead to increased morbidity/mortality (compared to the CNI arm). Long-term follow-up data from the SCHEDULE trial showed similar improvements in GFR and CAV in the everolimus group [33].

The optimal time frame to attempt to include PSI in chronic maintenance immunosuppression after a HTx is unknown. Recent ISHLT guidelines indicate that PSI use with CNI-reduced based maintenance immunosuppression can be considered cautiously if done after 3 months of HTx [2]. For low-risk patients with chronic kidney disease, substitution of PSI for CNI can be considered to reduce CNI-related nephrotoxicity. Due to the risk of proteinuria with PSI-based chronic immunosuppression, regular assessment of proteinuria should be completed [34]. PSI-based regimens (CNI-free) have shown increased rates of cellular rejection in clinical trials, so doses of MMF < 500 mg BID should be minimized, and patients in CNI-free maintenance immunosuppression regimens should have close monitoring of rejection [35].

## Tacrolimus Monotherapy to Minimize Immunosuppression

A different approach to immunosuppression minimization shown to be feasible is to use tacrolimus as monotherapy. In the TICTAC trial, 150 adult de novo HTx recipients were enrolled in a prospective, randomized, controlled, open-label study [16]. Induction therapy was, for the most part, not utilized. All patients received tacrolimus and MMF immediately after HTx. In the tacrolimus alone arm, MMF was weaned to off by 2 weeks post HTx. All patients received steroids post-transplant, which were weaned off by 8–9 weeks post-transplant. Tacrolimus trough levels were targeted in the 8–10 mg/dL range. MMF target dose was 1000 mg twice daily if tolerated. There were no significant differences in a composite biopsy score at 6 months, CAV by angiography and IVUS, or survival at 3 years. Angiography was completed at 3–6 months and yearly thereafter. Recently published long-term outcomes of the TICTAC trial revealed comparable post-transplant survival rates at 5, 10, and 15 years in the Tacrolimus monotherapy group and patients randomized to tacrolimus / MMF (84.5, 66.9, and 52.7, and 94.4, 78.2% and 56.1, respectively, $p=0.19$ log-rank). Similar rates of CAV and kidney failure were also recorded [36]. The TICTAC trial showed that tacrolimus without MMF or steroids was feasible in the prespecified tacrolimus target range. Tacrolimus monotherapy can be considered in patients with intolerable side effects with anti-metabolic agents, severe infection, or significant corticosteroid side effects [37]. In the TACTFUL trial, Pearston et al. evaluated the outcomes among patients converted to tacrolimus monotherapy compared with those maintained on combination immunosuppression. Leukopenia, infection, and gastrointestinal distress were the most common reasons for conversion. No differences in mortality or acute cellular rejection rates were noticed between groups [38].

## Personalizing Immunosuppression

### T Cell Immune Function Assay

To further individualize maintenance immunosuppression, the T cell immune function assay (ImmuKnow, Viracor Eurofins, Lee's Summit, MO, USA) is approved by the Food and Drug Administration (FDA) of the United States for monitoring [39]. Lymphocytes are isolated, stimulated with phytohemagglutinin, lysed, and adenosine triphosphate (ATP) release measured via spectroscopic analysis. An overall sense of immune function can be quantified. The test is less reliable in patients with leukopenia. Per the manufacturer's guidelines, low values (<200 ng/ml) suggest higher risk of infection [40]. One study showed elevated early ImmunKnow values were associated with increased plaque progression by intravascular ultrasound, consistent with increased risk for cardiac allograft vasculopathy [40, 41]. A validation study demonstrated that a score of 380 ATP ng/ml reflected the intersection of the odds ratio curves for infection and rejection with 200–550 ATP ng/ml representing a therapeutic range for overall immunosuppression [42]. Immunosuppression is adjusted primarily with low T cell immune function values; one can individualize immunosuppression to each patient and consider lowering the dose of an immunosuppressant agent particularly in patients with infections and malignancies. Of note, immunosuppression trough levels do not correlate well with ImmunKnow values, supporting the concept that additional data can be used to refine our immunosuppressive management of individual patients.

### Role of Precision Medicine and Artificial Intelligence to Minimize Maintenance Immunosuppression

The potential for personalized precision medicine could further refine and minimize each HTx recipient's immunosuppression. Currently, patients have their maintenance immunosuppression adjusted based on a pre-dose trough concentration level ($C_0$) of individual drugs. Monitoring of cyclosporine levels 2 h post-administration ($C_2$) was observed to allow lower CNI dosing while maintaining adequate immunosuppression in stable HTx recipients over a year post-HTx and in de novo HTx patients with basiliximab induction [43, 44]. However, the timing of obtaining $C_2$ blood samples is not always practical. There is the possibility for further precision medicine refinements in this area in the future [45]. Pharmacogenetic testing of a HTx recipient's cytochrome p450 system, specifically CYP3A5 and CYP3A4 can influence initial tacrolimus dosing to facilitate earlier time to therapeutic tacrolimus levels after HTx. Novel pharmacodynamic biomarkers, including nuclear factor of activated T cells (NFAT)-regulated gene expression and intracellular gamma-interferon, may be useful to guide CNI dosing and therapy. Furthermore, using evolutionary algorithms, neural networks, and other artificial intelligence (AI) techniques that have been trained in predicting drug levels and outcomes in transplant patients can play a potential role in predicting and adjusting dosages of immunosuppressive agents [46].

## Future Directions to Minimize Immunosuppression

Future directions to minimize and optimize maintenance immunosuppression after HTx may include other T cell-directed therapies and non-T cell maintenance immunosuppression with novel therapeutics. Belatacept is a selective T-cell co-stimulation blocker formed by the fusion of the Fc component of human IgG1 to the extracellular portion of human CTLA-4. Based on the use of belatacept in renal transplant patients and limited experience in HTx recipients, there are ongoing clinical trials with belatacept in HTx recipients [47, 48]. Non-T cell targets of immunosuppression include aspects of both the innate and adaptive immune systems. Complement inhibition with the use of eculizumab in addition to ATG induction allows for HTx in highly sensitized HTx recipients with acceptable outcomes (49). Until more novel therapeutics are developed, there will continue to be a number of competing interests in individualizing and minimizing maintenance immunosuppression for each HTx recipient.

## References


1. Chang D, Kobashigawa J. The use of the calculated panel-reactive antibody and virtual crossmatch in heart transplantation. Curr Opin Organ Transplant. 2012;17(4):423–6.
2. Velleca A, Shullo MA, Dhital K, Azeka E, Colvin M, DePasquale E, et al. The International Society for Heart and Lung Transplantation (ISHLT) guidelines for the care of heart transplant recipients. J Heart Lung Transplant. 2023;42(5):e1-141.
3. Nelson J, Alvey N, Bowman L, Schulte J, Segovia MC, McDermott J, et al. Consensus recommendations for use of maintenance immunosuppression in solid organ transplantation: endorsed by the American College of Clinical Pharmacy, American Society of Transplantation, and the International Society for Heart and Lung Transplantation. Pharmacother: J Hum Pharmacol Drug Therapy. 2022;42(8):599–633.
4. White M, Haddad H, Leblanc MH, Giannetti N, Pflugfelder P, Davies R, et al. Conversion from cyclosporine microemulsion to tacrolimus-based immunoprophylaxis improves cholesterol profile in heart transplant recipients with treated but persistent dyslipidemia: the Canadian multicentre randomized trial of tacrolimus vs cyclosporine microemulsion. J Heart Lung Transplant. 2005;24(7):798–809.
5. Penninga L, Møller CH, Gustafsson F, Steinbrüchel DA, Gluud C. Tacrolimus versus cyclosporine as primary immunosuppression after heart transplantation: systematic review with meta-analyses and trial sequential analyses of randomised trials. Eur J Clin Pharmacol. 2010;66:1177–87.
6. Eisen HJ, Kobashigawa J, Keogh A, Bourge R, Renlund D, Mentzer R, et al. Three-year results of a randomized, double-blind, controlled trial of mycophenolate mofetil versus azathioprine in cardiac transplant recipients. J Heart Lung Transplant. 2005;24(5):517–25.
7. Hosenpud JD, Bennett LE. Mycophenolate mofetil versus azathioprine in patients surviving the initial cardiac transplant hospitalization: an analysis of the joint UNOS/ISHLT thoracic registry. Transplantation. 2001;72(10):1662–5.
8. Kobashigawa JA, Miller LW, Russell SD, Ewald GA, Zucker MJ, Goldberg LR, et al. Tacrolimus with mycophenolate mofetil (MMF) or sirolimus vs. cyclosporine with MMF in cardiac transplant patients: 1-year report. Am J Transplant. 2006;6(6):1377–86.
9. International Thoracic Organ Transplant (TTX) Registry data slides. Adult heart transplantation statistics [internet]. 2019. https://ishltregistries.org/registries/slides.asp?yearToDisplay=2019. Accessed 31 Mar 2024
10. Chang DH, Youn JC, Dilibero D, Patel JK, Kobashigawa JA. Heart transplant immunosuppression strategies at cedars-sinai medical center. Int J Heart Fail. 2021;3(1):15.
11. Lund LH, Khush KK, Cherikh WS, Goldfarb S, Kucheryavaya AY, Levvey BJ, et al. The Registry of the International Society for Heart and Lung Transplantation: thirty-fourth adult heart transplantation report—2017; focus theme:

allograft ischemic time. J Heart Lung Transplant. 2017;36(10):1037–46.
12. Söderlund C, Rådegran G. Immunosuppressive therapies after heart transplantation—the balance between under-and over-immunosuppression. Transplant Rev. 2015;29(3):181–9.
13. Danovitch GM. Immunosuppressive medications and protocols for kidney transplantation. Handb Kidney Transplant. 2005;5:77–126.
14. Srinivas TR, Meier-Kriesche HU. Minimizing immunosuppression, an alternative approach to reducing side effects: objectives and interim result. Clin J Am Soc Nephrol. 2008;3(Supplement_2):S101-16.
15. Kobashigawa J, Miller L, Renlund D, Mentzer R, Alderman E, Bourge R, et al. A randomized active-controlled trial of mycophenolate mofetil in heart transplant recipients1. Transplantation. 1998;66(4):507–15.
16. Baran DA, Zucker MJ, Arroyo LH, Camacho M, Goldschmidt ME, Nicholls SJ, et al. A prospective, randomized trial of single-drug versus dual-drug immunosuppression in heart transplantation: the tacrolimus in combination, tacrolimus alone compared (TICTAC) trial. Circul Heart Fail. 2011;4(2):129–37.
17. Perkel D, Czer LSC, Morrissey RP, Ruzza A, Rafiei M, Awad M, et al. Heart transplantation for end-stage heart failure due to cardiac sarcoidosis. In: Transplantation proceedings. Elsevier; 2013. p. 2384–6.
18. Rosenthal DG, Anderson ME, Petek BJ, Arnett DM, Bravo PE, Raghu G, et al. Invasive hemodynamics and rejection rates in patients with cardiac sarcoidosis after heart transplantation. Can J Cardiol. 2018;34(8):978–82.
19. Ojo AO, Held PJ, Port FK, Wolfe RA, Leichtman AB, Young EW, et al. Chronic renal failure after transplantation of a nonrenal organ. N Engl J Med. 2003;349(10):931–40.
20. Delgado DH, Miriuka SG, Cusimano RJ, Feindel C, Rao V, Ross HJ. Use of basiliximab and cyclosporine in heart transplant patients with pre-operative renal dysfunction. J Heart Lung Transplant. 2005;24(2):166–9.
21. Cantarovich M, Metrakos P, Giannetti N, Cecere R, Barkun J, Tchervenkov J. Anti-CD25 monoclonal antibody coverage allows for calcineurin inhibitor "holiday" in solid organ transplant patients with acute renal dysfunction1. Transplantation. 2002;73(7):1169–72.
22. Mattei MF, Redonnet M, Gandjbakhch I, Bandini AM, Billes A, Epailly E, et al. Lower risk of infectious deaths in cardiac transplant patients receiving basiliximab versus anti-thymocyte globulin as induction therapy. J Heart Lung Transplant. 2007;26(7):693–9.
23. Hamour IM, Lyster HS, Burke MM, Rose ML, Banner NR. Mycophenolate mofetil may allow cyclosporine and steroid sparing in de novo heart transplant patients. Transplantation. 2007;83(5):570–6.
24. Angermann CE, Störk S, Costard-Jäckle A, Dengler TJ, Siebert U, Tenderich G, et al. Reduction of cyclosporine after introduction of mycophenolate mofetil improves chronic renal dysfunction in heart transplant recipients—the IMPROVED multi-centre study. Eur Heart J. 2004;25(18):1626–34.
25. Moro JA, Almenar L, Martinez-Dolz L, Sánchez-Lázaro I, Agüero J, Salvador A. Tolerance profile of the proliferation signal inhibitors everolimus and sirolimus in heart transplantation. In: Transplantation proceedings. Elsevier; 2008. p. 3034–6.
26. Chang DH, Kittleson M, Patel J, Aintablian T, Arakawa L, Jamero G, et al. Side effects of proliferation signal inhibitors limit their practical use after heart transplantation. J Heart Lung Transplant. 2017;36(4):S301.
27. Groetzner J, Kaczmarek I, Landwehr P, Mueller M, Daebritz S, Lamm P, et al. Renal recovery after conversion to a calcineurin inhibitor-free immunosuppression in late cardiac transplant recipients. Eur J Cardiothorac Surg. 2004;25(3):333–41.
28. Hunt J, Lerman M, Magee MJ, Dewey TM, Herbert M, Mack MJ. Improvement of renal dysfunction by conversion from calcineurin inhibitors to sirolimus after heart transplantation. J Heart Lung Transplant. 2005;24(11):1863–7.
29. Kushwaha SS, Khalpey Z, Frantz RP, Rodeheffer RJ, Clavell AL, Daly RC, et al. Sirolimus in cardiac transplantation: use as a primary immunosuppressant in calcineurin inhibitor–induced nephrotoxicity. J Heart Lung Transplant. 2005;24(12):2129–36.
30. Gullestad L, Iversen M, Mortensen SA, Eiskjær H, Riise GC, Mared L, et al. Everolimus with reduced calcineurin inhibitor in thoracic transplant recipients with renal dysfunction: a multicenter, randomized trial. Transplantation. 2010;89(7):864–72.
31. Hunt J, Bedanova H, Starling RC, Rabago G, Banner NR, Kobashigawa J, et al. 398: Premature termination of a prospective, open label, randomized, multicenter study of sirolimus to replace calcineurin inhibitors (CNI) in a standard care regimen of CNI, MMF and corticosteroids early after heart transplantation. J Heart Lung Transplant. 2007;26(2):S203.
32. Andreassen AK, Andersson B, Gustafsson F, Eiskjaer H, Rådegran G, Gude E, et al. Everolimus initiation with early calcineurin inhibitor withdrawal in de novo heart transplant recipients: three-year results from the randomized SCHEDULE study. Am J Transplant. 2016;16(4):1238–47.
33. Bollano E, Andreassen AK, Eiskjaer H, Gustafsson F, Rådegran G, Gude E, et al. Long-term follow-up of the randomized, prospective Scandinavian heart transplant everolimus de novo study with early calcineurin inhibitors avoidance (SCHEDULE) trial. J

Heart Lung Transplant [Internet]. 2024. https://doi.org/10.1016/j.healun.2024.07.002.
34. Nelson LM, Andreassen AK, Andersson B, Gude E, Eiskjær H, Rådegran G, et al. Effect of calcineurin inhibitor–free, everolimus-based immunosuppressive regimen on albuminuria and glomerular filtration rate after heart transplantation. Transplantation. 2017;101(11):2793–800.
35. Zuckermann A, Eisen H, Tai SS, Li H, Hahn C, Crespo-Leiro MG. Sirolimus conversion after heart transplant: risk factors for acute rejection and predictors of renal function response. Am J Transplant. 2014;14(9):2048–54.
36. Baran DA, Kapoor S, Grewal J, Andries G, Camacho M. Long term follow-up of the tacrolimus in combination, tacrolimus alone compared (TICTAC) trial. J Heart Lung Transplant. 2023;42(6):838–45.
37. Kobashigawa JA. Strategies in immunosuppression after heart transplantation: is less better? Circul Heart Fail Am Heart Assoc. 2011;4:111–3.
38. Pearston AP, Ingemi AI, Shaeffer ZA, Cameron CM, Biagi KT, Gobble M, et al. Conversion to tacrolimus alone compared to full immunosuppression following cardiac transplantation (TACTFUL). Clin Transplant. 2023;37(12):e15140.
39. Kowalski R, Post D, Schneider MC, Britz J, Thomas J, Deierhoi M, et al. Immune cell function testing: an adjunct to therapeutic drug monitoring in transplant patient management. Clin Transplant. 2003;17(2):77–88.
40. Cheng R, Azarbal B, Yung A, Chang DH, Patel JK, Kobashigawa JA. Elevated immune monitoring early after cardiac transplantation is associated with increased plaque progression by intravascular ultrasound. Clin Transplant. 2015;29(2):103–9.
41. Kobashigawa JA, Kiyosaki KK, Patel JK, Kittleson MM, Kubak BM, Davis SN, et al. Benefit of immune monitoring in heart transplant patients using ATP production in activated lymphocytes. J Heart Lung Transplant. 2010;29(5):504–8.
42. Kowalski RJ, Post DR, Mannon RB, Sebastian A, Wright HI, Sigle G, et al. Assessing relative risks of infection and rejection: a meta-analysis using an immune function assay. Transplantation. 2006;82(5):663–8.
43. Cantarovich M, Elstein E, de Varennes B, Barkun JS. Clinical benefit of neoral dose monitoring with cyclosporine 2-hr post-dose levels compared with trough levels in stable heart transplant patients1. Transplantation. 1999;68(12):1839–42.
44. Cantarovich M, Ross H, Arizón JM, Gómez MA, Straatman L, Orús J, et al. Benefit of Neoral C2 monitoring in de novo cardiac transplant recipients receiving basiliximab induction. Transplantation. 2008;85(7):992–9.
45. Brunet M, Van Gelder T, Åsberg A, Haufroid V, Hesselink DA, Langman L, et al. Therapeutic drug monitoring of tacrolimus-personalized therapy: second consensus report. Ther Drug Monit. 2019;41(3):261–307.
46. Al Moussawy M, Lakkis ZS, Ansari ZA, Cherukuri AR, Abou-Daya KI. The transformative potential of artificial intelligence in solid organ transplantation. Front Transplant. 2024;3:1361491.
47. Vincenti F, Larsen C, Durrbach A, Wekerle T, Nashan B, Blancho G, et al. Costimulation blockade with belatacept in renal transplantation. N Engl J Med. 2005;353(8):770–81.
48. Magua W, Okoh AK, Pranav P, Wang J, Karadkhele G, Cole R, et al. Belatacept-based immunosuppression in heart transplant recipients: national trends with outcomes from a single center. J Heart Lung Transplant. 2023;42(4):S248.
49. Patel JK, Coutance G, Loupy A, Dilibero D, Hamilton M, Kittleson M, et al. Complement inhibition for prevention of antibody-mediated rejection in immunologically high-risk heart allograft recipients. Am J Transplant. 2021;21(7):2479–88.

# 15 Pre-transplant Screening and Post-transplant Infection Prevention in Heart Transplant Recipients

Jillian Oft and Phillip Zakowski

**Abstract**

In addition to advances in surgical techniques, recipient/donor selection, and immunosuppression, progress in preventing and managing infections after heart transplant (HTx) has dramatically improved patient outcomes. While preventing rejection is crucial for long-term allograft survival, immunosuppressive regimens compromise the recipient's immune system and confer an increased risk of infection. HTx candidates and recipients are at risk for a multitude of infections, including community and hospital-acquired infections, opportunistic infections, and reactivation of latent infections. In this chapter, we will provide an overview of the prevention of infections after HTx, which begins with donor and recipient pre-transplant screening and includes targeted prophylaxis and infection prevention.

**Keywords**

Heart transplantation · Prophylaxis · Bacterial infections · Viral infections · Protozoa

P. Zakowski (✉) · J. Oft
Division of Infectious Diseases, Cedars-Sinai Medical Center, Los Angeles, CA, USA
e-mail: phillip.zakowski@cshs.org

J. Oft
e-mail: jillian.oft@cshs.org

## Clinical Pearls

- Pre-transplant screening of donors and candidates for bacterial/fungal/viral/protozoal infections is used to risk-stratify and guide targeted post-transplant infection prophylaxis.
- With careful selection, hearts from donors with positive blood cultures can be utilized and achieve favorable clinical outcomes
- Hearts from anti-HBc-positive donors carry a negligible risk of transmission in recipients immune to HBV and can be transplanted successfully with monitoring post-transplant
- Hearts from hepatitis C viremic donors may be used with HCV-specific informed consent, treatment, and monitoring.
- The combination of donor and recipient CMV status enables risk stratification and guide prophylaxis and monitoring
- With careful organ selection, it may be safe and effective to transplant organs from COVID-19 PCR-positive donors
- The vaccination history of the transplant candidate should be reviewed and updated as much as possible prior to transplant.
- Transplant recipients should continue to receive vaccinations post-transplant (after 6 months to reduce activating a rejection episode) with the exception of live virus vaccines.


J. Kobashigawa (ed.), *Clinical Guide to Heart Transplantation*, https://doi.org/10.1007/978-3-031-88290-6_15

- Additional preventive measures against infection include handwashing, remaining physically active, and being aware of potential pathogens in and out of the hospital, including animal-borne, food, and travel-related exposures.

## Pre-transplant Screening of the Donor and Recipient

Organ donors represent a potential vector of disease transmission to the recipient. Appropriate donor serologic screening prior to transplantation is crucial to identify infections that would prohibit transplant or require directed treatment or prophylaxis. The goal of pre- heart transplant (HTx) screening is to reduce the risk of infectious exposure to the recipient without prohibitively limiting the number of available organ donors. Infectious disease screening includes serologic testing, nucleic acid amplification testing (NAAT,) and donor microbiology cultures. When a donor heart becomes available, the medical and social history available in the Organ Procurement and Transplant Network (OPTN) database should include relevant information on risk factors for infection, including prior hospitalizations, blood transfusions, and intravenous drug use, if known. Additionally, the Organ Procurement Organization (OPO) provides results from donor microbiology cultures, serum serologies, and NAAT. NAAT is performed within 96 h of donation, as close as possible but with sufficient time so that the results are available at the time of transplant. In the following section, we will cover donor screening for each group of micro-organisms in greater detail.

## Donor Screening

### Bacterial Transmission

Bacterial infections may be transmitted as a result of active infection in the door or through contamination of the heart during procurement or transport. Most commonly, the source is a donor bacterial infection with bloodstream involvement, such as line sepsis, pneumonia, intra-abdominal sepsis, genitourinary sepsis, or even post-traumatic skin/soft tissue infection. Blood cultures should, therefore, be routinely performed as part of the evaluation for a potential donor heart. While isolated cases report transmission of bacteria such as Staphylococc*us, Pseudomonas,* and *Escherichia coli* from donor to recipient causing serious infective complications and death, more recent and comprehensive data suggests that donors who die of severe community-acquired bacterial infections (e.g., bacterial meningitis, pneumonia, septic shock) should not be arbitrarily excluded [1] and that with careful selection, donors with positive blood cultures can be used and maintain quality clinical outcomes [2]. With this in mind, the International Society for Heart and Lung Transplantation (ISHLT) specifies that heart from donors with bacteremia can be used, provided that the following criteria are met: donor has received a minimum of 24 h of targeted antimicrobial therapy, ideally with clearance of cultures, donor myocardial function is normal, and there is no evidence of endocarditis on inspection of the heart [3]. Additionally, in cases where such hearts are used for transplantation, the recipient should undergo surveillance blood cultures on the first post-operative day. Recipients of hearts from bacteremia donors should receive an appropriate course of therapy targeting the donor isolate. A similar recommendation exists for cases in which the donor has a known history of untreated or incompletely treated latent tuberculosis infection (LTBI): recipients should be treated for LTBI. Patients with active *Mycobacterium tuberculosis* infection are not recommended for organ donation [4–6].

### Fungal Transmission

Active fungal infection in a donor is a contraindication to transplantation. Transmission of Histoplasma and Coccidioides via organ transplant have been reported, although more commonly, infection is the result of reactivation in a previously infected recipient. Universal donor screening for endemic mycoses is not required, but explanted organs that contain granulomas should be tested for fungal histopathology and culture. In such cases, antigen and serology screening for Histoplasma and Coccidioides should be performed on blood and any stored body fluid samples [7].

## Viral Transmission

### Hepatitis B

Hepatitis B (HBV) remains ubiquitous in the global population, with over 300 million people affected. Prevalence and endemicity vary significantly across different regions. In recent years, the prevalence of past or present hepatitis B infection in the United States was estimated at approximately 4% [8]. The incidence of chronic hepatitis has decreased with infection control practices and the availability of effective vaccination. HBV vaccine provides significant protection against HBV infection and should be given prior to transplantation when possible since post-transplant response rates are decreased owing to immunosuppression. Serologic testing for anti-HBs 4–8 weeks after completion of the vaccine series is recommended to confirm immunity.

Donor screening for HBV is performed by surface antigen testing (HBsAg), serologic testing for antibodies against Hepatitis B surface antigen (anti-HBs), as well as antibodies against core antigen (anti-HBc) and universal HBV NAAT [9]. Many transplant centers will not accept a donor organ that is HBV NAAT positive due to the risk of reactivation, fulminant hepatitis, hepatocellular carcinoma, and cirrhosis. In contrast, hearts from anti-HBc donors carry a negligible risk of transmission in recipients immune to HBV [10]. No antiviral prophylaxis is required if the recipient has evidence of natural (anti-HBc, anti-HBs) or vaccine induced (anti-HBs only) immunity when an isolated anti-HBc donor is used. However, for non-immune recipients of anti-HBc donor organs, antiviral prophylaxis should be provided with tenofovir or entecavir, particularly during the first 12 months. Hearts from HBsAg donors do carry a risk of transmission but may be considered on an individual case basis with informed consent and use of antiviral prophylaxis, potentially indefinitely [11].

### Hepatitis C

Hepatitis C (HCV) is an enveloped, single-stranded blood-borne RNA virus with tissue reservoirs in the body. Donor screening for HCV is performed by serology and universal HCV NAAT. Transplant centers historically excluded donors who were infected with HCV due to the high rate of transmission of HCV, accelerated cardiac allograft vasculopathy, cirrhotic liver disease, and increased mortality in those receiving HCV-infected hearts [12]. However, the widespread availability of NAAT and substantial advances in treatment have allowed for the expansion of the donor pool, with many centers now utilizing hearts from HCV seropositive and viremic donors to HCV-negative recipients. HTx using organs from HCV viremic donors has been associated with excellent short-term outcomes. Current ISHLT recommendations state that hearts from hepatitis C viremic donors may be used with HCV-specific informed consent and treatment and monitoring in accordance with guidelines [3, 13].

### Cytomegalovirus

Cytomegalovirus (CMV) is a ubiquitous b-herpesvirus and a common opportunistic infection in HTx recipients. The seroprevalence of CMV in US adults is approximately 50% and varies with age, geography, and socioeconomic status. Higher seroprevalence rates have been reported in the organ donor population. Donor screening for CMV is performed using CMV-IgG [14]. Ideally, blood should be drawn from the donor prior to any blood transfusions, but this may not be possible, particularly in cases of trauma. There is no role for CMV IgM or polymerase chain reaction (PCR) in donors unless acute CMV infection is suspected. It is generally accepted that CMV-IgG-positive donor hearts can be transplanted into CMV-negative recipients due to the demonstrated success of prophylaxis and treatment. Nevertheless, it is vital that all donors have CMV serological status determined, as the combination of donor and recipient CMV status enables risk stratification for prophylaxis and monitoring.

### Human Immunodeficiency Virus

There are several documented cases of Human Immunodeficiency Virus (HIV) transmission from donor to recipient in cardiac transplantation [15], most of which occurred prior to the introduction of routine screening in 1985. All potential transplant donors should be tested for HIV. Donor screening is performed using current fourth-generation HIV antibody / p24 antigen tests, as well as universal NAAT screening. Just as for HBV and HCV, NAAT testing for HIV is performed within 96 h pre-transplant to yield the most current result possible. HIV-positive hearts are not eligible for transplant to HIV-negative recipients. However, the 2013 HIV Organ Policy Equity Act allowed HIV-positive donor organs to be used in HIV-positive recipients, thus expanding the donor pool for this particular subset of patients. Such transplants are currently conducted in the context of multicenter clinical trials and are an area of evolving developments in the field [16].

### Human T-Lymphotropic Virus

Human T-Lymphotropic Virus I (HTLV-1) is endemic in parts of the world, including the Caribbean, Japan, and parts of Africa. Infection is more common in individuals from these areas and is often asymptomatic. HTLV-2 is more widespread but not clearly associated with any disease. Due to low seroprevalence in the United States and the poor predictive value of available screening assays, routine screening of donors for HTLV-1/2 is not recommended [7]. Individual OPOs may elect to perform testing on certain high-risk individuals. If serologic status is known, current OPTN policy recommends against the use of donors with HTLV-1 seropositivity due to the risk of transmission and subsequent development of adult T-cell leukemia and spastic paraparesis, with reports of myelopathy after solid organ transplantation [17].

### West Nile Virus

West Nile Virus (WNV) is a flavivirus which can cause neuroinvasive disease with meningoencephalitis and polio-like myelitis. It is transmissible by blood transfusion and organ transplantation, with reports of transmission and death in solid organ transplant recipients [18]. Serology and PCR for WNV are available but limited by cost, logistics, risk of false positive testing, and widely varying risk depending on geographic distribution and time of year. Thus, although living organ donors are screened for WNV, HTx donors are not uniformly tested for WNV. However, donors with known WNV should be avoided, as well as donors with unexplained meningoencephalitis, as this scenario could pose a risk of transmission of other central nervous system viral infections. Select OPOs may elect to perform testing in regions of high virus circulation, particularly during the summer months. However, WNV illustrates one of the many challenges of managing infections in this population, as not every infection can be definitively ruled out or treated pre-emptively. Transplant clinicians should remain vigilant in their awareness of possible infectious risks and counsel transplant candidates and their families about the possibility of infectious diseases being transmitted during HTx [18].

### SARS-CoV2

The COVID-19 pandemic resulting from the SARS-CoV-2 virus was disruptive to many areas of the medical system, including organ transplantation, and exacerbated an already significant national shortage of thoracic organs. Donors are screened via PCR from nasopharyngeal swabs. There was initial uncertainty about the risks of using organs from COVID-19-positive donors. However, increasing evidence suggests that with careful organ selection, it may be safe and effective to transplant organs from COVID-19 PCR-positive donors. There is no evidence that a transmissible virus exists in cardiac allografts, and there have been no reports of donor-derived infection outside of the lung [19]. Further discussion of COVID-19, including management of active COVID-19 acquired after transplant, is covered separately.

## Protozoal Transmission

### Toxoplasma Gondii, Trypanosoma Cruzi (Chagas Disease)

*Toxoplasma gondii* is a protozoan parasite prevalent in humans and food animals, causing worldwide zoonosis and may be transmitted by organ transplant or blood transfusion. Donors are screened via serologic testing for Toxoplasma IgG. T.gondii donor seropositivity is not a contraindication to transplant but is important for the purposes of risk stratification and subsequent prophylaxis and treatment. Data from the literature are mixed regarding outcomes from T.gondii donor-recipient mismatched cardiac transplants [20, 21]. HTx is a safe and effective treatment for patients with advanced heart failure caused by the Trypanosoma cruzi parasite better known as Chagas disease. Because the immunosuppression required for a HTx can reactivate the disease, it was once considered a contraindication for the procedure. However, HTx is now the preferred treatment for patients with end-stage Chagas disease in countries where it's available. Endemic areas are in the Southwest U.S. [22]. To prevent negative outcomes, it's important to carefully screen patients for Chagas disease before a transplant. Reactivation of Chagas disease can lead to serious complications, including: myocarditis, allograft dysfunction, congestive heart failure, graft failure, and sepsis. Two drugs, benznidazole and nifurtimox, are effective for treating Chagas disease [23].

## Recipient Screening

HTx candidates undergo mirrored evaluation for the same diseases as the donor via serologic screening. In addition to evaluation for exposure to prior infections, evaluation of the potential transplant candidate's infection risk should also include a thorough history of antibiotic allergies (with the nature of the reaction), a dental examination, and a routine assessment for active infection.

## Bacterial/Fungal/Viral Infections

Recipients with active or uncontrolled bacterial or fungal infections should generally delay transplant until the infection is controlled. Table 15.1 summarizes the routine infection screening recommended for a transplant candidate [7]. All candidates should be evaluated for latent tuberculosis infection with a tuberculin skin test (TST) or interferon-gamma release assay (IGRA). Candidates or recipients with latent TB infection (LTBI) should be treated prophylactically to avoid progression to active tuberculosis. Isoniazid is the mainstay of treatment. Shorter regimens using Rifampin, or Isoniazid and Rifapentine are alternative regimens which may confer an advantage for compliance and completion rates in the pre-transplant setting. These regimens are not preferred post-transplant due to drug-drug interactions and may not be ideal if the patient is likely to undergo transplantation while receiving treatment for LTBI. Treatment LTBI should be started prior to transplantation unless there is a contraindication. If isoniazid is started pre-transplant, it can be held in the early peri-transplant period and resumed when the patient is stable and tolerating oral medications. The presence of a pre-existing infection such as HIV or Hepatitis B/C is not an absolute contraindication to transplant, but these patients should be treated appropriately prior to transplant. In the case of active or acute viral infection in a candidate, the transplant should be delayed, if possible, until the infection resolves or is controlled. Timing of transplant of candidates with acute community-acquired viral infections depends on urgency of transplant, severity of infection, and available treatment options. Vaccine-preventable infections are a common source of morbidity post-cardiac transplantation. The vaccination history and serostatus of the transplant candidate should be reviewed and updated prior to transplant, including those for diphtheria, tetanus, varicella zoster virus (VZV), hepatitis A/B, influenza A/B, *Hemophilus influenza* B, polio, meningococcus,

**Table 15.1** Recommended pathogenic screening in transplant candidates

| |
|---|
| • Antibiotic/medication allergies, adverse reactions |
| • Chest radiograph (to look for infiltrates, granulomas, scarring) |
| • Dental assessment |
| • Social/sexual history; high-risk behaviors, intravenous drug use, communicable diseases |
| • IGRA, history of tuberculosis risk factors |
| • Serologies for tetanus, diphtheria, measles, mumps and pneumococcal titers are recommended and may guide pretransplant immunization recommendations |
| • Routine serologic testing |
| - HIV Ab/Ag (4th generation HIV screening test) |
| - CMV IgG |
| - Hepatitis B screening: HBsAg, anti-HBc, anti-HBs |
| - HCV IgG |
| - EBV antibody panel (EBV VCA IgG, IgM) |
| - HSV IgG antibody |
| - VZV IgG antibody |
| - Syphilis screening- RPR, FTA-ABS, TP-EIA, TPPA, or VDRL |
| - *Toxoplasma* IgG |
| • Special serologic testing based on epidemiologic risk factors or exposure history |
| - Coccidioides IgM and IgG antibody |
| - Histoplasma immunodiffusion antibody or urine antigen |
| - HTLV-I/II antibody |
| - *Strongyloides* IgG |
| - *Trypanosoma cruzi* IgG |

*Abbreviations* IGRA: interferon-gamma release assay; HIV: human immunodeficiency virus; CMV: cytomegalovirus; Hepatitis B surface antigen; anti-HBc: hepatitis B core antibody; anti-HBs: hepatitis B surface antibody; HCV: hepatitis C; EBV: Epstein-Barr Virus; HSV: Herpes Simplex Virus; VZV: Varicella Zoster Virus; HTLV: Human T-Cell Lymphotropic Virus

SARS-CoV2, measles, mumps and rubella (MMR). VZV and MMR screening are of particular importance, so that seronegative candidates can be vaccinated if possible. Vaccination should be administered prior to any desensitization protocol to preserve the antibody response. Live vaccines like MMR can only be given before transplant and are contraindicated after transplant [7].

## Preventive Measures

In addition to antimicrobial prophylaxis and appropriate vaccination prior to transplantation, the usual infection control measures should be enacted after transplant. During hospitalization, hand-washing procedures by both staff and visitors are mandatory. Healthcare providers with air-transmissible diseases should also refrain from direct contact with the patient. As outpatients, caution should be exercised to minimize the risk of environmental or occupational exposures to potential pathogens, as well as pet-related exposures (birds, certain reptiles, livestock, stray animals), certain types of food should be avoided (raw or undercooked meat, unpasteurized dairy products), and the patient should be aware of possible travel-related exposures (including endemic or communicable diseases if traveling to a new area, as well as exposures related to exposure to natural bodies of water or caves, for instance). There is disagreement about the need for antibiotic prophylaxis, but there is a strong agreement that maintenance of good dental health is important. Despite diligent efforts at prevention, infections remain common after transplant. The next chapter will discuss the management of infections after HTx.

## References

1. Kubak BM, Gregson AL, Pegues DA, Leibowitz MR, Carlson M, Marelli D, et al. Use of hearts transplanted from donors with severe sepsis and infectious deaths. J Heart Lung Transplant. 2009;28(3):260–5.

2. Siddiqi U, Blitzer D, Lirette S, Patel A, Hoang R, Mohammed A, et al. Positive donor blood cultures are not associated with worse heart transplant survival. Clin Transplant. 2023.
3. Velleca A, Shullo MA, Dhital K, Azeka E, Colvin M, DePasquale E, et al. The International Society for Heart and Lung Transplantation (ISHLT) guidelines for the care of heart transplant recipients. J Heart Lung Transplant. 2023;42(5):e1-141.
4. Morris MI, Daly JS, Blumberg E, Kumar D, Sester M, Schluger N, et al. Diagnosis and management of tuberculosis in transplant donors: a donor-derived infections consensus conference report. Am J Transplant. 2012:2288–300.
5. Malinis M, LaHoz RM, Vece G, Annambhotla P, Aslam S, Basavaraju SV, et al. Donor-derived tuberculosis among solid organ transplant recipients in the United States—2008 to 2018. Transplant Infect Dis. 2022;24(2):e13800.
6. Subramanian AK, Theodoropoulos NM. Mycobacterium tuberculosis infections in solid organ transplantation: guidelines from the infectious diseases community of practice of the American Society of Transplantation. Clin Transplant. 2019;33(9):e13513.
7. Malinis M, Boucher HW. Practice ASTIDC of Screening of donor and candidate prior to solid organ transplantation—guidelines from the American Society of Transplantation Infectious Diseases Community of Practice. Clin Transplant. 2019;33(9):e13548.
8. Kruszon-Moran D, Paulose-Ram R, Martin CB, Barker LK, Mcquillan G. Prevalence and trends in Hepatitis B virus infection in the United States, 2015–2018 key findings data from the national health and nutrition examination survey [internet]. 2015. https://www.cdc.gov/nchs/products/index.htm.
9. Te H, Doucette K. Viral hepatitis: guidelines by the American Society of Transplantation Infectious Disease Community of Practice. Clin Transplant. 2019;33(9):e13514.
10. Pinney SP, Cheema FH, Hammond K, Chen JM, Edwards NM, Mancini D. Acceptable recipient outcomes with the use of hearts from donors with hepatitis-B core antibodies. J Heart Lung Transplant. 2005;24(1):34–7.
11. Yost CC, Jimenez DC, Weber MP, Belden KA, Tchantchaleishvili V, Massey HT, et al. Hepatitis B in heart transplant donors and recipients: a systematic review. J Heart Lung Transplant. 2021;40(4):S272.
12. Carbone M, Mutimer D, Neuberger J. Hepatitis C virus and nonliver solid organ transplantation. Transplantation. 2013;95:779–86.
13. Aslam S, Grossi P, Schlendorf KH, Holm AM, Woolley AE, Blumberg E, et al. Utilization of hepatitis C virus–infected organ donors in cardiothoracic transplantation: an ISHLT expert consensus statement. J Heart Lung Transplant. 2020;39(5):418–32.
14. Razonable RR, Humar A. Cytomegalovirus in solid organ transplant recipients—guidelines of the American Society of Transplantation Infectious Diseases Community of Practice. Clin Transplant. 2019;33(9):e13512.
15. Erice A, Rhame FS, Heussner RC, Dunn DL, Balfour HH. Human immunodeficiency virus infection in patients with solid-organ transplants: report of five cases and review. Rev Infect Dis. 1991;13(4):537–47.
16. Malani PN. New law allows organ transplants from deceased HIV-infected donors to HIV-infected recipients [internet]. 2013. www.sciencesource.com.
17. Ramanan P, Deziel PJ, Norby SM, Yao JD, Garza I, Razonable RR. Donor-transmitted HTLV-1-associated myelopathy in a kidney transplant recipient-case report and literature review. Am J Transplant. 2014;14:2417–21.
18. Soto RA, McDonald E, Annambhotla P, Velez JO, Laven J, Panella AJ, et al. West Nile virus transmission by solid organ transplantation and considerations for organ donor screening practices, United States. Emerg Infect Dis. 2022;28(2):403–6.
19. Eichenberger EM, Coniglio AC, Milano C, Schroder J, Bryner BS, Spencer PJ, et al. Transplanting thoracic COVID-19 positive donors: an institutional protocol and report of the first 14 cases. J Heart Lung Transplant. 2022;41(10):1376–81.
20. Kittleson MM, Kobashigawa JA. Toxoplasma gondii exposure in the heart transplant recipient: good, bad, or indifferent? Transplantation. 2013;96:1025.
21. Barge-Caballero E, Almenar-Bonet L, Crespo-Leiro MG, Brossa-Loidi V, Rangel-Sousa D, Gómez-Bueno M, et al. Preoperative Toxoplasma gondii serostatus does not affect long-term survival of cardiac transplant recipients. Analysis of the Spanish heart transplantation registry. Int J Cardiol. 2018;250:183–7.
22. da Consolação Vieira Moreira M, Renan Cunha-Melo J. Chagas disease infection reactivation after heart transplant. Trop Med Infect Dis. 2020;5(3):106.
23. Gray EB, La Hoz RM, Green JS, Vikram HR, Benedict T, Rivera H, et al. Reactivation of Chagas disease among heart transplant recipients in the United States, 2012–2016. Transpl Infect Dis. 2018;20(6):e12996.

# Managing Infections After Heart Transplantation

16

Jillian Oft and Phillip Zakowski

**Abstract**

Heart Transplant (HTx) recipients are at risk for a multitude of infections, including community and hospital-acquired infections, opportunistic infections, and reactivation of latent infections. In this chapter, we will provide an overview of the management of infections after HTx. We will discuss common pathogens, unique challenges, and general clinical approaches to managing infections in HTx recipients.

**Keywords**

Heart transplantation · Prophylaxis · Bacterial infections · Viral infections · Protozoa

## Clinical Pearls

- Bacterial organisms of importance that may cause infection post-transplant include Staphylococci, Enterococci, Streptococci, Listeria, Nocardia, C. difficile, Pseudomonas, H. influenzae and Legionella.
- Prophylaxis against CMV and/or HSV should be provided for all recipients using valganciclovir or acyclovir post-transplant. Selection and duration of prophylaxis depend on donor and recipient's history of infection.
- Viral infections are common in transplant recipients, including reactivation or newly acquired CMV, HSV, and VZV, as well as community respiratory and gastrointestinal viruses.
- Post-transplant prophylaxis against Pneumocystis includes trimethoprim-sulfamethoxazole as first-line treatment (typically for 1 year after transplant).
- Candida and Aspergillus are common fungal infections post-transplant.
- Transplant recipients are less likely to present with typical features of infection, including fever and leukocytosis, and more likely to present with organ dysfunction.
- The clinical approach to management of a suspected infection in a transplant recipient should take into account the time elapsed since transplant, donor/recipient infectious history, recent exposures, history of rejection and current immunosuppression regimen including induction or recently augmented immunosuppression.
- Generally speaking, for the assessment of pulmonary infiltrates, bacterial and viral infections tend to present acutely, whereas

J. Oft · P. Zakowski (✉)
Division of Infectious Diseases, Cedars-Sinai Medical Center, Los Angeles, CA, USA
e-mail: phillip.zakowski@cshs.org

J. Oft
e-mail: jillian.oft@cshs.org



J. Kobashigawa (ed.), *Clinical Guide to Heart Transplantation*, https://doi.org/10.1007/978-3-031-88290-6_16

fungal and parasitic infections are more insidious in onset. Judicious use of microbial cell-free DNA testing may aid in noninvasive diagnosis. A definitive diagnosis can often be obtained via histology from BAL and/or transbronchial lung biopsy.

## Bacterial Infections

Bacterial infections remain the most common cause of infectious morbidity in patients at all stages following HTx. Bacterial infections rise in the early post-transplantation period as recipients undergo induction of immunosuppression, presenting as wound infections, pneumonia, urinary tract infections (UTIs), bacteremia from catheter-associated infections, and, rarely, infective endocarditis [1]. Broadly speaking, pathogens in the early post-transplant period are similar to those causing infections in non-transplant surgical patients, including *Staphylococci,* as well as gram-negative bacilli and *Candida* spp.

## Peri-Operative Prophylaxis

Perioperative bacterial prophylaxis should include activity against skin flora with a cephalosporin, with or without vancomycin. If a chronically infected device (i.e., left ventricular assist device infection or infected ECMO circuit) is present at the time of transplant, perioperative antibiotics are directed to the involved pathogens. Duration depends on the extent of infection and whether source control is established [2].

## Gram-Positive Organisms

### Staphylococci

*Staphylococcus* species are the most common Gram-positive organisms causing infections after HTx, especially early post-transplant [3, 4]. *S. aureus* is the most common of these. Common manifestations include surgical site infections, line infections, pneumonia, or UTI. Rarely, S. *aureus* has been associated with endocarditis shortly after transplant. Methicillin-sensitive *S. aureus* (MSSA) may be treated with oxacillin or cefazolin. For methicillin-resistant *S. aureus* (MRSA), vancomycin is the first-line drug, although other antibiotics with MRSA activity may be preferred depending on allergy, intolerance, or the source and severity of the infection. In severe staphylococcal infections, combination therapy may be necessary. Coagulase-negative *staphylococci (CoNS)* are another group that commonly cause infection after HTx. Nearly all cases are nosocomial. Because these bacteria reside on human skin and mucous membranes, they are commonly found in the cultures of wound environments and may represent surface colonizers with or without involvement in a deeper infection. CoNS may also cause line-associated bloodstream infections in patients after HTx, like other surgical patients. Because of their potential as colonizers, attribution of infection requires consideration of the overall clinical picture. There is a high rate of methicillin resistance among the coagulase-negative staphylococci, making Vancomycin the recommended first-line drug pending susceptibilities.

### Enterococci

Enterococci are part of the normal gut flora but take on increased significance in the immunocompromised host. Like staphylococci, enterococcal infections commonly occur early after cardiac transplantation and manifest as wound or line infections, gastrointestinal, biliary, and urinary tract infections. Enterococci engage in synergistic relationships with other gut flora and are often involved in polymicrobial infections, although they may be the sole cause of line-associated bloodstream infections or urinary tract infections. For sensitive enterococci, the treatment of choice is ampicillin or vancomycin. However, in recent years, the emergence of vancomycin-resistant enterococci (VRE) has been a major source of morbidity and mortality [5]. VRE are a rising cause of resistant gram-positive infections in transplant recipients, exceeding MRSA in some patient cohorts [6]. Immunosuppressive agents may also contribute to alterations in the gut microbiome over time and influence risk of enterococcal infections [7]. Linezolid and daptomycin are preferred treatment options for ampicillin-resistant VRE. Infected lines or devices should be removed, and any urinary or biliary obstruction should be addressed.

## Streptococcus Pneumoniae

HTx recipients are at increased risk of *Streptococcus pneumoniae* infection compared to non-transplanted individuals [8], presenting with pneumonia, bacteremia, or meningitis. Pneumococcal infection is often community-acquired and tends to present later after transplantation (beyond one year). HTx recipients and close contacts should maintain current pneumococcal vaccines, which protect against many but not all serotypes. The treatment of choice is penicillin when sensitive. In cases of pneumococcal sepsis, vancomycin should be administered empirically while sensitivities are pending.

## Listeria Monocytogenes

*Listeria monocytogenes* is an important pathogen in the immunocompromised host. Risk correlates with the degree of immunosuppression, typically presenting early after transplantation or during treatment of rejection when boluses of immunosuppression are required. In the immunocompetent host, *Listeria* generally causes mild gastroenteritis, but transplant recipients commonly present with more invasive diseases, including bacteremia and meningitis [9]. HTx recipients with neurologic symptoms should undergo prompt lumbar puncture for cerebrospinal fluid (CSF) analysis and should be treated empirically with broad-spectrum antibiotics, including ampicillin, the treatment of choice for listeriosis. *L. monocytogenes* is known to be associated with unpasteurized meat and dairy products, and patients are advised to avoid them.

## Nocardia

*Nocardia* spp. are ubiquitous gram-positive rods that cause infections in immunocompromised individuals and are particularly associated with defective cell-mediated immunity. Despite the implementation of trimethoprim-sulfamethoxazole prophylaxis, *Nocardia* infections have been on the rise over the past two decades, likely due to increased detection as well as a growing immunocompromised population, with more recipients living longer. Nocardiosis may present at any time post-transplant, particularly when presenting with pulmonary or central nervous system (CNS) symptoms soon after intensified immunosuppression. Anti-lymphocyte globulin, high calcineurin inhibitor or cyclosporine levels, or high-dose corticosteroids are associated with increased risk, as well as cytomegalovirus disease in the preceding six months [10]. In HTx recipients, nocardiosis typically presents as subacute pneumonia with pulmonary nodular lesions. Up to 50% of pulmonary cases may be complicated by extrapulmonary spread [10] with brain abscess, skin and subcutaneous tissue infections, and bone and eye involvement reported [11]. The diagnosis of Nocardia pulmonary infection should prompt consideration of disseminated disease, with MRI to evaluate for brain abscess. Initial treatment should include antibiotic therapy with trimethoprim-sulfamethoxazole, and combination therapy with imipenem should be used for severe or CNS disease. Alternatives include imipenem, linezolid, or ceftriaxone. Immunosuppression should be reduced if possible. Definitive treatment may require surgical debridement, and the duration of antibiotics is generally at least 6–12 months [10].

## Rhodococcus Equi

A Gram-positive coccobacillus, *R. equi,* typically causes infection in animals but can also affect immunocompromised humans, causing pulmonary infection later after transplantation [12, 13]. It typically presents with nodular or cavitary pneumonia and empyema and may be confused with tuberculosis [14]. Treatment options include Vancomycin (nearly all isolates are susceptible), as well as macrolides, carbapenems, and ciprofloxacin. Combination therapy with two antibiotics is generally recommended, but the resolution may lag behind clinical improvement. Patients who have received a reasonable course with a clinical response may finish antibiotic therapy and then be monitored, even if lesions are not completely resolved [15].

### Mycobacteria

Both mycobacterium tuberculosis (MTB) and non-tuberculous mycobacteria (NTM) are potential causes of serious infections after HTx. Reactivation of tuberculosis may occur from donor-derived infections [16] or in individuals who resided in or visited a country with a high prevalence of MTB. HTx recipients may not present with typical symptoms of cough, hemoptysis, night sweats, and fever. Necrotizing granulomas in biopsy sites are a key finding, and disseminated infection, including involvement of skin, bone, and CNS, may also occur. Approximately 30% of MTB cases after solid organ transplant are extra-pulmonary [17]. Treatment for active MTB in HTx recipients is largely the same as for an immunocompetent host. Initial treatment should consist of isoniazid, rifampin (or rifabutin due to drug-drug interactions), pyrazinamide, and ethambutol [17]. Both isoniazid and rifampin affect the cytochrome P-450 enzyme system, requiring close monitoring of immunosuppressive levels.

## Gram-Negative Organisms

### Aerobic Gram-Negative Bacilli

Aerobic gram-negative bacilli are common causes of infection in post-transplant patients, causing pneumonia, mediastinitis, wound infections, UTIs, intra-abdominal sepsis, bacteremia, and rarely endocarditis. Infections often present within the first 1–2 months, similar to other post-surgical patients. Antibiotic resistance of these pathogens is an increasing problem globally. HTx recipients are at risk for infection from multidrug-resistant (MDR) organisms. Bacterial infection within the first year post-HTx has been associated with a higher risk of mortality, increasing further among patients with extensive drug resistance [6]. The usual sources for these pathogens are the gut and the respiratory tract. Respiratory tract gram-negative bacilli of note include *Haemophilus influenzae, Pseudomonas aeruginosa, Burkholderia cepacia, Stenotrophomonas maltophilia; Enteric Gram-negative bacilli* include *Escherichia coli, Pseudomonas spp., Enterobacter spp., Serratia spp., Klebsiella spp., Proteus spp.,* and *Citrobacter spp*. Treatment for gram-negative bacilli is based on susceptibility patterns per institution, and empiric therapy for hospitalized patients should include a broad-spectrum penicillin or carbapenem and consideration of an aminoglycoside for severe infections. Because many of these infections are nosocomial and the epidemiology of gram-negative infections varies between institutions, optimizing care for HTx recipients requires continued attention to infection prevention and control practices and tracking local antimicrobial susceptibility patterns.

### Legionella

HTx recipients are at increased risk of infections due to *Legionella spp*. The most common species are *L. pneumophilia* and *L. micdadei*, which usually cause pneumonia but may cause extrapulmonary infections [18]. In rare cases, *Legionella* may be transmitted to the patient via a contaminated water source within the hospital [19]. The clinical presentation may be non-specific, with fever, myalgias, non-productive cough, pleuritic chest pain, and diarrhea in half of all cases. Sputum culture using special media, direct-fluorescent testing of sputum or bronchoalveolar fluid, and urinary antigen testing are definitive diagnostic methods. When legionellosis is suspected, empiric treatment should be started, as delayed treatment corresponds with increased mortality. Even with treatment, legionella mortality ranges from 9 to 25%, including non-transplant patients. Fluoroquinolones and macrolides have similar efficacy [20]. The choice of drug may depend on allergies, side effect profile, and drug interactions. Importantly, macrolides can increase blood levels of calcineurin inhibitors.

### Clostridium Difficile

Diarrhea is relatively common in all stages following HTx and may be due to infection or medication effects. *Clostridium difficile* infection (CDI) is the most common infectious diarrhea and is typically nosocomial, with broad-spectrum antibiotics an exacerbating factor. Patients who have recently been treated for rejection may also be at risk. Potential complications of *C. difficile* infection include pseudomembranous colitis, intestinal perforation, and toxic megacolon. Additionally, severe diarrhea can lead to electrolyte abnormalities and malabsorption of immunosuppressive agents. The first step in the treatment of CDI is the cessation or narrowing of broad-spectrum systemic antibiotics. Oral vancomycin or fidaxomicin are recommended for the treatment of an initial episode of CDI. For cases of severe-complicated or fulminant CDI, high-dose vancomycin (500 mg orally QID) may be combined with intravenous metronidazole and possibly vancomycin retention enemas. Timely surgical evaluation is essential in cases of fulminant CDI in HTx recipients. Treatment options for recurrent CDI include fidaxomicin, vancomycin taper, or vancomycin followed by rifaximin. Additionally, Bezlotoxumab, a monoclonal antibody against *C difficile* toxin B, is recommended for solid organ transplant recipients at risk for recurrent CDI. Data on the use of fecal microbiota restoration therapy (FMT) in immunocompromised individuals are limited, but retrospective analyses suggest that outcomes for FMT for recurrent CDI are similar to those in immunocompetent individuals [21].

## Viral Infections

Viral infections are common after HTx, second only to bacterial infections in frequency. They commonly occur within six months post-transplantation but may occur at any stage following transplantation.

### Peri-Operative Prophylaxis

ISHLT guidelines recommend perioperative anti-viral prophylaxis in all transplant recipients against Cytomegalovirus (CMV) and Herpes simplex virus (HSV). Intravenous ganciclovir or oral valganciclovir is administered to patients in the highest risk category (i.e., CMV seropositive donor to CMV seronegative recipients), whereas patients at low risk for CMV infection may only receive anti-HSV prophylaxis with acyclovir. Some centers may also add CMV immunoglobulin in high-risk patients. Dosages of these drugs are given in Table 16.1, while recommendations for the duration of viral prophylaxis in HTx recipients according to risk category are summarized in Table 16.2 [2, 22].

### Cytomegalovirus

CMV is a ubiquitous DNA virus that commonly infects humans, establishing lifelong latency after primary infection. It is a pathogen of significant importance in transplant recipients. Transmission occurs through close contact, blood or tissue exposure, and perinatally. Seroprevalence is as high as 90% in certain regional populations around the world and over 50% in adults in the United States [23]. In the non-transplant host, CMV infection stimulates the development of cellular and antibody-mediated immunity, which controls viral persistence. After HTx, latent CMV may become reactivated. Alternatively, denovo CMV infection may be acquired during a transplant from a seropositive donor. Primary donor-derived CMV infection occurs when a CMV-seronegative recipient receives a CMV-positive donor organ (considered "high-risk" for CMV infection), whereas secondary CMV infection represents infection in a previously seropositive host, caused by reactivation of latent virus or additional infection with a new viral strain. Risk for CMV disease

**Table 16.1** Antiviral drugs for CMV prevention and treatment in heart transplant recipients

| Drug | Treatment[1] | Prophylaxis | Comments on use and toxicity |
|---|---|---|---|
| Valganciclovir | 900-mg[2] po twice daily | 900 mg[2] po once daily | Ease of administration<br>Leukopenia is major toxicity |
| IV Ganciclovir | 5 mg/kg IV every 12 h | 5 mg/kg IV once daily | Intravenous access and complications<br>Leukopenia is major toxicity |
| Valacyclovir | NOT recommended | 2 g po four times daily | Use in kidney transplant recipients only<br>NOT recommended for heart, liver, pancreas, lung, intestinal and composite tissue transplant recipients<br>High pill burden<br>Neurotoxicity<br>NOT recommended for treatment of CMV disease or asymptomatic infection |
| Foscarnet | 60 mg/kg IV every 8 h (or 90 mg/kg every 12 h) | NOT recommended | Second-line alternative for treatment<br>Highly nephrotoxic<br>Used for UL97-mutant ganciclovir-resistant CMV infection or disease<br>NOT recommended for preemptive therapy |
| Cidofovir | 5 mg/kg once weekly × 2 then every 2 weeks thereafter | NOT recommended | Third-line agent<br>Highly nephrotoxic<br>Used for UL97-mutant ganciclovir-resistant CMV infection or disease<br>NOT recommended for preemptive therapy |

Intravenous or CMV-immune globulin has been used by some centers as an adjunct to antiviral prophylaxis, especially in heart, lung, and intestinal transplant recipients. The efficacy of this approach is debated

The doses of the antiviral drugs are for adults and should be adjusted based on renal function

[1]These treatment doses are also recommended for preemptive therapy of asymptomatic CMV replication. Foscarnet, valacyclovir, oral ganciclovir and cidofovir are not recommended for preemptive therapy. Letermovir is not approved for treatment of CMV in solid organ transplant recipients but is approved for prophylaxis in high-risk kidney transplant recipients

*Abbreviations* CMV: cytomegalovirus; mg: milligrams; p.o.: per os; kg; kilogram; IV: intravenous; BSA: body surface area. Reused with permission from Razonable RR, Humar A. Cytomegalovirus in solid organ transplant recipients—Guidelines of the American Society of Transplantation Infectious Diseases Community of Practice. Clin Transplant. 2019 Sep 1; 33 (9). John Wiley and Sons

after HTx depends on the dose and duration of immunosuppression, particularly lymphodepleting agents. Mammalian target of rapamycin (mTOR) inhibitors are associated with a lower risk of CMV disease [22]. Overall, CMV risk is determined by net immunosuppression, which is a complex function of age, elements of the innate and adaptive immune system, prior exposure, organ dysfunction, co-infections, induction, and maintenance immunosuppression. The combination of a CMV-positive donor with a CMV-negative recipient, if untreated, will lead to CMV infection in most patients and is associated with increased rates of rejection, cardiac allograft vasculopathy, and death [24]. CMV infection contributes to immune

**Table 16.2** Recommendations for CMV prevention in heart transplant recipients

| Risk category | Recommendation | Evidence |
|---|---|---|
| D+/R− | Antiviral prophylaxis is preferred, initiated within 10 days of HTx | Strong, high, moderate (12 months prophylaxis) |
| | Ganciclovir 5 mg/kg IV daily or Valganciclovir 900 mg po daily | |
| | Duration: 12 months | |
| | Some transplant centers with add CMV immune globulin for high-risk patients | Weak, low |
| | Preemptive therapy is an option but generally not preferred (below) | Weak, low |
| R+ | Ganciclovir 5 mg/kg IV daily or Valganciclovir 900 mg po daily. Some centers add adjunctive CMV immune globulin | Strong, moderate<br>Weak, low (immune globulin) |
| | Duration: 3–6 months | |
| | Preemptive therapy is an alternative to universal prophylaxis | Strong, moderate |
| | Weekly CMV PCR or pp65 antigenemia for 12 weeks after transplantation, and if a positive CMV threshold is reached, treat with (1) valganciclovir 900-mg[1]p.o. BID, or (2) IV ganciclovir 5-mg/kg IV every 12 h until negative test | |

The above recommendations do not represent an exclusive course of action. Several factors may influence the precise nature and duration of prophylaxis or preemptive therapy

Antiviral prophylaxis should be started as soon as possible, and within 10 days after transplantation. Preemptive therapy is NOT recommended for heart–lung allograft transplantation

[1]Pediatric valganciclovir Dose is mg = 7 × BSA × Creatinine clearance

*Notes* CMV D−/R− heart transplant recipients do not require anti-CMV prophylaxis. Instead, CMV D–/R– should receive anti-Herpes Simplex Virus (HSV) prophylaxis (acyclovir) during the early period after transplantation. If blood transfusion is required, CMV D–/R– SOT patients should receive CMV-seronegative or leuko-reduced blood products

*Abbreviations* D+: donor seropositive; R−: recipient seronegative; D−: donor seronegative; R+: recipient seropositive; CMV: cytomegalovirus; PCR: polymerase chain reaction; IV: intravenous; mg: milligram; p.o.: per os; BID: twice a day; kg: kilogram; BSA: body surface area. Reused with permission from Razonable RR, Humar A. Cytomegalovirus in solid organ transplant recipients—Guidelines of the American Society of Transplantation Infectious Diseases Community of Practice. Clin Transplant. 2019 Sep 1; 33 (9). John Wiley and Sons

dysregulation [25] and has also been demonstrated to predispose transplant recipients to acquire other viral, fungal, and bacterial diseases [26]. The two main preventative strategies for CMV disease are antiviral prophylaxis or preemptive therapy. Each approach has advantages and disadvantages, and preference varies depending on the recipient population and transplant center. Prophylaxis has been demonstrated to decrease CMV-associated early morbidity and mortality [27]. However, universal prophylaxis with ganciclovir or valganciclovir has the drawbacks of increased cost, cytopenias, and increased rates of post-prophylaxis disease [28]. The duration of prophylaxis depends on several factors, including donor seropositivity and other known risk factors for CMV reinfection. Letermovir is a novel terminase complex inhibitor for CMV, which is not myelosuppressive and is approved for prophylaxis in hematopoietic cell transplantation (HCT) and kidney transplant recipients [28, 29]. It is likely to be used in the future in HTx recipients but is limited by cost and total pill burden. It does not have activity against other herpes viruses, so additional prophylaxis is needed with acyclovir. Active CMV infection may be symptomatic or asymptomatic. Clinical symptoms include a syndrome of fever, chills, and malaise with leukopenia and thrombocytopenia. CMV end-organ disease manifests as pneumonitis, hepatitis, retinitis, or colitis/enteritis but can involve nearly any organ system. Rarely, invasive CMV disease may also include the myocardium (necrotizing myocarditis). For rapid and quantitative diagnosis of acute disease, CMV quantitative nucleic acid testing (NAT) with polymerase chain reaction (PCR) is the test of choice. PCR is highly sensitive in the diagnosis of CMV disease and useful for monitoring response to therapy. CMV PCR may be performed on whole blood, plasma, or body fluid along with viral staining of tissue specimens to diagnose end-organ disease. Treatment for active CMV disease utilizes valganciclovir to clear CMV viremia in mild to moderate cases. In more severe cases (pneumonia, gastrointestinal infection, CNS infection, or high viral load), intravenous ganciclovir should be administered. Treatment should continue until the viral load is undetectable, clinical improvement is achieved, and a sufficient course of therapy is completed. At this point, the treating physician can decide to stop therapy or reduce to prophylaxis dosing for a total of three months if CMV disease occurred soon after augmented immunosuppression.

Common adverse effects of both ganciclovir and valganciclovir include myelosuppression, rash, and liver enzyme abnormalities. Since CMV disease itself may also present with cytopenias, it can be confusing whether CMV or the treatment is the culprit. Persistent or worsening leukopenia despite down-trending CMV PCR is likely therapy-related and may require support with a granulocyte colony-stimulating factor. The development of ganciclovir-resistant CMV is uncommon but may occur after prolonged courses of administration, under-dosing, or due to missed doses or poor absorption. Increasing viral load on treatment for more than two weeks should prompt consideration of resistance. In cases of suspected antiviral resistance, genotypic testing for resistance should be performed. While awaiting the results of viral resistance testing, possible solutions include switching to one of the other three classes of medications approved for the treatment of CMV in solid organ transplant recipients. Foscarnet, cidofovir, and maribavir are alternatives for CMV treatment. While foscarnet and cidofovir are limited by the risk of nephrotoxicity, maribavir has lower rates of nephrotoxicity and myelosuppression [30]. Clinical experience with maribavir is more limited, however, and there have been reports of resistance while on treatment, so the role of maribavir in HTx recipients is likely to be shaped by additional real-world experience.

## Herpes Simplex Virus

Herpes simplex virus (HSV) infection generally develops early after transplantation and predominantly affects mucosal surfaces, although dissemination can occur to the esophagus, liver, lungs, and brain. Most cases of active HSV infection after HTx are reactivation in previously infected patients. Diagnosis is based on the visual appearance of typical vesicular lesions, PCR, or positive immunofluorescent staining. In cases of suspected HSV encephalitis, CSF should be obtained for fluid analysis, and HSV PCR and high-dose IV acyclovir should be started empirically.

## Varicella Zoster Virus

Herpes zoster is caused by the reactivation of the varicella-zoster virus (VZV). In transplant recipients, active infection is often caused by reactivation of latent disease and typically presents as a dermatomal vesicular rash, although disseminated disease may occur. Symptoms typically present later than 3 months after transplantation, and diagnosis can usually be made clinically, with laboratory confirmation where necessary to differentiate between VZV and HSV. Oral valacyclovir is the agent of choice for milder cases, with intravenous acyclovir warranted for disseminated or CNS zoster [31].

## Epstein Barr Virus

Epstein-Barr Virus (EBV) is a gamma herpesvirus that causes acute mononucleosis. It is estimated that 90% of the Western population has been exposed to EBV by the fourth decade of life. In the transplant patient, EBV infection may be caused by the reactivation of latent virus or donor-to-recipient transmission [32]. EBV is responsible for more than 90% of early post-transplant lymphoproliferative disorders (PTLD), a potentially devastating complication after transplant. Clinically, PTLD encompasses a wide range of syndromes, from uncomplicated mononucleosis syndromes to life-threatening malignancies. All PTLD episodes are characterized by lymphoproliferation. Interestingly, EBV-negative PTLD is increasingly common in late post-transplant cases (>1 year) [32]. Acyclovir and ganciclovir have no effect on latent EBV infection, and treatment of mild EBV reactivation generally requires only supportive care and a reduction in immunosuppression. Treatment of EBV-associated clinically significant PTLD involves a reduction in immunosuppression to the lowest tolerated level, as well as rituximab for progressive disease. Antiviral therapy and IVIg may be used as adjuncts to B-cell-depleting chemotherapy. Serial monitoring of EBV viral load is not recommended, whether recovering from a mild infection or undergoing treatment for EBV-associated PTLD [32].

## Community Respiratory Viruses

Community respiratory viruses, including but not limited to influenza, parainfluenza, respiratory syncytial virus (RSV), and coronaviruses, may cause significant morbidity and mortality in HTx recipients. They are transmitted by respiratory droplets and aerosols via direct person-to-person contact or contaminated surfaces. The usual presentation is upper respiratory tract symptoms combined with fever, arthralgias, and mucosal inflammation. However, transplant patients may present with mild or atypical symptoms, particularly early in the course of the disease. Additionally, there is the potential for secondary bacterial complications, fungal pneumonia, and CMV reactivation [33]. Diagnosis is clinical, and identification of specific viruses may be performed via serology, viral culture, antigen detection, and nucleic acid testing. If there is clinical or radiologic evidence of lower tract involvement, bronchoalveolar lavage (BAL) should be considered [33].

Regarding treatment for influenza viruses (A and B), neuraminidase inhibitors may shorten symptom duration if commenced promptly. Influenza vaccine should be administered to all HTx recipients and household members. Oseltamivir may also be used for post-exposure prophylaxis for HTx recipients or for pre-exposure prophylaxis during influenza season in patients who are unable to receive the influenza vaccine or who may not respond due to high-level immunosuppression [33].

RSV infection is a significant cause of severe respiratory tract infections in HTx recipients. Aerosolized ribavirin is the only drug FDA-approved for the treatment of lower respiratory tract RSV infections. IV and oral preparations are often used for easier administration. An RSV vaccine was recently approved for use in older adults, which may be a great benefit to HTx recipients [34], pending additional studies and observational experience. For parainfluenza, there is no currently proven treatment, but ribavirin has demonstrated in vitro activity. Some centers also use IVIg and corticosteroids for severe RSV and parainfluenza infections [33].

## Hepatitis B

HTx recipients may acquire hepatitis B virus (HBV) pre-transplant or post-transplant from HBsAg-positive donors, de novo infection after HTx, or even endomyocardial biopsy, in which transmission was suspected to have occurred via an infected probe [35]. Left untreated, there is the potential for chronic liver disease or fulminant hepatitis. Clinical hepatitis post-transplant should be assessed for de novo HBV infection. Newly acquired cases of HBV should be treated with a nucleoside analog (NA), entecavir, or tenofovir. Recipients with a history of prior infection (HBsAg positive) should also be treated with a NA post-transplant to prevent reactivation. In cases of HBsAg-positive donors, hep B immune recipients should be monitored with serial liver enzymes, HBsAg, and HBV DNA every three months for at least 12 months post-transplant with initiation of antiviral therapy if HBsAg or HBV DNA becomes detectable. Recipients with low anti-HBs titers < 100 IU/mL should receive prophylaxis for a minimum of 6–12 months post-transplant [36].

### Hepatitis C

HTx recipients may be chronically infected with hepatitis C (HCV) due to infection acquired prior to transplant, donor-derived infection from a positive organ, or de novo infection acquired after transplantation. Only a small fraction of HTx donors are HCV positive, but expanding the donor pool to these donors increases the availability of valuable organs without sacrificing safety. All solid organ transplant recipients with HCV should be treated with DAA therapy [37]. The focus of this section is the treatment of donor-derived HCV infection when an HCV NAT-positive organ is transplanted to an HCV-negative recipient. Prior to the availability of pan-genotypic direct-acting antivirals (DAAs), HCV-positive hearts were generally not accepted due to limited treatment options with unacceptably high rates of toxicity and treatment failure. However, in the current era, hearts from donors with HCV viremia may be used with appropriate informed consent, monitoring, and treatment [2]. Accumulating evidence in thoracic organs has demonstrated excellent results with high rates of cure of HCV, comparable graft function, and one-year survival [38, 39]. For treatment of HCV acquired from a HCV-positive donor, blood is collected from the donor for HCV genotype testing. Following a transplant, HCV DNA testing is performed on the recipient beginning from day 0 post-transplant and continuing weekly until treatment is started. Treatment for HCV should begin as soon as possible, including immediately pre-transplant or day 0 post-transplant, but often within the first week post-transplant [37]. The feasibility of starting treatment depends on several factors: clinical stability, ability to tolerate enteral medications, availability of the medications, and insurance approval to verify that treatment will not be interrupted mid-course.

The choice of regimen will depend on local formulary, drug interactions, and renal function. Patients should undergo regular monitoring of HCV DNA for up to 12 weeks following completion of treatment to verify sustained virologic response (SVR12) and, at that time, be considered cured.

### Other Viruses

Other notable viral infections occurring after transplantation include the human herpesviruses HHV-6 and HHV-8, BK virus, adenovirus, parvovirus B19, human papillomavirus (HPV), and West Nile Virus. The approaches to treatment for these viruses in the post-transplantation patient are similar to the approach in the non-transplant patient, mostly owing to limited treatment options. However, the availability of PCR, as well as next-generation sequencing techniques, facilitates earlier detection of viral infections [40] and may direct future treatment prospects, including necessary adjustments in immunosuppression.

## Fungal Infections

Fungal infections remain a significant cause of morbidity and mortality after cardiac transplantation, presenting as locally invasive or disseminated disease. Breaching of skin and mucosal barriers via urinary catheterization, intravascular lines, and endotracheal intubation, combined with immunosuppression and administration of broad-spectrum antibiotics, creates an opportunistic environment for these pathogens.

## Peri-Operative Prophylaxis

Anti-fungal prophylaxis to prevent mucocutaneous candidiasis is initiated post-transplant, [2] commonly using nystatin or clotrimazole lozenges. Prophylaxis against *Pneumocystis jiroveci* pneumonia (PJP) should be initiated early after HTx (within ten days post-transplant), with trimethoprim/sulfamethoxazole preferred (Table 16.3).

## Candida Spp.

Candidiasis is the most common invasive fungal infection following HTx. Nosocomial infections are prevalent, often within the first month. The sub-species of *C. albicans* and *C. tropicalis* are the most observed in the cardiac transplant population [41]. Local infections may involve mucosal surfaces or skin, even the sternal wound. Disseminated candidiasis has the potential to involve all the major organ systems. Blood cultures are a reliable method of diagnosis, provided they are collected properly and of adequate volume. Isolation of *Candida* species from stool, wounds, drains, respiratory secretions, and urine does not necessarily indicate infection but may be a clue to patients at higher risk for developing an infection due to colonization. Echinocandins are the empiric drug of choice for invasive candidiasis due to increasing rates of non-albicans *Candida* spp as well as their lack of drug interactions, in contrast to azoles. Therapy can be tailored once speciation and sensitivities are available. Fluconazole remains the drug of choice for *Candida albicans* [41] although close monitoring is necessary for drug interactions.

## Aspergillus

*Aspergillus* species are ubiquitous soil-dwelling molds, of which *A. fumigatus, A. flavus, A. niger,* and *A. terreus* are the most common. *Aspergillus* is acquired via inhalation and commonly presents with pulmonary and sinus symptoms. Invasive *aspergillus* can disseminate to the central nervous system (CNS), causing abscess and angioinvasion and resulting in altered mental status or focal deficits. Chest x-ray or CT may show cavitating nodules with infiltrates. Blood cultures are rarely positive, and serologic assays are limited in utility, with high rates of false positive results. Bronchoalveolar galactomannan is more specific, but the most definitive test is histological evidence of tissue invasion by separating *Aspergillus* from the involved tissue. Newer strategies, including the detection of plasma microbial cell-free DNA, may facilitate earlier diagnosis, which is crucial for successful treatment [42]. Treatment has traditionally been amphotericin B, although recent solid organ transplant studies have demonstrated superior efficacy of voriconazole and isavuconazole [43].

## Pneumocystis Jiroveci

Well-known as fungal pneumonia infecting patients living with HIV and other immunocompromised populations, *Pneumocystis jirovecii* pneumonia *(PJP)* also represents a potential threat in HTx patients. *P. jiroveci* is an organism that usually has relatively low virulence and is found in the lungs of humans and other animals, but it can cause severe infection after HTx. Patients with PJP present with fever, dry cough, dyspnea, and progressive hypoxemia. Chest radiographs typically demonstrate diffuse interstitial infiltrates, sometimes with cavitary lesions. Histologic diagnosis is definitive; characteristic helmet-shaped organisms are seen on BAL or transbronchial biopsy [44]. Yield

**Table 16.3** Specific prophylactic agents for prevention of *Pneumocysitis* in heart transplant recipients, listed by preference

| Agents | Dosing | Comments |
|---|---|---|
| Trimethoprim-sulfamethoxazole (TMP-SMX, cotrimoxazole) | 80 mg TMP/400 mg SMX (single strength) **or** 160 mg TMP/800 mg SMX po (double strength) daily **or** three times weekly | • TMP-SMX remains the **drug of choice** for PJP prophylaxis<br>• Daily regimens may be required to have efficacy for other forms of post-transplant infections<br>• Continue for 1 year |
| Dapsone (4, 4′-diaminodiphenyl-sulfone) | 50–100 mg po qd | • Dapsone is considered a second-line agent for the prophylaxis of PCP<br>• Hematologic side effects may be more common among solid organ transplant recipients<br>• Avoid in G6PD deficiency, methemoglobin reductase deficiency<br>• Uncommon allergy to sulfone or sulfa-containing agents<br>• Generally not recommended in with history of severe sulfa reactions |
| Atovaquone | 1500 mg po qd (as single dose) | • Clinical trial data in HIV patients who could not tolerate TMP-SMX showed atovaquone to be equivalent to dapsone in preventing PJP<br>• Data in solid organ transplant recipients show it to be well-tolerated<br>• Failures of atovaquone have been reported at doses of 1000 mg or less daily |
| Pentamidine | 300 mg administered through aerosolized nebulizer q 3–4 weeks | • Pentamidine requires administration by experienced personnel with a nebulizer producing droplets of 1–3 μ<br>• Pentamidine is well-tolerated with minimal side effects other than cough and bronchospasm<br>• There is a higher incidence of breakthrough infection compared to TMP-SMX or dapsone<br>• Reports of disseminated infection involving the thyroid in HIV cases receiving inhaled pentamidine as prophylaxis |
| Clindamycin and pyrimethamine | Up to 300 mg of clindamycin po qd with 15 mg of pyrimethamine po qd (some clinicians have administered this regimen 3 times weekly instead of daily) | • Somewhat efficacious in patients with AIDS, though less effective than TMP-SMX or dapsone<br>• Failure rate higher than for aerosolized pentamidine<br>• Gastrointestinal intolerance may be limiting |

AIDS = acquired immunodeficiency syndrome; HIV = human immunodeficiency virus; PCP = Pneumocystis pneumonia; TMP-SMX = trimethoprim-sulfamethoxazole

*Dosing abbreviations* mg: milligrams; po: per os; qd: once a day

may vary with other methods, and PCR testing is used increasingly. Beta-D-glucan may be elevated, though it is not specific for *P. jiroveci* [44]. Routine prophylaxis reduces rates of active *P. jiroveci* infection. However, when active infection does occur, trimethoprim-sulfamethoxazole is also effective as a first-line treatment [44].

### Opportunistic Molds and Yeasts

Other significant opportunistic fungal infections seen in the cardiac transplant population include *Cryptococcus neoformans, Rhizopus spp., Histoplasma capsulatum, Blastomyces Dermatitis,* and *Coccidioides immitis*. Treatment of these infections is with fluconazole for endemic mycoses and Amphotericin B or triazole for mold infections, with close monitoring for drug interactions between azoles and immunosuppressive medications. On rare occasions these opportunistic molds or yeasts can be transmitted with an allograft and clinicians should maintain awareness when organs are received from highly endemic areas, particularly for coccidioidomycosis.

## Protozoa

### Toxoplasma Gondii

*Toxoplasma gondii* is a common protozoal parasite that causes disease in immunocompromised individuals, including HTx recipients. Two forms of toxoplasmosis infection occur in HTx recipients: acute and reactivation. Transmission may occur from seropositive donors or from contact with oocysts in cat feces or tissue cysts in improperly prepared meat [45]. Acute disease tends to occur early post-transplant (within the first 6 months), whereas reactivation disease tends to occur later. The disease commonly manifests as fever, lymphadenopathy, and leukopenia, but encephalitis, pneumonitis, and myocarditis are also seen. Cases of toxoplasma-related myocarditis may present similarly to acute rejection. Histopathological changes include an inflammatory cell infiltrate with eosinophils, lymphocytes, plasma cells, and macrophages. Tissue immunostaining for *T. gondii* and parasitic DNA detection are available. Seroconversion is also useful to support the diagnosis, particularly early after transplant.

If left untreated, toxoplasmosis can be fatal in the cardiac transplant recipient. The recommended regimen for solid organ transplant recipients is pyrimethamine with sulfadiazine, combined with folinic acid, but trimethoprim/sulfamethoxazole is also effective [45]. Prophylaxis against Toxoplasma gondii in high-risk cases (seropositive donor and/or seropositive recipient) should also be initiated in the early postoperative period. The first-line regimen is the same as for prophylaxis against PJP: trimethoprim/sulfamethoxazole [2].

### Trypanosoma Cruzi

Trypanosoma cruzi is the etiologic parasite for Chagas disease or American trypanosomiasis. It is common in rural Mexico, Central America and South America. Transplant-related Chagas disease in the United States is most prevalent in the Southwestern U.S. due to proximity to these endemic areas and infection may occur via reactivation or rare donor-derived infection. HTx candidates at risk for prior exposure include residents or travelers to endemic areas, or whose mothers lived in endemic area. These candidates should be screened via serology pre-transplant. Post-transplant, at-risk individuals (confirmed recipient or donor antibody test) should undergo monitoring for parasitemia with PCR testing weekly for the first two months post-transplant, every two weeks in the third month, and then monthly until six months post-transplant [2]. Detection of increasing parasitemia is indicative of infection and should be treated with an antitrypanosomal agent. Benznidazole is the first-line treatment, mostly owing to superior tolerance profile, although nifurtimox is also effective [46]. HTx candidates undergoing transplantation for known Chagas cardiomyopathy can be successfully transplanted using this approach and have outcomes similar to the general heart transplant population.

The parasite is trophic to muscle and heart cells as well as the neurologic system. While proactive monitoring with PCR may detect reactivation infection prior to onset of symptoms, clinical presentations include fever, malaise, myocarditis or decreased cardiac function, and may mimic acute rejection [47]. Additional presentations include hepatosplenomegaly, skin lesions, and less commonly CNS infection. These symptoms should prompt additional PCR testing if beyond six months post-transplant or following an increase in immunosuppression.

## Clinical Approach to Infectious Features

Many of the infections described above present with similar clinical syndromes in the immunocompromised population. A precise and timely diagnosis of infection in the HTx recipient is both more difficult and vital for successful treatment, preservation of graft function, and protection from morbidity and mortality. A general approach to these clinical aspects is summarized below.

### Fever

After the initial post-operative period, a new fever generally indicates an underlying infection and is frequently the first symptom. A systematic approach to fever requires consideration of risk factors for specific infections to identify the causative pathogen and guide appropriate empirical therapy. The timing of the fever in relation to the transplant is one of the first factors considered. Many bacterial infections occur in the first month after transplantation, often related to invasive devices or surgical complications. In the first six months, induction of immunosuppression increases susceptibility to opportunistic infections and reactivation of latent viral infections. After six months, infections are likely to be community-acquired and overlap with the non-transplant population, along with an accumulated risk for opportunistic infections as time goes on. Next, the total immunosuppression of the patient is considered, with attention to any recent history of rejection or augmented immunosuppression. Leukocyte differentials, immunoglobulin levels, and T-cell assays also help quantify the net immune status to some degree.

The infectious history of both the donor and recipient is important, particularly for fever occurring within the first three months after transplant. Both donor and recipient serologies prior to transplant should be reviewed, as well as the patient's occupational, recreational, and travel history. Overall, these principles can be used to aid in the evaluation of not just fever but many of the other clinical features of infection after transplant.

### Pulmonary Infiltrates

Pulmonary infiltrates in HTx patients occur due to bacterial, viral, fungal, or protozoal infections and may also be due to non-infectious causes, including pulmonary edema and neoplasm. Like fever, timing of onset is important. The nature of pulmonary symptoms may also offer a clue: generally speaking, bacterial and viral infections tend to present acutely, whereas fungal and parasitic infections are more insidious in onset. Sputum cultures should be performed along with chest X-rays or CT. Judicious use of microbial cell-free DNA testing may aid in non-invasive diagnosis. Lastly, definitive diagnosis can often be obtained via histology from BAL and/or transbronchial lung biopsy. Empiric treatment is warranted while awaiting the testing results.

### Wound Infections

Wound infections generally occur within the first month after transplantation and may lead to mediastinitis. Mediastinitis typically presents with fever, wound drainage, and sternal instability. Wound cultures should be collected to optimize antibiotic therapy. The most common causative pathogens are *Staphylococci,* and debridement should be performed if possible [48].

## Urinary Tract Infections

Urinary tract infections (UTIs) are common after HTx due to perioperative catheterization. The incidence and treatment are the same as the non-transplant surgical population. Treatment should be adjusted based on urine culture. Colonized catheters should be replaced, and treatment is not indicated to eradicate colonizing organisms. In the later post-transplant stages (> 6 months), in sexually active transplant recipients, a complaint of genitourinary symptoms or disclosure of high-risk behavior should trigger an appropriate evaluation for sexually transmitted infections [2].

## CNS Infection

While CNS infections after HTx are relatively rare, they are potentially fatal if left untreated. Common CNS syndromes include meningitis, focal deficits, and/or encephalitis. Typical symptoms are headache, altered mental state, fever, seizures, or focal symptoms. The timing of the onset of symptoms may offer clues to the potential pathogen. A useful principle is that early onset symptoms are likely due to bacteria, *Aspergillus, or Candida* (due to their capacity for hematogenous spread), whereas later symptoms tend to be due to opportunistic infections. Focal disease presenting within the first month may be due to a brain abscess. Later disease may be due to progressive multifocal leukoencephalopathy from JC virus, *Nocardia* or *Rhizopus* abscesses or meningoencephalitis from listeria, cryptococcus, VZV, HHV-6, or even CMV [49]. Brain imaging with CT and MRI should be performed, along with lumbar puncture for CSF analysis.

## GI and Liver Infections

Many of the opportunistic infections described may disseminate to the gastrointestinal (GI) and hepatobiliary systems. Symptoms such as abdominal pain, bleeding, and diarrhea are nonspecific and may also be caused by peptic ulceration, pancreatitis, or drug toxicities. There is a low threshold for performing endoscopy/colonoscopy with biopsy to aid in the identification of the responsible pathogen.

## References


1. Sherman-Weber S, Axelrod P, Suh B, Rubin S, Beltramo D, Manacchio J, et al. Infective endocarditis following orthotopic heart transplantation: 10 cases and a review of the literature. Transplant Infect Dis. 2004;6:165–70.
2. Velleca A, Shullo MA, Dhital K, Azeka E, Colvin M, DePasquale E, et al. The International Society for Heart and Lung Transplantation (ISHLT) guidelines for the care of heart transplant recipients. J Heart Lung Transplant. 2023;42(5):e1-141.
3. Perrault LP, Kirkwood KA, Chang HL, Mullen JC, Gulack BC, Argenziano M, et al. A prospective multi-institutional cohort study of mediastinal infections after cardiac operations. Ann Thorac Surg. 2018;105(2):461–8.
4. Pons S, Sonneville R, Bouadma L, Styfalova L, Ruckly S, Neuville M, et al. Infectious complications following heart transplantation in the era of high-priority allocation and extracorporeal membrane oxygenation. Ann Intensiv Care. 2019;9(1).
5. Bucheli E, Kralidis G, Boggian K, Cusini A, Garzoni C, Manuel O, et al. Impact of enterococcal colonization and infection in solid organ transplantation recipients from the Swiss Transplant Cohort Study. Transpl Infect Dis. 2014;16(1):26–36.
6. Bhatt PJ, Ali M, Rana M, Patel G, Sullivan T, Murphy J, et al. Infections due to multidrug-resistant organisms following heart transplantation: epidemiology, microbiology, and outcomes. Transplant Infect Dis. 2020;22(1).
7. Gibson CM, Childs-Kean LM, Naziruddin Z, Howell CK. The alteration of the gut microbiome by immunosuppressive agents used in solid organ transplantation. Transplant Infect Dis. 2021;23(1).
8. Amber IJ, Gilbert EM, Schiffman G, Jacobson JA. Increased risk of pneumococcal infections in cardiac transplant recipients. Transplantation. 1990;49(1):122–5.

9. Wiesmayr S, Tabarelli W, Stelzmueller I, Nachbaur D, Boesmueller C, Wykypiel H, et al. Listeria meningitis in transplant recipients. Vol. 117. Wiener Klinische Wochenschrift. 2005. p. 229–33.
10. Restrepo A, Clark NM. Nocardia infections in solid organ transplantation: guidelines from the Infectious Diseases Community of Practice of the American Society of Transplantation. Clin Transplant. 2019;33(9).
11. Majeed A, Beatty N, Iftikhar A, Mushtaq A, Fisher J, Gaynor P, et al. A 20-year experience with nocardiosis in solid organ transplant (SOT) recipients in the Southwestern United States: a single-center study. Transplant Infect Dis. 2018;20(4).
12. Kwak EJ, Strollo DC, Kulich SM, Kusne S. Cavitary pneumonia due to Rhodococcus equi in a heart transplant recipient. Transplant Infect Dis. 2003;5(1):43–6.
13. Rose R, Nord J, Lanspa M. Rhodococcus empyema in a heart transplant patient. Respirol Case Rep. 2014;2(1):42–4.
14. da Silva P, Barreto Santos AC, Nakamura Sato D, Otero Silva J, Cazentini Medeiros MI, Machado Carneiro AM, et al. Phenotypic and genotypic characterization of Rhodococcus equi isolated from sputum. Braz J Infect Dis. 2012;16(5):409–15.
15. Lin W V., Kruse RL, Yang K, Musher DM. Diagnosis and management of pulmonary infection due to Rhodococcus equi. In: Clinical microbiology and infection. Vol. 25. Elsevier B.V.; 2019. p. 310–5.
16. Malinis M, LaHoz RM, Vece G, Annambhotla P, Aslam S, Basavaraju SV, et al. Donor-derived tuberculosis among solid organ transplant recipients in the United States—2008 to 2018. Transplant Infect Dis. 2022;24(2).
17. Subramanian AK, Theodoropoulos NM. Mycobacterium tuberculosis infections in solid organ transplantation: guidelines from the infectious diseases community of practice of the American Society of Transplantation. Clin Transplant. 2019;33(9).
18. Guyot S, Goy JJ, Gersbach P, Jaton K, Blanc DS, Zanetti G. Legionella pneumophila aortitis in a heart transplant recipient. Transplant Infect Dis. 2007;9(1):58–9.
19. Knirsch CA, Jakob K, Schoonmaker D, Kiehlbauch JA, Wong SJ, Della-Latta P, et al. An outbreak of Legionella micdadei pneumonia in transplant patients: evaluation, molecular epidemiology, and control. Am J Med. 2000;108(4):290–5.
20. Jasper AS, Musuuza JS, Tischendorf JS, Stevens VW, Gamage SD, Osman F, et al. Are fluoroquinolones or macrolides better for treating legionella pneumonia? A systematic review and meta-analysis. Clin Infect Dis. 2021;72(11):1979–89.
21. Mullane KM, Dubberke ER. Management of Clostridioides (formerly Clostridium) difficile infection (CDI) in solid organ transplant recipients: guidelines from the American Society of Transplantation Community of Practice. Clin Transplant. 2019;33(9).
22. Razonable RR, Humar A. Cytomegalovirus in solid organ transplant recipients—guidelines of the American Society of Transplantation Infectious Diseases Community of Practice. Clin Transplant. 2019;33(9).
23. Fowler K, Mucha J, Neumann M, Lewandowski W, Kaczanowska M, Grys M, et al. A systematic literature review of the global seroprevalence of cytomegalovirus: possible implications for treatment, screening, and vaccine development. BMC Public Health. 2022;22(1).
24. Delgado JF, Reyne AG, De Dios S, López-Medrano F, Jurado A, Juan RS, et al. Influence of cytomegalovirus infection in the development of cardiac allograft vasculopathy after heart transplantation. J Heart Lung Transplant. 2015;34(8):1112–9.
25. Vietzen H, Jaksch P, Puchhammer-Stöckl E. The human cytomegalovirus-specific and UL40-mediated imprint in the natural killer cell repertoire is associated with antibody-mediated rejection in lung transplant recipients. J Heart Lung Transplant. 2023;42(3):305–14.
26. Singh N. Interactions between viruses in transplant recipients. Clin Infect Dis. 2005;40.
27. Potena L, Holweg CTJ, Chin C, Luikart H, Weisshaar D, Narasimhan B, et al. Acute rejection and cardiac allograft vascular disease is reduced by suppression of subclinical cytomegalovirus infection. Transplantation. 2006;82(3):398–405.
28. Haidar G, Boeckh M, Singh N. Cytomegalovirus infection in solid organ and hematopoietic cell transplantation: state of the evidence. J Infect Dis. 2021;221:S23-31.
29. Limaye AP, Budde K, Humar A, Vincenti F, Kuypers DRJ, Carroll RP, et al. Letermovir vs valganciclovir for prophylaxis of cytomegalovirus in high-risk kidney transplant recipients: a randomized clinical trial. JAMA. 2023;330(1):33–42.
30. Avery RK, Alain S, Alexander BD, Blumberg EA, Chemaly RF, Cordonnier C, et al. Maribavir for refractory cytomegalovirus infections with or without resistance post-transplant: results from a phase 3 randomized clinical trial. Clin Infect Dis. 2022;75(4):690–701.
31. Pergam SA, Limaye AP. Varicella zoster virus in solid organ transplantation: guidelines from the American Society of Transplantation Infectious Diseases Community of Practice. Clin Transplant. 2019;33(9).
32. Allen UD, Preiksaitis JK. Post-transplant lymphoproliferative disorders, Epstein-Barr virus infection, and disease in solid organ transplantation: guidelines from the American Society of Transplantation Infectious Diseases Community of Practice. Clin Transplant. 2019;33(9).
33. Manuel O, Estabrook M. RNA respiratory viral infections in solid organ transplant

recipients: guidelines from the American Society of Transplantation Infectious Diseases Community of Practice. Clin Transplant. 2019;33(9).
34. Walsh EE, Pérez Marc G, Zareba AM, Falsey AR, Jiang Q, Patton M, et al. Efficacy and safety of a bivalent RSV prefusion F vaccine in older adults. N Engl J Med. 2023;388(16):1465–77.
35. Richard JFC;, Franck D;, Vincent G;, Martino DI. Nosocomial transmission of hepatitis B virus associated with endomyocardial biopsy. Gastroenterol Clin Biol. 2006;30.
36. Te H, Doucette K. Viral hepatitis: guidelines by the American Society of Transplantation Infectious Disease Community of Practice. Clin Transplant. 2019;33(9).
37. Bhattacharya D, Aronsohn A, Price J, Lo Re V, Heald J, Demisashi G, et al. Hepatitis C Guidance 2023 update: American Association for the Study of Liver Diseases– Infectious Diseases Society of America recommendations for testing, managing, and treating hepatitis C virus infection. Clin Infect Dis. 2023.
38. Aslam S, Grossi P, Schlendorf KH, Holm AM, Woolley AE, Blumberg E, et al. Utilization of hepatitis C virus–infected organ donors in cardiothoracic transplantation: an ISHLT expert consensus statement. J Heart Lung Transplant. 2020;39(5):418–32.
39. Villegas-Galaviz J, Anderson E, Guglin M. Clinical outcomes of heart transplantation using hepatitis c-viremic donors: a systematic review with meta-analysis. J Heart Lung Transplant. 2022;41(4):538–49.
40. Shishido AA, Noe M, Saharia K, Luethy P. Clinical impact of a metagenomic microbial plasma cell-free DNA next-generation sequencing assay on treatment decisions: a single-center retrospective study. BMC Infect Dis. 2022;22(1).
41. Aslam S, Rotstein C. Candida infections in solid organ transplantation: guidelines from the American Society of Transplantation Infectious Diseases Community of Practice. Clin Transplant. 2019;33(9).
42. Heldman MR, Ahmed AA, Liu W, Vo A, Keane-Candib J, Stevens-Ayers T, et al. Serial quantitation of plasma microbial cell-free DNA before and after diagnosis of pulmonary invasive mold infections after hematopoietic cell transplant. J Infect Dis. 2023.
43. Husain S, Camargo JF. Invasive Aspergillosis in solid-organ transplant recipients: Guidelines from the American Society of Transplantation Infectious Diseases Community of Practice. Clin Transplant. 2019;33(9).
44. Fishman JA, Gans H. Pneumocystis jiroveci in solid organ transplantation: guidelines from the American Society of Transplantation Infectious Diseases Community of Practice. Clin Transplant. 2019;33(9).
45. Schwartz BS, Mawhorter SD. Parasitic infections in solid organ transplantation. Am J Transplant. 2013;13:280–303.
46. Gray EB, La Hoz RM, Green JS, Vikram HR, Benedict T, Rivera H, et al. Reactivation of Chagas disease among heart transplant recipients in the United States, 2012–2016. Transplant Infect Dis. 2018;20(6).
47. Kransdorf EP, Zakowski PC, Kobashigawa JA. Chagas disease in solid organ and heart transplantation. Curr Opin Infect Dis. 2014;27(5):418–24.
48. Strecker T, Rösch J, Horch RE, Weyand M, Kneser U. Sternal wound infections following cardiac surgery: risk factor analysis and interdisciplinary treatment. Heart Surg Forum. 2007;10(5):E366-71.
49. Wright AJ, Fishman JA. Central nervous system syndromes in solid organ transplant recipients. Clin Infect Dis. 2014;59(7):1001–11.

# 17 COVID-19 Considerations in Heart Transplantation

Yael Peled

**Abstract**

While much of the knowledge accumulated for COVID-19 is relevant to the general population and immunosuppressed patients alike, some of the particular characteristics of heart transplant (HTx) recipients warrant tailored approaches to patient management and to prevention and treatment. Although there are several pharmacologic therapies available for HTx recipients, it should be remembered that this is a rapidly evolving field, further emphasizing the crucial roles of transplant team in managing the patients according to the most up-to-date guidelines. Particularly important in the crystallization of a vaccination policy was to encourage vaccination as soon as vaccines became available. The impact of the accumulated data on SARS-CoV-2 will extend beyond protection from COVID-19 into the implementation of new vaccine technologies for various other infectious disease targets, improving preparedness for future health crises, and into applications for oncology, metabolic diseases, gene therapy, and gene editing. This chapter will explore the management of COVID-19 in HTx patients and vaccination strategies.

**Keywords**

Heart transplant · COVID-19 · Immunosuppression · Pharmacotherapy · Immunocompromised · Cytokine storm · Vaccines

## Clinical Pearls

- Heart transplant recipients are at risk for more severe COVID-19 and mortality compared with the general population.
- Medical comorbidities that have been associated with more severe COVID-19 and a greater risk of mortality include older age, chronic kidney disease, cardiac allograft vasculopathy/graft dysfunction, diabetes mellitus, obesity, frailty, and chronic lung disease.
- Heart transplant recipients, characterized by a failure to mount a sufficient recall response, are at risk for prolonged infection with SARS-CoV-2 and could constitute a reservoir of divergent escape variants that can spread in the general community.

Y. Peled (✉)
Leviev Heart and Vascular Center, Sheba Medical Center, Tel Hashomer, Ramat Gan, Israel
e-mail: yael.peled-potashnik@sheba.health.gov.il

Y. Peled
Faculty of Medical and Health Sciences, Tel Aviv University, Tel Aviv, Israel



J. Kobashigawa (ed.), *Clinical Guide to Heart Transplantation*, https://doi.org/10.1007/978-3-031-88290-6_17

- Pharmacotherapy targeted against the virus holds the greatest promise when administered early in the course of the illness (be aware of potential drug-drug interactions), whereas immunomodulatory agents to reduce systemic inflammation may be considered in the advanced inflammatory response phase.
- The relevant professional bodies encourage COVID-19 vaccination due to real-world data on the efficacy and safety of mRNA-based vaccines in transplant recipients.

## Introduction

On December 31, 2019, a cluster of pneumonia cases of unknown etiology was reported in Wuhan, China. On January 9, 2020, the novel Severe Acute Respiratory Coronavirus 2 (SARS-CoV-2) was identified as the causative agent of this outbreak. This was the start of what would become the coronavirus disease 2019 (COVID-19) pandemic, with over 774 million confirmed cases and over 7 million deaths reported globally as of March 3, 2024 [1, 2]. The global response to the COVID-19 pandemic has been a complex and multifaceted effort, leading to the introduction of a wide range of non-pharmaceutical interventions and the rapid development of pharmaceuticals (antivirals, monoclonal antibodies, and, most importantly, COVID-19 vaccines) to control the outbreak. The COVID-19 pandemic has constituted a particular challenge for heart transplant (HTx) recipients: Immunocompromised people, in general, have been over-represented in breakthrough infections, corresponding to 44% of post-vaccination infections despite accounting for only 2.7% of the population (in the pre-delta era) [3, 4]. For solid organ transplant recipients (SOTRs), the risk of contracting COVID-19 infection was 80-fold higher, and the risk of hospitalization and death was 485-fold higher compared to the general population [5]. SOTRs, being characterized by a failure to mount a sufficient recall response, are at risk for prolonged infection with SARS-CoV-2 and could constitute a reservoir of divergent escape variants that could spread in the general community. Prolonged viral replication in the context of an inadequate immune response facilitates viral evolution, which could lead to the evolution of new variants of concern (VOCs) [6, 7].

## COVID-19 in Heart Transplant Recipients

The specific characteristics of the SARS-CoV-2 virus pose a significant challenge in the care of HTx patients with COVID-19: The zoonotic origin of the virus limits pre-existing human immunity to SARS-CoV-2. In addition, the high affinity of the spike protein for the angiotensin-converting enzyme 2 (ACE2) receptor and the novel 4 amino acid insertion facilitate facile entry of the virus into host cells, and the ensuing replication in the host leads to high viral loads and efficient spread [8, 9]. SARS-CoV-2 undergoes a high degree of genomic mutation, and variants with more extensive mutations have been shown to be associated with higher transmissibility, higher viral infectivity, and greater immune evasion potential [10]. For HTx recipients, the consequences are more severe COVID-19 and a greater risk of mortality [11, 12] since the above challenges are exacerbated by coexisting medical comorbidities, increased exposure to SARS-CoV-2 (given their frequent contact with the health-care system), reduced immune responses following vaccination and, paradoxically, exclusion from clinical trials (calling into question the effectiveness of vaccination). Early in the pandemic [13–15], mortality of HTx recipients from COVID-19 was shown to be between 20 and 40%, which was significantly higher than the percentage mortality in the general population [16–18]. Transplant recipients with COVID-19 had a 30% increased risk of death or mechanical ventilation compared with matched controls (Table 17.1) [19–31]. From the onset of the pandemic to May 2021, the odds of being diagnosed with COVID-19 were more than five times higher in HTx recipients versus the general population, and the chances of hospitalization in HTx recipients

**Table 17.1** Clinical outcomes of heart transplant recipients with COVID-19[1]

| Study/Country | Organ (# recipients) | Time from HTx to COVID-19 | Reported clinical events | Predictors of adverse outcome |
|---|---|---|---|---|
| Rivinius et al. [19]/Germany | Heart (#21) | 95 months (median) | Mortality rate: 33%<br>In-hospital mortality rate: 36%<br>Hospitalized: 90%<br>Reduced RV function: 28%<br>Elevated pulmonary artery pressure: 28%<br>Moderate-to-severe tricuspid regurgitation: 19%<br>ECG abnormalities: 19%<br>New thromboembolic events: 19%<br>Severe COVID-19: 38% | RV dysfunction<br>↑ Pulmonary artery pressure<br>Tricuspid valve regurgitation<br>Thromboembolic events<br>Severe COVID-19<br>↑ Older age<br>↑ LDH, troponin-T, NT-proBNP, D-dimer<br>↓ absolute lymphocyte count |
| Latif et al. [20]/USA | Heart (#28) | 8.6 years (4.2–14.5) | Mortality rate: 25%<br>In-hospital mortality rate: 32%<br>Hospitalized: 79%<br>Evidence of myocardial injury: 77%<br>Severe COVID-19: 25% | NA |
| Ketcham et al. [21]/USA | Heart (#13) | 9.6 years (median) | Mortality rate: 15%<br>In-hospital mortality rate: 25%<br>Hospitalized: 61.5%<br>Acute kidney injury: 84%<br>Dialysis: 38%<br>Severe COVID-19: 46% | NA |
| Iacovoni et al. [22]/Italy | Heart (#26) | 6 years (median) | Mortality rate: 27%<br>In-hospital mortality rate: 41%<br>Hospitalized: 65%<br>Severe COVID-19: 31%<br>New thromboembolic events: 7% | Age (>65)<br>Higher incidence of CKD and diabetes<br>Higher respiratory rate and lower oxygen saturation at the first clinical evaluation<br>↑Procalcitonin.↑ CRP |

(continued)

**Table 17.1** (continued)

| Study/Country | Organ (# recipients) | Time from HTx to COVID-19 | Reported clinical events | Predictors of adverse outcome |
|---|---|---|---|---|
| Genuardi et al. [23]/USA | Heart (#99 recipients at 11 centers) | 5.6 years (2.0–13.7) | Mortality rate: 15%<br>In-hospital mortality rate: 25%<br>Hospitalized: 67%<br>Severe COVID-19: 25% | CNI + PSI > CNI + antimetabolite<br>PSI use was associated with a 6.8-fold risk of severe COVID-19<br>Prednisone use associated with a 7.3-fold risk of severe COVID-19 and17.8-fold increased risk of death |
| Bottio et al. [24]/7 HTx centers in Northern Italy | Heart (#47) | 10.5 ± 8.7 years | Mortality rate: 29.7%<br>Hospitalized: 17%<br>In-hospital stay: 17.8 days<br>ICU stay: 4(9) days<br>Severe COVID-19: 25% | ↑age, diabetes mellitus, extracardiac arteriopathy, previous PCI, CAV score, ↓ GFR, and ↑ NYHA functional classes were all significantly associated with in-hospital mortality |
| Soriano et al. [25]/Brazil | Heart (#5) | 3–264 months | Mortality rate: 40%<br>Hospitalized: 100%<br>20% Vasopressors and mechanical ventilation<br>ICU length of stay 4–21days | NA |
| Waleed Al-Darzi et al. [26]/USA | 5 Heart (#5)<br>Heart and Lung (#1) | 6.5 years (4.25–12.5) | Mortality rate: 0%<br>In-hospital mortality rate:0<br>Hospitalized: 100%<br>Mild-moderate COVID-19: 100% | NA |
| Taghavi et al. [27]/Iran | Heart (#22) | 3.1 years | Mortality rate: 13.6%<br>In-hospital mortality rate:<br>Hospitalized: 86.4%<br>Moderate-severe RV dysfunction: 27.3% | NA |
| Ahluwalia et al. [28]/USA | Heart (#5) | 21 years (6–25) | Mortality rate: 20% (prior hospitalization)<br>Hospitalized:100%<br>Moderate-severe COVID-19: 80% | NA |

(continued)

**Table 17.1** (continued)

| Study/Country | Organ (# recipients) | Time from HTx to COVID-19 | Reported clinical events | Predictors of adverse outcome |
|---|---|---|---|---|
| Ballout et al. [29]/USA | Heart (#3)<br>Heart and kidney (#1) | 2.2 years | Mortality rate: 0<br>In-hospital mortality rate: 0<br>Hospitalized: 100%<br>Mild-moderate COVID-19:100% | NA |
| Carraffa et al. [30]/Italy | Heart (#6) | 12 years (4.0–17.5) | Mortality rate: 33%<br>In-hospital mortality rate: 40%<br>Hospitalized: 83%<br>ARDS: 17%<br>ICU hospitalization: 33%<br>ICU stay: 18 days<br>Mechanical ventilation: 17%<br>Stroke: 17%<br>Moderate-severe RV dysfunction: 27.3% | NA |
| Lima et al. [31]/USA | Heart (#5) | 7.9 months (3 within 2 months post-HTx) | Mortality rate within 30 days of admission: 0<br>Hospitalized: 100%<br>Moderate COVID-19: 60%<br>Severe COVID-19: 40%<br>Mechanical ventilation: 40% | NA |

*Abbreviations* ARDS, acute respiratory distress syndrome; BNP, B-type natriuretic peptide; CAV, cardiac allograft vasculopathy; CKD, chronic kidney disease; CNI, calcineurin inhibitor; CRP, C-reactive protein; GFR, glomerular filtration rate; LDH, lactate dehydrogenase; NA, not available; PCI, percutaneous coronary intervention; PSI, proliferation signal inhibitor; RV, right ventricular

[1]Studies are pre-vaccination; not included are studies reporting SOTRs other than heart; also not included are single case reports.

with COVID-19 were approximately 80% [14]. Immunosuppressive therapy and the high burden of comorbidities in HTx patients were—and still are—major contributors to the poor COVID-19 prognosis. Factors associated with higher COVID-19 mortality include older age, diabetes mellitus, obesity, frailty, and chronic heart, kidney, and lung disease. In terms of laboratory values, lymphopenia and higher levels of C-reactive protein, ferritin, procalcitonin, IL-6, D-dimer, and lactate dehydrogenase have been reported to be predictors for mortality. Mortality was also higher among patients with lower incomes and those who live in more densely populated areas [32]. Social disparities may negatively affect outcomes, even in the highly selected population of HTx recipients, characterized by access to specialized care and close follow-up [33]. As the pandemic progressed, ongoing excess deaths of SOTRs were reported despite the advent of vaccinations and new therapeutics. COVID-19 likely caused over 5000 excess deaths among SOTRs in the USA in the 13-month period from March 2020 to March 2021 (representing 1 in 75 SOTRs) and a substantial proportion of all deaths among SOTRs during that time [34]. Thereafter, the susceptibility of HTx recipients to COVID-19 did not change, even for less virulent variants; for example, among hospitalized adult HTx recipients with omicron infection in two French transplant centers, there were 56% ICU admissions and 44% deaths versus 47% ICU admissions and 26% deaths among delta cases [12].

## Management of COVID-19-Positive Heart Transplant Patients

The viral evasion of immune responses and cytokine storm play essential roles in the pathogenesis, clinical manifestation, and outcomes of COVID-19 [35]. When determining therapy for COVID-19 in HTx recipients, clinicians must consider patient, vaccination, and virus characteristics (Table 17.2). Optimal timing of the therapeutic intervention in relation to the disease phase may maximize the therapeutic benefit (Fig. 17.1) [36]. Thus, involvement of the transplant team in treating COVID-19 and in keeping up to date with novel targeted therapies and vaccinations are of crucial value.

## Adjusting Chronic Immunosuppressive Therapies

Immunosuppressive medications have opposite effects in the early viral response phase versus the advanced host inflammatory response phase of COVID-19 progression [36]. In the early stage of COVID-19, immunosuppressive drugs reduce the innate/adaptive immune response needed to suppress SARS-CoV-2 viral replication. At advanced stages, immunosuppressive agents have been successfully used to prevent and treat the cytokine storm triggered by the virus and have been effective in reducing mortality and the need for mechanical ventilation in patients with COVID-19 [54–57]. Thus, a tailored phase-specific therapy approach should be pursued according to the potential benefit versus the risk of reducing immunosuppression (Fig. 17.1). Standard practice in most centers is to discontinue the anti-proliferative agent, mycophenolate, promptly after the diagnosis of COVID-19, the rationale being the possibilities of causing the viral infection to worsen, the development of leukopenia, or increasing the risk of secondary bacterial infection. Nevertheless, the actual effect of antirejection drugs on viral diseases is a complex issue that has not yet been fully elucidated. Mycophenolate is an anti-proliferative agent that impairs the synthesis of guanosine, which is essential for DNA and RNA synthesis during the replication of immune cells and viruses [58]. In-vitro studies have demonstrated that mycophenolate has antiviral activity against different viruses, such as dengue virus, coxsackievirus, and West Nile virus, and against coronaviruses, including MERS-CoV, and human coronaviruses HCoV-OC43 and HCoV-NL63 [56, 59, 60]. Clinical observations that mycophenolate was well tolerated in patients who were already being treated

**Table 17.2** Management of HTx patients with COVID-19: general guidance and special considerations

| Variable | Special consideration |
|---|---|
| **Patient characteristics** | |
| Underlying disease | Medical comorbidities that have been associated with more severe COVID-19 and a greater risk of mortality include older age, chronic kidney disease, cardiac allograft vasculopathy/graft dysfunction, diabetes mellitus, obesity, frailty and chronic lung disease [37] |
| Duration and severity of the illness | Pharmacotherapy tailored to the disease phase (early viral response phase versus advanced host inflammatory response phase; Fig. 17.1). Pharmacotherapy targeted against the virus applied early in the course of the illness has been consistently demonstrated to be associated with the best outcome [38], but its usefulness in advanced stages may be doubtful [36, 39, 40]. It is necessary to implement supportive measures for pulmonary disease and localized inflammation (i.e., supplemental oxygen, low-molecular-weight heparin) according to local guidelines, active surveillance for secondary bacterial and opportunistic fungal and viral infections (such as *Aspergillus* or cytomegalovirus), and consideration of specific prevention and treatment of acute respiratory distress syndrome (ARDS) and subsequent lung fibrosis. Immunomodulatory agents to reduce systemic inflammation in the advanced inflammatory response phase may be considered (corticosteroids, cytokine inhibitors; Fig. 17.1) [36, 41, 42]<br>Immunocompromised patients with mild to moderate COVID-19 are at high risk of progressing to severe disease and should receive anti-SARS-CoV-2 therapies early in the disease course [37]. For severe COVID-19, hospital care (versus ambulatory setting) is recommended [38] |
| Immunosuppressant protocol | Since immunosuppressive agents modulate several aspects of the immune response, the severity of COVID-19 could potentially be affected by the type and intensity of the immunosuppressive effect of the agent, as well as by specific combinations of immunosuppressive agents. Notably, prolonged infections, as have been reported in immunocompromised patients, can create evolutionary pressure for the emergence of variants that resist therapies or evade vaccine-induced immunity [7, 43, 44] |
| Donor specific antibodies (DSAs); time from HTx; rejection history | DSAs, rejection history, and early time from transplant are indications for more profound immunosuppression and hence a higher risk of severe COVID-19 and higher mortality. The overall degree of immunosuppression is one of the main predictors of poor humoral responses after vaccination |
| Overlapping toxicities | Special attention should be given to the potential for drug-drug interactions and overlapping toxicities between treatments for COVID-19 and concomitantly administered medications, such as immunosuppressants and antimicrobials used to prevent or treat opportunistic infections [37] |
| **Vaccination characteristics** | |
| Vaccination status | COVID-19 vaccination immune paresis in HTx recipients results in a high risk of breakthrough infections and mortality for vaccinated transplant recipients [5, 45, 46]. However, breakthrough infections in vaccinated versus non-vaccinated immunocompromised persons were less severe, suggesting that the SARS-CoV-2 vaccines mitigate disease severity. Risk factors for reduced antibody response include older age at vaccination, early time from transplant, type of vaccine (mRNA-based vaccines tend to elicit higher antibody responses than adenovirus vector vaccines), the interval between vaccine doses, and the type and intensity of immunosuppression [47–51]<br>HTx recipients and their close contacts are encouraged to maintain their COVID-19 vaccination status (vaccinations and boosters) according to the most up-to-date guidelines [37] |
| History of COVID-19 and timing of vaccination | Breakthrough infection after vaccination is immunogenic, eliciting a more robust immune response, and induces a cross-reactive humoral response to new VOCs [52] |

(continued)

**Table 17.2** (continued)

| Variable | Special consideration |
|---|---|
| Neutralization response | Determination of protective levels of antibodies is confounded by the wide variety of commercially available antibody tests. There is currently insufficient evidence to recommend either for or against the use of SARS-CoV-2 serologic testing to assess immunity or to guide clinical decisions. Preliminary data from a case–control study of HTx recipients is encouraging, suggesting that BNT162b2-vaccine-induced neutralizing antibodies conferred clinical protection against severe COVID-19 and related hospitalization [9]. Nevertheless, the complexity of neutralization studies limits their broad use in clinical practice |
| **Virus characteristics** | |
| VOCs; immune evasion; novel targeted therapies | SARS-CoV-2 undergoes a high degree of genomic mutations, and variants with more extensive mutations (VOCs) [7] have been shown to be associated with higher transmissibility, viral infectivity, and immune evasion potential [53]. The omicron variant has proven resilient to existing monoclonal antibodies and necessitates evaluating and creating novel prophylaxis and therapies. SARS-CoV-2 virus evolution is inherently unpredictable, and a likely future scenario is the emergence of a new VOC that is antigenically and, potentially, phenotypically distinct from the early forms of omicron. Ongoing clinical trials are evaluating variety of agents for treatment or prophylaxis of COVID-19 to guide future treatment recommendations; thus, ongoing updating is warranted |

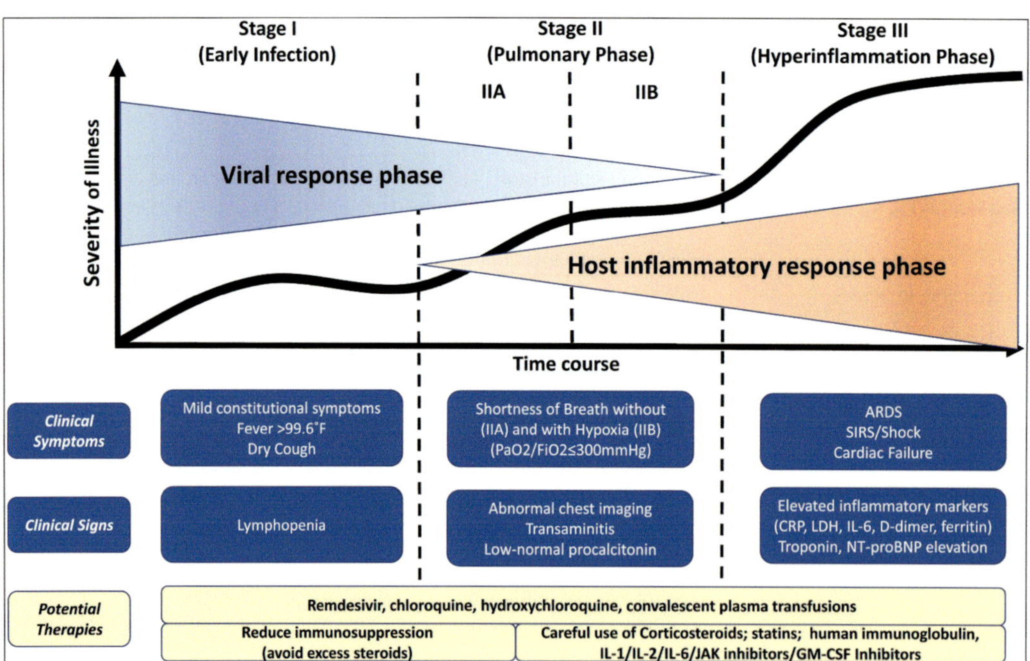


**Fig. 17.1** Stages of COVID-19 and potential therapeutic targets. The figure illustrates three escalating phases of COVID-19 progression, with associated signs, symptoms, and potential phase-specific therapies. *Abbreviations* ARDS, acute respiratory distress syndrome; CRP, C-reactive protein; JAK, Janus kinase; LDH, lactate dehydrogenase; NT-proBNP, N-terminal pro B-type natriuretic peptide; SIRS, systemic inflammatory response syndrome; GM-CSF, granulocyte macrophage colony stimulating factor. Reprinted from Publication title, [36], Hasan K. Siddiqi, Mandeep R. Mehra, COVID-19 illness in native and immunosuppressed states: A clinical–therapeutic staging proposal, 405–407, Copyright (2020), with permission from Elsevier

with mycophenolate before becoming ill with COVID-19 and continuing the drug during the illness with favorable outcomes suggest that it may be safe to continue mycophenolate during COVID-19 and that the drug may have a beneficial effect [56, 61]. A non-randomized prospective study revealed that the addition of mycophenolate sodium (360 mg orally once a day for one month) was associated with decreased mortality (1.9 vs. 17.9%, $p<0.001$) and reduced duration of hospital stay ($7.26 \pm 3.05$ days vs. $8.36 \pm 4.40$ days, $p=0.04$) compared to the standard of care in patients with COVID-19 [56]. Notably, in that study, a low dose of a single immunosuppressive was used, as it had previously been suggested that a low dose of mycophenolate was sufficient to inhibit replication of the SARS-CoV-2 virus [60], thus underscoring the importance of the overall degree of immunosuppression. Taken together, the above considerations suggest that it is reasonable to reduce immunosuppressive medications in the early viral response phase to prevent overt immunosuppression and its adverse effect on the innate response and to lessen the increased risk of secondary bacterial and opportunistic infections while augmenting immunomodulatory agents during the cytokine storm phase. The International Society for Heart and Lung Transplantation (ISHLT) COVID-19 Therapeutics Guidance recommends that alterations to baseline immunosuppressive therapy should be undertaken only in conjunction with the patient's transplant center, although potentially needed only in the inpatient setting in the case of severe/critical illness [39].

## Pharmacologic Therapies

### Ritonavir-Boosted Nirmatrelvir (Paxlovid)

In the EPIC-HR (Evaluation of Protease Inhibition for COVID-19 in High-Risk Patients) trial, ritonavir-boosted nirmatrelvir reduced the risk of hospitalization or death by 89% compared to placebo in unvaccinated, nonhospitalized adults with laboratory-confirmed SARS-CoV-2 infection [62]. In subsequent retrospective studies, some potential benefits of using ritonavir-boosted nirmatrelvir in people with various immunocompromising conditions have been observed [63, 64]. Notably, ritonavir is associated with serious drug-drug interactions with calcineurin inhibitors and mammalian target of rapamycin (mTOR) drugs, including fatal events [65], which limits its use in HTx recipients.

### Remdesivir

Remdesivir is a nucleotide prodrug of an adenosine analog that binds to the viral RNA-dependent RNA polymerase and inhibits SARS-CoV-2 replication by premature termination of viral RNA transcription. A double-blind, placebo-controlled (PINETREE) trial [66] of remdesivir for three days in high-risk, unvaccinated, nonhospitalized patients with mild-moderate COVID-19 showed that the drug resulted in an 87% relative reduction in the risk of hospitalization or death when compared to placebo. However, that trial included only a small number of immunocompromised participants. A retrospective study demonstrated that immunocompromised patients who received remdesivir were at lower risk for mortality than patients who did not receive remdesivir [67]. The optimal duration of treatment with remdesivir in immunocompromised patients is unknown. Given the increased likelihood of prolonged viral replication in transplant patients, some clinicians may choose to extend the course of antiviral therapy past 5–10 days in immunocompromised patients. Remdesivir can be used without dose adjustment in patients with an estimated glomerular filtration rate of $<30$ mL/min, including those on dialysis [68–71].

### Molnupiravir

Molnupiravir is the oral prodrug of beta-D-N4-hydroxycytidine, a ribonucleoside that has shown antiviral activity against SARS-CoV-2 in vitro and in some clinical trials [72, 73]. Molnupiravir appears to have lower clinical efficacy than ritonavir-boosted nirmatrelvir and remdesivir. The MOVe-OUT trial, which was conducted before the emergence of the omicron variant, enrolled high-risk, unvaccinated, nonhospitalized adults and reported that molnupiravir reduced the rate of hospitalization or death among those patients by 31% compared to placebo [74]. A large, multicenter, open-label, adaptive platform trial study (PANORAMIC trial) conducted during the period when the omicron variant was circulating [75] evaluated the use of molnupiravir in nonhospitalized adults who were at high risk of progressing to severe COVID-19; 8.5% of the patients in the trial were immunocompromised. The study found that the use of molnupiravir plus usual care did not reduce the primary composite outcome of hospitalization or death compared to usual care alone. Patients who are severely immunocompromised can experience prolonged periods of SARS-CoV-2 replication, which may lead to rapid viral evolution. There are theoretical concerns that using a single antiviral agent in these patients can produce antiviral-resistant viruses. Additional studies are needed to assess this risk. The ISHLT COVID-19 Therapeutics Guidance does not recommend molnupiravir, as data regarding its efficacy is not robust, and the drug increases the risk of viral mutations [38].

## COVID-19 Convalescent Plasma

There is insufficient evidence to recommend either for or against the use of high-titer COVID-19 convalescent plasma (CCP) for the treatment of COVID-19 in hospitalized immunocompromised patients [37]. Three key randomized trials that evaluated the use of CCP for the treatment of COVID-19 [RECOVERY (Randomised Evaluation of COVID-19 Therapy), CONCOR-1, and REMAP-CAP (Randomized Embedded Multifactorial Adaptive Platform for Community-acquired Pneumonia) did not report any evidence of a benefit of CCP in hospitalized patients with COVID-19. However, most of the patients enrolled in these trials were not immunocompromised [76–78]. Data from other case series, retrospective studies and meta-analyses are limited by their study design and the heterogeneity of the patient populations, and thus their findings are difficult to interpret [79–84].

## Corticosteroids

Unless otherwise indicated, corticosteroids should not be used for the treatment of COVID-19 in patients who are not receiving oxygen. HTx recipients may experience delayed development of favorable adaptive responses and a prolonged period of viral replication. For immunocompromised patients who are earlier in the course of COVID-19, and are receiving minimal levels of conventional oxygen, the preferred approach may be enhancing supportive care, using antiviral therapy, and avoiding corticosteroids. This strategy may reduce the duration of viral replication and the risk of secondary infections. Dexamethasone should be added if the patient has escalating oxygen requirements [37]. The RECOVERY trial demonstrated a survival benefit for dexamethasone in inpatients with COVID-19 who were receiving oxygen, high-flow nasal cannula oxygen, non-invasive ventilation, or mechanical ventilation, but no survival benefit was observed for dexamethasone in patients who did not require supplemental oxygen at enrollment. No specific data regarding the subgroup of patients who were immunocompromised are available [15]. In an observational cohort study of U.S. veterans, the use of dexamethasone was associated with higher mortality in hospitalized patients with COVID-19 who did not require supplemental oxygen [85].

## Interleukin-6 Inhibitors and Janus Kinase Inhibitors

For immunocompromised patients, adding anti-IL-6 receptor monoclonal antibodies (tocilizumab and sarilumab) or Janus kinase inhibitors (baricitinib and tofacitinib) to dexamethasone is reasonable for those who are hypoxemic and experiencing clinical progression and may provide a clinical benefit similar to the benefit seen in the general population, although the relevant trials were not representative of the immunocompromised population [86–89]. However, when using these additional immunomodulating agents, the associated risk of serious bacterial, invasive fungal, or parasitic infections is unknown and should be taken into consideration for risk versus benefit decisions [90–92].

## COVID-19 Vaccine Efficacy Considerations

WHO-approved vaccines againstSARS-CoV-2—based on both established and emerging technologies—are shown in Table 17.3. Emerging vaccine technologies include those based on nucleic acids (such as mRNA and viral vectors), which mimic a viral infection without the need for a live virus [93]. In general, the three main effects that constitute the protection criteria important for devising vaccination strategies are: protection against clinical disease, hospitalization, and death; indirect protection due to the reduced infectivity of breakthrough infections in vaccinated individuals relative to natural infections in unvaccinated individuals; and infection-blocking properties whereby vaccinated individuals are protected against any, even sub-clinical, infection. For the general population, COVID-19 vaccine trials, including more than 80,000 participants worldwide, demonstrated remarkable efficacy of mRNA vaccines (95% prevention of symptomatic COVID-19 and 100% efficacy against severe disease) and a low rate of serious adverse events [94–108] (Table 17.3). Transplant recipients were excluded from all SARS-CoV-2 vaccine clinical trials, so there was no information on vaccine efficacy, durability, or safety for this patient subpopulation. Nonetheless, because immunosuppressed solid organ transplant recipients (SOTRs) were far more likely to suffer a severe outcome from COVID-19 than from the vaccine, the relevant professional societies encouraged COVID-19 vaccination despite the uncertainty as to its clinical efficacy or possible adverse responses [109], leading to rapidly evolving real-world data on the efficacy and safety of mRNA-based vaccines in transplant recipients.

## COVID-19 Vaccination Immune Paresis in Heart Transplant Recipients

In contrast to the general population, immune responses to COVID-19 vaccines in HTx recipients were markedly attenuated. Indeed, COVID-19 vaccination immune paresis was demonstrated for a broad range of immunocompromising conditions. Compared with non-immunocompromised healthcare workers, who demonstrated 92.4% seropositive humoral responses to two doses of the BNT162b2 or the mRNA-1273 vaccines, SOTRs demonstrated the lowest seropositivity (30.7%), followed by patients with hematological malignancies (50.0%), solid tumors (78.7%), autoimmune conditions (79.1%), and the human immunodeficiency virus (HIV) (79.8%) [110]. Seropositivity in lung, heart, or kidney transplant recipients was significantly lower than that in liver transplant recipients (for lung or HTx recipients, the odds for seropositivity were 79 and 74% lower than the odds for liver transplant recipients, respectively). The odds for seropositivity in SOTRs who were vaccinated within the first year vs. > 1 year post-transplantation and for those receiving two or more immunosuppressive drugs versus those receiving only one drug were 55 and 72% lower, respectively [110]. These observations underscore the importance of the overall degree of immunosuppression as the main predictor of poor humoral responses after vaccination. Other clinical factors, including advanced age, sex, race, and vaccine type (BNT162b2 vs. mRNA-1273), showed comparatively weaker associations with the antibody response [111]. Antimetabolite immunosuppression has also been associated with a reduced likelihood of developing a humoral response to COVID-19 vaccines [47, 112–115]. It soon became evident that the COVID-19 vaccination immune paresis of SOTRs translated into a clinical picture that included an unacceptably increased risk of breakthrough infections and mortality in vaccinated transplant recipients [5, 45, 46]. The increased risk of breakthrough infections varied with the underlying immunocompromising diagnosis and occurred substantially faster in individuals with immune dysfunction than in the general population [4, 116, 117]. There was, nonetheless, a decrease in disease severity and hospitalizations in vaccinated immunocompromised persons who experienced a breakthrough infection compared to those infected with SARS-CoV-2 before vaccination. This finding emphasizes that SARS-CoV-2 vaccines mitigated disease severity in immunosuppressed individuals.

## Correlates of Protection

At present, a significant impairment to our understanding of COVID-19 immune responses is a lack of immune correlates of protection. Whether antibodies elicited by disease or vaccination confer clinical immunity and whether the vaccine immune paresis in HTx recipients means that antibodies elicited by vaccines may be less protective in certain subgroups of seropositive immunocompromised individuals compared to non-immunocompromised individuals are unknown, suggesting that clinicians should be cautious when counseling patients who are indeed seropositive after vaccination, since the presence of antibodies need not necessarily imply protection. The HTx caregiver community has, however, made some progress in this direction. For example, in a case–control study of HTx recipients, BNT162b2-vaccine-induced neutralizing antibodies conferred clinical protection against severe disease and COVID-19-related hospitalization. Importantly, the optimal variant-specific cut-off values for vaccine-induced neutralization titers that are predictive of COVID-19-related hospitalization were defined [9]. Nonetheless, many open questions remain before we can implement routine monitoring of SARS-CoV-2 antibody testing as a measure of vaccine effectiveness or as a decision-making tool. Identifying correlates of protection for new viral variants, for new populations, including previously infected people, for new vaccine classes, for different immunosuppression mechanisms, and for various aspects of COVID-19 disease (e.g., symptom types, durations, and severities) [118] still remains to be achieved.

## Waning Immunity and Variant Evolution

It has been shown that the vaccine immune paresis that renders transplant patients vulnerable to severe infection, even after vaccination, is further exacerbated by mutations in epitopes and by waning immunity, limiting viral recognition by the immune system and the durability of protection against infection [119–122]. SARS-CoV-2 undergoes a high degree of genomic mutations, and variants with extensive mutations in the S protein escape many facets of the vaccine-induced immune response. In addition, rapid viral evolution in immunocompromised patients may be an important factor in the emergence of VOCs. Organ transplant recipients may have prolonged SARS-CoV-2 infection and could thereby constitute a reservoir of divergent escape variants that could spread in the general community. In other words, prolonged viral replication in the context of an inadequate immune response can facilitate the emergence of highly mutated, more pathogenic, or more transmissible, SARS-CoV-2 variants [7]. Compared to the ancestral strain, VOCs are characterized by an increase in transmissibility and virulence and by a decrease in the effectiveness of vaccination and treatment measures [123]. It is known that immunity wanes over time. For HTx recipients, significant waning of the humoral response within the 6 months after the second and third homologous BNT162b2 vaccine dose was demonstrated, with the loss of immunity being more profound against the VOCs [124, 125]. Nonetheless, waning antibody protection after

**Table 17.3** WHO-approved vaccines for use against SARS-CoV-2[1]

| Vaccine trade names and other names | Manufacturer | Efficacy in preventing symptomatic COVID-19[2] | Efficacy in preventing severe COVID-19[2] | References |
|---|---|---|---|---|
| Established vaccine technologies | | | | |
| **Inactivated whole SARS-CoV-2 vaccines**: use a virus inactivated by heat, ultraviolet light, or chemical treatment and provide a safer approach with a simplified development path | | | | |
| Covaxin (BBV152) | Bharat biotech | 77.8% | 93.4% | [94] |
| Covilo (BBIBP-CorV) | Beijing Institute of Biological PRODUCTS/ Sinopharm | 78.1% | 100% | [95] |
| CoronaVac (PiCoVacc) | Sinovac biotech | 50.7% | 100% | [96] |
| **Recombinant protein subunit vaccines**: focus on the immune response only against the key viral proteins of interest | | | | |
| Nuvaxovid (NVXCoV2373) | Novavax | 89.7% | 100% | [97] |
| COVOVAX (Novavax formulation)[3] | Serum Institute of India | | | |
| **Emerging vaccine technologies** | | | | |
| **mRNA vaccines**: consist of viral antigen-encoding messenger RNA (mRNA) encapsulated in and stabilized by lipid nanoparticles. Once delivered to cells, they drive transient expression of antigens that are then recognized by the immune system | | | | |
| Spikevax ancestral; monovalent index virus; (elasomeran, mRNA-1273) | Moderna | 93.2% | 98.2% | [98] |
| Spikevax variant-adapted vaccines; bivalent variant-containing; bivalent original/omicron[4] | Moderna | | | |
| Spikevax 2023–2024 formula; monovalent variant-containing; monovalent omicron XBB.1.5.[4] | Moderna | | | |
| Comirnaty ancestral; monovalent index virus; (tozinameran, BNT162b2) | Pfizer/BioNTech | 91.3% | 96.7% | [99] |
| Comirnaty variant-adapted vaccines; bivalent variant-containing; bivalent, original/omicron[4] | Pfizer/BioNTech | | | |
| Comirnaty monovalent variant-containing; updated antigen, omicron XBB.1.5[4] | Pfizer/BioNTech | | | |
| **Viral vector vaccines**: employ unrelated, modified viruses as vaccine vectors to deliver antigen-coding genes into the host cells to stimulate an immune response | | | | |
| Jcovden (Ad26.COV2.S) | Janssen (Johnson and Johnson) | 52.4% | 74.6% | [100] |
| Vaxzevria (ChAdOx1nCoV-19, AZD1222) | Oxford/AstraZeneca | 79% | 100% | [101, 102] |
| Covishield (Oxford/AstraZeneca formulation)[5] | Serum Institute of India | | | |
| Convidecia (AD5-nCoV) | CanSino biologics | 57.5% | 91.7% | [103] |

[1] Data based on References [93, 104, 105]

[2] Efficacy relates to controlled trials for the general population and for primary series, not including immunocompromised patients

[3] NVX-CoV2373 marketed as Covovax by Serum Institute of India

[4] In the context of high infection- and vaccine-derived immunity in the population, vaccine effectiveness estimates for the "updated vaccines" are mostly relative (rVE), rather than absolute (comparing vaccinated to unvaccinated individuals) and demonstrate the added protection of a vaccine over and above pre-existing infection- and vaccine-derived immunity. Estimates of rVE against currently circulating SARS-CoV-2 variants, including XBB or JN.1 descendent subclades, are limited in terms of the number of studies, geographic diversity, vaccine platforms evaluated, populations assessed, duration of follow-up, and comparative estimates for monovalent XBB.1.5 vaccines versus other formulations delivered at the same time

[5] Vaxzevria (AZD1222, ChAdOx1 nCoV-19, or ChAdOx1) is a vaccine designed by the University of Oxford and produced by AstraZeneca. The vaccine is also produced by the Serum Institute of India under the name Covishield

vaccination may not necessarily lead to complete susceptibility to severe disease because SARS-CoV-2 specific T-cell responses are an important factor in the development of protective immunity against viral infection [126]. Vaccine-induced spike-specific T cells are multispecific and can recognize different regions of the spike protein [127, 128]. Thus, despite the ability of emerging variants to alter T-cell specificity, these variants do not escape the entire repertoire of spike-specific T cells. Indeed, it has been demonstrated that, for most vaccinated individuals, VOCs are recognized by the spike-specific T cells induced by mRNA vaccines [129, 130].

## Strategies to Mitigate COVID-19 Vaccine Immune Paresis in Heart Transplant Recipients

The reduced vaccine-immune response and the increased risk of a poor outcome following COVID-19 for SOTRs stimulated the need to explore whether alternative vaccination strategies could be more immunogenic. Alternative potential vaccination strategies to increase the immunogenicity of COVID-19 vaccination include (1) additional booster doses; (2) the use of different combinations of vaccines (heterologous vaccination); (3) higher doses, as has been shown for hepatitis B and influenza vaccines in immunocompromised patients [131]; (4) vaccination of candidates before transplant; (5) temporary immunosuppression reduction or discontinuation around the time of vaccination; (6) prophylactic administration of monoclonal antibodies; and (7) updated vaccine formulations aiming to overcome the immune-evasive omicron and other variants.

In HTx recipients, four versus three doses of mRNA vaccine reduced the hazard risk for infection in approximately 50% of vaccinated individuals, but effectiveness against the omicron variant was reduced [132]. The incomplete immunological response and reduced effectiveness support efforts to find supplementary approaches to the prevention of SARS-CoV-2 infection that are different from—and can be used in conjunction with—the sole strategy of repeated booster doses to protect this high-risk population. In the context of repeated COVID-19 vaccination in patients treated with immunosuppressive drugs, increasing the dose of the mRNA-1273 vaccine had no beneficial effect [133]. Data indicates that lengthening the time interval between mRNA COVID-19 vaccine doses may improve the immune response and vaccine effectiveness. A tendency toward higher neutralization inhibition was seen for a longer interval between the first and second BNT doses in SOTRs [134]. Therefore, follow-up studies must be conducted to determine the optimal vaccination interval for better vaccine efficacy in immunocompromised SOTRs, who are expected to have reduced vaccine-induced immunogenicity. Patients on the transplant waiting list show a slightly reduced response to vaccination, compared to the healthy population, but a significantly better response than transplant recipients [135, 136]. HTx recipients vaccinated with two doses of the BNT162b2 vaccine prior to transplant demonstrated a high and durable immune response at 12 weeks after HTx [137]. Similarly, the anti-SARS-CoV2 antibody titers in kidney recipients vaccinated prior to transplant were persistently higher than those in recipients vaccinated after transplant. Thus, it is recommended that all transplant candidates receive a full SARS-Cov-2 vaccine cycle before transplant. The net benefit of reducing or withdrawing immunosuppressive drugs aiming to improve the response to SARS-CoV2 vaccination is still under investigation, and currently, the strategy cannot be recommended or excluded in this context. Passive immunization with preformed single-conformation monoclonal antibodies can potentially support an immune defense against SARS-CoV2 in SOTRs. However, due to the specificity of the immune support provided by monoclonal antibodies, caution must be exercised in applying such a strategy in light of the evolution of novel VOCs characterized by high degree of genomic mutations associated with evasion. Findings to date support updating COVID-19 vaccines to match antigenically divergent variants and to exclude the ancestral spike-antigen due to the potential for immune imprinting (i.e., on subsequent exposures, reactivity toward the original strain is maintained at higher levels than reactivity toward newer strains).

**In summary**: While much of the knowledge accumulated for COVID-19 is relevant to the general population and immunosuppressed patients alike, some of the particular characteristics of HTx recipients warrant tailored approaches to patient management and to prevention and treatment. Although there are several pharmacologic therapies available for HTx recipients, it should be remembered that this is a rapidly evolving field, further emphasizing the crucial roles of transplant team in managing the patients according to the most up-to-date guidelines. Particularly important in the crystallization of a vaccination policy was to encourage vaccination as soon as vaccines became available. It was this approach that led to the generation of rapidly accumulating real-world data that confirmed the efficacy and safety of mRNA-based vaccines. The impact of the accumulated data on SARS-CoV-2 will extend beyond protection from COVID-19 into the implementation of new vaccine technologies for various other infectious disease targets, improving preparedness for future health crises, and into applications for oncology, metabolic diseases, gene therapy, and gene editing [93].

## References

1. Ecdc. Lessons from the COVID-19 pandemic. 2023. www.ecdc.europa.eu. Accessed 10 Oct 2024
2. Weekly epidemiological update on COVID-19 - 20 April 2023 [Internet]. https://www.who.int/publications/m/item/weekly-epidemiological-update-on-covid-19---20-april-2023. Accessed 10 Oct 2024
3. Kent SJ, Khoury DS, Reynaldi A, Juno JA, Wheatley AK, Stadler E, et al. Disentangling the relative importance of T cell responses in COVID-19: leading actors or supporting cast? Nat Rev Immunol. 2022;22(6):387–97.
4. Tenforde MW, Patel MM, Ginde AA, Douin DJ, Talbot HK, Casey JD, et al. Effectiveness of severe acute respiratory syndrome coronavirus 2 messenger RNA vaccines for preventing coronavirus disease 2019 hospitalizations in the United States. Clin Infect Dis. 2022;74(9):1515–24.
5. Qin CX, Moore LW, Anjan S, Rahamimov R, Sifri CD, Ali NM, et al. Risk of breakthrough SARS-CoV-2 infections in adult transplant recipients. Transplantation. 2021;105(11):e265-6.
6. Markov PV, Ghafari M, Beer M, Lythgoe K, Simmonds P, Stilianakis NI, et al. The evolution of SARS-CoV-2. Nat Rev Microbiol. 2023;21(6):361–79.
7. Corey L, Beyrer C, Cohen MS, Michael NL, Bedford T, Rolland M. SARS-CoV-2 variants in patients with immunosuppression. N Engl J Med. Mass Med Soc. 2021;385:562–6.
8. Forni D, Cagliani R, Clerici M, Sironi M. Molecular evolution of human coronavirus genomes. Trends Microbiol. 2017;25(1):35–48.
9. Peled Y, Patel JK, Raanani E, Eilon R, Fardman A, Beigel R, et al. BNT162b2-vaccine-induced neutralization responses are immune correlates of clinical protection against SARS-CoV-2 in heart transplant recipients. Clin Transplant. 2023;37(11):e15091.
10. Hu W, Yen YT, Singh S, Kao CL, Wu-Hsieh BA. SARS-CoV regulates immune function-related gene expression in human monocytic cells. Viral Immunol. 2012;25(4):277–88.
11. Aslam S, Ison MG. SARS-CoV-2 vaccination in heart transplantation: what we do and do not know. J Heart Lung Transplant. 2022;41(2):158–60.
12. Hazan F, Verdonk C, Coutance G, Ferré VM, Marot S, Melo VDD, et al. Severity of SARS-CoV-2 omicron variant infection in heart transplant recipients. J Heart Lung Transplant. 2023;42(5):558–61.
13. Andersen KM, Mehta HB, Palamuttam N, Ford D, Garibaldi BT, Auwaerter PG, et al. Association between chronic use of immunosuppresive drugs and clinical outcomes from coronavirus disease 2019 (COVID-19) hospitalization: a retrospective cohort study in a large US health system. Clin Infect Dis. 2021;73(11):e4124-30.
14. Ahmed F, Abid M, Maniya T, Usman MS, Fudim M. Incidence and prognosis of COVID-19 amongst heart transplant recipients: a systematic review and meta-analysis. Eur J Prev Cardiol. 2022;29(6):e224-6.
15. Group RC. Dexamethasone in hospitalized patients with Covid-19. N Engl J Med. 2021;384(8):693–704.
16. Marcondes-Braga FG, Murad CM, Belfort DSP, Dantas RCT, Lira MTSS, Aragão CAS, et al. Characteristics and outcomes of heart transplant recipients with coronavirus-19 disease in a high-volume transplant center. Transplantation. 2022;106(3):641–7.
17. Nair V, Jandovitz N, Hirsch JS, Nair G, Abate M, Bhaskaran M, et al. COVID-19 in kidney transplant recipients. Am J Transplant. 2020;20(7):1819–25.

18. Aversa M, Benvenuto L, Anderson M, Shah L, Robbins H, Pereira M, et al. COVID-19 in lung transplant recipients: a single center case series from New York City. Am J Transplant. 2020;20(11):3072–80.
19. Rivinius R, Kaya Z, Schramm R, Boeken U, Provaznik Z, Heim C, et al. COVID-19 among heart transplant recipients in Germany: a multicenter survey. Clin Res Cardiol. 2020;109:1531–9.
20. Latif F, Farr MA, Clerkin KJ, Habal MV, Takeda K, Naka Y, et al. Characteristics and outcomes of recipients of heart transplant with coronavirus disease 2019. JAMA Cardiol. 2020;5(10):1165–9.
21. Ketcham SW, Adie SK, Malliett A, Abdul-Aziz AA, Bitar A, Grafton G, et al. Coronavirus disease-2019 in heart transplant recipients in southeastern Michigan: a case series. J Card Fail. 2020;26(6):457–61.
22. Iacovoni A, Boffini M, Pidello S, Simonato E, Barbero C, Sebastiani R, et al. A case series of novel coronavirus infection in heart transplantation from 2 centers in the pandemic area in the North of Italy. J Heart Lung Transplant. 2020;39(10):1081–8.
23. Genuardi MV, Moss N, Najjar SS, Houston BA, Shore S, Vorovich E, et al. Coronavirus disease 2019 in heart transplant recipients: risk factors, immunosuppression, and outcomes. J Heart Lung Transplant. 2021;40(9):926–35.
24. Bottio T, Bagozzi L, Fiocco A, Nadali M, Caraffa R, Bifulco O, et al. COVID-19 in heart transplant recipients: a multicenter analysis of the Northern Italian outbreak. Heart Fail. 2021;9(1):52–61.
25. Soriano RV de M, Rossi Neto JM, Finger MA, Santos CC. COVID-19 in heart transplant recipients in Sao Paulo: a case series. Arq Bras Cardiol. 2021;116:1–3.
26. Al-Darzi W, Aurora L, Michaels A, Cowger J, Grafton G, Selektor Y, et al. Heart transplant recipients with confirmed 2019 novel coronavirus infection: the Detroit experience. Clin Transplant. 2020;34(12):e14091.
27. Taghavi S, Jelodar HR, Rafati A, Naderi N, Mirtajaddini M, Amin A, et al. COVID-19 in heart transplant recipients. J Cardiovasc Thorac Res. 2022;14(4):258.
28. Ahluwalia M, Givertz MM, Mehra MR. A proposed strategy for management of immunosuppression in heart transplant patients with COVID-19. Clin Transplant. 2020;34(11):e14032.
29. Ballout JA, Ahmed T, Kolodziej AR. COVID-19 and heart transplant: a case series and review of the literature. In: Transplantation proceedings. Elsevier; 2021. p. 1219–23.
30. Caraffa R, Bagozzi L, Fiocco A, Bifulco O, Nadali M, Ponzoni M, et al. Coronavirus disease 2019 (COVID-19) in the heart transplant population: a single-centre experience. Eur J Cardiothorac Surg. 2020;58(5):899–906.
31. Lima B, Gibson GT, Vullaganti S, Malhame K, Maybaum S, Hussain ST, et al. COVID-19 in recent heart transplant recipients: clinicopathologic features and early outcomes. Transpl Infect Dis. 2020;22(5):e13382.
32. Azzi Y, Bartash R, Scalea J, Loarte-Campos P, Akalin E. COVID-19 and solid organ transplantation: a review article. Transplantation. 2021;105(1):37–55.
33. Kullar R, Marcelin JR, Swartz TH, Piggott DA, Macias Gil R, Mathew TA, et al. Racial disparity of coronavirus disease 2019 in African American communities. J Infect Dis. 2020;222(6):890–3.
34. Massie AB, Werbel WA, Avery RK, Chiang TPY, Snyder JJ, Segev DL. Quantifying excess deaths among solid organ transplant recipients in the COVID-19 era. Am J Transplant. 2022;22(8):2077–82.
35. Rizk JG, Kalantar-Zadeh K, Mehra MR, Lavie CJ, Rizk Y, Forthal DN. Pharmaco-immunomodulatory therapy in COVID-19. Drugs. 2020;80:1267–92.
36. Siddiqi HK, Mehra MR. COVID-19 illness in native and immunosuppressed states: a clinical–therapeutic staging proposal. J Heart Lung Transplant. 2020;39(5):405–7.
37. COVID-19 treatment guidelines 2. https://www.covid19treatmentguidelines.nih.gov/. Accessed 10 Oct 2024
38. Ging P, Ison M, Patel J, Campos SV, Vos R, Aslam S. New ISHLT COVID-19 therapeutics guidance. https://www.fda.gov/emergency-preparedness-and-. Accessed 10 Oct 2024
39. Wang M, Cao R, Zhang L, Yang X, Liu J, Xu M, et al. Remdesivir and chloroquine effectively inhibit the recently emerged novel coronavirus (2019-nCoV) in vitro. Cell Res. 2020;30(3):269–71.
40. Cao B, Wang Y, Wen D, Liu W, Wang J, Fan G, et al. A trial of lopinavir–ritonavir in adults hospitalized with severe Covid-19. N Engl J Med. 2020;382(19):1787–99.
41. Hermine O, Mariette X, Porcher R, Djossou F, Nguyen Y, Arlet JB, et al. Tocilizumab plus dexamethasone versus dexamethasone in patients with moderate-to-severe COVID-19 pneumonia: a randomised clinical trial from the CORIMUNO-19 study group. EClinicalMedicine. 2022;46.
42. Salama C, Han J, Yau L, Reiss WG, Kramer B, Neidhart JD, et al. Tocilizumab in patients hospitalized with Covid-19 pneumonia. N Engl J Med. 2021;384(1):20–30.
43. Kemp SA, Collier DA, Datir RP, Ferreira IATM, Gayed S, Jahun A, et al. SARS-CoV-2 evolution during treatment of chronic infection. Nature. 2021;592(7853):277–82.
44. Leung WF, Chorlton S, Tyson J, Al-Rawahi GN, Jassem AN, Prystajecky N, et al. COVID-19 in an immunocompromised host: persistent shedding of viable SARS-CoV-2 and emergence of multiple mutations: a case report. Int J Infect Dis. 2022;114:178–82.

45. Ali NM, Alnazari N, Mehta SA, Boyarsky B, Avery RK, Segev DL, et al. Development of COVID-19 infection in transplant recipients after SARS-CoV-2 vaccination. Transplantation. 2021;105(9):e104-6.
46. Embi PJ. Effectiveness of 2-dose vaccination with mRNA COVID-19 vaccines against COVID-19–associated hospitalizations among immunocompromised adults—nine states, January–September 2021. MMWR Morb Mortal Wkly Rep. 2021;70.
47. Boyarsky BJ, Werbel WA, Avery RK, Tobian AAR, Massie AB, Segev DL, et al. Antibody response to 2-dose SARS-CoV-2 mRNA vaccine series in solid organ transplant recipients. JAMA. 2021;325(21):2204–6.
48. Haidar G, Agha M, Bilderback A, Lukanski A, Linstrum K, Troyan R, et al. Prospective evaluation of COVID-19 vaccine responses across a broad spectrum of immunocompromising conditions: the COVICS study. Clin Infect Dis. 2022;75(1):e630-44.
49. Narasimhan M, Mahimainathan L, Clark AE, Usmani A, Cao J, Araj E, et al. Serological response in lung transplant recipients after two doses of SARS-CoV-2 mRNA vaccines. Vaccines (Basel). 2021;9(7):708.
50. Havlin J, Svorcova M, Dvorackova E, Lastovicka J, Lischke R, Kalina T, et al. Immunogenicity of BNT162b2 mRNA COVID-19 vaccine and SARS-CoV-2 infection in lung transplant recipients. J Heart Lung Transplant. 2021;40(8):754–8.
51. COVID-19 vaccination and pre-exposure prophylaxis in heart and lung transplant candidates and recipients.
52. Peled Y, Afek A, Patel JK, Raanani E, Segev A, Ram E, et al. Neutralization of SARS-CoV-2 variants elicited by the combination of vaccination and natural infection in heart transplant recipients. Clin Transplant. 2023;37(11):e15092.
53. Ao D, Lan T, He X, Liu J, Chen L, Baptista-Hon DT, et al. SARS-CoV-2 omicron variant: immune escape and vaccine development. MedComm (Beijing). 2022;3(1):e126.
54. Saghazadeh A, Rezaei N. Towards treatment planning of COVID-19: rationale and hypothesis for the use of multiple immunosuppressive agents: Anti-antibodies, immunoglobulins, and corticosteroids. Int Immunopharmacol. 2020;84:106560.
55. Karki R, Sharma BR, Tuladhar S, Williams EP, Zalduondo L, Samir P, et al. Synergism of TNF-α and IFN-γ triggers inflammatory cell death, tissue damage, and mortality in SARS-CoV-2 infection and cytokine shock syndromes. Cell. 2021;184(1):149–68.
56. Sajgure A, Kulkarni A, Joshi A, Sajgure V, Pathak V, Melinkeri R, et al. Safety and efficacy of mycophenolate in COVID-19: a nonrandomised prospective study in western India. Lancet Reg Health-Southeast Asia. 2023;11.
57. Thakur M, Datusalia AK, Kumar A. Use of steroids in COVID-19 patients: a meta-analysis. Eur J Pharmacol. 2022;914: 174579.
58. Ritter ML, Pirofski L. Mycophenolate mofetil: effects on cellular immune subsets, infectious complications, and antimicrobial activity. Transpl Infect Dis. 2009;11(4):290–7.
59. Cheng KW, Cheng SC, Chen WY, Lin MH, Chuang SJ, Cheng IH, et al. Thiopurine analogs and mycophenolic acid synergistically inhibit the papain-like protease of Middle East respiratory syndrome coronavirus. Antiviral Res. 2015;115:9–16.
60. Kato F, Matsuyama S, Kawase M, Hishiki T, Katoh H, Takeda M. Antiviral activities of mycophenolic acid and IMD-0354 against SARS-CoV-2. Microbiol Immunol. 2020;64(9):635–9.
61. Sajgure AD, Sajgure VA, Date GV, Kulkarni AP. Safety of mycophenolate in covid-19 infection: a case series.
62. Hammond J, Leister-Tebbe H, Gardner A, Abreu P, Bao W, Wisemandle W, et al. Oral nirmatrelvir for high-risk, nonhospitalized adults with Covid-19. N Engl J Med. 2022;386(15):1397–408.
63. Najjar-Debbiny R, Gronich N, Weber G, Khoury J, Amar M, Stein N, et al. Effectiveness of paxlovid in reducing severe coronavirus disease 2019 and mortality in high-risk patients. Clin Infect Dis. 2023;76(3):e342-9.
64. Qian G, Wang X, Patel NJ, Kawano Y, Fu X, Cook CE, et al. Outcomes with and without outpatient SARS-CoV-2 treatment for patients with COVID-19 and systemic autoimmune rheumatic diseases: a retrospective cohort study. Lancet Rheumatol. 2023;5(3):e139-50.
65. Fda, Cder. March 16, 2023 Meeting of the Antimicrobial Drugs Advisory Committee Meeting. 2023.
66. Gottlieb RL, Vaca CE, Paredes R, Mera J, Webb BJ, Perez G, et al. Early remdesivir to prevent progression to severe covid-19 in outpatients. N Engl J Med. 2022;386(4):305–15.
67. Mozaffari E, Chandak A, Gottlieb RL, Kalil AC, Read SH, Jiang H, et al. Remdesivir reduces mortality in immunocompromised patients hospitalized for COVID-19 poster #557 background. Clin Infect Dis. 2023;383(11):2881–92.
68. Sunny S, Samaroo-Campbell J, Abdallah M, Luka A, Quale J. Is remdesivir safe in patients with renal impairment? Experience at a large tertiary urban medical center. Infection. 2023;51(1):247–52.
69. Shah MK, Parikh M, Prajapati D, Kute VB, Bhende P, Prajapati A, et al. Safety and tolerability of remdesivir in patients with end-stage renal disease on maintenance hemodialysis. Indian J Crit Care Med. 2022;26(5):619.
70. Davoudi-Monfared E, Ahmadi A, Karimpour-Razkenari E, Shahrami B, Najmeddin F, Mojtahedzadeh M. Remdesivir administration in COVID-19 patients with renal impairment: a systematic review. Am J Ther. 2022;29(5):e520-33.
71. Aiswarya D, Arumugam V, Dineshkumar T, Gopalakrishnan N, Lamech TM, Nithya G, et al. Use of remdesivir in patients with COVID-19 on hemodialysis: a study of safety and tolerance. Kidney Int Rep. 2021;6(3):586–93.

72. Fischer WA, Eron Jr JJ, Holman W, Cohen MS, Fang L, Szewczyk LJ, et al. A phase 2a clinical trial of molnupiravir in patients with COVID-19 shows accelerated SARS-CoV-2 RNA clearance and elimination of infectious virus. Sci Transl Med. 2021;14(628):eabl7430.
73. Zou R, Peng L, Shu D, Zhao L, Lan J, Tan G, et al. Antiviral efficacy and safety of molnupiravir against omicron variant infection: a randomized controlled clinical trial. Front Pharmacol. 2022;13:939573.
74. Jayk Bernal A, Gomes da Silva MM, Musungaie DB, Kovalchuk E, Gonzalez A, Delos Reyes V, et al. Molnupiravir for oral treatment of covid-19 in nonhospitalized patients. N Engl J Med. 2022;386(6):509–20.
75. Butler CC, Hobbs FDR, Gbinigie OA, Rahman NM, Hayward G, Richards DB, et al. Molnupiravir plus usual care versus usual care alone as early treatment for adults with COVID-19 at increased risk of adverse outcomes (PANORAMIC): an open-label, platform-adaptive randomised controlled trial. The Lancet. 2023;401(10373):281–93.
76. Group RC. Convalescent plasma in patients admitted to hospital with COVID-19 (RECOVERY): a randomised controlled, open-label, platform trial. Lancet. 2021;397(10289):2049.
77. Bégin P, Callum J, Jamula E, Cook R, Heddle NM, Tinmouth A, et al. Convalescent plasma for hospitalized patients with COVID-19: an open-label, randomized controlled trial. Nat Med. 2021;27(11):2012–24.
78. Abdelhady H, Abdelrazik M, Abdi Z, Abdo D, Abdulle A, Abel L, et al. Effect of convalescent plasma on organ support–free days in critically ill patients with COVID-19: a randomized clinical trial. JAMA. 2021;326(17):1690–702.
79. Thompson MA, Henderson JP, Shah PK, Rubinstein SM, Joyner MJ, Choueiri TK, et al. Association of convalescent plasma therapy with survival in patients with hematologic cancers and COVID-19. JAMA Oncol. 2021;7(8):1167–75.
80. Lanza F, Monaco F, Ciceri F, Cairoli R, Sacchi MV, Guidetti A, et al. Lack of efficacy of convalescent plasma in COVID-19 patients with concomitant hematological malignancies: an Italian retrospective study. Hematol Oncol. 2022;40(5):857–63.
81. Lang-Meli J, Fuchs J, Mathé P, Ho H en, Kern L, Jaki L, et al. Case series: convalescent plasma therapy for patients with COVID-19 and primary antibody deficiency. J Clin Immunol. 2022;42(2):253–65.
82. Rodionov RN, Biener A, Spieth P, Achleitner M, Hölig K, Aringer M, et al. Potential benefit of convalescent plasma transfusions in immunocompromised patients with COVID-19. Lancet Microbe. 2021;2(4): e138.
83. Franchini M, Focosi D, Percivalle E, Beccaria M, Garuti M, Arar O, et al. Variant of concern-matched COVID-19 convalescent plasma usage in seronegative hospitalized patients. Viruses. 2022;14(7):1443.
84. Ljungquist O, Lundgren M, Iliachenko E, Månsson F, Böttiger B, Landin-Olsson M, et al. Convalescent plasma treatment in severely immunosuppressed patients hospitalized with COVID-19: an observational study of 28 cases. Infect Dis. 2022;54(4):283–91.
85. Crothers K, DeFaccio R, Tate J, Alba PR, Goetz MB, Jones B, et al. Dexamethasone in hospitalised COVID-19 patients not on intensive respiratory support. Eur Respir J. 2022;60(1).
86. Investigators RC. Interleukin-6 receptor antagonists in critically ill patients with covid-19. N Engl J Med. 2021;384(16):1491–502.
87. Group RC. Tocilizumab in patients admitted to hospital with COVID-19 (RECOVERY): a randomised, controlled, open-label, platform trial. Lancet. 2021;397(10285):1637.
88. Marconi VC, Ramanan AV, de Bono S, Kartman CE, Krishnan V, Liao R, et al. Efficacy and safety of baricitinib for the treatment of hospitalised adults with COVID-19 (COV-BARRIER): a randomised, double-blind, parallel-group, placebo-controlled phase 3 trial. Lancet Respir Med. 2021;9(12):1407–18.
89. Kalil AC, Patterson TF, Mehta AK, Tomashek KM, Wolfe CR, Ghazaryan V, et al. Baricitinib plus remdesivir for hospitalized adults with covid-19. N Engl J Med. 2021;384(9):795–807.
90. Charan J, Dutta S, Kaur R, Bhardwaj P, Sharma P, Ambwani S, et al. Tocilizumab in COVID-19: a study of adverse drug events reported in the WHO database. Expert Opin Drug Saf. 2021;20(9):1125–36.
91. Peng J, Fu M, Mei H, Zheng H, Liang G, She X, et al. Efficacy and secondary infection risk of tocilizumab, sarilumab and anakinra in COVID-19 patients: a systematic review and meta-analysis. Rev Med Virol. 2022;32(3):e2295.
92. Shah R, Shah J, Gohil J, Revathi G, Surani S. Secondary infections in patients with COVID-19 pneumonia treated with tocilizumab compared to those not treated with tocilizumab: a retrospective study at a tertiary hospital in kenya. Int J Gen Med. 2022;2415–25.
93. Edwards AM, Baric RS, Saphire EO, Ulmer JB. Stopping pandemics before they start: lessons learned from SARS-CoV-2. Science (1979). 2022;375(6585):1133–9.
94. Ella R, Reddy S, Blackwelder W, Potdar V, Yadav P, Sarangi V, et al. Efficacy, safety, and lot-to-lot immunogenicity of an inactivated SARS-CoV-2 vaccine (BBV152): interim results of a randomised, double-blind, controlled, phase 3 trial. The Lancet. 2021;398(10317):2173–84.

95. Al Kaabi N, Zhang Y, Xia S, Yang Y, Al Qahtani MM, Abdulrazzaq N, et al. Effect of 2 inactivated SARS-CoV-2 vaccines on symptomatic COVID-19 infection in adults: a randomized clinical trial. JAMA. 2021;326(1):35–45.
96. Palacios R, Patiño EG, de Oliveira PR, Conde MTRP, Batista AP, Zeng G, et al. Double-blind, randomized, placebo-controlled phase III clinical trial to evaluate the efficacy and safety of treating healthcare professionals with the adsorbed COVID-19 (inactivated) vaccine manufactured by sinovac–PROFISCOV: a structured summary of a study protocol for a randomised controlled trial. Trials. 2020;21:1–3.
97. Heath PT, Galiza EP, Baxter DN, Boffito M, Browne D, Burns F, et al. Safety and efficacy of NVX-CoV2373 covid-19 vaccine. N Engl J Med. 2021;385(13):1172–83.
98. El Sahly HM, Baden LR, Essink B, Doblecki-Lewis S, Martin JM, Anderson EJ, et al. Efficacy of the mRNA-1273 SARS-CoV-2 vaccine at completion of blinded phase. N Engl J Med. 2021;385(19):1774–85.
99. Thomas SJ, Moreira ED Jr, Kitchin N, Absalon J, Gurtman A, Lockhart S, et al. Safety and efficacy of the BNT162b2 mRNA Covid-19 vaccine through 6 months. N Engl J Med. 2021;385(19):1761–73.
100. Sadoff J, Gray G, Vandebosch A, Cárdenas V, Shukarev G, Grinsztejn B, et al. Final analysis of efficacy and safety of single-dose Ad26. COV2. S. N Engl J Med. 2022;386(9):847–60.
101. Falsey AR, Frenck RW Jr, Walsh EE, Kitchin N, Absalon J, Gurtman A, et al. SARS-CoV-2 neutralization with BNT162b2 vaccine dose 3. N Engl J Med. 2021;385(17):1627–9.
102. Polack FP, Thomas SJ, Kitchin N, Absalon J, Gurtman A, Lockhart S, et al. Safety and efficacy of the BNT162b2 mRNA covid-19 vaccine. N Engl J Med. 2020;383(27):2603–15.
103. Halperin SA, Ye L, MacKinnon-Cameron D, Smith B, Cahn PE, Ruiz-Palacios GM, et al. Final efficacy analysis, interim safety analysis, and immunogenicity of a single dose of recombinant novel coronavirus vaccine (adenovirus type 5 vector) in adults 18 years and older: an international, multicentre, randomised, double-blinded, placebo-controlled phase 3 trial. The Lancet. 2022;399(10321):237–48.
104. Chi WY, Li YD, Huang HC, Chan TEH, Chow SY, Su JH, et al. COVID-19 vaccine update: vaccine effectiveness, SARS-CoV-2 variants, boosters, adverse effects, and immune correlates of protection. J Biomed Sci. 2022;29(1):82.
105. Abufares HI, Oyoun Alsoud L, Alqudah MAY, Shara M, Soares NC, Alzoubi KH, et al. COVID-19 vaccines, effectiveness, and immune responses. Int J Mol Sci. 2022;23(23):15415.
106. Voysey M, Clemens SAC, Madhi SA, Weckx LY, Folegatti PM, Aley PK, et al. Safety and efficacy of the ChAdOx1 nCoV-19 vaccine (AZD1222) against SARS-CoV-2: an interim analysis of four randomised controlled trials in Brazil, South Africa, and the UK. The Lancet. 2021;397(10269):99–111.
107. WHO Target Product Profiles for COVID-19 Vaccines. Revised version April 2022 [Internet]. https://www.who.int/publications/m/item/who-target-product-profiles-for-covid-19-vaccines. Accessed 10 Oct 2024
108. Fda, Cber. Vaccines and related biological products advisory committee December 17, 2020 meeting briefing document-FDA. 2020.
109. Aslam S, Goldstein DR, Vos R, Gelman AE, Kittleson MM, Wolfe C, et al. COVID-19 vaccination in our transplant recipients: the time is now. J Heart Lung Transplant. Elsevier. 2021;40:169–71.
110. Haidar G, Agha M, Bilderback A, Lukanski A, Linstrum K, Troyan R, et al. Prospective evaluation of coronavirus disease 2019 (COVID-19) vaccine responses across a broad spectrum of immunocompromising conditions: the COVID-19 vaccination in the immunocompromised study (COVICS). Clin Infect Dis. 2022;75(1):e630-44.
111. Alejo JL, Mitchell J, Chiang TPY, Chang A, Abedon AT, Werbel WA, et al. Predicting a positive antibody response after 2 SARS-CoV-2 mRNA vaccines in transplant recipients: a machine learning approach with external validation. Transplantation. 2022;106(10):e452-60.
112. Boyarsky BJ, Werbel WA, Avery RK, Tobian AAR, Massie AB, Segev DL, et al. Immunogenicity of a single dose of SARS-CoV-2 messenger RNA vaccine in solid organ transplant recipients. JAMA. 2021;325(17):1784–6.
113. Peled Y, Ram E, Lavee J, Segev A, Matezki S, Wieder-Finesod A, et al. Third dose of the BNT162b2 vaccine in heart transplant recipients: immunogenicity and clinical experience. J Heart Lung Transplant. 2022;41(2):148–57.
114. Osmanodja B, Ronicke S, Budde K, Jens A, Hammett C, Koch N, et al. Serological response to three, four and five doses of SARS-CoV-2 vaccine in kidney transplant recipients. J Clin Med. 2022;11(9):2565.
115. Peled Y, Ram E, Lavee J, Sternik L, Segev A, Wieder-Finesod A, et al. BNT162b2 vaccination in heart transplant recipients: clinical experience and antibody response. J Heart Lung Transplant. 2021;40(8):759–62.
116. Sun J, Zheng Q, Madhira V, Olex AL, Anzalone AJ, Vinson A, et al. Association between immune dysfunction and COVID-19 breakthrough infection after SARS-CoV-2 vaccination in the US. JAMA Intern Med. 2022;182(2):153–62.
117. Brosh-Nissimov T, Orenbuch-Harroch E, Chowers M, Elbaz M, Nesher L, Stein M, et al. BNT162b2 vaccine breakthrough: clinical characteristics of 152 fully vaccinated hospitalized COVID-19 patients in Israel. Clin Microbiol Infect. 2021;27(11):1652–7.

118. Gilbert PB, Donis RO, Koup RA, Fong Y, Plotkin SA, Follmann D. A Covid-19 milestone attained—a correlate of protection for vaccines. N Engl J Med. 2022;387(24):2203–6.
119. Greaney AJ, Loes AN, Crawford KHD, Starr TN, Malone KD, Chu HY, et al. Comprehensive mapping of mutations in the SARS-CoV-2 receptor-binding domain that affect recognition by polyclonal human plasma antibodies. Cell Host Microbe. 2021;29(3):463–76.
120. Yewdell JW. Antigenic drift: understanding COVID-19. Immunity. 2021;54(12):2681–7.
121. Rouzine IM, Rozhnova G. Evolutionary implications of SARS-CoV-2 vaccination for the future design of vaccination strategies. Commun Med. 2023;3(1):86.
122. Greaney AJ, Starr TN, Gilchuk P, Zost SJ, Binshtein E, Loes AN, et al. Complete mapping of mutations to the SARS-CoV-2 spike receptor-binding domain that escape antibody recognition. Cell Host Microbe. 2021;29(1):44–57.
123. Zhou Z, Zhu Y, Chu M. Role of COVID-19 vaccines in SARS-CoV-2 variants. Front Immunol. 2022;13:898192.
124. Peled Y, Afek A, Kreiss Y, Rahav G, Nemet I, Kliker L, et al. Kinetics of cellular and humoral responses to third BNT162B2 COVID-19 vaccine over six months in heart transplant recipients–implications for the omicron variant. J Heart Lung Transplant. 2022;41(10):1417–25.
125. Peled Y, Ram E, Mandelboim M, Lavee J, Sternik L, Segev A, et al. Waning humoral immune response to the BNT162b2 vaccine in heart transplant recipients over 6 months. Am J Transplant. 2022;22(7):1931–2.
126. Chen J, Liu X, Zhang X, et al. Decline in neutralising antibody responses, but sustained T-cell immunity, in COVID-19 patients at 7 months post-infection. Clin Transl Immunology. 2021;10(7):e1319. Published 2021 Jul 26.https://doi.org/10.1002/cti2.1319.
127. Tarke A, Sidney J, Methot N, Yu ED, Zhang Y, Dan JM, et al. Impact of SARS-CoV-2 variants on the total CD4+ and CD8+ T cell reactivity in infected or vaccinated individuals. Cell Rep Med. 2021;2(7).
128. Woldemeskel BA, Garliss CC, Blankson JN. SARS-CoV-2 mRNA vaccines induce broad CD4+ T cell responses that recognize SARS-CoV-2 variants and HCoV-NL63. J Clin Invest. 2021;131(10).
129. Reynolds CJ, Pade C, Gibbons JM, Butler DK, Otter AD, Menacho K, et al. Prior SARS-CoV-2 infection rescues B and T cell responses to variants after first vaccine dose. Science (1979). 2021;372(6549):1418–23.
130. Redd AD, Nardin A, Kared H, Bloch EM, Abel B, Pekosz A, et al. Minimal crossover between mutations associated with Omicron variant of SARS-CoV-2 and CD8+ T-cell epitopes identified in COVID-19 convalescent individuals. mBio. 2022;13(2):e03617–21.
131. Mombelli M, Rettby N, Perreau M, Pascual M, Pantaleo G, Manuel O. Immunogenicity and safety of double versus standard dose of the seasonal influenza vaccine in solid-organ transplant recipients: a randomized controlled trial. Vaccine. 2018;36(41):6163–9.
132. Masetti M, Scuppa MF, Aloisio A, Giovannini L, Borgese L, Manno S, et al. Effect of a fourth dose of mRNA vaccine and of immunosuppression in preventing SARS-CoV-2 breakthrough infections in heart transplant patients. Microorganisms. 2023;11(3):755.
133. Kho MML, Messchendorp AL, Frölke SC, Imhof C, Koomen VJCH, Malahe SRK, et al. Alternative strategies to increase the immunogenicity of COVID-19 vaccines in kidney transplant recipients not responding to two or three doses of an mRNA vaccine (RECOVAC): a randomised clinical trial. Lancet Infect Dis. 2023;23(3):307–19.
134. Kang JM, Lee J, Huh KH, Joo DJ, Lee JG, Kim HR, et al. Matched versus mixed COVID-19 vaccinations in Korean solid organ transplant recipients: an observational study. Transplantation. 2022;106(9):e392-403.
135. Akyol M, Çevik E, Ucku D, Tanrıöver C, Afşar B, Kanbay A, et al. Immunogenicity of SARS-CoV-2 mRNA vaccine in dialysis and kidney transplant patients: a systematic review. Tuberk Toraks. 2021;69(4):547–60.
136. Calleri A, Saracco M, Pittaluga F, Cavallo R, Romagnoli R, Martini S. Seroconversion after coronavirus disease 2019 vaccination in patients awaiting liver transplantation: fact or fancy? Liver Transplant. 2022;28(2):180–7.
137. Peled Y, Ram E, Sternik L, Segev A, Wieder-Finesod A, Mandelboim M, et al. BNT162b2 vaccination before heart transplantation: kinetics of the antibody response. Transplantation. 2022;106(3):e190-1.

# 18 Cardiac Allograft Rejection Surveillance

David H. Chang and Yosef Manla

**Abstract**

Heart transplant rejection has sharply declined with the introduction of effective immunosuppression, including calcineurin inhibitors. Improvement in survival rates has permitted cardiac transplantation to become, arguably, the most durable option for end-stage heart disease. The risk of rejection persists significantly, particularly in the early period following transplantation, and if untreated, is associated with poor clinical outcomes. Therefore, routine surveillance for both acute cellular rejection and antibody-mediated rejection is critical. This chapter will discuss forms of surveillance for cardiac allograft rejection, including standard and emerging diagnostic methods.

**Keywords**

Heart failure · Heart transplantation · Acute cellular rejection · Antibody-mediated rejection · Endomyocardial biopsy · Molecular diagnostics · Cardiac allograft vasculopathy

D. H. Chang (✉) · Y. Manla
Cedars-Sinai Smidt Heart Institute, Los Angeles, CA, USA
e-mail: David.chang2@cshs.org

Y. Manla
e-mail: Yosef.manla@cshs.org

## Clinical Pearls

- Surveillance, diagnosis, and grading of rejection are based on histologic examination of scheduled protocol endomyocardial biopsies which have been reduced in frequency among many heart transplant programs due to decreasing rejection episodes and the availability of non-invasive testing.
- Concordance among pathologists to call biopsy-proven rejection is only 67% so other modalities to aid in the detection of rejection may be considered such as results of cardiac imaging (e.g. echocardiography, cardiac MRI), clinical presentation and blood testing.
- As an adjunct to the interpretation of endomyocaridial biopsies, the use of intragraft mRNA transcripts has emerged to classify a biopsy sample as acute cellular rejection, acute antibody-mediated rejection, injury pattern, or normal tissue, and could inform guiding appropriate treatment.
- Non-invasive methods to detect rejection have been developed, such as solid-phase assays for donor-specific antibodies, gene expression profiling and donor-derived cell-free deoxyribonucleic acid (dd-cfDNA) blood tests. Clinical trials to assess utility (outcomes benefit) for heart transplant patients are underway.



J. Kobashigawa (ed.), *Clinical Guide to Heart Transplantation*, https://doi.org/10.1007/978-3-031-88290-6_18

## Introduction

Heart transplant (HTx) rejection has sharply declined with the introduction of effective immunosuppression, including calcineurin inhibitors. Improvement in survival rates has permitted cardiac transplantation to become, arguably, the most durable option for end-stage heart disease. The risk of rejection persists significant, particularly in the early period following transplantation, leading to routine surveillance for both acute cellular rejection (ACR) and antibody-mediated rejection (AMR). If left untreated, acute rejection is reported to lead to cardiac allograft vasculopathy (CAV) [1], one of the main barriers to long-term survival, making surveillance and diagnosis of acute rejection episodes critical.

## Pathology and Diagnosis of Cardiac Allograft Rejection

### The Endomyocardial Biopsy (EMB)

At this time, the EMB, first described by Caves [2], remains the gold-standard method for detecting rejection following HTx (see Fig. 18.1). Indeed, diagnosis and grading of rejection are based on histologic examination of the biopsy, which may be combined with clinical observations but cannot be made by clinical observations alone.

#### Procedural Technique

EMB is commonly performed by a percutaneous technique using the internal jugular or femoral vein with fluoroscopic guidance, 2-dimensional echocardiography, or both. Since the introduction of more flexible bioptomes, however, such as the Argon Jawz bioptome, the preferred site of access is now the right internal jugular vein for access to the right ventricle. Biopsies should be taken from the interventricular septum. The right ventricular free wall is thin, and right ventricular perforation and pericardial tamponade can occur when sampling the free wall. Right heart catheterization often follows EMB when rejection is clinically suspected as it provides cardiac pressures and cardiac output/index and can guide therapeutic interventions in the setting of acute rejection [1].

#### Procedural Limitations

Due to its invasive nature, the test may provoke anxiety and discomfort for the patient and remains particularly challenging in the pediatric population, often requiring the use of general anesthesia. A major drawback to the EMB is that it samples only a limited area of the endocardium. Inflammatory changes may be sporadic through the myocardium or may predominantly affect the sub-endomyocardium; in these cases, the biopsy may miss the diagnosis. The diagnosis of rejection also relies on the clinical presentation and echocardiographic findings, which may or may not be supported by histology [3, 4]. Furthermore, biopsy utilizes significant resources, including physician time and cardiac catheterization lab time, and is associated with substantial costs.

#### Potential Complications

Although the procedure is considered safe, with a complication rate well below 6% [5], there is a risk of injury. Such reported complications include transient right bundle branch block, tricuspid regurgitation, access site hematoma or vascular injury, transient arrhythmias, and occult pulmonary embolism [5]. More rarely (<1%), right ventricular perforation has been reported [5]. Generally speaking, only those who undergo repeated biopsies are at risk of long-term complications, which may include severe tricuspid regurgitation and coronary artery to right ventricular fistula.

#### Scheduling of EMB

As the transplanted heart is denervated, symptoms resulting from graft rejection may remain silent and may not be recognized until late during the course of a rejection episode. Consequently, surveillance biopsies are traditionally performed at standard intervals from the time of transplantation. There has been a trend

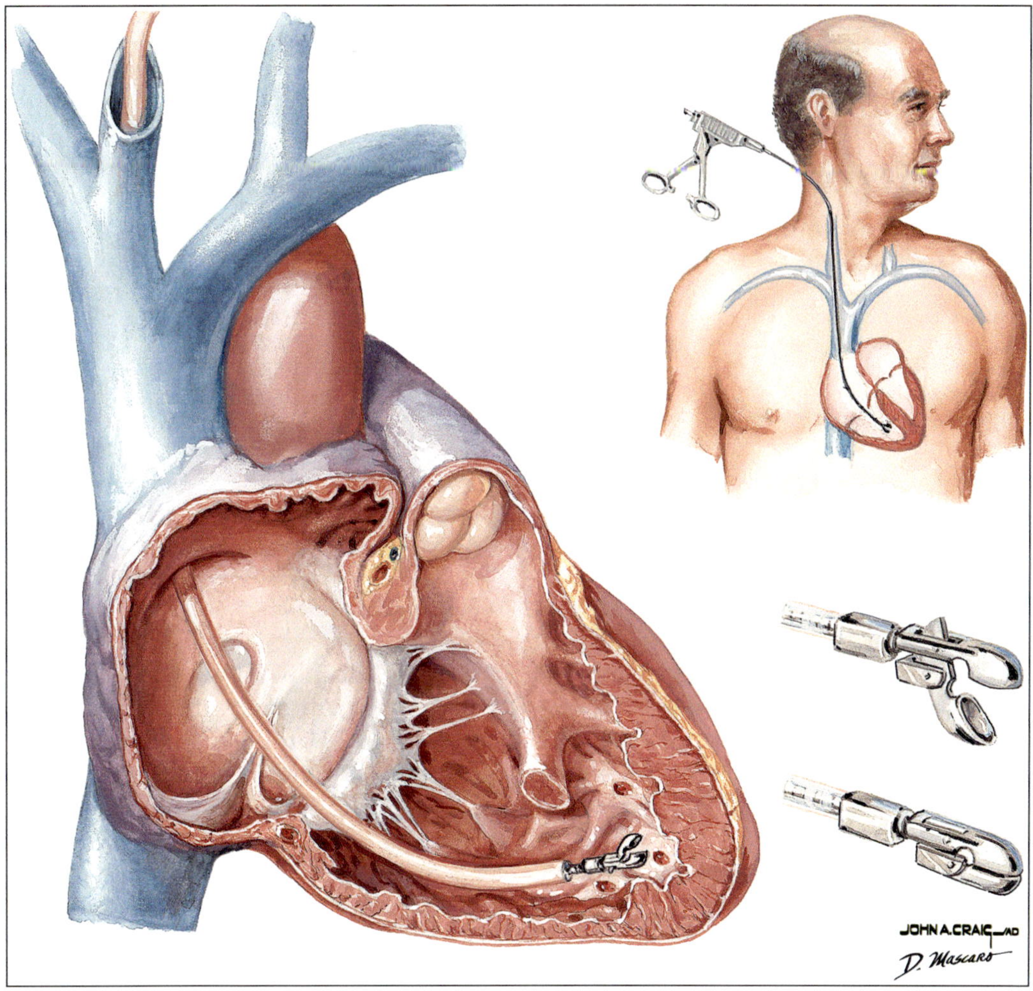

**Fig. 18.1** Overview of the endomyocardial biopsy. Used with permission of Elsevier. All rights reserved

toward a reduction in protocol-based surveillance biopsies in asymptomatic patients, as the chance of moderate to severe ACR is <2% [1]. The development of alternative, non-invasive surveillance methods has further decreased the use of biopsy at many centers. For high-risk patients, a biopsy schedule may consist of performing the procedure weekly during the first month, every two weeks for another month, monthly until six months, and then every two or three months until the end of the first postoperative year. This schedule is intended to reflect the general risk of allograft rejection, which is highest in the first 6 months post-transplant. After the first year, any additional protocol biopsies are likely not to be of clinical significance, given the very low rates of rejection observed in this period [6]. However, biopsies are performed anytime in cases of clinically suspected rejection.

## Histological Features of Allograft Rejection

By histology, acute rejection is observed as an inflammatory response of the host to the transplanted organ. Though T-cell-mediated mechanisms leading to ACR were initially described, there is now consensus that host antibody

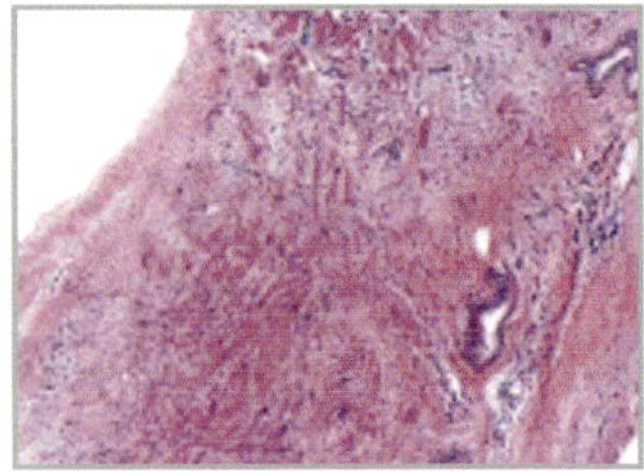
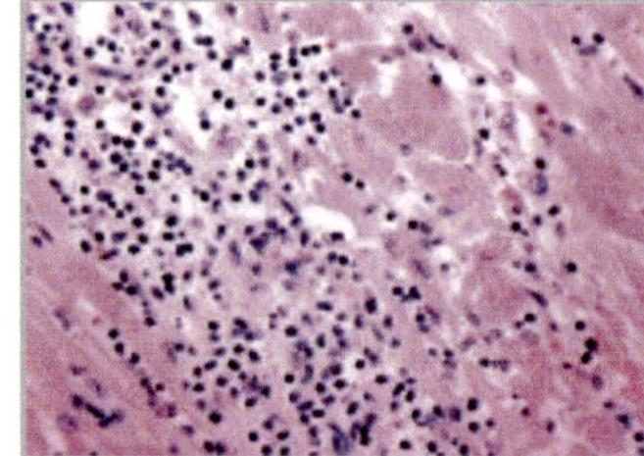
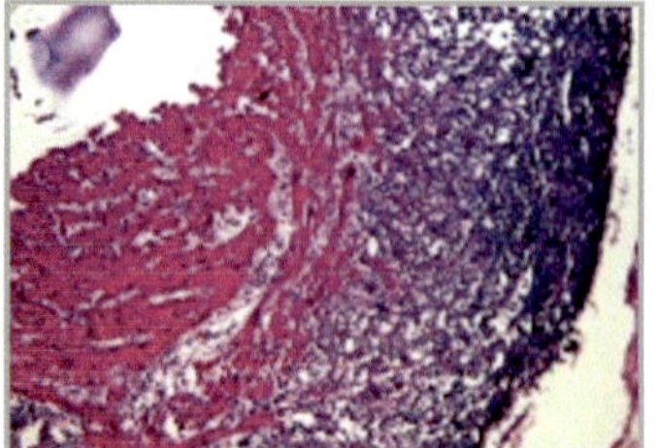



**Fig. 18.2** Common histological artifacts that mimic rejection

responses play an equally important role and may result in AMR. The diagnosis of AMR remains technically more challenging but is now a pathologic definition by consensus opinion [7]. As rejection is a histologic diagnosis, there are cases where the patient may remain asymptomatic, especially with milder forms of rejection.

There are common histological artifacts that may mimic rejection (Fig. 18.2) [8]. It is common for bioptomes to be guided to the same site of previous biopsies, creating scar tissue. In some of these cases, B and T cells may infiltrate the area, leading to an inaccurate diagnosis of rejection. In addition, certain infections, such as cytomegalovirus or Toxoplasma, may show lymphocytic infiltration. Another encountered artificat could be due to the Quilty effect, whereby patients treated with cyclosporine can develop subendothelial infiltrates resembling rejection.

## Intragraft mRNA Transcript Diagnostics to Augment the EMB

An example of the use of intragraft mRNA transcripts is the Molecular Microscope Diagnostic System (MMDx) which is a central biopsy diagnostic system that measures gene expression in intact RNA with high precision (>99%) using genome-wide microarrays. It incorporates ensembles of predefined machine learning-derived algorithms to compare the biopsy to a reference set and can classify samples as consistent with ACR, AMR, injury pattern, or normal tissue and subsequently influence clinical decision-making in guiding appropriate treatment [1, 9, 10]. At the time of obtaining tissue for a standard EMB, an additional endomyocardial tissue sample may be sent for MMDx to help potentially increase the accuracy of surveillance of rejection. This technology is primarily used in North America at this time and is not currently routinely used for diagnostic purposes. It may be utilized more in the future for the diagnosis of AMR, particularly in cases of biopsy negative rejection. Other intragraft mRNA transcript systems such as the use of the NanoString Platform are in development.

## Non-invasive Diagnostic Methods in Cardiac Allograft Rejection

While EMB-derived histology remains the gold standard for rejection diagnosis, the potential complications and disadvantages- in particular, patient discomfort, sampling error, and poor inter-pathologist concordance- are notable. Concordance in the reading of significant ACR may be only 67% among expert pathologists and maybe even less in the reading of AMR [11].

Furthermore, the pathological finding of rejection is a relatively late phenomenon, with diagnosis only made once myocardial damage has already taken place. An ideal test would be non-invasive, utilize less resources and allow early detection for the onset of rejection before any significant myocardial necrosis has occurred. Many non-invasive modalities have been investigated for this purpose, with the aim of minimizing biopsies if possible.

## Clinical Evaluation and Antibody Surveillance

The patient is clinically evaluated for symptoms of rejection at every biopsy appointment, ensuring a regular surveillance schedule. In addition to clinical evaluation and in the light of emergent knowledge of the mechanisms of AMR, many centers now regularly assess post-transplant circulating antibodies, given their increased association with the incidence of AMR and poor subsequent outcomes, including CAV [12]. The ISHLT now recommends that solid-phase assays (including Luminex single antibody) and or cell-based assays to assess for presence of DSA, along with quantification if antibody is present. Quantification may further help stratify risk in patients with circulating antibodies. For low-risk patients, at minimum, the recommended schedule post-transplant includes testing at weak 2, and months 1, 3, 6, and 12, or when rejection is clinically suspected [13]. Testing for DSA testing should also occur at regular intervals for patients at higher risk of rejection.

## Gene Expression Profiling

This innovative technique involves screening for genetic markers to determine a gene expression profile that may be representative of the process of ACR. Microarray technology was used to screen for a number of candidate genes that were expressed in cardiac allograft cellular rejection as determined by routine EMB. The selected genes were then examined in peripheral leukocytes using polymerase chain reaction from blood samples obtained at the time of EMB [14]. An algorithm that factors in the level of expression in each of these genes via blood sample is used to produce a score (0–40) that predicts rejection. In general, a score of ≥34 at 6 months or more post-transplant or ≥30 at 2–6 months post-transplant is considered predictive.

In the multicenter IMAGE (Invasive Monitoring Attenuation through Gene Expression) trial [15], 602 patients between 6 months and 5 years post-transplant were randomized to either routine surveillance EMBs or gene expression profiling, with the study powered to determine non-inferiority between the two groups. The study concluded that a strategy of monitoring for rejection that involved gene expression profiling, as compared with routine biopsies, was not associated with an increased risk of serious adverse outcomes and resulted in the performance of significantly fewer biopsies. A subsequent, 60-patient follow-up study-the EIMAGE (Early Invasive Monitoring Attenuation through Gene Expression) trial-initiated gene expression profiling starting at 2 months post-transplant [16], also demonstrating similar outcomes, with no difference in 12-month death, hemodynamic compromise, or intimal thickening between the biopsy and gene expression groups. The technique was shown to have a high negative predictive value for the diagnosis of ACR but a low positive predictive value. A low score was highly associated with a low risk of rejection, demonstrating that the test may be useful in identifying low-risk patients who may safely avoid the need for surveillance biopsy. However, both these studies demonstrated a selection bias towards stable, low-risk patients, with most of those in the IMAGE trial greater than 1-year post-transplant. Indeed, many centers typically do not perform routine surveillance EMB after the first year in such patients, as the risk of allograft rejection is very low. However, gene expression profiling is now used at many centers in low-risk patients in lieu of biopsy, starting at 2 months post-transplant. Thus, while there is evidence that gene expression profiling can be used in low-risk patients starting at 2-months post-transplant while using biopsy only sparingly, the test is only validated with regard to ACR and is not applicable for the monitoring of AMR, which can occur in up to 15% of patients. Thus, in high-risk sensitized populations, gene expression profiling alone is not considered a viable strategy. Nevertheless, to date, it remains the only non-invasive test for the detection of cardiac allograft cellular rejection that has reached routine clinical use and is approved by the Federal Drug Administration in the United States.

## Donor-Derived Cell-Free DNA

An additional serum test that can aid in the non-invasive surveillance of ACR and AMR is donor-derived cell-free DNA (dd-cfDNA) [1]. These are small fragments of donor DNA that can be detected in the HTx recipient's blood. During acute rejection with cell apoptosis, necrosis, and graft injury, increased levels of dd-cfDNA are released into the bloodstream. Through shotgun whole-genome sequencing, using single nucleotide polymorphisms (SNPs), there can be differentiation between donor and recipient DNA [17]. One multicenter study of dd-cfDNA as compared to EMB was completed in 171 patients post-HTx, followed out to a median of 17 months [18]. dd-cfDNA fell to basal levels 28 days post-HTx. An increase of dd-cfDNA appeared 0.5–3.2 months prior to an episode of acute ACR and AMR, respectively. After that time, with the use of a $\geq 0.25\%$ ratio of dd-cfDNA, the negative predictive value was 99% and would have avoided 81% of surveillance biopsies. In this study, the area under the receiver operator curve for acute rejection was 0.92. dd-cfDNA levels were 5-fold higher in AMR compared to ACR. Another single-center study of dd-cfDNA has allowed low-risk patients to convert from a surveillance strategy of EMB to dd-cfDNA [19]. At this time, different centers use different thresholds of dd-cfDNA in surveillance testing to prompt a "safety" EMB. Safety EMBs are done with abnormal gene expression profile testing and/or abnormal dd-cfDNA results. The advent of competing invasive (MMDx) and non-invasive (dd-cfDNA) tests expands the landscape for surveillance of allograft rejection [20]. It remains to be seen what the best combination of tests is and when to appropriately utilize the numerous diagnostic modalities for the surveillance of HTx rejection.

## Electrocardiogram (ECG)

Intramyocardial electrocardiograms and ventricular evoked response monitoring for rejection surveillance are no longer recommended per the most recent ISHLT guidelines [1].

## Echocardiography

While echocardiography remains a vital tool for assessment of graft function in routine management of transplant patients, systolic dysfunction is generally detected relatively late in the course of allograft rejection. Other echocardiographic parameters, such as diastolic function and tissue Doppler imaging, have also been investigated to determine their potential utility in detecting rejection earlier during the course of the disease [21, 22]. Studies have demonstrated low specificity but high negative predictive value, which may allow a significant reduction in the number of biopsies needing to be performed. Echocardiogram alone can be considered for surveillance testing in low-risk patients with difficult vascular access or tricuspid valve replacement. In these instances, use of other non-invasive testing strategies can be considered to augment the findings on echocardiography.

## Cardiac Magnetic Resonance Imaging (CMRI)

CMRI has been investigated and shows promise for the detection of allograft rejection with high sensitivity [23, 24]. In various single-center studies, the separate combinations of myocardial contrast enhancement/edema and right ventricular end-diastolic volume index (RVEDVI)/T2 relaxation time have been found to correlate with biopsy-proven rejection with good accuracy, and high sensitivity and specificity. One study even showed that the combination of RVEDV/T2 relaxation time is more sensitive than biopsy in predicting clinical rejection [25]. Another single-center study used multi-parametric mapping (without the use of gadolinium contrast) in validation and derivation phases that showed CMR-based surveillance starting 4 weeks after HTx was feasible and favorably compared with an EMB-based surveillance protocol [26]. Overall, this technique has the potential to detect early changes that accompany allograft rejection and may be helpful in cases where the biopsy is negative, but much larger studies are needed for validation.

## Biomarkers

Predictably, the traditional biomarkers used in myocardial infarction (troponin) and congestive heart failure (B-type natriuretic peptide and NT-pro BNP) have also been investigated for the purposes of rejection detection post-transplant. Logically, myocardial necrosis may be a consequence of the inflammation accompanying allograft rejection, resulting in the release of ultra-structural proteins, including creatine phosphokinase and cardiac troponin. However, in practice, troponin has been found to be non-specific and only detected in episodes of severe rejection [27]. Similarly, while natriuretic peptides are produced in response to cardiac stress, as is reasonably expected to occur during rejection, the significant variability of BNP levels in the early post-transplant period limits its utility in detecting rejecting patients or identifying those at low risk of rejection, although BNP change over longer periods of time can predict significant rejection [28–30].

## Future Directions

There has been significant development and progress in both invasive and non-invasive tests for surveillance of HTx rejection. Another new (invasive) modality under active research consideration is the NanoString nCounter technology to assess EMB tissue for ACR or AMR [31, 32]. The time is near when low-risk patients after HTxs may have surveillance for allograft rejection, predominantly not including EMB. Recent trials suggest low-risk patients one month after HTx can be followed by a number of equivalent strategies for allograft rejection surveillance, including dd-cfDNA, cMRI, or a combination of non-invasive tests [33]. The EMB will likely remain the gold standard (perhaps augmented by intragraft mRNA transcript assessment) for patients with sufficiently abnormal non-invasive findings to prompt tissue-level assessment for rejection.

## References

1. Velleca A, Shullo MA, Dhital K, Azeka E, Colvin M, DePasquale E, et al. The International Society for Heart and Lung Transplantation (ISHLT) guidelines for the care of heart transplant recipients. J Heart Lung Transplant. 2023;42(5):e1-141.
2. Caves PK, Stinson EB, Graham AF, Billingham ME, Grehl TM, Shumway NE. Percutaneous transvenous endomyocardial biopsy. JAMA. 1973;225(3):288–91.
3. Kirklin JK, Naftel DC, Bourge RC, White-Williams C, Caulfield JB, Tarkka MR, et al. Rejection after cardiac transplantation. A time-related risk factor analysis. Circulation. 1992;86(5 Suppl):II236-41.
4. Kobashigawa JA, Kirklin JK, Naftel DC, Bourge RC, Ventura HO, Mohanty PK, et al. Pretransplantation risk factors for acute rejection after heart transplantation: a multiinstitutional study. The transplant cardiologists research database group. J Heart Lung Transplant. 1993;12(3):355–66.

5. From AM, Maleszewski JJ, Rihal CS. Current status of endomyocardial biopsy. In: Mayo clinic proceedings. Elsevier; 2011. p. 1095–102.
6. Mehra MR, Parameshwar J. Gene expression profiling and cardiac allograft rejection monitoring: is IMAGE just a mirage? J Heart Lung Transplant Elsevier. 2010;29:599–602.
7. Berry GJ, Burke MM, Andersen C, Bruneval P, Fedrigo M, Fishbein MC, et al. The 2013 International Society for Heart and Lung Transplantation Working Formulation for the standardization of nomenclature in the pathologic diagnosis of antibody-mediated rejection in heart transplantation. J Heart Lung Transplant Elsevier. 2013;32:1147–62.
8. Pullen LC. Diagnosing cardiac rejection. Am J Transplant [Internet]. 2017;17(11):2751–2. https://www.sciencedirect.com/science/article/pii/S1600613522251892.
9. Kobashigawa J, Hall S, Shah P, Fine B, Halloran P, Jackson AM, et al. The evolving use of biomarkers in heart transplantation: consensus of an expert panel. Am J Transplant. 2023;23(6):727–35.
10. Alam A, Van Zyl J, McKean S, Abdelrehim A, Patel R, Milligan G, et al. Rejection! Or is it? Correlation among molecular microscope diagnostic system, histopathology and clinical judgement following heart transplantation. Transpl Immunol. 2023;81:101924.
11. Kobashigawa JA. Continuing the pursuit of heart transplant antibody-mediated rejection. J Heart Lung Transplant. 2015;34(9):1134–5.
12. Tambur AR, Pamboukian SV, Costanzo MR, Herrera ND, Dunlap S, Montpetit M, et al. The presence of HLA-directed antibodies after heart transplantation is associated with poor allograft outcome. Transplantation. 2005;80(8):1019–25.
13. Colvin MM, Cook JL, Chang P, Francis G, Hsu DT, Kiernan MS, et al. Antibody-mediated rejection in cardiac transplantation: emerging knowledge in diagnosis and management: a scientific statement from the American Heart Association. Circulation. 2015;131(18):1608–39.
14. Deng MC, Eisen HJ, Mehra MR, Billingham M, Marboe CC, Berry G, et al. Noninvasive discrimination of rejection in cardiac allograft recipients using gene expression profiling. Am J Transplant. 2006;6(1):150–60.
15. Pham MX, Teuteberg JJ, Kfoury AG, Starling RC, Deng MC, Cappola TP, et al. Gene-expression profiling for rejection surveillance after cardiac transplantation. N Engl J Med. 2010;362(20):1890–900.
16. Kobashigawa J, Patel J, Azarbal B, Kittleson M, Chang D, Czer L, et al. Randomized pilot trial of gene expression profiling versus heart biopsy in the first year after heart transplant: early invasive monitoring attenuation through gene expression trial. Circul Heart Fail. 2015;8(3):557–64.
17. Benck L, Sato T, Kobashigawa J. Molecular diagnosis of rejection in heart transplantation. Circul J. 2022;86(7):1061–7.
18. Agbor-Enoh S, Shah P, Tunc I, Hsu S, Russell S, Feller E, et al. Cell-free DNA to detect heart allograft acute rejection. Circulation. 2021;143(12):1184–97.
19. Teszak T, Bödör C, Hegyi L, Levay L, Nagy B, Fintha A, et al. Local laboratory-run donor-derived cell-free DNA assay for rejection surveillance in heart transplantation—first six months of clinical experience. Clin Transplant. 2023;37(9):e15078.
20. Alam A, Van Zyl J, Paul Milligan G, Michelle McKean S, Patel R, Anne HS. Evolving the surveillance and workup of heart transplant rejection: a real-world analysis of the Molecular Microscope Diagnostic System. Am J Transplant. 2022;22(10):2443–50.
21. Behera SK, Trang J, Feeley BT, Levi DS, Alejos JC, Drant S. The use of Doppler tissue imaging to predict cellular and antibody-mediated rejection in pediatric heart transplant recipients. Pediatr Transplant. 2008;12(2):207–14.
22. Dandel M, Hummel M, Müller J, Wellnhofer E, Meyer R, Solowjowa N, et al. Reliability of tissue Doppler wall motion monitoring after heart transplantation for replacement of invasive routine screenings by optimally timed cardiac biopsies and catheterizations. Circulation. 2001;104(suppl_1):1–184.
23. Butler CR, Thompson R, Haykowsky M, Toma M, Paterson I. Cardiovascular magnetic resonance in the diagnosis of acute heart transplant rejection: a review. J Cardiovasc Magn Reson. 2009;11(1):7.
24. Taylor AJ, Vaddadi G, Pfluger H, Butler M, Bergin P, Leet A, et al. Diagnostic performance of multisequential cardiac magnetic resonance imaging in acute cardiac allograft rejection. Eur J Heart Fail. 2010;12(1):45–51.
25. Butler CR, Savu A, Bakal JA, Toma M, Thompson R, Chow K, et al. Correlation of cardiovascular magnetic resonance imaging findings and endomyocardial biopsy results in patients undergoing screening for heart transplant rejection. J Heart Lung Transplant. 2015;34(5):643–50.
26. Anthony C, Imran M, Pouliopoulos J, Emmanuel S, Iliff J, Liu Z, et al. Cardiovascular magnetic resonance for rejection surveillance after cardiac transplantation. Circulation. 2022;145(25):1811–24.
27. Gleissner CA, Klingenberg R, Nottmeyer W, Zipfel S, Sack F, Schnabel PA, et al. Diagnostic efficiency of rejection monitoring after heart transplantation with cardiac troponin T is improved in specific patient subgroups. Clin Transplant. 2003;17(3):284–91.
28. Kittleson MM, Skojec DV, Wittstein IS, Champion HC, Judge DP, Barouch LA, et al. The change in B-type natriuretic peptide levels over time predicts

significant rejection in cardiac transplant recipients. J Heart Lung Transplant. 2009;28(7):704–9.
29. Hammerer-Lercher A, Mair J, Antretter H, Ruttmann E, Poelzl G, Laufer G, et al. B-type natriuretic peptide as a marker of allograft rejection after heart transplantation. J Heart Lung Transplant. 2005;24(9):1444-e5.
30. Avello N, Molina BD, Llorente E, Bernardo MJ, Prieto B, Alvarez FV. N-terminal pro-brain natriuretic peptide as a potential non-invasive marker of cardiac transplantation rejection. Ann Clin Biochem. 2007;44(2):182–8.
31. Shannon CP, Hollander Z, Dai DLY, Chen V, Assadian S, Lam KK, et al. HEARTBiT: a transcriptomic signature for excluding acute cellular rejection in adult heart allograft patients. Can J Cardiol. 2020;36(8):1217–27.
32. Goldberg JF, Truby LK, Agbor-Enoh S, Jackson AM, Defilippi CR, Khush KK, et al. Selection and interpretation of molecular diagnostics in heart transplantation. Circulation. 2023;148(8):679–94.
33. Fang JC, Wever-Pinzon O. Allograft rejection surveillance in heart transplantation: is there a better way? Circul Am Heart Assoc. 2022;145:1825–8.

# 19 Cardiac Allograft Rejection Treatment

David H. Chang and Yosef Manla

**Abstract**

Although the incidence of significant rejection post-heart transplant (HTx) has decreased in time, over 10% of patients continue to have an episode of treated rejection in the first year after an HTx. This chapter provides a comprehensive overview of acute cellular, antibody-mediated, mixed, and biopsy-negative rejection. It also addresses the management of hyperacute rejection and late rejection. The treatment landscape for HTx rejection will continue to evolve and improve and will require further research to reduce the risk of long-term complications and improve clinical outcomes.

**Keywords**

Heart transplant · Asymptomatic rejection · Acute cellular rejection · Recurrent cellular rejection · Hyperacute rejection · Acute antibody-mediated rejection · Mixed rejection · Biopsy negative rejection · Late acute rejection · Outcomes

D. H. Chang (✉) · Y. Manla
Cedars-Sinai Smidt Heart Institute, Los Angeles, CA, USA
e-mail: David.chang2@cshs.org

Y. Manla
e-mail: Yosef.manla@cshs.org

## Clinical Pearls

- Rejection can be asymptomatic or symptomatic in which the patient may present with symptoms of dyspnea, edema, syncope, tachyarrhythmias or dizziness.
- Acute cellular rejection (ACR) is divided into the following grades of severity based on histologic criteria: 0R (no rejection), 1R (mild rejection), 2R (moderate rejection) and 3R (severe rejection). Rejection treatment is usually indicated for biopsy grades 2R, 3R.
- Antibody-mediated rejection (AMR) is divided into the following grades of severity based on immunologic and histopathologic criteria: pAMR 0 (no rejection), pAMR 1 (Histology+, 1h) or pAMR 1 (Immunopathology+, 1i), pAMR 2, and pAMR 3. Rejection treatment is usually indicated for biopsy grades pAMR 2, 3.
- Treatment options for asymptomatic biopsy grade pAMR 2 or greater consist of corticosteroids and maintenance immunosuppression modification; if symptomatic, treatment is empiric and consideration of additional agents such as intravenous immunoglobulin (IVIG), rituximab, bortezomib or plasmapheresis is warranted
- Empiric aggressive treatment is required in the scenario of acute cardiogenic shock due to clinically severe rejection, including corticosteroids, ATG, IVIG, plasmapheresis,



J. Kobashigawa (ed.), *Clinical Guide to Heart Transplantation*, https://doi.org/10.1007/978-3-031-88290-6_19

inotropes, and potential initiation of short-term mechanical circulatory support.

- For recurrent or recalcitrant rejection, photopheresis (for ACR) and tocilizumab or belatacept (for AMR) may be considered.
- Patients with biopsy-negative rejection suggested by clinical signs and symptoms, along with echocardiographic findings of systolic dysfunction (defined as left ventricular ejection fraction < 40%), should be aggressively treated for HTx rejection.

## Introduction

Although the incidence of significant rejection post-heart transplant (HTx) has decreased in time, over 10% of patients continue to have an episode of treated rejection in the first year after a HTx [1]. Most rejection episodes are asymptomatic and diagnosed from the surveillance endomyocardial biopsy. In recent times, non-invasive testing for rejection may suggest rejection which triggers an endomyocardial biopsy to be performed. Treatment is usually administered for ISHLT biopsy grades greater than or equal to 2R (for acute cellular rejection) and pAMR 2 (for antibody-mediated rejection) [2, 3]. Given the possibility of asymptomatic rejection, surveillance remains important, particularly in the first year after an HTx. The most critical time frame and highest risk of rejection encompass the first three months post-HTx. Higher-risk patients may require a period of surveillance and testing over one year to evaluate for rejection. Patients who require treatment for HTx rejection require higher levels of surveillance post-treatment as they are at increased risk of morbidity, including CAV and mortality.

Symptomatic HTx rejection requires more aggressive treatment [4, 5]. When symptomatic, clinical manifestations of HTx rejection can include symptoms of congestion and a low cardiac output state. Congestive symptoms include shortness of breath, dyspnea on exertion, orthopnea, paroxysmal nocturnal dyspnea, nausea, bloating, lower extremity edema, and fluid weight gain. Low cardiac output state can present with cognitive slowing, decreased urine output, hypotension, and pre-syncope/syncope. Additional signs and symptoms experienced with HTx rejection include palpitations, which may reflect supraventricular tachycardia with atrial fibrillation and/or atrial flutter or ventricular ectopy. Patients with clinical signs and symptoms most consistent with HTx rejection should have an urgent evaluation. This evaluation would include endomyocardial biopsy (EMB) if the patient is stable for this procedure. If necessary, empiric treatment for rejection should not be delayed if the clinical suspicion is high [5]. Serum biomarkers, including natriuretic peptides and troponin, may be abnormal in the context of rejection but are not sufficient to confirm the diagnosis. If possible, serum testing for de novo donor specific antibodies (dnDSA) should be sent prior to the initiation of treatment. Results of antibody testing will take time and similarly, should not delay the start of treatment for HTx rejection. Echocardiographic findings demonstrating ventricular systolic dysfunction can be a late finding in HTx rejection; acute systolic dysfunction would support the diagnosis of rejection [5]. Patients with acute systolic dysfunction (without presumed infectious cause) should begin empiric treatment for HTx rejection. Emerging molecular imaging diagnostic modalities, including, but not limited to, the molecular microscope diagnostic system (MMDx) test and cardiac MRI (discussed in Chap. 18), can augment the EMB in the assessment of HTx rejection.

## Acute Cellular Rejection (ACR)

### Definition

ACR, the most common form of rejection post-HTx, is characterized by a predominantly T-cell mediated response with infiltration of macrophages and lymphocytes, which in turn can lead to myocyte necrosis (see Table 19.1, Fig. 19.1). Diagnosis of ACR is classically made by EMB; the first standardized grading scale

**Table 19.1** Revised 2004 International Society of Heart and Lung Transplantation (ISHLT) standardized cardiac biopsy grading for acute cellular rejection

| Rejection grade | Comments |
|---|---|
| Grade 0R | No rejection |
| Grade 1R—mild | Interstitial and/or perivascular infiltrate with up to 1 focus of myocyte damage |
| Grade 2R—moderate | ≥2 foci of infiltrate with associated myocyte damage |
| Grade 3R—severe | Diffuse infiltrate with multifocal myocyte damage ± edema ± hemorrhage ± vasculitis |

Reprinted from The Journal of Heart and Lung Transplantation, 24(11) Susan Stewart, Gayle L. Winters, Michael C. Fishbein, Henry D. Tazelaar, Jon Kobashigawa, Jacki Abrams, Claus B. Andersen, Annalisa Angelini, Gerald J. Berry, Margaret M. Burke, Anthony J. Demetris, Elizabeth Hammond, Silviu Itescu, Charles C. Marboe et al., Revision of the 1990 Working Formulation for the Standardization of Nomenclature in the Diagnosis of Heart Rejection, 1710–1720, Copyright (2005), with permission from Elsevier

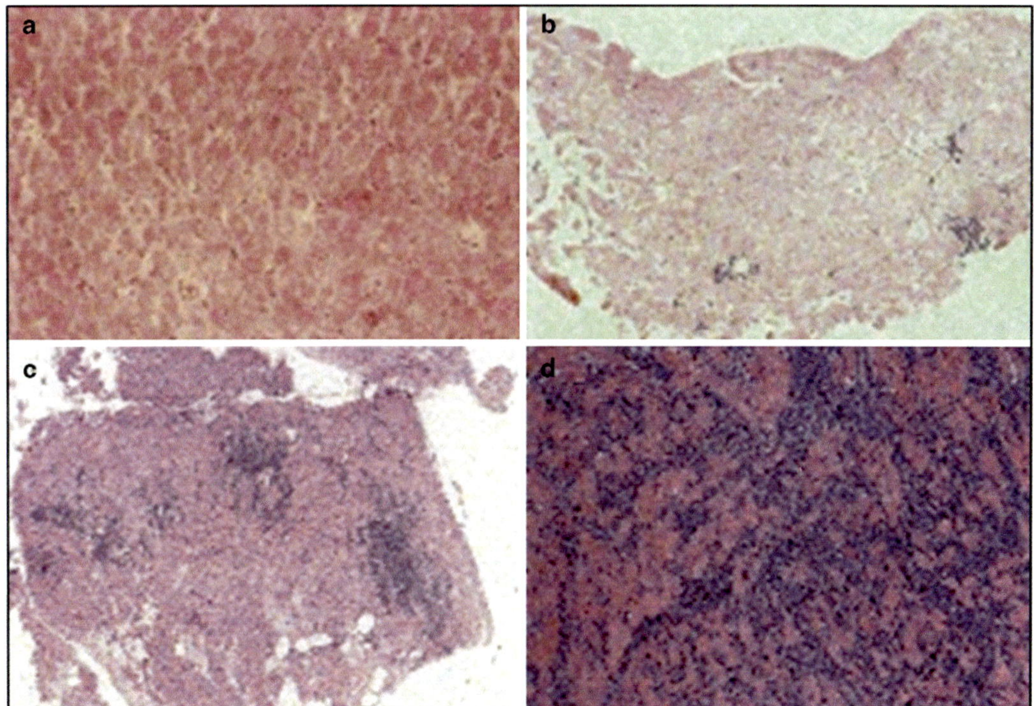


**Fig. 19.1** Panel **a** Grade 0R: Normal endomyocardial biopsy showing no evidence of cellular infiltration (H&E stain). Panel **b** Grade 1R: Low power view of endomyocardial biopsy showing three focal, perivascular infiltrates without myocyte damage (H&E). Panel **c** Grade 2R: Low power view showing three foci of damaging mononuclear cell infiltrate with normal myocardium intervening (H&E). Panel **d**: Grade 3R: Diffuse damaging infiltrates with encroachment of myocytes and disruption of normal architecture (H&E). Reprinted from The Journal of Heart and Lung Transplantation, 24(11) Susan Stewart, Gayle L. Winters, Michael C. Fishbein, Henry D. Tazelaar, Jon Kobashigawa, Jacki Abrams, Claus B. Andersen, Annalisa Angelini, Gerald J. Berry, Margaret M. Burke, Anthony J. Demetris, Elizabeth Hammond, Silviu Itescu, Charles C. Marboe et al., Revision of the 1990 Working Formulation for the Standardization of Nomenclature in the Diagnosis of Heart Rejection, 1710–1720, Copyright (2005), with permission from Elsevier

was proposed by Billingham in 1990 [6], which was later revised in 2004 to accommodate for the reporting of antibody-mediated rejection (AMR) [2]. The most recent ACR grading scale, which classifies rejection into mild (1R), moderate (2R), or severe (3R) grades, has allowed standardization of reporting, although the variability of interpretation and discordance between pathologists remains, particularly for lower grades of rejection [7]. The main benefit of the new grading scale is that it allows improved guidance for appropriate therapy in conjunction with clinical assessment.

## Risk Factors for ACR

A number of risk factors have been identified for ACR: younger age of recipients, female gender (donor and recipients), a higher number of HLA mismatches, black recipients, and induction therapy [9, 10]. The development of acute rejection requiring treatment leads to a higher incidence of CAV and mortality [11].

## Treatment of ACR

Patients may be asymptomatic or symptomatic with ACR. Generally speaking, mild grades of rejection (ISHLT Grade 1R) do not require augmentation of immunosuppressive therapy as the vast majority of these episodes resolve spontaneously, without increased risk of poor subsequent outcomes. Patients with grade 2R and 3R cellular rejection on EMB require treatment for HTx rejection. For asymptomatic grade 2R cellular rejection, an oral Prednisone bolus (50 mg po bid × 3 days) with taper over 2 weeks is commonly administered. Asymptomatic patients with grade 3R cellular rejection should receive high dose intravenous corticosteroids (commonly given as 500 mg IV solumedrol × 3 days with an oral Prednisone taper over 2 weeks).

Symptomatic patients with ACR should be hospitalized for treatment. Overall, due to the small number of HTx recipients treated for rejection, there is no set standard treatment for cellular rejection. Moreover, this scenario makes clinical trial design in this area challenging. Though potentially dynamic, hemodynamics from right heart catheterization can help determine the appropriate hospital setting for treatment of HTx rejection. Critically ill patients with hemodynamic compromise rejection (HCR) have elevated filling pressures and low cardiac output/cardiac index and should be cared for in an intensive care unit (ICU). These patients may need inotropes to maintain adequate cardiac output/cardiac index and may require vasopressors to maintain adequate blood pressure. High dose intravenous (IV) corticosteroids are the first line of treatment for symptomatic ACR. For patients with HCR, the addition of cytolytic therapy with anti-thymocyte globulin (ATG) is recommended. Maintaining or raising the target calcineurin inhibitor (CNI) trough goal should be considered in conjunction with treatment of ACR. Once the acute phase of treatment with IV corticosteroids (±IV cytolytic therapy) is completed, an oral steroid taper should follow. Consideration of the change of anti-metabolite to proliferation signal inhibitor (PSI) can occur in the hospital or at outpatient discharge follow-up, depending on a number of clinical factors. After the initiation of high dose IV corticosteroids, appropriate antibiotic prophylaxis should be prescribed for approximately 3 months. Trimethoprim-sulfamethoxazole (Bactrim) can be prescribed to prevent pneumocystis jiroveci and nocardia infections. Valganciclovir (Valcyte) can be prescribed to prevent viral infections, including cytomegalovirus (CMV). Clotrimazole (Mycelex) can be used to prevent fungal infections, including oral thrush. Repeat surveillance EMB should follow in 2–4 weeks after the diagnosis and initiation of treatment for ACR.

## Recurrent Cellular Rejection

For patients with recurrent (or steroid-resistant) cellular rejection, further immunosuppressive therapy is required. Maintenance immunosuppression should be optimized, with consideration for CNI+PSI in combination and reassessment of target immunosuppressive goals. Assessment of ACR and AMR should occur with follow-up EMB. If resolution or improvement in the grade of cellular rejection is not present on repeat EMB, cytolytic therapy with ATG can be administered. For patients who do not respond to cytolytic therapy, additional modalities of immunomodulation should be considered, such as photopheresis. Photopheresis involves the treatment of blood with a photosensitizing agent and subsequent ultraviolet exposure with specified wavelengths of light to alter the function of T cells. Photopheresis takes place over a six-month period of time. Patients can be treated twice weekly for one month and then twice monthly for the remaining 5 months of this six-month period. Patients treated for recurrent or resistant cellular rejection should have close clinical follow up with more frequent graft assessment by echocardiography.

## Hyperacute Rejection

Although now uncommon, the development of hyperacute rejection was the most feared complication prior to the advent of effective immunosuppressive therapy. It can present in the minutes to hours after the release of cross-clamp at the time of orthotopic HTx. Hyperacute rejection is mediated by preformed antibodies to predominantly HLA antigens, although the phenomenon has also been observed in cases of ABO incompatibility [8]. It is characterized by thrombotic occlusions and hemorrhage of the graft vasculature that begins minutes to hours after the graft is placed. Antigen recognition activates the complement system, along with an influx of neutrophils. Endothelial cells and platelets are induced to shed lipid particles from their membrane that promote coagulation; the resulting inflammation prevents vascularization of the graft, which suffers irreversible damage from ischemia. While this is the most drastic consequence of preformed antibodies to the graft, the presence of donor-specific antibodies (DSA) is also associated with adverse outcomes even after successful engraftment [12]. Hyperacute rejection is likely a rare entity at this time with use of pre-transplant immune compatibility testing including the virtual crossmatch [13, 14]. However, there are limitations to the virtual crossmatch and the assessment of recipient serum, including the prozone effect, so when appropriate, complete assessment of recipient serum, including dilutional testing, should be considered. Though time and resource-intensive, when needed, a complement-dependent cytotoxic prospective crossmatch with donor cells (from spleen or lymph nodes) and recipient serum can be checked to assess for immunologic risk. Highly sensitized patients, including patients who have undertaken desensitization, are potential candidates for use of the prospective crossmatch [15, 16]. Patients with hyperacute rejection may need initiation of mechanical circulatory support (MCS) and immunologic therapies that begin in the operating room after HTx. IV inotropes and vasopressor agents can be used to maintain cardiac contractility and left ventricular ejection with blood flow across the aortic valve, as well as maintain adequate mean arterial pressure. Heparin can be used to aid in vascular flow and prevent thrombotic complications in the heart allograft [17, 18]. Potential immunologic therapies that can be used together include IV corticosteroids, IV calcineurin inhibitor (tacrolimus preferred over cyclosporine) and IV antimetabolite agent (mycophenolate mofetil preferred over azathioprine), plasmapheresis, IV cytolytic therapy, IV immunoglobulins (IVIG), Eculizumab and Rituximab [19]. Of note, antibody therapies should be timed after completion of a plasmapheresis session as plasmapheresis removes antibodies present in the HTx recipient's serum.

## Antibody-Mediated Rejection (AMR)

### Definition

While the role of antibodies in mediating acute myocardial injury has been appreciated since the early days of cardiac transplantation when sub-optimal immunosuppressive regimens and unidentified preformed circulating antibodies led to early post-operative graft failure from hyperacute rejection, only in recent years has there been an acknowledgment of the role of humoral (antibody) responses in causing allograft rejection in the later phases post-transplantation [20].

It is now known that AMR develops when recipient antibody is directed against donor-HLA antigens on the donor heart endothelium. The recipient antibody initiates fixation and activation of the complement cascade, resulting in donor tissue injury. This complement activation results in activation of the innate and adaptive immune responses. Complement and immunoglobulin are deposited within the allograft microvasculature, resulting in an inflammatory process characterized by endothelial cell activation, macrophage infiltration, cytokine upregulation, increased vascular permeability, and microvascular thrombosis [21]. This process ultimately manifests clinically as allograft dysfunction. In 2005, the ISHLT revised the 1990 working formulation for the standardization of HTx rejection to officially recognize AMR as a distinct rejection entity alongside ACR. The new scale established immunohistologic criteria for reporting AMR [2]. It was defined by histopathological changes consisting of capillary endothelial changes, macrophage (in particular CD68-expressing) and neutrophil infiltration, interstitial edema, and linear accumulations of immunoglobulins and complement, especially complement component C4d (see Fig. 19.2). Additional clinical and serological findings of DSA support the diagnosis of AMR [5]. However, in subsequent years, the phenomenon

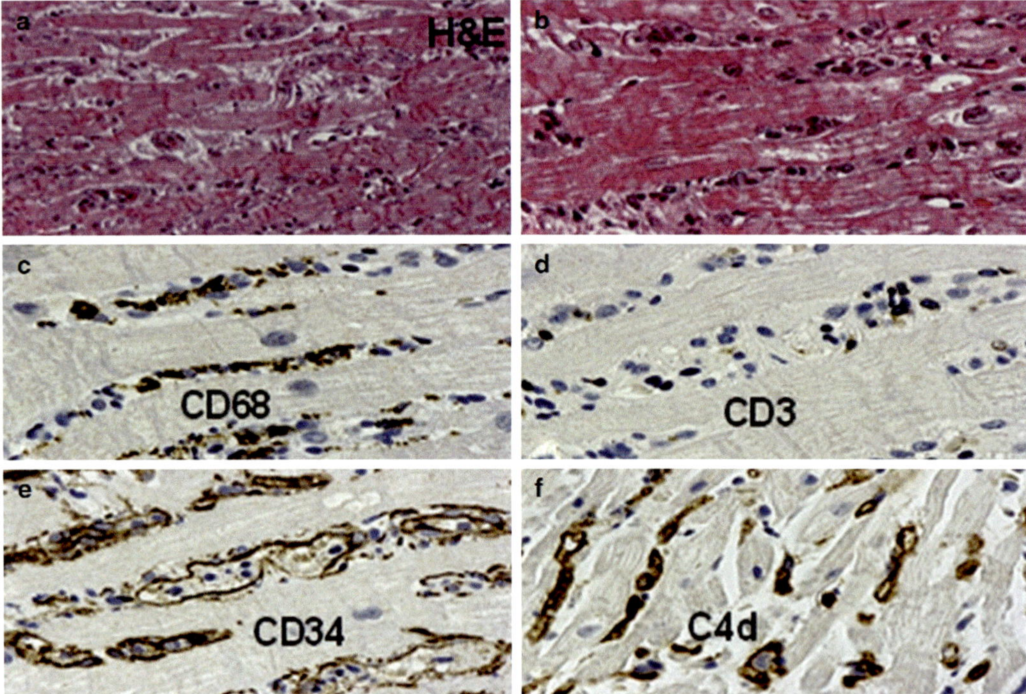


**Fig. 19.2** Histologic findings of AMR are typified by the presence of macrophages (CD68+) within capillaries with a relative paucity of lymphocytes (CD3+). Additionally there is evidence of myocyte degeneration on hematoxylin and eosin (H&E) stain and complement deposition (C4D+). **a**, **b**, **h**, **e** stain, **c**=CD68 (macrophages), **d**=CD3 (T cells), **e**=CD34 (endothelial cells), **f**=C4d (Complement). Reprinted from The Surgeon, 9(3), Jignesh K. Patel, Michelle Kittleson, Jon A. Kobashigawa, Cardiac allograft rejection, 160–167, Copyright (2011), with permission from Elsevier

**Table 19.2** The 2013 ISHLT working formulation for pathology diagnosis of cardiac antibody-mediated rejection

| Grade | Definition | Substrates |
|---|---|---|
| pAMR 0 | Negative for pathologic AMR | Histologic and immunopathologic studies are both negative |
| pAMR 1 (H+) | Histopathologic AMR alone | Histologic findings are present and immunopathologic findings are negative |
| pAMR 1 (I+) | Immunopathologic AMR alone | Histologic findings are negative and immunopathologic findings are positive (CD68+ and/or C4d+) |
| pAMR 2 | Pathologic AMR | Histologic and immunopathologic findings are both present |
| pAMR 3 | Severe pathologic AMR | Interstitial hemorrhage, capillary fragmentation, mixed inflammatory infiltrates, endothelial cell pyknosis, and/or karyorrhexis, and marked edema and immunopathologic findings are present. These cases may be associated with profound hemodynamic dysfunction and poor clinical outcomes |

*Abbreviations* pAMR = pathology Antibody-Mediated Rejection, CD = Cluster of Differentiation. Reprinted from The Journal of Heart and Lung Transplantation, 32(12), Gerald J. Berry, Margaret M. Burke, Claus Andersen, Patrick Bruneval, Marny Fedrigo, Michael C. Fishbein, Martin Goddard, Elizabeth H. Hammond, Ornella Leone, Charles Marboe, Dylan Miller, Desley Neil, Doris Rassl, Monica P. Revelo, Alexandra Rice et al., The 2013 International Society for Heart and Lung Transplantation Working Formulation for the standardization of nomenclature in the pathologic diagnosis of antibody-mediated rejection in heart transplantation, 1147–1162, Copyright (2013), with permission from Elsevier

of asymptomatic AMR associated with worse outcomes was raised [22–24], and the sensitivity and specificity of the immunohistologic features and C4d staining were questioned [25–30]. Furthermore, surveys revealed a variety of approaches to the biopsy specimen investigation and considerable discordance between pathologists in the diagnosis of AMR, with opinion growing that AMR should be classified by severity analogous to ACR [26, 30–32]. Thus, in 2013, following expert discussions and consensus of expert opinion [33], further revisions were made by the ISHLT to the diagnostic criteria for AMR in an attempt to further standardize diagnosis and acknowledge that AMR evolves along a worsening spectrum of pathologic changes similar to ACR [3]. The new system specifies that AMR is divided into 3 degrees of severity (see Table 19.2) and is diagnosed from a combined histologic and immunopathologic review of the EMB. The histopathologic features of AMR include intravascular macrophage accumulation within distended capillaries/venules, enlarged nuclei, and expanded cytoplasmic projections within endothelial cells that may narrow or even occlude the vessel lumen. For more severe cases, there may be signs of hemorrhage, interstitial edema, myocyte degeneration and necrosis, mixed inflammatory infiltrates, and endothelial cell pyknosis/karyorrhexis. The immunopathologic component of AMR comprises applying a panel for various antibodies (including C4d, CD68, and anti-HLA-DR) using immunohistochemistry from paraffin sections or immunofluorescence from frozen graft sections. Based on the combination of these findings, an overall pAMR grade is assigned to the biopsy (Table 19.2).

## Risk Factors for AMR

Risk factors associated with the development of AMR include elevated pre-transplant panel-reactive antibodies (PRAs), positive donor-specific crossmatch, development of dnDSA post-transplant, multiparous female, CMV seropositivity, prior implantation of ventricular assist device, and/or retransplantation [5, 20, 34–38]. There is no established therapeutic treatment regimen for acute AMR. Similarly, there is no set treatment protocol for dnDSA. However, expert consensus opinions and guideline statements have been published to help move this treatment area forward [3, 5]. Ongoing and future research into the treatment of acute AMR and dnDSA is needed to determine optimal therapies and help reduce morbidity and mortality from these processes.

## Treatment of AMR

There is a wide range of clinical presentations for acute AMR with a variable clinical course. A patient may be asymptomatic with AMR. Alternatively, a patient may present with cardiogenic shock with findings similar to delayed hyperacute rejection. Treatment for AMR will proceed based on the patient's clinical presentation and severity of findings on EMB (Table 19.3). If possible, the HTx patient's blood should be sent for the presence, quantity, specificity, and compliment-binding ability of pathologic antibodies prior to initiating treatment for AMR [39]. In cases of high suspicion for AMR, blood can be sent for assessment of non-HLA antibodies, including angiotensin type 1 receptor antibody (AT1R), anti-endothelial cell antibody (AECA), major histocompatibility complex Class I chain-related A antibody (MICA) and other non-HLA antibodies [40]. In general, patients with pAMR 1I with no prior history of treated rejection, normal graft function by echocardiogram, normal hemodynamics by right heart catheterization, and no evidence of dnDSA may continue with close clinical follow-up and surveillance. Patients with pAMR 1 h may be considered for treatment if there is clinical suspicion for rejection. Patients with pAMR 2 or pAMR3 should be treated. Multiple modalities for treatment are possible based on the severity of the illness. Patients should have optimization

**Table 19.3** Treatment options for acute cellular and antibody-mediated rejection

<table>
<tr><th></th><th>Asymptomatic</th><th>Reduced EF</th><th>Heart failure/ shock</th></tr>
<tr><td>Cellular Rejection (ACR grade ≥ 2R)</td><td>• Target higher CNI levels<br>• Oral steroid bolus + taper<br>• MMF → PSI</td><td>• Oral steroid bolus/taper<br>or<br>• IV pulse steroids</td><td rowspan="3">Treat based on clinical presentation; do not await biopsy findings<br>• IV pulse steroids<br>• Cytolytic therapy (ATG)<br>• Plasmapheresis (before ATG dose)<br>• IV immune globulin<br>• Inotropic therapy<br>• IV heparin<br>• IABP or ECMO support</td></tr>
<tr><td>Antibody-Mediated Rejection (pAMR grade ≥ 2) with no/↓ DSA</td><td>• Target higher CNI levels<br>• MMF → PSI</td><td>• IV pulse steroids<br>• Consider IV immune globulin</td></tr>
<tr><td>Antibody-Mediated Rejection (pAMR grade ≥ 2) with ↑DSA</td><td>• Oral steroid bolus + taper<br>• MMF → PSI</td><td>• IV pulse steroids<br>• IV immune globulin<br>• Consider ATG, rituximab, bortezomib</td></tr>
</table>

*Abbreviations* DSA = Donor-specific Antibody, CNI = Calcineurin Inhibitor, MMF = mycophenolate mofetil, PSI = Proliferation Signal Inhibitor, ATG = Anti-thymocyte Globulin, IV = intravenous, IABP = Intra-Aortic Balloon Pump, ECMO = Extra-corporeal Membrane Oxygenation

Immunosuppression Following Heart Transplantation: Prospects and Challenges, David H Chang, Michelle M Kittleson, Jon A Kobashigawa, Immunotherapy, Feb 3, 2014, reprinted by permission of the publisher (Taylor & Francis Ltd, http://www.tandfonline.com).

of maintenance immunosuppression, including the use of CNI. There should be consideration for replacement of antimetabolite with proliferation signal inhibitor. Clinicians should consider higher target trough levels of maintenance immunosuppression. IV (or PO) corticosteroids should be administered depending on severity of AMR, generally at high doses with subsequent corticosteroid taper. Antibody removal can be achieved with plasmapheresis or immune apheresis (immunoadsorption). IVIG can be used to neutralize and decrease the activity of pathologic antibodies. Other immunomodulating treatments can alter the adaptive or innate immune systems. In the adaptive immune system, T cell depletion can be accomplished with cytolytic therapy (ATG), CD-20 expressing B cells can be depleted with Rituximab [41], and plasma cells can be reduced with Bortezomib [42, 43] or Carfilzomib (Table 19.4). For patients with cardiogenic shock, the terminal complement inhibitor Eculizumab can be used to prevent the formation of the membrane attack complex and other downstream complement-mediated effects. Anticoagulation, including heparin, can be used to prevent thrombosis in the macro- and microvascular trees [17, 18]. In addition to strong immunomodulatory therapies, inotropes can be used to help contractility, vasopressors may be required to

**Table 19.4** Specific medications for AMR

| Therapy | Mechanism of action | Immune effects | Major adverse effects |
|---|---|---|---|
| Alemtuzumab | CD52 monoclonal antibody | Depletes circulating lymphocytes, macrophages, and monocytes | Leukopenia, thrombocytopenia, infusion related reactions |
| Bortezomib | Proteasome inhibitor | Depletes plasma cells | Peripheral neuropathy, thrombocytopenia, neutropenia |
| Carfilzomib | Proteasome inhibitor | Depletes plasma cells | AKI, thrombocytopenia, cardiotoxicity |
| Eculizumab | Complement C5 inhibitor | Inhibits formation of terminal complement C5b-9 | Meningococcal infection (vaccination recommended) |
| Intravenous immunoglobulin | Immunomodulatory effects | Neutralize circulating antibody, inhibit complement, inhibit B cells | Infusion-related reactions, hemolysis, interference with antibody assays |
| Plasmapheresis | Extracorporeal plasma antibody filtration | Removes circulating immunoglobulins | Access and line related complications, coagulopathy |
| Rituximab | CD20 monoclonal antibody | Depletes circulating B cells | Infusion-related reactions |

Transplantation grading system for heart transplant biopsy specimens: clarification and commentary. J Heart Lung Transplant. 1998;17(8):754–60.
7. Kim IC, Youn JC, Kobashigawa JA. The past, present and future of heart transplantation. Korean Circul J. 2018;48(7):565–90.
8. Pikul FJ, Bolman RM, Saffitz JE, Chaplin H. Anti-B-mediated rejection of an ABO-incompatible cardiac allograft despite aggressive plasma exchange transfusion. Transplant Proc. 1987;19(6):4601–4.
9. Kobashigawa JA, Kirklin JK, Naftel DC, Bourge RC, Ventura HO, Mohanty PK, et al. Pretransplantation risk factors for acute rejection after heart transplantation: a multiinstitutional study. The transplant cardiologists research database group. J Heart Lung Transplant. 1993;12(3):355–66.
10. Jarcho J, Naftel DC, Shroyer TW, Kirklin JK, Bourge RC, Barr ML, et al. Influence of HLA mismatch on rejection after heart transplantation: a multiinstitutional study. The cardiac transplant research database group. J Heart Lung Transplant. 1994;13(4):583–95.
11. Lund LH, Edwards LB, Kucheryavaya AY, Benden C, Dipchand AI, Goldfarb S, et al. The registry of the International Society for Heart and Lung Transplantation: thirty-second official adult heart transplantation report—2015; focus theme: early graft failure. J Heart Lung Transplant. 2015;34(10):1244–54.
12. Ratkovec RM, Hammond EH, O'Connell JB, Bristow MR, Dewitt CW, Richenbacher WE, et al. Outcome of cardiac transplant recipients with a positive donor-specific crossmatch—preliminary results with plasmapheresis. Transplantation. 1992;54(4):651–5.
13. Kiernan JJ, Ellison CA, Tinckam KJ. Measuring alloantibodies: a matter of quantity and quality. Curr Opin Organ Transplant. 2019;24(1):20–30.
14. Chang D, Kobashigawa J. The use of the calculated panel-reactive antibody and virtual crossmatch in heart transplantation. Curr Opin Organ Transplant. 2012;17(4):423–6.
15. Chang DH, Kobashigawa JA. Desensitization strategies in the patient awaiting heart transplantation. Curr Opin Cardiol. 2017;32(3):301–7.
16. Chang DH, Youn JC, Dilibero D, Patel JK, Kobashigawa JA. Heart transplant immunosuppression strategies at cedars-Sinai medical center. Int J Heart Fail. 2021;3(1):15.
17. Arbustini E, Roberts WC. Morphological observations in the epicardial coronary arteries and their surroundings late after cardiac transplantation (allograft vascular disease). Am J Cardiol. 1996;78(7):814–20.
18. Fishbein MC, Kobashigawa J. Biopsy-negative cardiac transplant rejection: etiology, diagnosis, and therapy. Curr Opin Cardiol. 2004;19(2):166–9.
19. Montgomery RA, Loupy A, Segev DL. Antibody-mediated rejection: new approaches in prevention and management. Am J Transplant. 2018;18:3–17.
20. Michaels PJ, Espejo ML, Kobashigawa J, Alejos JC, Burch C, Takemoto S, et al. Humoral rejection in cardiac transplantation: risk factors, hemodynamic consequences and relationship to transplant coronary artery disease. J Heart Lung Transplant. 2003;22(1):58–69.
21. Colvin MM, Cook JL, Chang P, Francis G, Hsu DT, Kiernan MS, et al. Antibody-mediated rejection in cardiac transplantation: emerging knowledge in diagnosis and management: a scientific statement from the American Heart Association. Circulation. 2015;131(18):1608–39.
22. Kfoury AG, Hammond MEH, Snow GL, Stehlik J, Reid BB, Long JW, et al. Early screening for antibody-mediated rejection in heart transplant recipients. J Heart Lung Transplant. 2007;26(12):1264–9.
23. Wu GW, Kobashigawa JA, Fishbein MC, Patel JK, Kittleson MM, Reed EF, et al. Asymptomatic antibody-mediated rejection after heart transplantation predicts poor outcomes. J Heart Lung Transplant. 2009;28(5):417–22.
24. Kfoury AG, Hammond MEH, Snow GL, Drakos SG, Stehlik J, Fisher PW, et al. Cardiovascular mortality among heart transplant recipients with asymptomatic antibody-mediated or stable mixed cellular and antibody-mediated rejection. J Heart Lung Transplant. 2009;28(8):781–4.
25. Hammond MEH, Stehlik J, Snow G, Renlund DG, Seaman J, Dabbas B, et al. Utility of histologic parameters in screening for antibody-mediated rejection of the cardiac allograft: a study of 3,170 biopsies. J Heart Lung Transplant. 2005;24(12):2015–21.
26. Angelini A, Andersen CB, Bartoloni G, Black F, Bishop P, Doran H, et al. A web-based pilot study of inter-pathologist reproducibility using the ISHLT 2004 working formulation for biopsy diagnosis of cardiac allograft rejection: the European experience. J Heart Lung Transplant. 2011;30(11):1214–20.
27. Gupta S, Mitchell JD, Lavingia B, Ewing GE, Feliciano MN, Kaiser PA, et al. Utility of routine immunofluorescence staining for C4d in cardiac transplant recipients. J Heart Lung Transplant. 2009;28(8):776–80.
28. Smith RN, Brousaides N, Grazette L, Saidman S, Semigran M, Disalvo T, et al. C4d deposition in cardiac allografts correlates with alloantibody. J Heart Lung Transplant. 2005;24(9):1202–10.
29. Rodriguez ER, Skojec DV, Tan CD, Zachary AA, Kasper EK, Conte JV, et al. Antibody-mediated rejection in human cardiac allografts: Evaluation of immunoglobulins and complement activation products C4d and C3d as markers. Am J Transplant. 2005;5(11):2778–85.
30. Tan CD, Sokos GG, Pidwell DJ, Smedira NG, Gonzalez-Stawinski GV, Taylor DO, et al. Correlation of donor-specific antibodies, complement and its regulators with graft dysfunction in cardiac antibody-mediated rejection. Am J Transplant. 2009;9(9):2075–84.

31. Tan CD, Rodriguez ER. Diagnosis of antibody-mediated rejection in cardiac transplantation: a call for standardization. Curr Opin Organ Transplant. 2010;15(6):769–73.
32. Kfoury AG, Hammond MEH. Controversies in defining cardiac antibody-mediated rejection: need for updated criteria. J Heart Lung Transplant. 2010;29(4):389–94.
33. Kobashigawa J, Crespo-Leiro MG, Ensminger SM, Reichenspurner H, Angelini A, Berry G, et al. Report from a consensus conference on antibody-mediated rejection in heart transplantation. J Heart Lung Transplant. 2011;30(3):252–69.
34. Reed EF, Demetris AJ, Hammond E, Itescu S, Kobashigawa JA, Reinsmoen NL, et al. Acute antibody-mediated rejection of cardiac transplants. J Heart Lung Transplant. 2006;25(2):153–9.
35. Hammond EH, Wittwer CT, Jay G, Knape WA, Yowell RL, Menlove RL, et al. Relationship of OKT3 sensitization and vascular rejection in cardiac transplant patients receiving OKT3 rejection prophylaxis. Transplantation. 1990;50(5):776–82.
36. Leech SH, Rubin S, Eisen HJ, Mather PJ, Goldman BI, McClurken JB, et al. Cardiac transplantation across a positive prospective lymphocyte cross-match in sensitized recipients. Clin Transplant. 2003;17:17–26.
37. Toyoda M, Petrosian A, Jordan SC. Immunological characterization of anti-endothelial cell antibodies induced by cytomegalovirus infection1. Transplantation. 1999;68(9):1311–8.
38. Hodges AM, Lyster H, McDermott A, Rice AJ, Smith JD, Rose ML, et al. Late antibody-mediated rejection after heart transplantation following the development of de novo donor-specific human leukocyte antigen antibody. Transplantation. 2012;93(6):650–6.
39. Zeevi A, Lunz J, Feingold B, Shullo M, Bermudez C, Teuteberg J, et al. Persistent strong anti-HLA antibody at high titer is complement binding and associated with increased risk of antibody-mediated rejection in heart transplant recipients. J Heart Lung Transplant. 2013;32(1):98–105.
40. Reinsmoen NL, Lai CH, Mirocha J, Cao K, Ong G, Naim M, et al. Increased negative impact of donor HLA-specific together with non-HLA–specific antibodies on graft outcome. Transplantation. 2014;97(5):595–601.
41. Waiser J, Budde K, Schütz M, Liefeldt L, Rudolph B, Schönemann C, et al. Comparison between bortezomib and rituximab in the treatment of antibody-mediated renal allograft rejection. Nephrol Dial Transplant. 2012;27(3):1246–51.
42. Morrow WR, Frazier EA, Mahle WT, Harville TO, Pye SE, Knecht KR, et al. Rapid reduction in donor-specific anti-human leukocyte antigen antibodies and reversal of antibody-mediated rejection with bortezomib in pediatric heart transplant patients. Transplantation. 2012;93(3):319–24.
43. Patel J, Everly M, Chang D, Kittleson M, Reed E, Kobashigawa J. Reduction of alloantibodies via proteosome inhibition in cardiac transplantation. J Heart Lung Transplant. 2011;30(12):1320–6.
44. Coutance G, Ouldamar S, Rouvier P, Saheb S, Suberbielle C, Bréchot N, et al. Late antibody-mediated rejection after heart transplantation: mortality, graft function, and fulminant cardiac allograft vasculopathy. J Heart Lung Transplant. 2015;34(8):1050–7.
45. Patel JK, Kittleson M, Kobashigawa JA. Cardiac allograft rejection. The Surgeon. 2011;9(3):160–7.
46. Loupy A, Toquet C, Rouvier P, Beuscart T, Bories MC, Varnous S, et al. Late failing heart allografts: pathology of cardiac allograft vasculopathy and association with antibody-mediated rejection. Am J Transplant. 2016;16(1):111–20.
47. Kittleson MM, Patel JK, Moriguchi JD, Kawano M, Davis S, Hage A, et al. Heart transplant recipients supported with extracorporeal membrane oxygenation: outcomes from a single-center experience. J Heart Lung Transplant. 2011;30(11):1250–6.
48. Anthony C, Imran M, Pouliopoulos J, Emmanuel S, Iliff J, Liu Z, et al. Cardiovascular magnetic resonance for rejection surveillance after cardiac transplantation. Circulation. 2022;145(25):1811–24.
49. Kewcharoen J, Kim J, Cummings MB, Leitner KB, Suzuki EMB, Banerjee D, et al. Initiation of noninvasive surveillance for allograft rejection in heart transplant patients> 1 year after transplant. Clin Transplant. 2022;36(3):e14548.
50. Xie Y, Dilibero D, Chang DH. Review of major drug-drug interactions in thoracic transplantation. Curr Transplant Rep. 2018;5:220–30.
51. Foster BJ, Dahhou M, Zhang X, Dharnidharka V, Ng V, Conway J. High risk of graft failure in emerging adult heart transplant recipients. Am J Transplant. 2015;15(12):3185–93.
52. Tumin D, McConnell PI, Galantowicz M, Tobias JD, Hayes D Jr. Reported nonadherence to immunosuppressive medication in young adults after heart transplantation: a retrospective analysis of a national registry. Transplantation. 2017;101(2):421–9.
53. McGovern E, Hosking MCK, Balbacid E, Voss C, Berger F, Schubert S, et al. Optical coherence tomography for the early detection of coronary vascular changes in children and adolescents after cardiac transplantation: findings from the international pediatric OCT registry. JACC Cardiovasc Imaging. 2019;12(12):2492–501.
54. Hammond MEH, Kfoury AG. Antibody-mediated rejection in the cardiac allograft: diagnosis, treatment and future considerations. Curr Opin Cardiol. 2017;32(3):326–35.
55. Pober JS, Chih S, Kobashigawa J, Madsen JC, Tellides G. Cardiac allograft vasculopathy: current review and future research directions. Cardiovasc Res. 2021;117(13):2624–38.
56. Vincenti F, Charpentier B, Vanrenterghem Y, Rostaing L, Bresnahan B, Darji P, et al. A phase

III study of belatacept-based immunosuppression regimens versus cyclosporine in renal transplant recipients (BENEFIT study). Am J Transplant. 2010;10(3):535–46.
57. Vincenti F, Rostaing L, Grinyo J, Rice K, Steinberg S, Gaite L, et al. Belatacept and long-term outcomes in kidney transplantation. N Engl J Med. 2016;374(4):333–43.
58. Miller CL, Madsen JC. IL-6 directed therapy in transplantation. Curr Transplant Rep. 2021;8(3):191–204.
59. Van den Bosch TPP, Kannegieter NM, Hesselink DA, Baan CC. Targeting the monocyte–macrophage lineage in solid organ transplantation. Front Immunol. 2017;8:243275.
60. Vo AA, Choi J, Kim I, Louie S, Cisneros K, Kahwaji J, et al. A phase I/II trial of the interleukin-6 receptor–specific humanized monoclonal (tocilizumab)+ intravenous immunoglobulin in difficult to desensitize patients. Transplantation. 2015;99(11):2356–63.
61. Choi J, Aubert O, Vo A, Loupy A, Haas M, Puliyanda D, et al. Assessment of tocilizumab (anti–interleukin-6 receptor monoclonal) as a potential treatment for chronic antibody-mediated rejection and transplant glomerulopathy in HLA-sensitized renal allograft recipients. Am J Transplant. 2017;17(9):2381–9.

# Part IV
# Long-Term Management of Heart Transplant Recipients

# 20 Medical Adherence and Outcomes After Heart Transplant

Andriana P. Nikolova

**Abstract**

Recent innovations in transplantation, such as tailored immunosuppressive regimens, thorough preoperative psychosocial evaluations, and the emergence of non-invasive graft monitoring strategies through novel molecular technologies, have led to increased longevity and quality of life of the recipients. However, heart transplant (HTx) recipients face numerous challenges in the post-operative setting. In particular, patients are expected to adhere to a complex multi-drug medication regimen, including maintenance immunosuppression to prevent rejection, as well as prophylactic medications for infectious, coronary vasculopathy, and general health protection. In this chapter, we discuss adherence with medical and lifestyle habits post-HTx, its association with outcomes, and outline current interventional strategies to improve adherence in HTx recipients.

**Keywords**

Calcineurin inhibition · Anti-metabolite · Corticosteroid · Prednisone wean · Proliferation signal inhibitor · Precision medicine · Co-stimulation blockade

## Clinical Pearls

- Medication adherence rate in heart transplant patients is reported between 50 and 80%.
- Non-adherence has been associated with rejection, cardiac allograft vasculopathy, and graft loss.
- Socio-demographic, behavioral, medication-obtaining support, mental/emotional well-being, and health/transplant-related factors are among the factors associated with medication adherence in heart transplant patients.
- Impediments to medical adherence include the intensity of the surveillance schedule encompassing medical appointments and invasive procedures (biopsies and angiograms), which pose a significant burden on heart transplant recipients and their caregivers.
- Interventional strategies (electronic monitoring feedback, pharmacist-led interventions,

A. P. Nikolova (✉)
Cedars-Sinai Smidt Heart Institute, Los Angeles, CA, USA
e-mail: andriana.nikolova@csmc.edu



J. Kobashigawa (ed.), *Clinical Guide to Heart Transplantation*, https://doi.org/10.1007/978-3-031-88290-6_20

and cognitive education) have shown to be modestly associated with improved adherence metrics.

- Digital visits are feasible in heart transplant patients. However, technological infrastructure, reimbursement, and limited patient digital literacy, can hinder the adoption of remote care.

## Introduction

Recent innovations in transplantation, such as tailored immunosuppressive regimens, thorough preoperative psychosocial evaluations, and the emergence of non-invasive graft monitoring strategies through novel molecular technologies, have led to increased longevity and quality of life of the recipients [1]. Despite these advances, however, heart transplant (HTx) recipients face numerous challenges in the postoperative setting. In particular, the intensity of the surveillance schedule encompassing medical appointments and invasive procedures, such as endomyocardial biopsies and angiograms, poses a significant burden on the recipient and their support system of caregivers. Additionally, the patients are expected to adhere to a complex multi-drug medication regimen including maintenance immunosuppression as well as prophylactic medications for infectious, coronary vasculopathy and general health protection. For certain immunosuppressive medications with twice daily dosing, the recipient needs to be cognizant of the timing of the medication intake to prevent low trough blood levels that can be associated with increased rejection risk. Each component of the care of the transplant recipients is associated with costs, issues with access to medical care and transportation as well as lost productivity for the patients themselves as well as their caregivers due to the need for medical leave from work to attend appointments or during periods of hospitalizations.

## Metrics of Compliance and Associated Challenges

Findings from several studies have indicated that immunosuppressant non-adherence is a pervasive problem among solid organ recipients [2]. Non-adherence can be either deliberate or unintentional and include such events as not taking the medication as often as required, not in the exact dose and/or at the correct times. However, non-adherence surveillance metrics for HTx recipients are not well defined, and there is an evolving need to refine and standardize these tools. Proposed methods in the literature have included measuring blood immunosuppression levels, electronic pill bottle monitoring, or, most commonly, a variety of validated self-report questionnaires, each associated with shortcomings and advantages [3]. Self-reports are practical and inexpensive tools for adherence assessment but are highly susceptible to errors, such as memory bias. Electronic monitoring of medication refills can be labor intensive but lends a more objective lens onto patterns of adherence behavior. Given its cost, it is less frequently applied in this setting. Variability in blood trough levels of relevant immunosuppressive medications is also frequently applied as an adherence measure, given their proven association with rejection and mortality in HTx recipients [3]. To increase sensitivity, some studies also use a combination of measurement methods to assess non-adherence, which mostly results in detecting very high non-adherence rates.

A further complicating factor in this area of research is the uncertainty surrounding what rate of adherence constitutes an acceptable threshold. Currently, there is no clear target value identified, and as such, there is a wide variability in the cut-off for non-adherence used in studies on solid-organ transplant recipients, ranging from $\geq$80% up to <98% [4]. The stringier cut-off limits stem from the established correlation between even subclinical noncompliance to immunosuppression and increased incidence of late acute rejections, as reported by De Geest et al. [5].

## Adherence and Heart Transplant Outcomes

Depending on the definition of adherence and the metrics employed, studies have provided wide ranges of adherence estimates in organ transplant recipients. A recent systematic review on the topic in HTx recipients provides an overview of this heterogeneity in reporting [4]. The authors demonstrate that adherence was reported to be 25% in 1 study, between 25 and 40% in 5 studies, and the majority of studies (9 of them) noted an adherence rate between 50 and 80% [4]. Non-adherence is widely recognized to impact various post-transplant outcomes. A study by De Geest et al. stratified patients into different "compliance" groups based on several compliance-related variables into "excellent compilers" (84%), "minor subclinical noncompliers" (7%), and "moderate subclinical noncompliers" (9%), which showed a 1.19, 14.28, and 22.22% incidence of late acute rejections, respectively [5]. Dobbels et al. found that non-adherence was significantly associated with the development of cardiac allograft vasculopathy (CAV) [3]. Farmer et al. showed a significant association between both moderate and high adherence and improved mortality rates at 5–10 years [6]. Similarly, a retrospective study using claims data from a single, large national pharmacy chain (claims data from 2013 to 2016) and post-transplant follow-up data from the OPTN database showed that after adjusting for covariates, the odds of having a surviving graft were almost double for adherent patients than for non-adherent patients (OR:1.94, 95% CI 1.58–2.37; $p<0.001$) [7]. Other notable factors associated with graft survival included having three or fewer post-index prescriptions for chronic conditions (OR: 4.33, 95% CI 3.55–5.27; $p<0.001$) and filling immunosuppressants digitally (OR: 2.25, 95% CI 1.13–4.48, $p<0.001$) [7].

## Factors Associated with Poor Medical Adherence

Various factors are associated with medication adherence rates, and Hussain et al. have broadly and aptly divided them into five categories: sociodemographic, behavioral, medication-obtaining support, mental/emotional well-being, and health/transplant-related factors [4]. In the *socio-demographic category*, factors associated with better adherence include older age and female gender, while longer time since transplant, African ancestry, and lower monthly income are associated with non-adherence [4]. In the *behavioral category*, non-compliance with other behavioral recommendations is a marker for poorer medical compliance [4]. Examples of such are the consumption of soft-boiled unpasteurized eggs and unpasteurized milk as well as being a current/recent smoker. In the *support category*, patients appear to demonstrate better adherence if they fill their medications digitally, have better social support, and improve their health literacy by getting help with reading health-related educational materials [4]. In the *mental/emotional status category*, lower adherence is observed in those with higher self-care disability, poorer psychosocial functioning, higher depression scores, avoidant attachments, and distrust of medications and healthcare systems [4]. Finally, in terms of *health/transplant-related factors*, improved medical compliance correlates with the need for fewer concomitant prescriptions for other chronic conditions [4].

## Compliance with Lifestyle Habits

In addition to medication adherence, lifestyle habits can also adversely affect organ survival [8–10]. Oftentimes, due to time limits, these factors are not adequately reviewed during post-transplant follow-up appointments, and as such, emphasis on their importance is lost. Studies have shown that among solid organ transplant patients, HTx recipients exhibit some of the highest non-adherence rates to physical exercise, with estimated rates of 34–49% [8–11]. Similar trends are reported for non-adherence to dietary recommendations (rates 23–46%) and missed or canceled appointment rates (up to the astronomical 94%) [9]. Alcohol and tobacco use has been reported in approximately 4.9–27.8% and 3.2–9.1% of HTx recipients, respectively [12]. Helmy et al. further revealed that up to 39.9% of HTx recipients did not apply sun protection as recommended to prevent skin cancer [8]. However, there is a paucity of studies on how these various risk categories interact, co-exist, and influence one another.

## Interventional Strategies to Improve Adherence in Heart Transplant Recipients

Multiple interventional strategies have been explored with the goal of improving transplant recipients' adherence. These have included mobile health strategies (mHealth) with electronic monitoring feedback, pharmacist-led interventions, and cognitive education [13]. They have been modestly associated with improved compliance metrics [4]. A small single-center randomized control trial of 137 HTx recipients (mHeart trial) tested an mHealth-based tool vs conventional follow-up to improve patient adherence [14]. Metrics assessed included patients' experience of therapeutic regimens (including the degree of inconvenience related to taking medication, patients' knowledge of their regimen intakes, drug names, drug doses, and drug indications [14]. This small pilot study showed that an mHealth-based strategy significantly improved adherence in HTx recipients [14]. Additionally, the study showed a significant reduction in the number of patients needing to travel to the clinic for follow-up appointments with the clinical pharmacist [14]. Similarly, findings from a systematic review by Marcelino indicated that a psycho-educational intervention program exerted a positive impact on adherence in HTx recipients [15]. Such strategy was tested in a randomized control trial (The MAESTROTx trial), which included 205 heart, liver, and lung transplant recipients who were randomized to a control vs interventional group [16]. The intervention group received staged multicomponent tailored behavioral interventions (visits 2–4) based on social cognitive theory and the transtheoretical model (e.g., electronic monitoring feedback, motivational interviewing) [16]. The control group received usual care and attended visits 1–5 only. The intervention group had a 16% higher dosing adherence post-intervention (95.1 vs. 79.1%; $p<0.001$), resulting in odds of adherence being five times higher [16]. This effect was sustained at the end of follow-up (similar results for timing adherence). The 5-year clinical event-free survival was 82.5 versus 72.5% in the intervention vs control groups ($p=0.18$) [16]. A systematic review focusing on renal, heart, and liver transplant recipients revealed that a combination of interventions may be effective for long-term immunosuppressant adherence of solid organ recipients [17]. A study by Shi et al. reviewed interventions tested by randomized controlled trials to improve adherence in solid organ transplant recipients and found that such tools significantly improved the pooled risk ratios for overall adherence, dosing adherence, and timing adherence compared to controls [13]. Interestingly, these interventions lead to no significant improvement in immunosuppressant blood concentration [13].

The COVID-19 pandemic ushered in the greater utilization of telehealth as healthcare professionals were forced to limit face-to-face in-person visits. The adoption of this technology was specifically important for the HTx recipients who were more vulnerable to higher morbidity and mortality consequences due to CVOID-19 infections. Multiple small single-center studies showed the feasibility of his strategy in the transplant population [18]. Despite increasing telehealth utilization, several factors, such as technological infrastructure, reimbursement, and limited patient digital literacy, can hinder the adoption of remote care. Future studies are needed to determine the impact of this modality on post-HTx outcomes.

## Future Directions

Although preliminary findings from small studies demonstrate promising data on the effectiveness of some interventions to improve patient adherence, further large-scale studies are needed in this realm. While some adherence tools have been associated with good patient satisfaction, others have been shown to suffer from a high attrition rate [4]. Additionally, none of the interventions tested have been shown to improve patient survival or other medical outcomes [4]. Future studies should carefully evaluate the ongoing adherence rate to these novel tools over time.

## References


1. Velleca A, Shullo MA, Dhital K, Azeka E, Colvin M, DePasquale E, et al. The International Society for Heart and Lung Transplantation (ISHLT) guidelines for the care of heart transplant recipients. J Heart Lung Transplant. 2023;42(5):e1-141.
2. De Bleser L, Dobbels F, Berben L, Vanhaecke J, Verleden G, Nevens F, et al. The spectrum of nonadherence with medication in heart, liver, and lung tranplant patients assessed in various ways. Transpl Int. 2011;24(9):882–91.
3. Dobbels F, De Geest S, Van Cleemput J, Droogne W, Vanhaecke J. Effect of late medication noncompliance on outcome after heart transplantation: a 5-year follow-up. J Heart Lung Transplant. 2004;23(11):1245–51.
4. Hussain T, Nassetta K, O'Dwyer LC, Wilcox JE, Badawy SM. Adherence to immunosuppression in adult heart transplant recipients: a systematic review. Transplant Rev. 2021;35(4):100651.
5. De Geest S, Abraham I, Moons P, Vandeputte M, Van Cleemput J, Evers G, et al. Late acute rejection and subclinical noncompliance with cyclosporine therapy in heart transplant recipients. J Heart Lung Transplant. 1998;17(9):854–63.
6. Farmer SA, Grady KL, Wang E, McGee EC Jr, Cotts WG, McCarthy PM. Demographic, psychosocial, and behavioral factors associated with survival after heart transplantation. Ann Thorac Surg. 2013;95(3):876–83.
7. Boghani S, Kirkham H, Witt EA, Hira N, Cherikh WS, Wilk AR, et al. Medication adherence and graft survival among kidney transplant recipients. J Drug Assess. 2019;8(sup1):6.
8. Helmy R, Duerinckx N, De Geest S, Denhaerynck K, Berben L, Russell CL, et al. The international prevalence and variability of nonadherence to the nonpharmacologic treatment regimen after heart transplantation: findings from the cross-sectional BRIGHT study. Clin Transplant. 2018;32(7):e13280.
9. De Geest S, Dobbels F, Martin S, Willems K, Vanhaecke J. Clinical risk associated with appointment noncompliance in heart transplant recipients. Prog Transplant. 2000;10(3):162–8.
10. Duerinckx N, Burkhalter H, Engberg SJ, Kirsch M, Klem ML, Sereika SM, et al. Correlates and outcomes of posttransplant smoking in solid organ transplant recipients: a systematic literature review and meta-analysis. Transplantation. 2016;100(11):2252–63.
11. Brocks Y, Zittermann A, Grisse D, Schmid-Ott G, Stock-Gießendanner S, Schulz U, et al. Adherence of heart transplant recipients to prescribed medication and recommended lifestyle habits: a single-center experience. Prog Transplant. 2017;27(2):160–6.
12. Lieb M, Weyand M, Seidl M, Erim Y. Protocol: prospective single-centre clinical observational study on electronically monitored medication non-adherence, its psychosocial risk factors and lifestyle behaviours after heart transplantation: a study protocol. BMJ Open. 2020;10(10):e038637.
13. Shi YX, Liu CX, Liu F, Zhang HM, Yu MM, Jin YH, et al. Efficacy of adherence-enhancing interventions for immunosuppressive therapy in solid organ transplant recipients: a systematic review and meta-analysis based on randomized controlled trials. Front Pharmacol. 2020;11:578887.
14. Gomis-Pastor M, Mirabet Perez S, Roig Minguell E, Brossa Loidi V, Lopez Lopez L, Ros Abarca S, et al. Mobile health to improve adherence and patient experience in heart transplantation recipients: the mHeart trial. In: Healthcare. MDPI; 2021. p. 463.
15. Marcelino CAG, Díaz LJR, da Cruz DM. The effectiveness of interventions in managing treatment adherence in adult heart transplant patients: a systematic review. JBI Evid Synth. 2015;13(9):279–308.
16. Dobbels F, De Bleser L, Berben L, Kristanto P, Dupont L, Nevens F, et al. Efficacy of a medication adherence enhancing intervention in transplantation: the MAESTRO-Tx trial. J Heart Lung Transplant. 2017;36(5):499–508.
17. De Bleser L, Matteson M, Dobbels F, Russell C, De Geest S. Interventions to improve medication-adherence after transplantation: a systematic review. Transpl Int. 2009;22(8):780–97.
18. Wang CW, Ha N, Duarte M, Sherman CB. Telemedicine implementation in Solid Organ Transplant (SOT) clinics is associated with satisfaction among patients and providers but increased burden on staff. Am J Transplant. 2022;868–9

# Cardiac Allograft Vasculopathy

# 21

Lily Stern, Evan Kransdorf, and Yosef Manla

**Abstract**

Cardiac allograft vasculopathy (CAV) is one of the major complications after heart transplantation (HTx) that contributes to graft failure and significant morbidity and mortality. This chapter explores the epidemiology, pathophysiology, and clinical features, as well as diagnosis, medical and surgical management of CAV. Advancements in post-HTx immunosuppression, imaging technology, and risk stratification techniques will lead to improved quality of life and longevity after transplant.

**Keywords**

Heart failure · Heart transplantation · Chronic rejection · Cardiac allograft vasculopathy · Surveillance · Trajectory score

L. Stern · E. Kransdorf (✉) · Y. Manla
Cedars-Sinai Smidt Heart Institute, Los Angeles, CA, USA
e-mail: Evan.kransdorf@cshs.org

L. Stern
e-mail: Lily.stern@cshs.org

Y. Manla
e-mail: Yosef.manla@cshs.org; Yosef.manla1@gmail.com

## Clinical Pearls

- Cardiac allograft vasculopathy (CAV) is one of the major causes of death limiting the long-term survival after heart transplantation
- CAV is a chronic form of rejection, best characterized as a diffuse immune-mediated pan-arteritis with non-immune factors also contributing to risk.
- CAV often remains asymptomatic due to denervation of the donor heart, which blunts angina pain. Symptomatic CAV may present with dyspnea, left ventricular dysfunction, restrictive physiology, or even sudden cardiac death.
- The gold standard for diagnosis of CAV is the coronary angiogram, with surveillance protocols varying from annually to protocols at specific year marks.
- Intravascular ultrasound (IVUS) during a baseline and 1-year angiogram is performed at some centers. The change in first-year IVUS measurement of maximal intimal thickness (MIT) is a predictor for subsequent angiographic development of CAV and other poor outcomes at 5 years.
- Through the use of artificial intelligence and machine learning, a CAV trajectory score was developed and can be calculated at 1-year post-heart transplant to assist with risk stratification of patients for the development of



J. Kobashigawa (ed.), *Clinical Guide to Heart Transplantation*, https://doi.org/10.1007/978-3-031-88290-6_21

CAV and the need for protocol-scheduled coronary angiograms. In this assessment, donor age, donor male sex, donor tobacco consumption, recipient dyslipidemia, class II anti-HLA DSAs, and acute cellular rejection (> 2R), are independently associated with higher CAV risk trajectories.
- Medical strategies to abrogate CAV include the administration of statins and targeted use of proliferation signal inhibitors (PSIs) such as sirolimus/everolimus.
- Interventional options for CAV include the placement of drug-eluting stents, but these are usually temporary measures; the only definitive solution is re-transplantation.

## Epidemiology

Cardiac allograft vasculopathy (CAV), known as chronic allograft rejection, imposes a significant long-term morbidity and mortality burden on heart transplant (HTx) recipients and is one of the leading causes of death post-transplant [1]. The incidence of CAV increases in a progressive manner over time. Per the latest registry report from the ISHLT [1], for adult HTx recipients, the prevalence of CAV is 7.7% at 1-year post-transplant, 29% at 5 years post-transplant, and 46.8% at 10 years post-transplant. Younger recipient age is associated with an increased risk of CAV, possibly due to more robust immune systems or the lack of CAV screening with angiography in older recipients who have a propensity for renal dysfunction [1]. Older donor age has been associated with the development of CAV [2]. In a 2019 ISHLT registry study, donors over age 49 were noted to have a higher prevalence of traditional cardiac risk factors, and the risk of CAV was higher at 5 and 10-year follow-ups [3]. Additionally, the female sex of either donor or recipient is associated with decreased risk for development of CAV within 5 years post-transplant. The hazard ratio for the development of CAV with the female donor-female recipients is 0.72 when compared to the male donor-male recipients [1].

## Pathophysiology

CAV is generally thought to be a diffuse pan arteritis with concentric, longitudinal intimal thickening of the epicardial coronary arteries [4]. It can involve the coronary microvasculature as well. While CAV is generally a diffuse process, it can manifest in ways similar to native coronary artery disease with focal stenosis. The pathophysiology and molecular basis for CAV include contributions from immune responses to the donor heart including atherosclerotic mechanisms, ischemia–reperfusion injury, and particular infections [5] (Fig. 21.1). Non-immune mechanisms include atherosclerotic mechanisms and traditional risk factors for coronary atherosclerosis, which are frequent after HTx and include hypertension, hyperlipidemia, obesity, renal dysfunction, and glucose intolerance (diabetes). Tissue damage may occur during the process of HTx and include donor physiologic changes due to the processes of brain death, cardiac arrest, heart procurement, and ischemia–reperfusion at the time of heart implantation. Elements of the adaptive and innate immune systems likely contribute to the development of CAV. Human leukocyte antigen (HLA) shedding during heart implantation can lead to indirect allorecognition with internalization and processing of donor-soluble HLA by recipient antigen-presenting cells, leading to T-cell stimulation. Heat shock proteins may be detected by toll-like receptors and promote the maturation of dendritic cells. Complement deposition, namely C3d and C4d deposition, are associated with antibody-mediated rejection and CAV [6]. Over time, alloimmune interactions will lead to T and B cell stimulation, the release of pro-inflammatory cytokines, and a state of vascular inflammation. Endothelial cells that line transplanted coronary arteries are the main point of contact and communication between the recipient blood and the transplanted graft and, thus, maybe the primary antigenic stimulus for the initiation and progression of CAV. Donor-specific antibodies (DSA) can develop in the transplanted graft, particularly after episodes of cellular and/

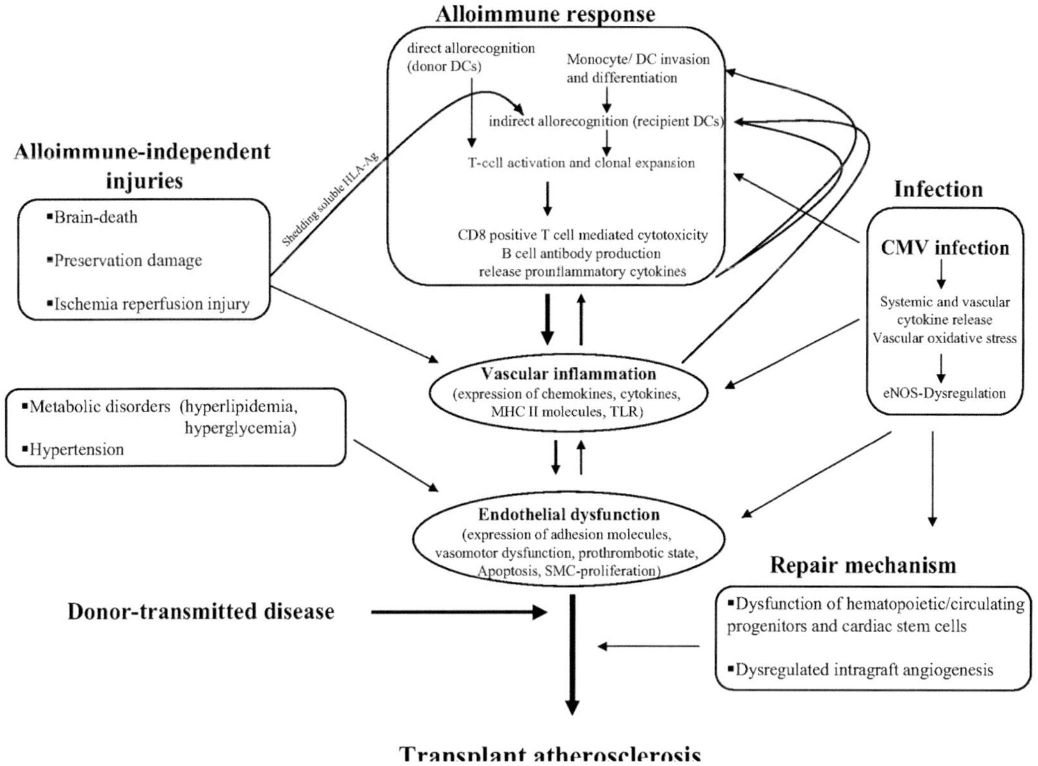

**Fig. 21.1** A diagram demonstrating the collaboration and interaction of alloimmune-dependent and independent factors that influence the pathogenesis of transplant vasculopathy. *Abbreviations* Ag antigen, CD cluster of differentiation, eNOS endothelial nitric oxide synthase, and SMC smooth muscle cell. Reused with permission Daniel Schmauss, Michael Weis, Cardiac Allograft Vasculopathy: Recent Developments, Circulation, 117(16), 2131–214, https://doi.org/10.1161/CIRCULATIONAHA.107.711911; American Heart Association

or antibody-mediated rejection. The presence of DSA, particularly in major histocompatibility complex (MHC) type II antigens, is associated with CAV and poor outcomes after HTx [7–10]. In addition to DSA, non-HLA antibodies, many of which are expressed on endothelial cells, are likely involved in the development of CAV and include anti-angiotensin II type I receptor [11], anti-MHC class I chain-related A [12], MHC class I chain-related B, as well as adhesion and trafficking receptors. In addition, vimentin is also expressed on endothelial cells thus anti-vimentin antibodies have been associated with CAV [13]. Moreover, inflammatory modulators may influence cytokine signaling and the development of CAV [14, 15]. Infections, such as breakthrough cytomegalovirus (CMV) infections despite prophylactic antiviral treatment, may also influence the development of CAV [16, 17].

## Clinical Features

As the process of HTx causes denervation of the transplanted graft, cardiac angina is typically absent, and CAV may present insidiously. Shortness of breath or atypical symptoms may accompany CAV, but CAV may be asymptomatic. CAV may present with left ventricular systolic dysfunction, but even with severe CAV, left ventricular systolic function may be preserved. Significant CAV is often accompanied by restrictive allograft physiology, defined as symptomatic heart failure with either echocardiographic or hemodynamic abnormalities on right heart catheterization. This form of CAV with restrictive cardiac physiology is felt secondary to microvascular disease [18]. Echocardiographic parameters consistent with restrictive allograft physiology in adults include E to A velocity ratio > 2, decreased isovolumic relaxation time < 60 ms, and shortened mitral valve deceleration time < 150 ms. Restrictive hemodynamics on right heart catheterization include right atrial pressure > 12 mmHg, pulmonary capillary wedge pressure > 25 mmHg, and cardiac index < 2 L/minute/square meter. A consensus statement was published in 2011 by the International Society for Heart and Lung Transplant (ISHLT) that established a working formulation of standardized nomenclature for CAV (Table 21.1). By this form of classification, CAV can be divided into non-significant (CAV0), mild (CAV1), moderate (CAV2), and severe (CAV3) disease, which includes significant restrictive cardiac physiology due to microvascular disease [19].

## Diagnosis

### Invasive Assessment of Cardiac Allograft Vasculopathy

Due to the usually silent progression and increased morbidity and mortality associated with CAV, surveillance, and diagnosis of this disease process is critical. The gold standard test for diagnosis of CAV continues to be the conventional coronary angiogram. Interpretation of lumen patency by conventional coronary angiography may give a false sense of security as the lumen of the coronary artery may not be compromised until intimal thickening encroaches and causes focal stenosis (Fig. 21.2). For this reason, many institutions utilize intravascular ultrasound (IVUS) or optical coherence tomography (OCT) in addition to conventional coronary angiography for the assessment of CAV [20, 21]. Although a number of IVUS-based parameters have been analyzed post-transplant, change in maximal intimal thickness (MIT) of a matched cross-sectional area of a coronary

**Table 21.1** The International Society for Heart and Lung Transplantation nomenclature of cardiac allograft vasculopathy

| Grade of CAV | Disease severity | Angiographic findings |
|---|---|---|
| CAV0 | No disease | No detectable angiographic lesion |
| CAV1 | Mild | Angiographic LM <50%, or primary vessel with maximum lesion of <70%, or any branch stenosis <70% (including diffuse narrowing) without allograft dysfunction |
| CAV2 | Intermediate | Angiographic LM <50%; a single primary vessel >70%, or isolated branch stenosis >70% in branches of 2 systems, without allograft dysfunction |
| CAV3 | Severe | Angiographic LM >50%, or ≥2 primary vessels >70% stenosis, or isolated branch stenosis >70% in all 3 systems; or ISHLT CAV1 or CAV2 with allograft dysfunction (defined as LVEF <45%, usually in the presence of regional wall motion abnormalities) or evidence of significant restrictive physiology |

*Abbreviations* CAV: cardiac allograft vasculopathy; ISHLT: International Society of Heart and Lung Transplantation; LM: left main; LVEF: left ventricular ejection fraction

Reprinted from The Journal of Heart and Lung Transplantation, 29(7), Mandeep R. Mehra, Maria G. Crespo-Leiro, Anne Dipchand, Stephan M. Ensminger, Nicola E. Hiemann, Jon Kobashigawa, Joren Madsen, Jayan Parameshwar, Randall C. Starling, Patricia A. Uber, International Society for Heart and Lung Transplantation working formulation of a standardized nomenclature for cardiac allograft vasculopathy—2010, 717–727, Copyright (2010), with permission from Elsevier

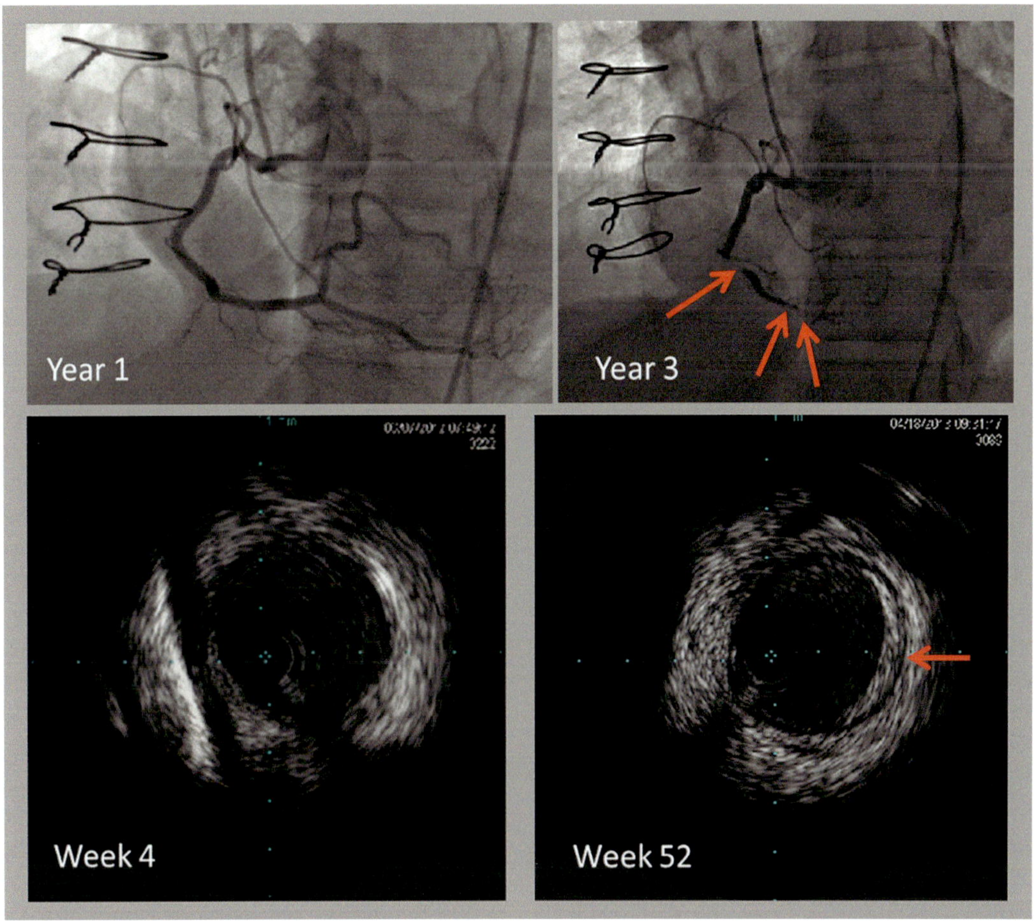

**Fig. 21.2** The top half demonstrates the progression of cardiac allograft vasculopathy as demonstrated by the right coronary artery angiogram at year 3 post-transplant compared to year 1. Note the multiple, diffuse stenoses (red arrows). The bottom half demonstrates the progression of intimal thickness (red arrow) as demonstrated by intravascular ultrasound at 52 weeks (1 year) post-transplant compared to baseline (week 4 post-transplant). There was a difference of greater than 0.5 mm change between baseline and 1 year. Such a finding is highly prognostic for poor long-term outcomes. Reused with permission from Author, Outpatient Management and Long-Term Complications in Heart Transplantation, Clinical guide to heart transplantation, 171–183, 2017, Springer Nature. https://doi.org/10.1007/978-3-319-43773-6_13

artery from baseline (approximately 6 weeks post-transplant) to 1-year post-transplant was a reliable surrogate marker for subsequent mortality, nonfatal major adverse cardiac events (MACE), and development of angiographic CAV through 5 years post HTx. Historically, patients with an MIT increase of 0.5 mm or greater in any matched site of a coronary artery had a significantly higher incidence of death or graft loss, nonfatal MACE, and a higher incidence of new angiographic CAV [22, 23]. A more recent, large single-center retrospective trial demonstrated that a baseline MIT of 0.64 mm at approximately 6 weeks post-transplant, consistent with donor-transmitted coronary artery disease, as well as a change in MIT of at least 0.27 mm within the first year, were independently associated with increased 5-year mortality and development of CAV [24]. This updated MIT threshold has been incorporated into the most recent HTx management guidelines (Class IIa, Level of Evidence B) [25].

A CAV trajectory model was recently developed to risk stratify patients for the development of clinically significant CAV and associated mortality over 10 years from transplant [26]. In an international multicenter study, 1301 HTx recipients were prospectively assessed for the presence of allograft coronary disease and stratified into 4 distinct CAV trajectories based on disease found on angiography with IVUS at baseline at 4–8 weeks and 1 year post HTx: (1) no CAV over time (2) mild and late-onset CAV, (3) early onset and progressive evolution of CAV and (4) early onset with rapid evolution of CAV. Recipient and donor characteristics, including donor age, donor male sex, donor tobacco consumption, recipient dyslipidemia, class II anti-HLA DSAs, and acute cellular rejection (>2R), were found to be independently associated with higher risk trajectories. The trajectory model was initially developed from patients in Europe and then was validated on patients in a large center in the United States. The model found that not only were higher CAV trajectories associated with higher rates of clinically significant CAV over time but also with higher mortality (Fig. 21.3). As such, patients with CAV trajectories 3 or 4 noted at 1-year post-transplant should undergo more intensive annual CAV surveillance. Recently, it was found in a single-center study of 102 patients that using an additive probability of >0.7 to be in CAV trajectory scores 1 and 2 appears safe and predictive to avoid annual angiograms within 5 years post-transplant [27]. Furthermore, the CAV trajectory has the potential to serve as an important surrogate for 10-year clinical outcomes in future trials.

## Non-invasive Assessment of Cardiac Allograft Vasculopathy

Procedures such as conventional coronary angiography and IVUS pose risks that accompany invasive tests. These risks include bleeding, infection, contrast-induced nephropathy, peripheral vascular disease, risk of myocardial infarction, dissection or damage of the coronary artery, stroke, and potential death from the invasive test(s). Due to patient discomfort and the inherent risks of invasive testing, non-invasive tests can be used to assess for CAV. Non-invasive tests for CAV include exercise or pharmacologic-based stress tests, positive emission tomography (PET) testing with myocardial blood flow (MBF) and myocardial flow reserve (MFR), cardiac magnetic resonance (CMR), and coronary computed tomographic angiography (CCTA). Dobutamine stress echocardiography and single photon emission computed tomography (SPECT) are less useful than other non-invasive modalities such PET with MBF/MFR, CMR, and CCTA for CAV surveillance and evaluation due to relatively lower sensitivity with high rates of false negative results [28–32]. The limited performance of SPECT may be due to the diffuse and balanced nature of CAV. Nevertheless, these modalities are still an option for patients who are unable to undergo invasive evaluation or other non-invasive modalities due to cost or imaging limitations from rapid heart rate in a denervated cardiac allograft due to the lack of parasympathetic nervous system tone (Class IIb, Level of Evidence B) [25]. In contrast, PET with MBF and MFR has shown promise for non-invasive surveillance and diagnosis of macro and microvascular CAV [33, 34]. A study evaluating patients who underwent PET

**Fig. 21.3** Overall, 10-year survival probability according to the CAV trajectory. Trajectories 3 and 4 were associated with higher mortality rates (10-year patient survival of 73.43% [95% CI, 65.18–80.02] and 51.89% [95% CI, 38.76–63.51], respectively) in comparison with trajectories 1 and 2 that were characterized by 10-year patient survival of 80.01 (95% CI, 76.38–84.82) and 83.49% (95% CI, 71.34–90.80), respectively (P<0.001). Reprinted with permission from Alexandre Loupy, Guillaume Coutance, Guillaume Bonnet, Jan Van Keer, et al., Identification and Characterization of Trajectories of Cardiac Allograft Vasculopathy After Heart Transplantation: A Population-Based Study, Circulation, 141(24), 1954–1967, and https://doi.org/10.1161/CIRCULATIONAHA.119.044924; American Heart Association

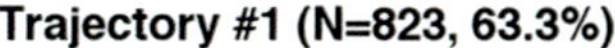


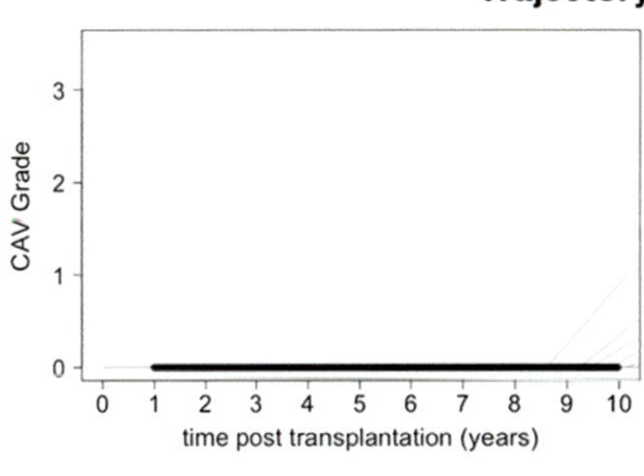


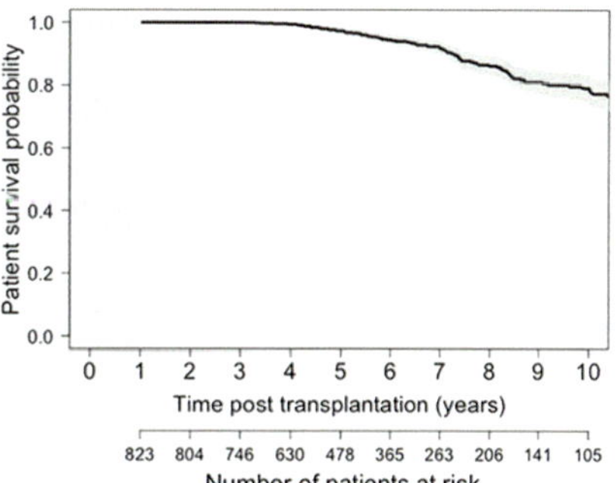


Trajectory #2 (N=79, 6.1%)

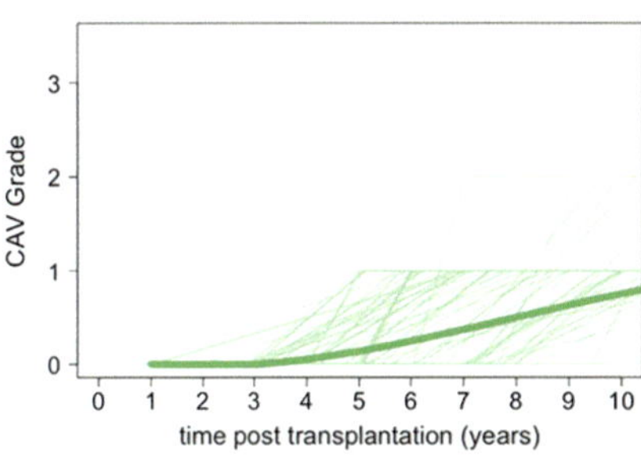


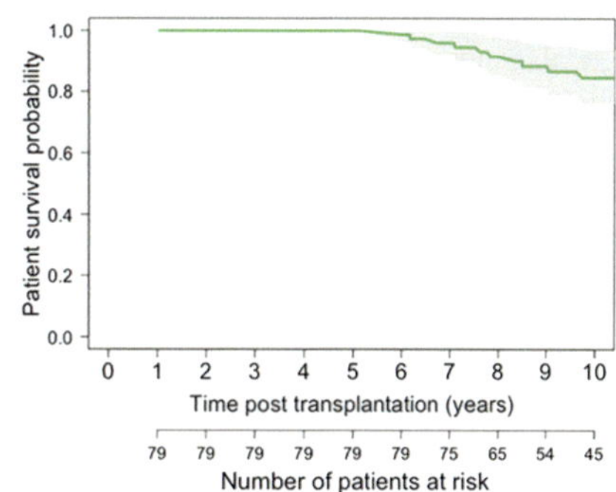


Trajectory #3 (N=261, 20.1%)

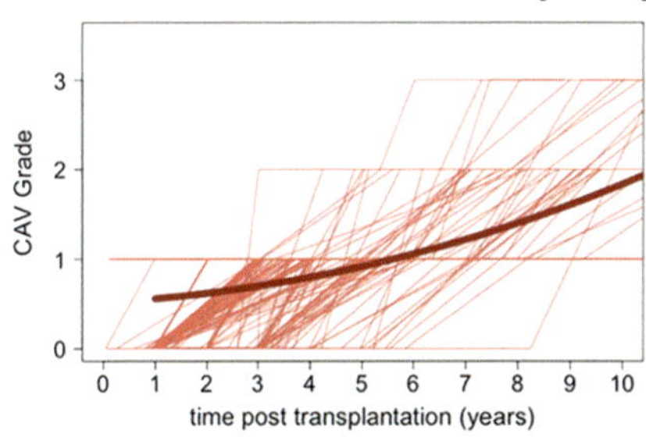


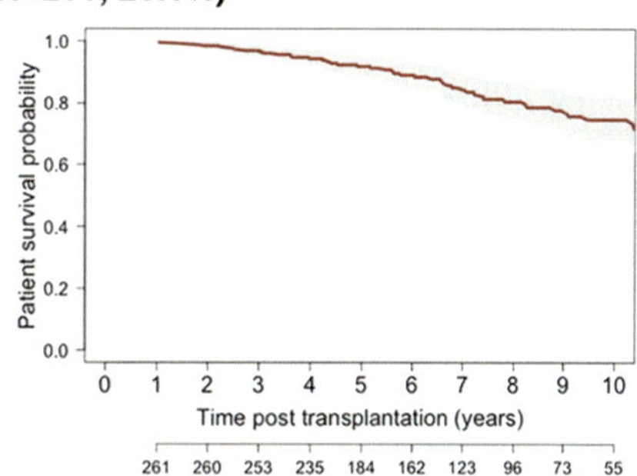


Trajectory #4 (N=138, 10.6%)

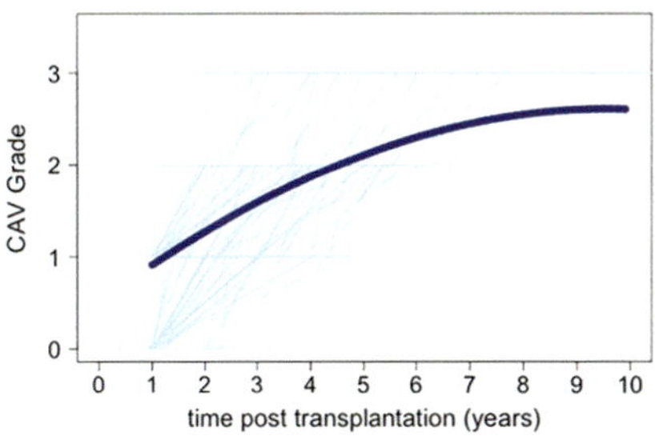


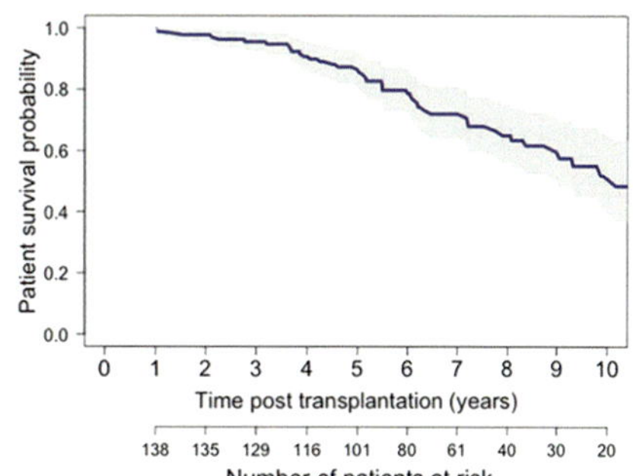

testing with MBR and MFR (both corrected and uncorrected) showed high diagnostic accuracy for detection of CAV grades 2 and 3, and uncorrected MFR > 2 identified low-risk patients with an annual mortality risk of less than 5%. Whereas left ventricular ejection fraction lower than 45% and MFR < 1.7 were associated with increased annual all-cause mortality (up to 51%). As such, the finding of high-risk features on PET imaging may prompt consideration of retransplantation before patients develop significant heart failure complications [35]. CMR, with the assessment of myocardial perfusion reserve, is also an accurate modality for detecting epicardial and microvascular CAV (Class IIb, Level of Evidence C) compared to invasive coronary angiography [36]. Additional CMR features, including increased T2 values, which are associated with myocardial edema, and increased extracellular volume and late gadolinium enhancement (LGE), which are associated with increased fibrosis, are associated with grade 2 or 3 CAV [37, 38]. Increased LGE is independently associated with increased mortality and major adverse cardiac events [38]. However, the utility of CMR for CAV surveillance is limited by cost, poor imaging quality with rapid heart rates in a denervated heart allograft, and concern for accumulation of gadolinium in the brain after repeated exposure [39]. Although there are limitations of CCTA, including limited visualization of vessels < 2 mm, it may be a reasonable alternative in patients who have had complications from conventional coronary angiography or for assessment of variant coronary anatomy (Class IIa, Level of Evidence B [25]). A meta-analysis of thirteen prospective CCTA studies of 615 HTx patients demonstrated a sensitivity of 94%, specificity of 92%, negative predictive value of 99%, and positive predictive value of 67% for detecting a stenosis ≥ 50% on an invasive coronary angiogram [40]. The addition of quantitative plaque has also been shown to improve sensitivity for the detection of CAV [41]. Historically, CCTA has been technically limited by higher resting heart rates post-transplant. However, newer generation CCTA scanners yield technically adequate results in the post-HTx population, and in fact, quality may even be better than for native hearts due to reduced heart rate variability of the denervated cardiac allograft [42].

## Management

### Medical

Prevention and treatment options for CAV include medical therapies, modulation of the immune system, mechanical therapies including percutaneous intervention, and redo-HTx. The 3-hydroxy-3 methylglutaryl coenzyme A reductase inhibitor, pravastatin, was shown in prospective clinical trials to reduce the incidence of CAV, reduce cholesterol levels, reduce cardiac rejection with hemodynamic compromise, and increase survival at 1-year post-transplant [43]. This study was supported by another prospective trial of simvastatin, a similar drug, which demonstrated superior 8-year survival and freedom from CAV compared to a control group [44]. Studies of PCSK9 inhibitors demonstrate safety and efficacy in stabilizing coronary intimal hyperplasia [45]. Most recently, outcomes of EVOLVD (Cholesterol lowering with EVOLocumab to prevent cardiac allograft vasculopathy in De-novo HTx recipients) trial have shown that treatment of HTx recipients with a PCSK9 inhibitor, evolocumab, for 1 year in addition to statin therapy, substantially reduced LDL cholesterol but did not reduce maximal coronary intimal thickness, suggesting that mechanisms other than dyslipidemia, including inflammation and low-grade rejection, should be addressed to mitigate CAV [46]. In another trial, the use of vitamins C and E showed no progression of CAV (compared to placebo-treated control patients) [47]. Given the risk of development of CAV and the likely contribution of traditional risk factors to the development of CAV, low-dose aspirin is generally advised post-transplant. The use of induction agents at the time of HTx, including T cell depleting agents and interleukin (IL)-2 receptor antagonists, may lead to reduced rates of CAV (see Chap. 13).

Anti-thymocyte globulin (ATG), a commonly used T cell depleting agent, has shown delayed onset of CAV [47] and decreased CAV progression by IVUS parameters between baseline and 1-year post-transplant [48]. Different approaches to maintenance immunosuppression have shown differences in the development of CAV. The purine inhibitor mycophenolate mofetil (MMF), in combination with the calcineurin inhibitor (CNI) cyclosporine, showed a decreased incidence of CAV [49]. Clinical trials using the proliferation signal inhibitors (PSI) sirolimus or everolimus in conjunction with CNI have shown reduced rates of CAV compared to maintenance immunosuppressive regimens with CNI in combination with purine antagonist. Everolimus, in combination with cyclosporine, showed lower rates of CAV compared to cyclosporine with azathioprine [50]. Sirolimus, in combination with cyclosporine, showed lower rates of CAV compared to cyclosporine in combination with azathioprine [51]. High-dose everolimus in combination with cyclosporine showed harm in one trial, but low-dose everolimus with cyclosporine showed decreased CAV progression by IVUS and similar mortality compared to cyclosporine with MMF [52]. Everolimus showed efficacy over MMF for CAV in subpopulations, including women, diabetics, patients over age 60, and patients with higher cholesterol levels [53]. Another study examined low-dose everolimus with reduced dose cyclosporine versus standard dose cyclosporine with MMF. Low-dose CNI was withdrawn, and PSI dose increased to target levels 7–11 weeks post-transplant. This study also demonstrated a lower CAV burden in the PSI arm [54, 55]. Immunomodulation with photopheresis may reduce rates of CAV due to the reduction of rejection episodes. Patients treated empirically with photopheresis for the first 6 months post-transplant had reduced rates of acute rejection without increased risk of infection. Using photopheresis in the treatment of patients with rejection with hemodynamic compromise or recurrent rejection decreased the risk of subsequent significant rejection episodes [56]. Reduction of rejection and the inflammatory state may lead to decreased rates of CAV, although this has not formally been studied in a clinical trial format.

## Interventional

CAV is generally a pan-arteritis, but it can present with focal stenosis. Percutaneous intervention and stent placement are generally temporary measures for CAV. Data with newer everolimus DES suggest durability of stented segments with low rates of target lesion revascularization [57, 58]. Prior attempts at revascularization by coronary artery bypass grafting (CABG) surgery resulted in high post-surgical mortality and low rates of survival one year after CABG [59, 60]. CAV is the main cause of need for redo-HTx. Annually, 2–3% of HTx recipients are redo HTx recipients. Unfortunately, survival after a redo HTx is reduced compared to an index HTx. For adult recipients, 1-year survival after redo HTx is approximately 70%, and 10-year survival is 38% [61]. Redo transplant for acute rejection results in poor post-transplant survival and is not recommended. However, patients undergoing redo HTx for stable CAV have comparable post-transplant survival to primary transplants [62].

**In summary**, CAV is one of the major complications after an HTx that contributes to graft failure and significant morbidity and mortality. Improvement in post-HTx immunosuppression, imaging technology, and risk stratification techniques will lead to improved quality of life and longevity after transplant. Investigations into other types of immunosuppressants, including targeting of interleukin (IL-6), down-regulation of the immune system by impairing T cell co-stimulation, and targeting components of the innate immune system may augment the current regimen of agents used in induction and maintenance immunosuppression. Furthermore, insights into the immune mechanisms of CAV may have an impact on native atherosclerosis as there may be an immune component to the development of native atherosclerosis in non-transplant patients.

## References


1. Khush KK, Hsich E, Potena L, Cherikh WS, Chambers DC, Harhay MO, et al. The International Thoracic Organ Transplant Registry of the International Society for Heart and Lung Transplantation: thirty-eighth adult heart transplantation report - 2021; focus on recipient characteristics. J Heart Lung Transplant. 2021;40(10):1035–49.
2. Axtell AL, Fiedler AG, Chang DC, Yeh H, Lewis GD, Villavicencio MA, et al. The effect of donor age on posttransplant mortality in a cohort of adult cardiac transplant recipients aged 18–45. Am J Transplant. 2019;19(3):876–83.
3. Bergenfeldt H, Lund LH, Stehlik J, Andersson B, Höglund P, Nilsson J. Time-dependent prognostic effects of recipient and donor age in adult heart transplantation. J Heart Lung Transplant. 2019;38(2):174–83.
4. Laks JA, Dipchand AI. Cardiac allograft vasculopathy: a review. Pediatr Transplant. 2022;26(3):e14218.
5. Schmauss D, Weis M. Cardiac allograft vasculopathy: recent developments. Circulation. 2008;117(16):2131–41.
6. Moseley EL, Atkinson C, Sharples LD, Wallwork J, Goddard MJ. Deposition of C4d and C3d in cardiac transplants: a factor in the development of coronary artery vasculopathy. J Heart Lung Transplant. 2010;29(4):417–23.
7. Barten MJ, Schulz U, Beiras-Fernandez A, Berchtold-Herz M, Boeken U, Garbade J, et al. The clinical impact of donor-specific antibodies in heart transplantation. Transplant Rev. 2018;32(4):207–17.
8. Kobashigawa J, Colvin M, Potena L, Dragun D, Crespo-Leiro MG, Delgado JF, et al. The management of antibodies in heart transplantation: an ISHLT consensus document. J Heart Lung Transplant. 2018;37(5):537–47.
9. Smith JD, Banner NR, Hamour IM, Ozawa M, Goh A, Robinson D, et al. De novo donor HLA-specific antibodies after heart transplantation are an independent predictor of poor patient survival. Am J Transplant. 2011;11(2):312–9.
10. Wang M, Patel NJ, Zhang X, Kransdorf EP, Azarbal B, Kittleson MM, et al. The effects of donor-specific antibody characteristics on cardiac allograft vasculopathy. Clin Transplant. 2021;35(12):e14483.
11. Yousufuddin M, Haji S, Starling RC, Tuzcu EM, Ratliff NB, Cook DJ, et al. Cardiac angiotensin II receptors as predictors of transplant coronary artery disease following heart transplantation. Eur Heart J. 2004;25(5):377–85.
12. Kauke T, Kaczmarek I, Dick A, Schmoeckel M, Deutsch MA, Beiras-Fernandez A, et al. Anti-MICA antibodies are related to adverse outcome in heart transplant recipients. J Heart Lung Transplant. 2009;28(4):305–11.
13. Rose ML. Role of anti-vimentin antibodies in allograft rejection. Hum Immunol. 2013;74(11):1459–62.
14. de Weger RA. Immune regulators regulated to prevent transplant reactions. J Am Coll Cardiol. 2014;63(1):30–2.
15. Qin L, Huang Q, Zhang H, Liu R, Tellides G, Min W, et al. SOCS1 prevents graft arteriosclerosis by preserving endothelial cell function. J Am Coll Cardiol. 2014;63(1):21–9.
16. Boutolleau D, Coutance G, Désiré E, Bouglé A, Bréchot N, Leprince P, et al. Association between cytomegalovirus infection and allograft rejection in a large contemporary cohort of heart transplant recipients. Transpl Infect Dis. 2021;23(4):e13569.
17. Klimczak-Tomaniak D, Roest S, Brugts JJ, Caliskan K, Kardys I, Zijlstra F, et al. The association between cytomegalovirus infection and cardiac allograft vasculopathy in the era of antiviral valganciclovir prophylaxis. Transplantation. 2020;104(7):1508–18.
18. Tsuji M, Patel JK, Kittleson MM, Chang DH, Kransdorf EP, Nikolova AP, et al. The outcome of restrictive cardiac allograft physiology in severe coronary allograft vasculopathy. The Journal of Heart and Lung Transplantation. 2024.
19. Mehra MR, Crespo-Leiro MG, Dipchand A, Ensminger SM, Hiemann NE, Kobashigawa JA, et al. International Society for Heart and Lung Transplantation working formulation of a standardized nomenclature for cardiac allograft vasculopathy-2010. J Heart Lung Transplant. 2010;29(7):717–27.
20. Mehra M. Contemporary concepts in prevention and treatment of cardiac allograft vasculopathy. Am J Transplant. 2006;6(6):1248–56.
21. Gao S-Z, Hunt SA, Schroeder JS, Alderman EL, Hill IR, Stinson EB. Early development of accelerated graft coronary artery disease: risk factors and course. J Am Coll Cardiol. 1996;28(3):673–9.
22. Kobashigawa JA, Tobis JM, Starling RC, Tuzcu EM, Smith AL, Valantine HA, et al. Multicenter intravascular ultrasound validation study among heart transplant recipients: outcomes after five years. J Am Coll Cardiol. 2005;45(9):1532–7.
23. Tuzcu EM, Kapadia SR, Sachar R, Ziada KM, Crowe TD, Feng J, et al. Intravascular ultrasound evidence of angiographically silent progression in coronary atherosclerosis predicts long-term morbidity and mortality after cardiac transplantation. J Am Coll Cardiol. 2005;45(9):1538–42.
24. Seguchi O, Azarbal B, Mirocha J, Youn J-C, Passano E, Patel J, et al. Change in first-year intravascular ultrasound results predicts adverse events in heart transplant recipients: implications for clinical trial endpoints. Transplantation. 2023;107(3):737–47.
25. Velleca A, Shullo MA, Dhital K, Azeka E, Colvin M, DePasquale E, et al. The International Society for Heart and Lung Transplantation (ISHLT)

guidelines for the care of heart transplant recipients. J Heart Lung Transplant. 2023;42(5):e1–141.
26. Loupy A, Coutance G, Bonnet G, Keer JV, Raynaud M, Aubert O, et al. Identification and characterization of trajectories of cardiac allograft vasculopathy after heart transplantation. Circulation. 2020;141(24):1954–67.
27. Kobashigawa J, Kittleson M, Chang D, Azarbal B, Lee M, Bhatnagar N, et al. Real world use of the Cardiac Allograft Vasculopathy (CAV) score to monitor for CAV after heart transplant. J Heart Lung Transplant. 2024;43(4):S194.
28. Aguilar J, Miller RJH, Otaki Y, Tamarappoo B, Hayes S, Friedman J, et al. Clinical utility of SPECT in the heart transplant population: analysis from a single large-volume center. Transplantation. 2022;106(3):623–32.
29. Chirakarnjanakorn S, Starling RC, Popović ZB, Griffin BP, Desai MY. Dobutamine stress echocardiography during follow-up surveillance in heart transplant patients: diagnostic accuracy and predictors of outcomes. J Heart Lung Transplant. 2015;34(5):710–7.
30. Clerkin KJ, Farr MA, Restaino SW, Ali ZA, Mancini DM. Dobutamine stress echocardiography is inadequate to detect early cardiac allograft vasculopathy. J Heart Lung Transplant. 2016;35(8):1040–1.
31. Elkaryoni A, Abu-Sheasha G, Altibi AM, Hassan A, Ellakany K, Nanda NC. Diagnostic accuracy of dobutamine stress echocardiography in the detection of cardiac allograft vasculopathy in heart transplant recipients: a systematic review and meta-analysis study. Echocardiography. 2019;36(3):528–36.
32. Thompson D, Koster MJ, Wagner RH, Heroux A, Barron JT. Single photon emission computed tomography myocardial perfusion imaging to detect cardiac allograft vasculopathy. Eur Heart J – Cardiovasc Imaging. 2011;13(3):271–5.
33. Bravo PE, Bergmark BA, Vita T, Taqueti VR, Gupta A, Seidelmann S, et al. Diagnostic and prognostic value of myocardial blood flow quantification as non-invasive indicator of cardiac allograft vasculopathy. Eur Heart J. 2017;39(4):316–23.
34. Chih S, Chong AY, Erthal F, deKemp RA, Davies RA, Stadnick E, et al. PET Assessment of epicardial intimal disease and microvascular dysfunction in cardiac allograft vasculopathy. J Am Coll Cardiol. 2018;71(13):1444–56.
35. Miller RJH, Manabe O, Tamarappoo B, Hayes S, Friedman JD, Slomka PJ, et al. Comparative prognostic and diagnostic value of myocardial blood flow and myocardial flow reserve after cardiac transplantation. J Nucl Med. 2020;61(2):249–55.
36. Miller CA, Sarma J, Naish JH, Yonan N, Williams SG, Shaw SM, et al. Multiparametric cardiovascular magnetic resonance assessment of cardiac allograft vasculopathy. J Am Coll Cardiol. 2014;63(8):799–808.
37. Abbasi MA, Blake AM, Sarnari R, Lee D, Anderson AS, Ghafourian K, et al. Multiparametric cardiac magnetic resonance imaging detects altered myocardial tissue and function in heart transplantation recipients monitored for cardiac allograft vasculopathy. J Cardiovasc Imaging. 2022;30(4):263–75.
38. Hughes A, Okasha O, Farzaneh-Far A, Kazmirczak F, Nijjar PS, Velangi P, et al. Myocardial fibrosis and prognosis in heart transplant recipients. Circul Cardiovasc Imaging. 2019;12(10):e009060.
39. Gulani V, Calamante F, Shellock FG, Kanal E, Reeder SB. Gadolinium deposition in the brain: summary of evidence and recommendations. Lancet Neurol. 2017;16(7):564–70.
40. Wever-Pinzon O, Romero J, Kelesidis I, Wever-Pinzon J, Manrique C, Budge D, et al. Coronary computed tomography angiography for the detection of cardiac allograft vasculopathy: a meta-analysis of prospective trials. J Am Coll Cardiol. 2014;63(19):1992–2004.
41. Miller RJH, Kwiecinski J, Shah KS, Eisenberg E, Patel J, Kobashigawa JA, et al. Coronary computed tomography-angiography quantitative plaque analysis improves detection of early cardiac allograft vasculopathy: A pilot study. Am J Transplant. 2020;20(5):1375–83.
42. Pergola V, Mattesi G, Cozza E, Pradegan N, Tessari C, Dellino CM, et al. New non-invasive imaging technologies in cardiac transplant follow-up: acquired evidence and future options. Diagnostics (Basel). 2023;13(17):2818.
43. Kobashigawa JA, Katznelson S, Laks H, Johnson JA, Yeatman L, Wang XM, et al. Effect of pravastatin on outcomes after cardiac transplantation. N Engl J Med. 1995;333(10):621–7.
44. Wenke K, Meiser B, Thiery J, Nagel D, von Scheidt W, Krobot K, et al. Simvastatin initiated early after heart transplantation: 8-year prospective experience. Circulation. 2003;107(1):93–7.
45. Sammour Y, Dezorzi C, Austin BA, Borkon AM, Everley MP, Fendler TJ, et al. PCSK9 inhibitors in heart transplant patients: safety, efficacy, and angiographic correlates. J Cardiac Fail. 2021;27(7):812–5.
46. Broch K, Lemström KB, Gustafsson F, Eiskjær H, Karason K, Gjesdal G, et al. Randomized trial of cholesterol lowering with evolocumab for cardiac allograft vasculopathy in heart transplant recipients. JACC: Heart Fail. 2024.
47. Fang JC, Kinlay S, Beltrame J, Hikiti H, Wainstein M, Behrendt D, et al. Effect of vitamins C and E on progression of transplant-associated arteriosclerosis: a randomised trial. Lancet. 2002;359(9312):1108–13.
48. Azarbal B, Cheng R, Vanichsarn C, Patel JK, Czer LS, Chang DH, et al. Induction therapy with antithymocyte globulin in patients undergoing cardiac transplantation is associated with decreased coronary plaque progression as assessed by intravascular ultrasound. Circul Heart Fail. 2016;9(1):e002252.

49. Kaczmarek I, Ertl B, Schmauss D, Sadoni S, Knez A, Daebritz S, et al. Preventing cardiac allograft vasculopathy: long-term beneficial effects of mycophenolate mofetil. J Heart Lung Transplant. 2006;25(5):550–6.
50. Eisen HJ, Tuzcu EM, Dorent R, Kobashigawa J, Mancini D, Valantine-von Kaeppler HA, et al. Everolimus for the prevention of allograft rejection and vasculopathy in cardiac-transplant recipients. N Engl J Med. 2003;349(9):847–58.
51. Keogh A, Richardson M, Ruygrok P, Spratt P, Galbraith A, O'Driscoll G, et al. Sirolimus in de novo heart transplant recipients reduces acute rejection and prevents coronary artery disease at 2 years: a randomized clinical trial. Circulation. 2004;110(17):2694–700.
52. Eisen HJ, Kobashigawa J, Starling RC, Pauly DF, Kfoury A, Ross H, et al. Everolimus versus mycophenolate mofetil in heart transplantation: a randomized, multicenter trial. Am J Transplant. 2013;13(5):1203–16.
53. Kobashigawa JA, Pauly DF, Starling RC, Eisen H, Ross H, Wang SS, et al. Cardiac allograft vasculopathy by intravascular ultrasound in heart transplant patients: substudy from the Everolimus versus mycophenolate mofetil randomized, multicenter trial. JACC Heart Fail. 2013;1(5):389–99.
54. Andreassen AK, Andersson B, Gustafsson F, Eiskjaer H, Radegran G, Gude E, et al. Everolimus initiation and early calcineurin inhibitor withdrawal in heart transplant recipients: a randomized trial. Am J Transplant. 2014;14(8):1828–38.
55. Gustafsson F, Andreassen AK, Andersson B, Eiskjær H, Rådegran G, Gude E, et al. Everolimus initiation with early calcineurin inhibitor withdrawal in De Novo heart transplant recipients: long-term follow-up from the randomized schedule study. Transplantation. 2020;104(1):154–64.
56. Kirklin JK, Brown RN, Huang ST, Naftel DC, Hubbard SM, Rayburn BK, et al. Rejection with hemodynamic compromise: objective evidence for efficacy of photopheresis. J Heart Lung Transplant. 2006;25(3):283–8.
57. Azarbal B, Arbit B, Ramaraj R, Kittleson M, Young A, Czer L, et al. Clinical and angiographic outcomes with everolimus eluting stents for the treatment of cardiac allograft vasculopathy. J Interv Cardiol. 2014;27(1):73–9.
58. Pyka Ł, Hawranek M, Szyguła-Jurkiewicz B, Desperak P, Szczurek W, Lekston A, et al. Everolimus-Eluting Second-Generation Stents for Treatment of De Novo lesions in patients with cardiac allograft vasculopathy. Ann Transplant. 2020;25:e921266.
59. Halle AA 3rd, DiSciascio G, Massin EK, Wilson RF, Johnson MR, Sullivan HJ, et al. Coronary angioplasty, atherectomy and bypass surgery in cardiac transplant recipients. J Am Coll Cardiol. 1995;26(1):120–8.
60. Musci M, Loebe M, Wellnhofer E, Meyer R, Pasic M, Hummel M, et al. Coronary angioplasty, bypass surgery, and retransplantation in cardiac transplant patients with graft coronary disease. Thorac Cardiovasc Surg. 1998;46(5):268–74.
61. Lund LH, Edwards LB, Kucheryavaya AY, Benden C, Christie JD, Dipchand AI, et al. The registry of the International Society for Heart and Lung Transplantation: thirty-first official adult heart transplant report–2014; focus theme: retransplantation. J Heart Lung Transplant. 2014;33(10):996–1008.
62. Barghash MH, Pinney SP. Heart retransplantation: candidacy, outcomes, and management. Curr Transplant Reports. 2020;7:12–7.

# 22 Long-Term Complications in Heart Transplantation

Lily Stern, Evan Kransdorf, and Yosef Manla

**Abstract**

Heart transplantation requires longitudinal follow-up to monitor for potential long-term complications. The focus of this chapter is the diagnosis and management of other potential long-term complications, including malignancy, hypertension, renal dysfunction, hyperlipidemia, diabetes, osteoporosis, and gastrointestinal complications.

**Keywords**

Heart failure · Heart transplantation · Rejection · Cardiac allograft vasculopathy · Malignancy · Outcomes · Infection

L. Stern · E. Kransdorf (✉) · Y. Manla
Cedars-Sinai Smidt Heart Institute, Los Angeles, CA, USA
e-mail: Evan.kransdorf@cshs.org

L. Stern
e-mail: Lily.stern@cshs.org

Y. Manla
e-mail: Yosef.manla@cshs.org; Yosef.manla1@gmail.com

## Clinical Pearls

- Malignancy due to chronic immunosuppression is a major limitation to long-term survival and is more than twice as common compared to the non-transplant population; more common malignancies post-heart transplant include skin cancer, lung cancer and post-transplant lymphoproliferative disease.
- Common medical problems after transplantation include calcineurin inhibitor-induced hypertension, diabetes and renal dysfunction; steroid-induced osteoporosis, peptic ulcer disease, and hyperlipidemia.
- Diarrhea, nausea, and leukopenia are common side effects from the anti-metabolite mycophenolate mofetil and may require dose reduction and, in severe cases, transition to an enteric-coated formulation.
- After the first three months post-transplant, proliferation signal inhibitors such as sirolimus or everolimus can be considered in place of anti-metabolites for recurrent rejection, donor-specific antibodies, cardiac allograft vasculopathy, malignancy, and cytomegalovirus infection. Side effects of these medications may limit general use.
- Proliferation signal inhibitors may be used in place of calcineurin inhibitors (along with mycophenolate mofetil) in carefully selected patients with significant renal dysfunction


J. Kobashigawa (ed.), *Clinical Guide to Heart Transplantation*, https://doi.org/10.1007/978-3-031-88290-6_22

(renal sparing immunosuppression) and metastatic malignancy, although with an increased risk of rejection.

## Outpatient Management

There are a number of factors that are important to the long-term management of heart transplant (HTx) patients. Generally, maintenance immunosuppression is most intense in the first months after transplant. The risk for rejection and infection is highest early post-transplant. Therefore, outpatient follow-up is the most intense. Patients generally require the involvement of caregivers to assist with medication administration, medication adherence, and transportation to frequent clinic visits. As the risk of rejection decreases over time, target trough levels of immunosuppressant medications are lowered. Decrement in cardiac function may be asymptomatic, and therefore, cardiac function and lab work, including echocardiography and renal function, are frequently assessed during follow-up [1]. Many programs use a combination of triple immunosuppressant medications, including a calcineurin inhibitor, anti-proliferative medications, and prednisone. If a patient avoids rejection, maintains normal left ventricular (LV) systolic function, and does not develop donor-specific antibodies, patients can start to wean prednisone off by 6 months, but usually are not weaned off until 12 months post transplant. After surgery, a patient's functional status often improves with cardiac rehabilitation. Nevertheless, complications often arise and are actively managed by the transplant team with close multidisciplinary involvement.

## Malignancy

The main limitations to long-term survival after an HTx are CAV, graft failure, infection, and malignancy [1]. The use of chronic immunosuppression after transplant to prevent allograft rejection increases the risk of malignancy in the long term. Recipients of HTx may have a pre-existing history of malignancy that, after transplant and on immunosuppression, predisposes them to recurrence of their primary malignancy. Youn et al. recently reported in their study of patients with pre-transplant malignancies that during a median follow-up of 8.6 years post-transplant, patients with pre-transplant malignancy compared to those without showed a significantly higher incidence of posttransplant malignancies (43.8 vs. 20.8%, $p<0.001$), including 9.6% ($n=7$) of cancer recurrence. However, comparable 10-year survival, 10-year freedom from rejection, CAV, or non-fetal major adverse cardiac events were recorded, underlying that a history of pre-transplant malignancy should not disqualify patients from HTx listing [2]. For patients with pre-existing cancer with a high risk of recurrence, HTx should be delayed for an adequate time, as opined by oncology, to ensure patients remain free from cancer recurrence. High-risk cancers include melanoma, breast and colorectal cancer. Although data is limited, there is possible transmission of malignant oncogenic cells from donor to recipient. Caution should be considered in donors with a history of renal cell carcinoma with vascular invasion, melanoma, choriocarcinoma, and sarcomas (3). Malignancy may be discovered in organ donors after the process or at the time of organ transplant. The rate of de novo malignancy is approximately two-fold higher in transplant recipients compared to the general population [4]. Common malignancies after HTx include skin cancer, lung cancer, and anogenital cancer, post-transplant lymphoproliferative disease (PTLD), and Kaposi's sarcoma. In a recent analysis of the International Society for Heart and Lung Transplantation registry, the risk of any de novo solid malignancy between years 1 and 5 after transplantation was 10.7%, with the cumulative incidence for skin cancer and non-skin solid cancers of 7.0 and 4.0%, respectively [5]. Proposed mechanisms for increased rates of de novo malignancy include direct effects of immunosuppression, reduced immune surveillance, and expansion of atypical cells. In addition, oncogenic viruses may proliferate in the setting of immunosuppression and contribute to the development of malignancy. Viruses including Epstein-Barr (EBV), human herpes virus 8 (HHV-8), human papillomavirus (HPV), human T-cell lymphotropic virus 1 (HTLV-1), and Merkel cell polyomavirus (MCV) have associations with specific malignancies. Survival after diagnosis of malignancy depends on many factors, including the size of the tumor, local or distant spread of the tumor, aggressiveness of the tumor, and ability of the patient to tolerate treatments directed against the tumor. Cardiac transplants may require more intense immunosuppression because of the risk of death with graft loss. Animal studies suggest that calcineurin inhibitors (CNI) may promote cancer through increased production of transforming growth factor (TGF) beta [6].

PTLD represents a heterogeneous group of lymphoproliferative disorders. EBV infection is associated with PTLD. EBV-seronegative recipients receiving transplants from EBV-seropositive donors are at elevated risk for the development of PTLD. With EBV infection, B cells incorporate EBV DNA into the cellular genome, decreasing the rate of apoptosis and leading to cellular proliferation. EBV DNA load is suggestive in the right clinical context for PTLD. Imaging studies, including fluorodeoxyglucose (FDG)-positron emission tomography, can assess hypermetabolic tissue, but ultimately, diagnosis of PTLD is made on histopathology. In a recent analysis of the ISHLT registry, it was reported that 3.8% of the patients developed PTLD within 10 years of transplantation. Independent risk factors of PTLD development within 3 years of transplantation included male recipient, EBV donor-positive–recipient-negative match, while maintenance therapy with cyclosporine vs tacrolimus at initial discharge was associated with a lower incidence. It was also observed that PTLD development within 3 years of transplantation set patients as a significant mortality risk (HR: 2.42 [95% CI: 2.01–2.91]; $P<0.001$) [7]. The risk of PTLD is highest in the first year after transplant when immunosuppression is most intense. Common sites of PTLD in HTx recipients include lung, GI tract, liver, lymph nodes, and disseminated disease. In heart–lung transplant recipients, PTLD is primarily found in the lung. Symptoms are variable with PTLD. PTLD can present with fever, fatigue, malaise, recurrent infections that do not respond to antibiotic therapy, lymphadenopathy, or with significant organ dysfunction. Low grade PTLD is generally treated with a significant reduction of immunosuppressive therapies. Reduction of EBV can be attempted with the antiviral agent acyclovir or ganciclovir. In high-risk patients, prophylaxis with anti-viral agents can be considered. For the treatment of neoplastic B cells, several approaches are possible, including the use of chemotherapy, anti-B cell therapy with rituximab, the use of proliferation signal inhibitors (PSI, and withdrawal of one immunosuppressant agent), and tumor resection [8]. When the reduction or withdrawal of immunosuppressant therapies is not effective, mortality from PTLD is high. Kaposi's sarcoma is associated with HHV-8 and occurs in men at rates 3-fold higher than is seen in women. Lesions typically affect the legs and cause lymphedema. Skin cancers include squamous cell and basal cell carcinomas, melanoma, and Merkel cell carcinoma. Factors that mitigate the risk of skin cancer development include ultraviolet radiation, fair skin, pre-transplant history of skin cancer or actinic keratosis, geographic location, intensity, duration, and type of immunosuppressant therapy. The use of voriconazole for the treatment of fungal infection has been associated with the development of aggressive squamous cell carcinomas [9]. Nicotinamide, an amide form of Vitamin B3, has been shown to prevent cutaneous skin cancer in animal studies [10] and in immunocompetent patients [11]. However, it was not demonstrated to be effective for the prevention of skin cancer or actinic keratosis in a randomized control trial of solid organ transplant recipients [12]. Lung cancer, particularly in patients with prior significant tobacco exposure, is increased in HTx recipients. Anogenital cancer occurs in 2–3% of transplant recipients. Lesions may be multiple and extensive and may resemble genital warts. Screening for the presence of malignancy after a HTx is critical. Dermatologic evaluation should be done to screen for skin cancer. There are no formal guidelines for cancer screening after a HTx, but regular health maintenance screening would be appropriate. As with CAV, the use of PSI instead of anti-metabolite may be favorable in the context of malignancy. Transition to PSI may decrease the risk of development of subsequent malignancies after a HTx [13]. Additional indications for the use of PSI in this context include the history of HTx rejection, development of donor-specific antibodies, and viral infection with CMV. Although PSI can cause proteinuria kidney disease, it can be used instead of CNI in a renal sparing effort; however, given concern for possible increased risk of rejection, CNI minimization with PSI may be a safer method [14]. The use of PSI instead of CNI may also be indicated for disseminated malignancies such as PTLD. PSI use should be made on an individual basis. Potential risks of PSI include increased risk of fungal infection, fluid retention, risk of venous thromboembolism, hypertriglyceridemia, oral ulcers, proteinuria renal disease, nausea, diarrhea, leukopenia, and pneumonitis.

## General Medical Management

### Cardiovascular Risk Factors

Risk factors for the development of heart disease are quite prevalent after a HTx. Within five years post-transplant, hypertension occurs in 92% of patients, and hyperlipidemia occurs in 88% of patients [15]. Hypertension is a known side effect of treatment with CNI [16] and steroids. Salt restriction is advisable, particularly at the earliest post-transplant, when steroid doses and CNI target trough levels are highest. Hypertension management using standard guidelines and directed targets can be done with a number of different anti-hypertensive agents. Calcium channel blockers in combination with angiotensin-converting enzyme inhibitors showed benefit by IVUS-based parameters of CAV assessment at one-year post-transplant [17]. Statin therapy is recommended post-transplant, in part for the treatment of hyperlipidemia. Due to drug-drug interactions, high-dose, high-intensity statin therapy is avoided. Hypertriglyceridemia can be caused by PSI therapy, at times requiring cessation of PSI therapy. Hypertriglyceridemia can usually be managed by agents, including fenofibrate or fish oil.

### Renovascular

As with hypertension, CNI is known to lead to gradual reduction of glomerular filtration rate and lead to renal dysfunction with long-term use. Renal dysfunction occurs in 52% of patients, with 15% on chronic dialysis [15]. CNI toxicity can lead to acute renal dysfunction, so trough levels of CNI are monitored closely. While the mainstay of chronic immunosuppressant therapy remains the use of CNI, usually in combination with an anti-metabolite immunosuppressant, CNI-free immunosuppressant regimens can be used to avoid the long-term nephrotoxic effects of CNI, although careful consideration of the risks of possible rejection [14]. Nephrotoxins, in particular, NSAIDS, should be avoided, if possible, post-transplant. The use of colchicine for the treatment of gout should be done with caution.

### Endocrine

Another common risk factor that is often present prior to and post-HTx is glucose intolerance and diabetes. Need for steroid use post-transplant requires adequate control of diabetes prior to listing for a HTx. Use of high-dose steroids post-transplant leads to diabetes in 30–40% of patient's post-transplant. Screening for ocular, renal, and podiatric complications of diabetes should continue per usual recommendation. Early high-dose steroids are weaned such that, in one approach, patients are reduced to 10 mg prednisone by three months post-transplant, 5 mg by six months post-transplant, and, if possible, weaned off the prednisone by one year post-transplant. Many patients will experience symptoms of steroid withdrawal, most often manifest in muscle or joint aches or fatigue.

Rarely will steroid withdrawal symptoms prevent steroid weaning. At times, patients with autoimmune disease may require higher than usual maintenance doses of prednisone. The presence of autoimmune disease does not appear to affect long-term outcomes after a HTx [18]. Bone complications after HTx include osteoporosis, fracture, and osteonecrosis [avascular necrosis (AVN)]. Risk factors for osteoporosis include pre-transplant bone state and post-transplant bone loss. Advanced heart failure, chronic heparin or loop diuretic use, chronic kidney disease, vitamin D deficiency, hyperparathyroidism, hypogonadism, and reduced physical activity can lead to low bone mineral density (BMD) prior to transplant[19]. Post-transplant, bone loss is greatest in the first year due to higher doses of steroids and possibly due to higher CNI target trough levels (when cyclosporine is used in maintenance immunosuppression). Steroids cause reduced bone formation and increased bone resorption. In one study of patients who had annual spinal radiographs, a vertebral fracture was reported in 27% of patients in the first two years after transplant [20]. Predictors of fracture included age and pre-transplant BMD. In another study, women with the lowest BMD pre-transplant were at the highest risk of fracture, with most fractures occurring in the first six months post-transplant [21]. Prevention of falls, smoking cessation, early mobilization after transplant, and regular weight-bearing exercise are recommended. Treatment with Vitamin D (particularly in those with Vitamin D deficiency) and calcium is recommended prior to and post-transplant. Bisphosphonate therapy to prevent bone loss should be considered in patients over age 65, patients with a history of prior fragility fracture, and those with BMD T scores below negative 1.0. If bisphosphonate therapy is not tolerated or if the patient has significant renal insufficiency, calcitriol is an alternate option. If calcitriol is prescribed, serum and urine calcium levels should be monitored [22]. Treatment with bisphosphonate therapy for osteoporosis may not be required for more than one year after transplant. The use of chronic steroids post-transplant is also associated with osteonecrosis. The risk of AVN is <3% in patients maintained on doses of prednisone less than 15 mg/day. Other risk factors for the development of AVN include excess alcohol intake, systemic lupus erythematosus, anti-phospholipid antibodies, trauma, sickle cell disease, Gaucher disease, and decompression disease. AVN often presents with weight-bearing pain but can occur at rest or with night symptoms. Plain films may yield the diagnosis, but magnetic resonance imaging (MRI) is the most sensitive test for diagnoses of AVN. Treatment options include non-operative and operative options. Early-stage AVN may benefit from medical therapy with bisphosphonates, statin therapy to reduce the transition of bone marrow pluripotent cells into fat cells, iloprost (prostacyclin) vasodilator therapy, and anticoagulation when AVN is related to thrombophilia. Electrical stimulation and hyperbaric oxygen were used for early-stage AVN. Operative approaches include joint preserving procedures or joint replacement.

## Gastrointestinal

Gastrointestinal issues can occur post-HTx. Early post-transplant, with the use of higher doses of steroids, peptic ulcer disease and gastritis symptoms can be reduced by the use of proton pump inhibition (PPI). PPI use is generally not required in the long term. Patients on mycophenolate mofetil can have diarrhea or nausea, which usually improves with dose reduction; however, if ineffective, it usually responds to transition to enteric-coated formulations. Patients maintained on azathioprine are at risk for pancreatitis. Patients post-transplant are at risk for cholelithiasis and diverticular disease.

In summary, major complications after HTx, in addition to infection, rejection, and CAV, include malignancy, hypertension, hyperlipidemia, renal disease, glucose intolerance, bone and gastrointestinal disease. Advances in techniques for immunosuppression minimization for renal disease, infection, or malignancy improve the quality of life and longevity of HTx patients. Potential alternative immunosuppression therapies, including T cell co-stimulation blockade and Interleukin-6 antagonism, may allow for further CNI minimization in the future that may mitigate renal dysfunction. Standardized schedules for assessment of symptoms and laboratory findings guide diagnosis and prompt treatment for complications post-HTx. Additionally, close collaboration with multidisciplinary teams, including the primary care physician, is critical for the health of the post-transplant patient.

## References


1. Velleca A, Shullo MA, Dhital K, Azeka E, Colvin M, DePasquale E, et al. The International Society for Heart and Lung Transplantation (ISHLT) guidelines for the care of heart transplant recipients. J Heart Lung Transplant. 2023;42(5):e1–141.
2. Youn J-C, Kim D, Kim KA, Kim J-J, Kim I-C, Lee HS, et al. Characteristics and outcomes of heart transplant recipients with a pretransplant history of malignancy. Am J Transplant. 2022;22(12):2942–50.
3. Buell JF, Trofe J, Hanaway MJ, Lo A, Rosengard B, Rilo H, et al. Transmission of donor cancer into cardiothoracic transplant recipients. Surgery. 2001;130(4):660–6; discussion 6–8.
4. Engels EA, Pfeiffer RM, Fraumeni JF Jr, Kasiske BL, Israni AK, Snyder JJ, et al. Spectrum of cancer risk among US solid organ transplant recipients. JAMA. 2011;306(17):1891–901.
5. Youn J-C, Stehlik J, Wilk AR, Cherikh W, Kim I-C, Park G-H, et al. Temporal trends of de novo malignancy development after heart transplantation. J Am Coll Cardiol. 2018;71(1):40–9.
6. Maluccio M, Sharma V, Lagman M, Vyas S, Yang H, Li B, et al. Tacrolimus enhances transforming growth factor-beta1 expression and promotes tumor progression. Transplantation. 2003;76(3):597–602.
7. Kim I-C, Kim SH, Youn J-C, Kim D, Lee S, Kim H, et al. Temporal trends, risk factors, and clinical outcomes of de novo lymphoproliferative disorders after heart transplantation. Heart Failure. 2024;12(2):395–405.
8. Mucha K, Foroncewicz B, Ziarkiewicz-Wróblewska B, Krawczyk M, Lerut J, Paczek L. Post-transplant lymphoproliferative disorder in view of the new WHO classification: a more rational approach to a protean disease? Nephrol Dial Transplant. 2010;25(7):2089–98.
9. Williams K, Mansh M, Chin-Hong P, Singer J, Arron ST. Voriconazole-associated cutaneous malignancy: a literature review on photocarcinogenesis in organ transplant recipients. Clin Infect Dis. 2014;58(7):997–1002.
10. Gensler HL, Williams T, Huang AC, Jacobson EL. Oral Niacin Prevents Photocarcinogenesis and Photoimmunosuppression in Mice. Nutr Cancer. 1999;34(1):36–41.
11. Chen AC, Martin AJ, Choy B, Fernández-Peñas P, Dalziell RA, McKenzie CA, et al. A Phase 3 Randomized Trial of Nicotinamide for Skin-Cancer Chemoprevention. N Engl J Med. 2015;373(17):1618–26.
12. Allen NC, Martin AJ, Snaidr VA, Eggins R, Chong AH, Fernandéz-Peñas P, et al. Nicotinamide for Skin-Cancer Chemoprevention in Transplant Recipients. N Engl J Med. 2023;388(9):804–12.
13. Rivinius R, Helmschrott M, Ruhparwar A, Schmack B, Klein B, Erbel C, et al. Analysis of malignancies in patients after heart transplantation with subsequent immunosuppressive therapy. Drug Des Devel Ther. 2015;9:93–102.
14. Barten MJ, Hirt SW, Garbade J, Bara C, Doesch AO, Knosalla C, et al. Comparing everolimus-based immunosuppression with reduction or withdrawal of calcineurin inhibitor reduction from 6 months after heart transplantation: The randomized MANDELA study. Am J Transplant. 2019;19(11):3006–17.
15. Lund LH, Edwards LB, Kucheryavaya AY, Benden C, Christie JD, Dipchand AI, et al. The registry of the International Society for Heart and Lung Transplantation: thirty-first official adult heart transplant report–2014; focus theme: retransplantation. J Heart Lung Transplant. 2014;33(10):996–1008.
16. Hoorn EJ, Walsh SB, McCormick JA, Zietse R, Unwin RJ, Ellison DH. Pathogenesis of calcineurin inhibitor-induced hypertension. J Nephrol. 2012;25(3):269–75.
17. Erinc K, Yamani MH, Starling RC, Crowe T, Hobbs R, Bott-Silverman C, et al. The effect of combined Angiotensin-converting enzyme inhibition and calcium antagonism on allograft coronary vasculopathy validated by intravascular ultrasound. J Heart Lung Transplant. 2005;24(8):1033–8.
18. Yabuno J, Patel J, Kittleson M, Luu M, Liou F, Siddiqui S, et al. Abstract 13688: Patients With Autoimmune Disease: Not a Contraindication for Heart Transplantation. Circulation. 2015;132(suppl_3):A13688-A.
19. Shane E, Mancini D, Aaronson K, Silverberg SJ, Seibel MJ, Addesso V, et al. Bone mass, vitamin D deficiency, and hyperparathyroidism in congestive heart failure. Am J Med. 1997;103(3):197–207.
20. Leidig-Bruckner G, Hosch S, Dodidou P, Ritschel D, Conradt C, Klose C, et al. Frequency and predictors of osteoporotic fractures after cardiac or liver transplantation: a follow-up study. Lancet. 2001;357(9253):342–7.
21. Shane E, Rivas M, Staron RB, Silverberg SJ, Seibel MJ, Kuiper J, et al. Fracture after cardiac transplantation: a prospective longitudinal study. J Clin Endocrinol Metab. 1996;81(5):1740–6.
22. Shane E, Addesso V, Namerow PB, McMahon DJ, Lo SH, Staron RB, et al. Alendronate versus calcitriol for the prevention of bone loss after cardiac transplantation. N Engl J Med. 2004;350(8):767–76.

# Part V
# Special Considerations

# Pediatric Cardiomyopathies

23

Juan C. Alejos and Majid Husain

**Abstract**

Pediatric cardiomyopathies are a rare but serious group of diseases. This chapter will explore dilated, hypertrophic, and restrictive cardiomyopathies with a focus on epidemiology, genetic factors, clinical features, diagnostic imaging modalities, and management strategies. Additionally, oncological cardiomyopathies will be discussed.

**Keywords**

Dilated cardiomyopathy · Hypertrophic cardiomyopathy · Restricted cardiomyopathy · Oncologic cardiomyopathies

## Clinical Pearls

- Dilated cardiomyopathy (DCM) is the most common cardiomyopathy in children and is also the most frequent indication for heart transplantation in children. An endomyocardial biopsy (EMB) can be important to determine the underlying pathologies of DCM.
- Outcome prediction in children with DCM include age at presentation, clinical symptoms, ventricular size/mass, severity of dysfunction, the presence of arrhythmias, high end-diastolic pressure, and endocardial fibroelastosis.
- Hypertrophic cardiomyopathy (HCM) is the second most common cardiomyopathy seen in children and is often found to be the underlying pathology in children and young adults who suffer from sudden cardiac death. Patient-centered shared decision-making for an implantable cardioverter defibrillator for the prevention of sudden cardiac death is warranted.
- Heart transplantation is not a first-line therapy for HCM and is only considered when there are ventricular arrhythmias refractory to treatment or when features of DCM or restrictive cardiomyopathy develop.
- Restrictive cardiomyopathy (RCM) is the least common cardiomyopathy seen in children and carries a poor prognosis related to a higher incidence of pulmonary hypertension, thromboembolic events, and sudden death.
- Chemotherapy-induced cardiomyopathy remains the most common cause of death among pediatric cancer survivors for which heart transplantation may be an option.

J. C. Alejos (✉) · M. Husain
UCLA Mattel Children's Hospital, Los Angeles, CA, USA
e-mail: jalejos@mednet.ucla.edu

M. Husain
e-mail: Majidhusain@mednet.ucla.edu



J. Kobashigawa (ed.), *Clinical Guide to Heart Transplantation*, https://doi.org/10.1007/978-3-031-88290-6_23

## Dilated Cardiomyopathy

Dilated cardiomyopathy (DCM) is the most common cardiomyopathy in children, accounting for more than half of the total cases. The overall incidence of DCM in the pediatric population is 0.57 per 100,000 per year, with boys being slightly more susceptible than girls [1]. DCM is also one of the leading causes of heart failure and the most frequent indication for heart transplantation (HTx) in children. Notably, in infants < 1 year of age, recipients with DCM have nearly doubled from 21% in 1988–2003 to 38% in the modern era [2]. In recipients > 1 year of age, DCM has remained the most common diagnosis for transplantation for the past few decades, accounting for 44–50% of pediatric HTx. Within the Pediatric Heart Transplant Study Group (PHTSG), patients affected by DCM represent 75% of the group of patients with cardiomyopathy receiving a HTx [3]. DCM is characterized by left ventricular or biventricular dilation with impaired systolic function in the absence of any coronary artery pathology. It can be congenital or acquired. Familial causes were previously thought to be rare, but it is now known that a majority of cases involve patients with an underlying genetic abnormality [4]. The causative genes encode proteins found in the cytoskeleton, sarcomere, desmosomes, sarcoplasmic reticulum, nuclear envelope, nucleus, ion channels, mitochondria, and the extracellular matrix. Novel candidate genes in various other loci are being actively discovered. Viruses, in particular, adenoviruses, Coxsackie A and B, cytomegalovirus, and Epstein-Barr, are a significant etiology. Of note is that DCM is secondary to anthracyclines, given that malignancy can be a contraindication to transplantation. DCM can also be related to neuromuscular diseases such as dystrophinopathies (including Duchenne and Becker muscular dystrophy), Friedreich's ataxia, and myotonic dystrophy. On rare occasions, metabolic and endocrine conditions, as well as infiltrative and autoimmune diseases, have been implicated in the development of DCM.

It is important to differentiate DCM from conditions with phenotypic overlap, including but not limited to ischemic cardiomyopathy, advanced hypertrophic cardiomyopathy, arrhythmogenic right ventricular cardiomyopathy (ARVC), noncompaction, and the well-defined Athlete's heart.

In DCM, the dilated ventricle increases the stress exerted on the chamber wall. Consequently, there is contractile impairment, functional mitral regurgitation, and arrhythmias due to enlargement of the cardiac chambers. Children may develop heart failure and present with anorexia and weight loss. Clinical signs include tachycardia, jugular venous distention, hepatomegaly, and a systolic murmur consistent with mitral regurgitation. The echocardiogram findings, as mentioned above, include left ventricular dilation with a decreased ejection fraction and fractional shortening, mitral regurgitation, and/or pericardial effusion. The electrocardiograph (ECG) may show sinus tachycardia, pathological Q waves, bundle-branch block, heightened QRS complexes, atrial fibrillation, or ventricular arrhythmias. Notably, the presence of persistent tachycardia should raise suspicion for tachycardia-induced cardiomyopathy, especially if there is recovery of ventricular function with rhythm control over a period of time. Left ventricular non-compaction (LVNC), a disease of increased and prominent endomyocardial trabeculations, can also present as DCM. The biomarker brain natriuretic peptide (BNP) or NT-proBNP can be useful when trying to distinguish lung disease from heart failure or for monitoring disease progression. An endomyocardial biopsy (EMB) may be performed to determine the etiology of DCM. This is especially necessary for identifying reversible underlying pathologies or requiring different management plans, such as sarcoidosis or glycogen storage diseases. The biopsy sample can additionally confirm or exclude viral myocarditis as the etiology by isolating viral genetic material via PCR testing since serologies are generally unhelpful because of high background seropositivity rates in the population [4]. Several studies have suggested a greater than 50% chance of resolution of myocarditis-related DCM within two years of presentation, with fulminant myocarditis having the highest likelihood of resolution [5]. Furthermore, cardiovascular magnetic resonance imaging (CMR) is increasingly becoming a widely used noninvasive modality for the diagnosis and evaluation of DCM as well as other cardiomyopathies. It can detect myocardial edema and late gadolinium enhancement (LGE), a maker of fibrosis due to prior myocardial injury that may be present in ischemic cardiomyopathy, muscular dystrophy, or previous myocarditis. Notably, CMR is the current gold standard for comprehensive biventricular assessment. Lastly, predictors of outcome in children with DCM are highly variable. The factors described in the literature range from ventricular size, mass, and severity of dysfunction to the presence of arrhythmias, high end-diastolic pressure, and endocardial fibroelastosis. Age at presentation and constellation of symptoms have similarly been implicated. However, none of the above predictors have been definitively shown to have better or worse outcomes. Nonetheless, for those with evidence of progressive or refractory heart failure, the use of ventricular assist devices or extracorporeal membrane oxygenation remains an option as a bridge to recovery or transplantation.

## Hypertrophic Cardiomyopathy

Hypertrophic cardiomyopathy (HCM) is the second most common cardiomyopathy seen in children, accounting for 30–50% of cases (6). The overall incidence of HCM in the pediatric Population is 0.24–0.47 per 100,000 per year [7]. HCM is the most common form of Mendelian inherited heart disease, and it is often found to be the underlying pathology in children and young adults who suffer from sudden cardiac death (SCD) [8]. Several gene mutations have been described, with most encoding for proteins found in the sarcomere. Unlike DCM and restrictive cardiomyopathy, no acquired forms of this disease have been found. Despite its incidence, HCM less often leads to transplantation, with only 5% of patients carrying the diagnosis pre-operatively [3, 6]. Pediatric HCM comprises a heterogeneous group of diseases with variable genotypes and phenotypic expression. As stated above, genetic mutations in the sarcomeric proteins lead to primary HCM. Pathogenic genes include MYH7, MYL2, MYL3, MYBPC3, TNNT2, TNNI3, TPM1, ACTC1, ACTN2, CSRP3 and PLN [9]. Like DCM, novel candidate genes are being actively discovered. Unlike DCM, the molecular mechanisms that lead to the variable HCM phenotype remain uncertain. Causes of secondary HCM include disease of glycogen storage (Pompe, Danon, Cori, or Forbes disease), lysosomal storage disorders (Mucopolysaccharidoses, Anderson-Fabry disease), syndromic pathology (Noonan, Costello, or Beckwith-Widemann syndrome), fatty acid oxidation disorders, mitochondrial diseases (Friedreich ataxia) and various endocrine disorders [10, 11]. There is also a coexistence of HCM with congenital heart disease, specifically in patients with Noonan syndrome who have valvular pulmonary stenosis.

By echocardiography, HCM is characterized by the presence of a hypertrophied and nondilated left ventricle in the absence of a hemodynamically significant physiologic or pathologic etiology. The hypertrophy is asymmetric and predominantly isolated to the interventricular septum. Primary diagnostic criteria for pediatric HCM require adjusting the maximum diastolic septal thickness for body surface area. According to the American College of Cardiology/American Heart Association guidelines on pediatric HCM published in 2020, a Z-score > 2.5 for the maximal end-diastolic wall thickness has been suggested to identify early HCM in asymptomatic children with no significant family history, and a Z-score of > 2 may be sufficient for a diagnosis of HCM in children with a positive family history or a positive genetic test [12]. Ventricular function is generally normal, although early diastolic dysfunction has been reported. There may be associated structural anomalies, including mitral valve abnormalities, myocardial crypts, or the presence of noncompaction. Electrocardiographically, there is LVH by well-defined voltage criteria, abnormal Q-waves, and repolarization abnormalities in patients with pathogenic genetic mutations. Consequently, children with HCM are prone to life-threatening malignant arrhythmias requiring screening, surveillance, and appropriate risk stratification with patient-centered shared decision-making for an implantable cardioverter defibrillator (ICD) for the prevention of SCD. On a microscopic level, cardiac myocytes are in disarray. Functionally, the collective anatomical changes may result in left ventricular outflow obstruction, termed hypertrophic obstructive cardiomyopathy (HOCM).

Like the diverse genetic origins of HCM, its clinical presentation is also highly variable. Most patients are asymptomatic, with some experiencing chest pain and dyspnea. Palpitations and pre-syncopal episodes can occur. Syncope is rare but is a prominent risk factor for SCD. Children under the age of 1 often present with congestive heart failure. HCM is infamous for its insidiousness and its tendency to present with SCD in young athletes. Therefore, it is imperative to screen and survey this population closely using electrocardiography, echocardiography, and CMR. Additionally, Holter monitoring is useful for identifying occult and pathologic arrhythmias, which carry an increased risk of SCD. Given the autosomal dominance of HCM, screening of parents, siblings, and 1st-degree relatives is advisable.

Treatment depends on the severity of symptoms and the presence of risk factors for SCD. Patients with chest pain and dyspnea are treated medically with beta-blockers and calcium channel antagonists. The detection of ventricular arrhythmias warrants the placement of an ICD. Patients with severe left ventricular outflow obstruction may undergo septal myectomy, although this is only for symptom relief and does not slow disease progression, nor does it prevent potentially fatal arrhythmias.

HTx is not a first-line therapy for HCM and is only considered when there are ventricular arrhythmias refractory to treatment or when features of DCM or restrictive cardiomyopathy develop. Risk factors for death or transplantation include age < 1 year, low presenting shortening fraction, and increased LV posterior wall thickness [6]. The 5-year survival rate for children with HCM ranges from 42% in children with an Associated inborn error of metabolism (IEM) to 94% in children with noninfantile idiopathic disease presenting after one year of age; the overall survival at 9 years across various other disease processes, including infantile presentation < 1 year of age, but excluding IEM is approximately 80% [7].

Recently, the EXPLORER-HCM [13] clinical trial showed that Mavacamten, a cardiac myosin inhibitor, was superior to placebo in improving the functional status and health status of patients with HOCM. Specifically, it was associated with a significant reduction in post-exercise left ventricular outflow tract gradient compared with placebo at 30 weeks, which was sustained to 48 weeks. CMR found that Mavacamten was also associated with favorable remodeling compared with placebo. Additionally, Mavacamten improved various measures of cardiopulmonary exercise testing, including peak $V_E/VCO_2$, METs, and peak circulatory power. Lastly, it was shown to be well tolerated with no significant long-term adverse events. The increasing use of pharmacologic therapy to treat HCM may slow the progression of the disease and further delay or potentially eliminate the need for transplantation.

## Restrictive Cardiomyopathy

Restrictive cardiomyopathy (RCM) is the least common cardiomyopathy seen in children and represents only 3% of pediatric cases [14]. The overall incidence of RCM in the pediatric population is unclear. Compared to other cardiomyopathies, pediatric RCM carries a poor prognosis related to a higher incidence of pulmonary hypertension, thromboembolic events, and sudden death. Despite being the rarest cardiomyopathy in children, sudden death occurs in approximately 25% of pediatric RCM patients, with an annual mortality of 7%. Medical and surgical treatment options are limited and not well supported by clinical studies in this patient population. Freedom from death was 68% at 5 years, with a transplant-free survival of 22% [15]. Due to these high mortality rates, transplantation is often the only therapeutic option. Not surprisingly, despite being the least common cardiomyopathy, patients affected by RCM represent 12% of transplant recipients within PHTSG [3].

Pediatric RCM is characterized by diastolic dysfunction due to restrictive filling with a normal ventricle wall thickness, chamber size, and ejection fraction. Like DCM and HCM, it represents a heterogeneous group of diseases with variable genotypes and phenotypic expression. The etiology of RCM includes inherited and acquired causes. Inherited causes involve defects in sarcomeric, cytoskeleton, and nuclear envelope genes. Among the aforementioned, mutations in the sarcomeric genes, including MYBPC3, MYH7, TTN, TNNI3, TNNT2, and ACTC, are the most commonly identified [16]. Other inherited etiologies include storage diseases (namely, Anderson Fabry and Danon disease), as well as infiltrative processes, such as cardiac amyloidosis and sarcoidosis. Iron overload cardiomyopathies related to beta-thalassemia, sickle-cell anemia, and hereditary hemochromatosis have also been implicated in the familial causes of RCM. Acquired RCM includes chemotherapy or radiotherapy-related cardiomyopathies.

Clinically, RCM often lacks symptoms early on and can present with decreased exercise tolerance, exertional chest pain, and syncope. Children with RCM may report a history of frequent respiratory infections. It can also present with acute right and/or left heart failure with pulmonary hypertension. Physical exam findings include jugular venous distension (possibly with Kussmaul sign), hepatomegaly, a prominent $S_2$ heart sound, a gallop rhythm, peripheral edema, and ascites in the setting of heart failure. Echocardiography shows markedly dilated atria with normal-sized ventricles and generally preserved ejection fraction. There are abnormal mitral inflow and tissue Doppler variables consistent with diastolic dysfunction. With disease progression, the estimated pulmonary artery pressure will be elevated. Notably, echocardiography is helpful in distinguishing RCM from constrictive pericarditis, which can present in a similar manner but carries a different outcome and is treated differently. The electrocardiogram is abnormal and most commonly shows right and/or left atrial enlargement. ST-T segments are elevated and notched, or biphasic T-waves are frequently present. ST-T segment depressions, prolonged PR, and wide QRS complex have also been reported and implicated as risk factors for SCD in this patient population [17, 18]. Holter evaluation is useful for detecting atrial or ventricular arrhythmias, WPW with SVT, or AV block. Cardiac catheterization is useful for confirming elevated pulmonary pressures seen on the echocardiogram, determining the severity of pulmonary vascular resistance, testing pulmonary vascular reactivity, and evaluating cardiac index. Hemodynamic assessment can further help distinguish restrictive and constrictive physiology beyond echocardiographic assessment. An endomyocardial biopsy (EMB) is only done to exclude etiologies such as amyloidosis or sarcoidosis, which more commonly cause RCM in adults. Lastly, CMR can be used to obtain detailed structural, functional, and tissue characteristics of the myocardium to aid in clarifying the etiology of RCM. Once the diagnosis is established, first-degree relatives should be screened.

Pharmacological treatments for RCM are principally for palliative symptom relief. Diuretics are used to reduce venous congestion. Caution should be exercised, however, to ensure cardiac output is not compromised. Angiotensin-converting enzyme inhibitors (ACEi) and angiotensin receptor blockers (ARBs) may be used if there is associated systemic hypertension. Although beta-blockers and calcium channel blockers may theoretically provide relief to patients by prolonging the diastolic interval, allowing for better filling, these medications are generally not recommended in pediatric RCM since cardiac output is dependent on heart rate due to the compromised stroke volume in the setting of significant diastolic dysfunction. Similarly, digoxin, intravenous inotropes, and pulmonary vasodilators are not recommended unless they are being used to treat secondary complications of the disease. Given the risk of atrial fibrillation and the presence of abnormal hemodynamics, anticoagulants are sometimes used prophylactically to prevent the formation and embolization of mural thrombi. Due to the lack of studies and consensus on the efficacy and use of antiplatelet agents versus vitamin K antagonists versus low molecular weight heparin [19], the type and choice of antithrombotic or anticoagulation therapy varies by institution and professional experience.

Given that RCM is refractory to other therapies, patients are more likely to be considered for transplantation. In the United States, many centers advocate immediate listing for transplantation because of the rapid development of pulmonary hypertension, the high risk of thromboembolism, and a mean survival of approximately 2 years [20]. The use of mechanical circulatory support as a bridge to transplantation remains an option since many children with RCM would otherwise die on the waitlist due to the progression of their heart failure, resulting in multi-organ failure.

## Oncological Cardiomyopathy

Despite progress in cancer therapeutics over the past few decades in improving survival across most childhood malignancies, cardiac-related disease remains the most common non-oncologic cause of death among survivors [21]. Anthracycline chemotherapy agents such as doxorubicin, daunorubicin, and epirubicin, which are typically used for hematologic cancers and solid tumors, are cardiotoxic. One of the most detrimental side- effects of this class of drugs is the development of drug-induced cardiomyopathy, specifically DCM, with a restrictive physiology. The mechanism of action is thought to be free radical-induced oxidative damage to cardiac myocytes [22]. There is a dose-dependent relationship between the cumulative anthracycline dose and cardiotoxicity. At very high doses, cardiomyopathy develops in 36% of patients [23]. This number is negligible at the lowest doses. There can be a delay of up to 20 years after the completion of chemotherapy before cardiomyopathy becomes clinically apparent [24]. Radiotherapy can similarly result in radiation-induced restrictive cardiomyopathy as a result of biventricular fibrosis reducing myocardial compliance. An initial echocardiogram should be obtained prior to initiation of chemotherapy to delineate structural anatomy and establish baseline ventricular function. Follow-up studies should be performed routinely post-therapy to monitor ventricular function and survey for early signs, development, and progression of cardiomyopathy. A baseline ECG should also be obtained. ECG changes related to anthracycline therapy are non-specific and include sinus tachycardia, a flattened T wave, or a prolonged QT interval. Treatment options for this drug-induced cardiomyopathy are limited. It is refractory to usual regimens. Symptom relief can be provided by pharmacologic therapies highlighted in the RCM subsection, but there is no improvement in mortality. HTx remains the only therapeutic option if the malignancy is well-controlled or in remission. The decision to evaluate for transplant candidacy is made in concert with the patient's oncology team.

## References


1. Towbin JA, Lowe AM, Colan SD, Sleeper LA, Orav EJ, Clunie S, et al. Incidence, causes, and outcomes of dilated cardiomyopathy in children. JAMA. 2006;296(15):1867–76.
2. Rossano JW, Dipchand AI, Edwards LB, Goldfarb S, Kucheryavaya AY, Levvey Rn BJ, et al. The Registry of the International Society for Heart and Lung Transplantation: Nineteenth Pediatric Heart Transplantation Report-2016; Focus Theme: Primary Diagnostic Indications for Transplant. J Heart Lung Transplant. 2016;35(10):1185–95.
3. Canter CND. Recipient characteristics. In: Pediatric solid organ transplantation. Malden, Mass: Blackwell; 2007.
4. Japp AG, Gulati A, Cook SA, Cowie MR, Prasad SK. The Diagnosis and Evaluation of Dilated Cardiomyopathy. J Am Coll Cardiol. 2016;67(25):2996–3010.
5. English RF, Janosky JE, Ettedgui JA, Webber SA. Outcomes for children with acute myocarditis. Cardiol Young. 2004;14(5):488–93.

6. Canter CE, Shaddy RE, Bernstein D, Hsu DT, Chrisant MR, Kirklin JK, et al. Indications for heart transplantation in pediatric heart disease: a scientific statement from the American Heart Association Council on Cardiovascular Disease in the Young; the Councils on Clinical Cardiology, Cardiovascular Nursing, and Cardiovascular Surgery and Anesthesia; and the Quality of Care and Outcomes Research Interdisciplinary Working Group. Circulation. 2007;115(5):658–76.
7. Colan SD, Lipshultz SE, Lowe AM, Sleeper LA, Messere J, Cox GF, et al. Epidemiology and cause-specific outcome of hypertrophic cardiomyopathy in children: findings from the Pediatric Cardiomyopathy Registry. Circulation. 2007;115(6):773–81.
8. Maron BJ, Shirani J, Poliac LC, Mathenge R, Roberts WC, Mueller FO. Sudden death in young competitive athletes. Clinical, demographic, and pathological profiles. JAMA. 1996;276(3):199–204.
9. Nguyen MB, Mital S, Mertens L, Jeewa A, Friedberg MK, Aguet J, et al. Pediatric hypertrophic cardiomyopathy: exploring the genotype-phenotype association. J Am Heart Assoc. 2022;11(5):e024220.
10. Monda E, Rubino M, Lioncino M, Di Fraia F, Pacileo R, Verrillo F, et al. Hypertrophic cardiomyopathy in children: pathophysiology, diagnosis, and treatment of non-sarcomeric causes. Front Pediatr. 2021;9:632293.
11. Lipshultz SE, Law YM, Asante-Korang A, Austin ED, Dipchand AI, Everitt MD, et al. Cardiomyopathy in children: classification and diagnosis: a scientific statement from the American Heart Association. Circulation. 2019;140(1):e9–68.
12. Ommen SR, Mital S, Burke MA, Day SM, Deswal A, Elliott P, et al. 2020 AHA/ACC guideline for the diagnosis and treatment of patients with hypertrophic cardiomyopathy: a report of the American College of Cardiology/American Heart Association joint committee on clinical practice guidelines. Circulation. 2020;142(25):e558–631.
13. Olivotto I, Oreziak A, Barriales-Villa R, Abraham TP, Masri A, Garcia-Pavia P, et al. Mavacamten for treatment of symptomatic obstructive hypertrophic cardiomyopathy (EXPLORER-HCM): a randomised, double-blind, placebo-controlled, phase 3 trial. Lancet. 2020;396(10253):759–69.
14. Lipshultz SE, Sleeper LA, Towbin JA, Lowe AM, Orav EJ, Cox GF, et al. The incidence of pediatric cardiomyopathy in two regions of the United States. N Engl J Med. 2003;348(17):1647–55.
15. Webber SA, Lipshultz SE, Sleeper LA, Lu M, Wilkinson JD, Addonizio LJ, et al. Outcomes of restrictive cardiomyopathy in childhood and the influence of phenotype: a report from the Pediatric Cardiomyopathy Registry. Circulation. 2012;126(10):1237–44.
16. Ditaranto R, Caponetti AG, Ferrara V, Parisi V, Minnucci M, Chiti C, et al. Pediatric restrictive cardiomyopathies. Front Pediatr. 2021;9:745365.
17. Hayashi T, Tsuda E, Kurosaki K, Ueda H, Yamada O, Echigo S. Electrocardiographic and clinical characteristics of idiopathic restrictive cardiomyopathy in children. Circ J. 2007;71(10):1534–9.
18. Walsh MA, Grenier MA, Jefferies JL, Towbin JA, Lorts A, Czosek RJ. Conduction abnormalities in pediatric patients with restrictive cardiomyopathy. Circ Heart Fail. 2012;5(2):267–73.
19. Chen K, Williams S, Chan AK, Mondal TK. Thrombosis and embolism in pediatric cardiomyopathy. Blood Coagul Fibrinolysis. 2013;24(3):221–30.
20. Russo LM, Webber SA. Idiopathic restrictive cardiomyopathy in children. Heart. 2005;91(9):1199–202.
21. Lipshultz SE, Adams MJ, Colan SD, Constine LS, Herman EH, Hsu DT, et al. Long-term cardiovascular toxicity in children, adolescents, and young adults who receive cancer therapy: pathophysiology, course, monitoring, management, prevention, and research directions: a scientific statement from the American Heart Association. Circulation. 2013;128(17):1927–95.
22. Rosen GM, Halpern HJ. Spin trapping biologically generated free radicals: correlating formation with cellular injury. Methods Enzymol. 1990;186:611–21.
23. Lefrak EA, Pitha J, Rosenheim S, Gottlieb JA. A clinicopathologic analysis of adriamycin cardiotoxicity. Cancer. 1973;32(2):302–14.
24. Steinherz LJ, Steinherz PG, Tan CT, Heller G, Murphy ML. Cardiac toxicity 4 to 20 years after completing anthracycline therapy. JAMA. 1991;266(12):1672–7.

# Pediatric Heart Transplantation

# 24

Juan C. Alejos and Majid Husain

**Abstract**

Pediatric heart transplantation (HTx) is the ultimate option in the treatment of end-stage heart disease refractory to maximum medical therapy or surgical management. This chapter comprehensively overviews pediatric HTx indications, pre-transplant evaluation, donor selection, waitlist management, post-transplant management and surveillance, and long-term complications. In addition, the survival and outcomes of pediatric HTx were discussed.

**Keywords**

Pediatric heart transplantation · Infants · ABO-incompatible heart transplantation · Congenital heart disease

## Clinical Pearls

- Waitlist mortality in children is higher than in the adult population for heart transplantation due to donor shortages and the limited availability of VADs.
- Children can be transplanted safely with a pre-operative pulmonary vascular resistance index of up to 9 Woods units/m2
- Contrary to the adult population, ABO-incompatible heart transplantation is possible in infants and younger children with comparable outcomes.
- Pediatric patients with congenital heart disease and with palliative procedures have led to a higher risk of pre-transplant sensitization.
- Steroid-avoidance immunosuppressive regimens show good outcomes in children who are not sensitized.
- Children of minority race or ethnicity have been shown to have worse outcomes.
- Post-transplant survival in the pediatric population continues to improve with enhanced immunosuppression regimens, and advancement in invasive and non-invasive techniques for monitoring rejection

J. C. Alejos (✉) · M. Husain
UCLA Mattel Children's Hospital, Los Angeles, CA, USA
e-mail: jalejos@mednet.ucla.edu

M. Husain
e-mail: Majidhusain@mednet.ucla.edu





J. Kobashigawa (ed.), *Clinical Guide to Heart Transplantation*, https://doi.org/10.1007/978-3-031-88290-6_24

## Introduction

The first pediatric heart transplant (HTx) was performed by Adrian Kantrowitz at Maimonides Medical Center in Brooklyn, New York, on December 6, 1967 (Fig. 24.1). This was the first human HTx in the United States and followed the first-ever human HTx in only 3 days. The recipient was an 18-day-old male with Ebstein's anomaly and pulmonary atresia. The donor was an infant with anencephaly. Interestingly, the operation was performed under hypothermia rather than cardiopulmonary bypass. The patient survived for only six hours [1]. Poor survival and a lack of donors resulted in enthusiasm for pediatric HTx waning for over a decade until the success of immunosuppression in adults revived interest in the field. In 1983, Leonard Bailey

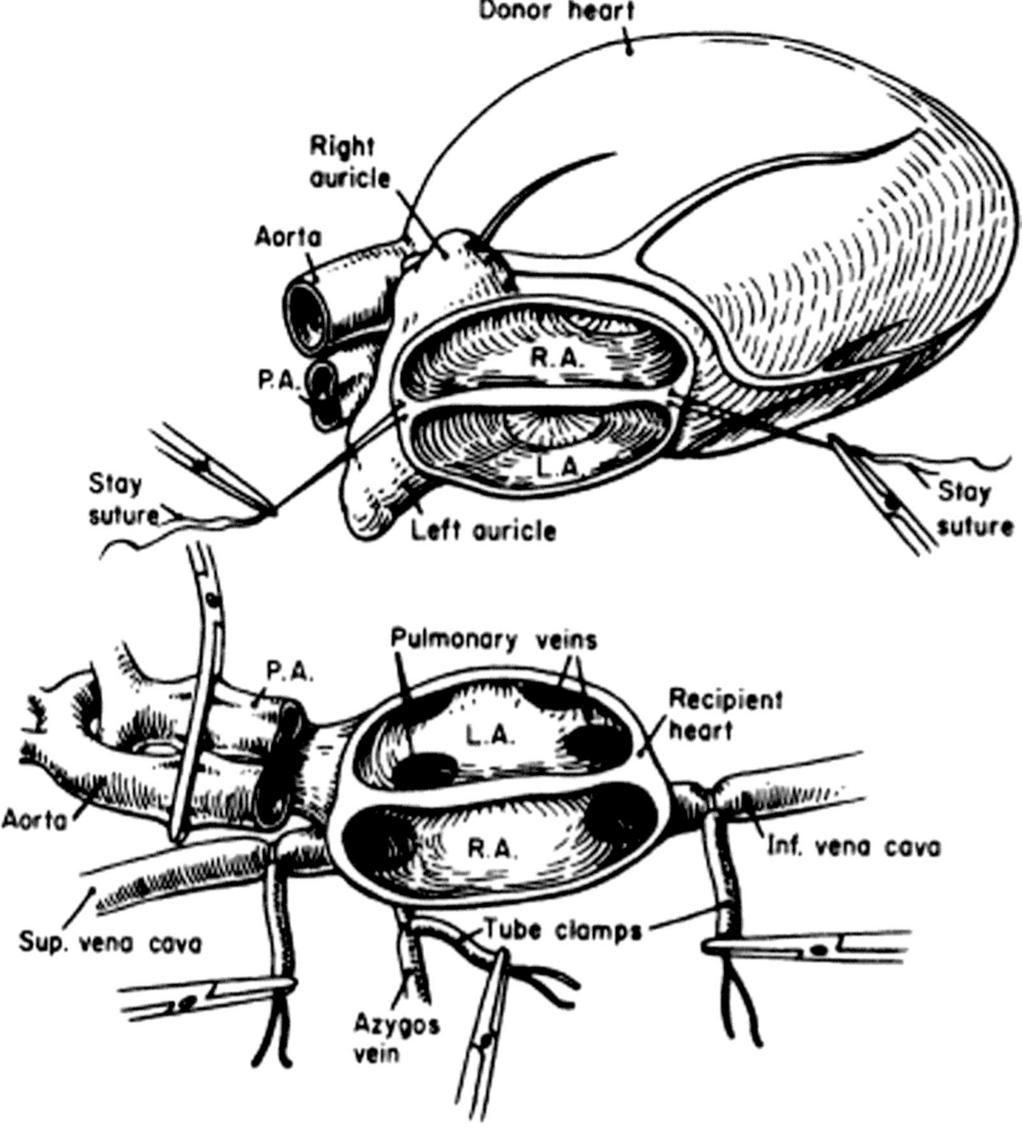


**Fig. 24.1** Surgical schematic of the first pediatric heart transplant performed by Adrian Kantrowitz on December 6, 1967. Reused with permission from Mendeloff EN. The history of pediatric heart and lung transplantation. Pediatric transplantation. 2002 Sep;6(4):270–9, published by JOHN WILEY AND SONS

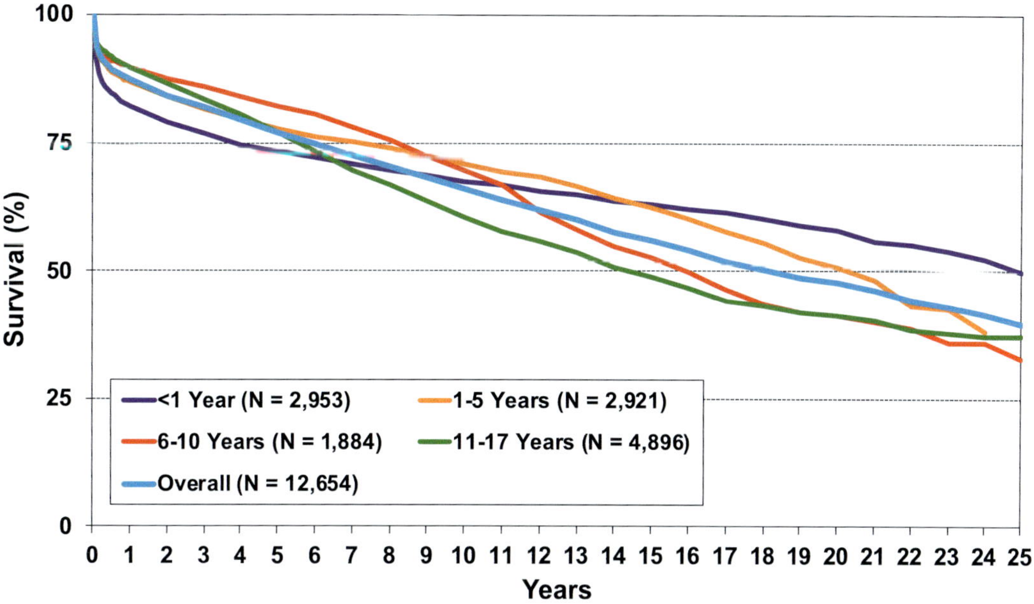


**Fig. 24.2** Kaplan–Meier survival curve in pediatric heart transplantation by age (January 1992- June 2017). *Source* Pediatric Heart Transplantation Statistics-2019 slides, JHLT. 2019 Oct; 38(10): 1015–1066, publicly available at: https://ishltregistries.org/downloadables/slides/2019/heart_pediatric.pptx

and his colleagues at Loma Linda attempted a xenotransplant between a baboon and a 12-day-old girl. The procedure was technically successful, although the recipient suffered severe acute rejection and died 20 days later [2]. The case was highly publicized and helped increase the availability of donor organs in the pediatric population. Bailey went on to perform human-to-human neonatal orthotopic HTx. Children who undergo HTx show excellent outcomes. Depending on the recipient's age, the median life expectancy is over 18 years after the first-year post-transplantation [3, 4]. (Fig. 24.2) Despite this, waitlist mortality is higher than for any other solid organ. The risk of death for infants less than 12 months of age in the USA is approximately 25%. The infants at higher risk were those on extracorporeal membrane oxygenation (ECMO) or requiring ventilator support, those with congenital heart disease, small infants with weight less than 3 kg, and infants of non-white race or ethnicity [5]. This is, in part, due to the lack of available mechanical circulatory support devices for this age group. However, there is a reduced waitlist mortality in children bridged with ventricular assist device (VAD) support as opposed to an earlier era during which this type of support was significantly less common. In general, centers performing HTx in pediatrics do not have sufficient cases to make statistically significant observations. For that reason, the Pediatric Heart Transplant Study (PHTS) was established in 1993 by six centers with the objective of advancing our understanding of the specialty by keeping an event-driven database that could be used for clinical research.

## Indications for Heart Transplantation

Pediatric HTx is the ultimate option in the treatment of end-stage heart disease refractory to maximum medical therapy or surgical management. Pediatric HTx comprise approximately 10% of total cases of HTx (Fig. 24.3) [6]. Cardiomyopathies and congenital heart defects collectively remain the most common indications for pediatric HTx. The primary diagnosis and indications, however, do vary significantly

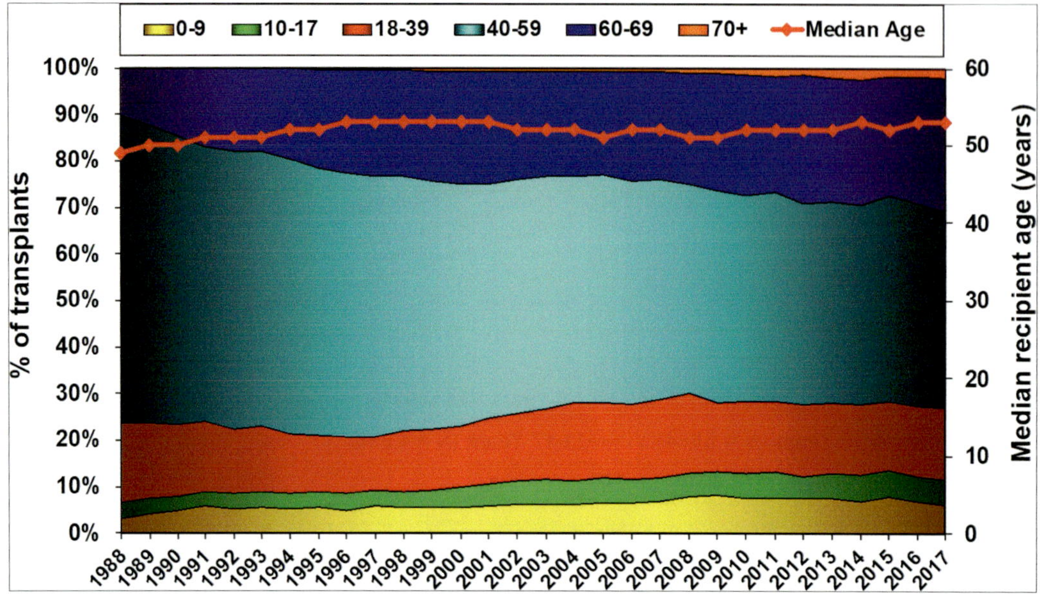


**Fig. 24.3** Total adult and pediatric heart transplantation by age and year. *Source* Pediatric Heart Transplantation Statistics-2019 slides, JHLT. 2019 Oct; 38(10): 1015–1066, publicly available at: https://ishltregistries.org/downloadables/slides/2019/heart_pediatric.pptx

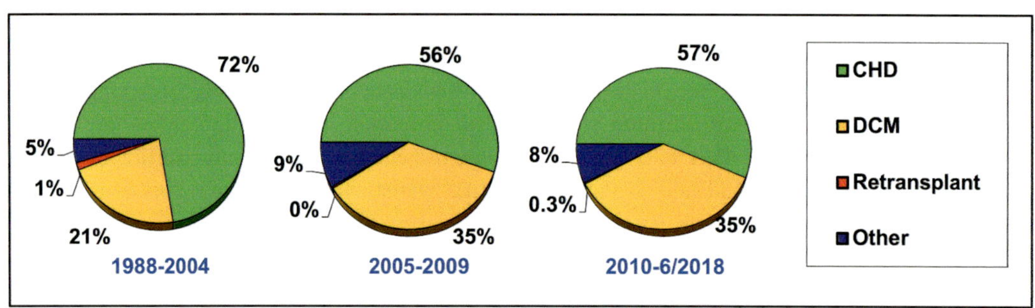


**Fig. 24.4** Pediatric heart transplant recipient diagnosis by age < 1 year. *Source* Pediatric Heart Transplantation Statistics-2019 slides, JHLT. 2019 Oct; 38(10): 1015–1066, publicly available at: https://ishltregistries.org/downloadables/slides/2019/heart_pediatric.pptx

by age. In infants < 1 year of age, repaired and unrepaired congenital heart disease is the most common underlying diagnosis (Fig. 24.4). In children > 1 year of age, cardiomyopathy, specifically dilated cardiomyopathy, becomes the most common underlying diagnosis, followed by congenital heart disease (Fig. 24.5) [7, 8]. The total annual number of pediatric HTx recorded by the registry of the International Society for Heart and Lung Transplantation (ISHLT) in the United States has remained relatively constant at between 400 and 600 from 1991 to 2017 (Fig. 24.6) [7]. However, the number of infants undergoing transplantation has increased over the past decade due to the growing availability of VAD, allowing longer waitlist times for small infants who would have otherwise died and broader acceptance of ABO incompatibility and donation after circulatory death (DCD), collectively allowing for more options. Nonetheless, the Pediatric Committee of the American Society of Transplantation [9] and a consensus

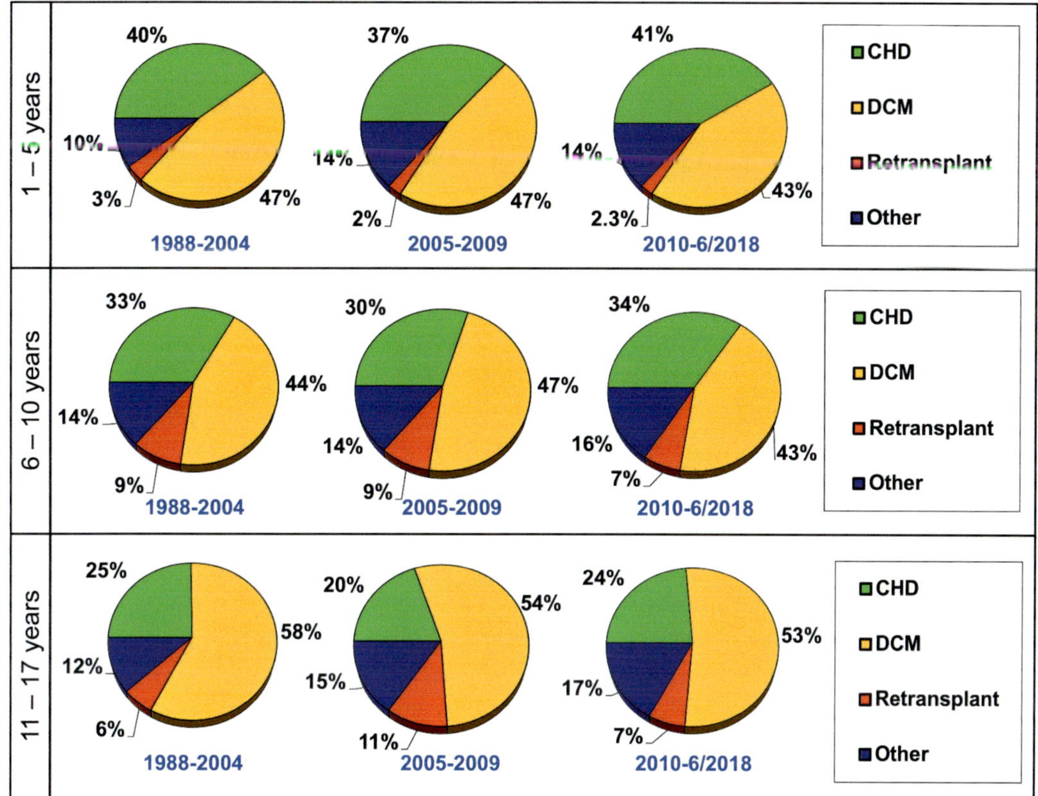


**Fig. 24.5** Pediatric heart transplant recipient diagnosis by age. *Source* Pediatric Heart Transplantation Statistics-2019 slides, JHLT. 2019 Oct; 38(10): 1015–1066, publicly available at: https://ishltregistries.org/downloadables/slides/2019/heart_pediatric.pptx

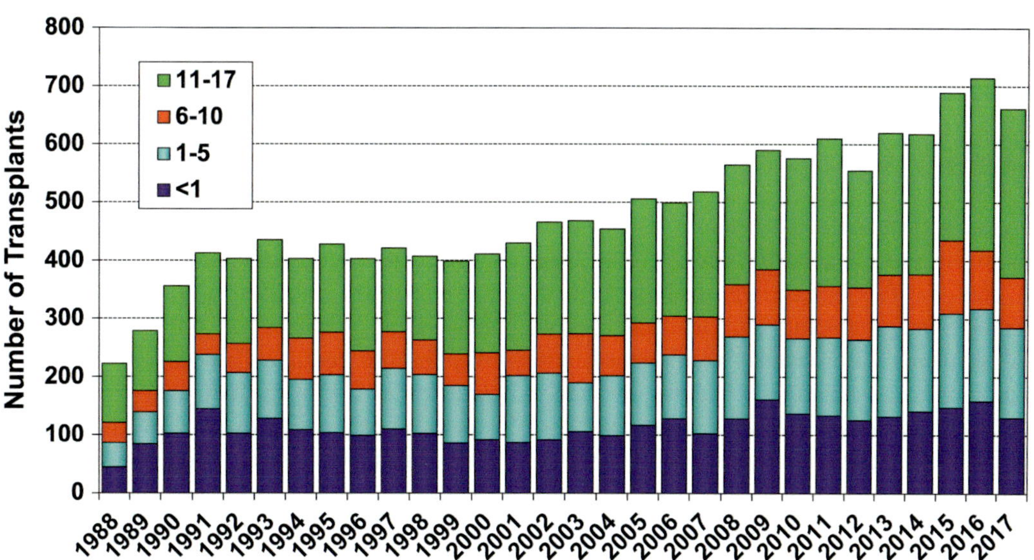


**Fig. 24.6** Pediatric heart transplantation—recipient age distribution by year. *Source* Pediatric Heart Transplantation Statistics-2019 slides, JHLT. 2019 Oct; 38(10): 1015–1066, publicly available at: https://ishltregistries.org/downloadables/slides/2019/heart_pediatric.pptx

group of the American Heart Association (AHA) [10] broadly agree on the indications as well as contraindications for HTx in children.

Congenital heart disease remains a common pre-operative diagnosis in the pediatric HTx population in the United States. It is the most common indication for transplantation during infancy (Fig. 24.4) [11]. However, cardiac transplantation as a primary therapy is becoming increasingly rare with advances and improved outcomes following palliative or corrective surgery. Instead, children are being referred, evaluated, and subsequently listed for end-stage cardiac disease and refractory heart failure without available medical or surgical options. The most common forms of congenital heart disease listed for transplantation are non-HLHS single-ventricle abnormalities (36%), followed by conditions in which the right ventricle functions as the systemic pump (20%) [10]. The failing Fontan population is another subset that is referred for transplantation. Primary cardiac transplantation is selectively recommended for severe systemic ventricular dysfunction, severe atrioventricular valve insufficiency, and occlusive coronary artery anomalies, particularly in those patients with pulmonary atresia with an intact ventricular septum. Notably, compared to survival following transplantation for cardiomyopathy, survival following transplantation for complex congenital heart disease is significantly lower [8].

## Candidate Evaluation

Evaluating pediatric candidates for HTx is similar to the process used for adults (see Chaps. 4 and 5). This chapter will examine considerations unique to children. Generally, potential recipients are evaluated for life expectancy, morbidity and weighing the relative advantages and disadvantages of alternative treatments. Due to the diverse pathologies leading to transplantation, special consideration must be given to the anatomy and hemodynamics. An assessment looking for chronic disease and the involvement of other organ systems is of particular importance in the pediatric population, given that heart failure etiologies such as inborn errors of metabolism will often have widespread effects. The issue of compatibility is somewhat different in children, as sensitization is not always preclusive. Genetic evaluation, particularly in neonates and infants, can be of critical importance in early assessment.

## Anatomy

The most important anatomical considerations relate to the systemic and pulmonary vasculature. Adequately developed, appropriately sized, and confluent pulmonary arteries are important for successful transplantation. Any anomalies of the venous return to the heart will also require special attention. If transplantation is being performed after previous palliative surgery, then caution is required in dealing with adhesions and anatomical distortions such as enlarged atria resulting from the Fontan procedure. The visceral anatomy of the heart is of minimal significance, given that it will be almost entirely removed. However, it does impact the sizing criteria when evaluating potential donor hearts.

## Pulmonary Vascular Resistance

An increase in pulmonary vascular resistance features in many forms of pediatric heart disease. Congenital heart disease is more strongly associated with pulmonary hypertension, particularly fixed forms. A recent retrospective study of the UNOS database [12] demonstrated that pulmonary vascular resistance was not an independent predictor of postoperative mortality in the pediatric population. The adult guideline is overly restrictive in the pediatric population, and patients with a PVRI of up to 9 Woods units/m$^2$ can safely undergo HTx [13]. In patients with a high PVRI, inotropes and vasodilators can be used intensively to reduce the PVRI pre-operatively. Strategies, including the pre-operative use of pulmonary vasodilators and the use of VADs, have pushed these boundaries. Inhaled nitric oxide, milrinone, and vasodilators may also be considered intra-operatively. A period of prolonged sedation and intubation may be warranted immediately following surgery. Delayed sternal closure is also an option postoperatively. Patients may also be started on oral, pulmonary vasodilators, including PDE-5 inhibitors (sildenafil, tadalafil), endothelium receptor antagonists (i.e., macitentan, ambrisentan), and prostacyclins. VADs are increasingly being used in the pediatric population as a bridge to transplant after their successful use in adults.

## ABO Incompatibility

The shortage of donors in the infant population led to ABO-incompatible (ABOi) transplantation on the basis that the immune system is underdeveloped in this age group. Infants with isohemagglutinin titers that show absent or low levels of antibodies can receive a heart from an ABOi donor with results comparable to ABO-compatible HTx [14]. Most recipients do not go on to form antibodies later in life despite no enhancements to their immunosuppressive therapy [15]. It has also been observed that post-HTx, these recipients were less likely to develop de novo donor-specific antibodies (particularly class II) or acute rejection [16, 17]. Even recipients who do form antibodies still have good outcomes [15]. In 2016 urgent candidates under one year of age were made eligible to be listed for ABOi donors regardless of the isohemagglutinin titer. In addition, patients between one and two years of age with isohemagglutinin titers less than or equal to 1:16 could be listed for these donors [18]. More recently, in March of 2023, the UNOS policy changed once again. At this time, patients who were status 1a, 1B, or 2 and under the age of 18 years could be listed for ABOi. More recently, older children have been successfully ABOi transplanted [19] All-cause mortality has been noted to be equivalent between ABO compatible and ABOi. One-, 5-, and 10-year survival rates among compatible vs. incompatible transplants were estimated to be 90 versus 88%, 82 versus 79%, and 77 versus 73%, respectively [18].

## Pre-transplant Sensitization

Sensitivity to human leukocyte antigen (HLA) and non-HLA donor antigens remains a significant factor in the already high waitlist mortality for children awaiting HTx. The presence of donor-specific antibodies (DSAs) carries the risk of allograft rejection and/or cardiac allograft vasculopathy (CAV) [20]. Sensitization can occur from blood products (especially platelets), palliative procedures for congenital heart disease, prior HTx, and the use of mechanical circulatory support devices (MCS) devices. It has also been suggested that preoperative treatment of allograft tissue used in congenital heart surgeries could prevent profound sensitization in patients requiring subsequent HTx [21]. Potential recipients are tested for panel reactive antibodies (PRA). Testing demonstrates preformed anti-HLA antibodies. Most centers now use Luminex® solid phase flow beads to detect alloantibodies. Patients with a PRA > 10% are considered sensitized and are at increased risk of graft loss [22]. However, data from the Clinical Trials in Organ Transplant-04 (CTOTC-04) suggest comparable 1-year survival among highly sensitized and non-sensitized pediatric HTx recipients [23]. Many centers perform HLA typing so that "virtual" cross-matching can be done once a potential donor is found. In an analysis of the 3914 patients enrolled in the Pediatric Heart Transplant Society Registry database for the years 2010–2021, a shorter time to first rejection was observed in patients with positive crossmatch compared to those with negative crossmatch with no between-group difference in 10 years mortality [24]. Moreover, clinicians should take into consideration that HLA antibodies may be high in the first 12–18 months after birth (passively acquired maternally) or be falsely low such as in pediatric patients following Fontan surgery who have protein-losing enteropathy [25]. Desensitization strategies were developed with the ultimate goal of increasing the available donor pool. These included mechanical removal of antibodies, intravenous immunoglobulins, and novel immunosuppressive agents targeting antibody production. However, the use of plasmapheresis/immunoadsorption in the pediatric population is hampered by low blood volume, vascular access limitations, side effects, as well as patient compliance [26].

## Infection

All potential recipients require serological evaluation for Epstein-Barr virus (EBV), cytomegalovirus (CMV), *Toxoplasma gondii*, HIV, varicella zoster virus (VZV), measles, hepatitis, and HIV. Positive results are now rarely an absolute contraindication for HTx but help determine necessary prophylactic treatments and perioperative management plans. HIV was once considered an absolute contraindication. With newer anti-retroviral therapies, survival is now over 90% at 10-years [27]. Good outcomes have been realized for HIV-positive adults who are compliant and have low or undetectable viral loads at the time of transplantation [28]. HTx recipients who are seropositive for hepatitis B show similar survival rates to those who are seronegative. However, the majority of deaths in seropositive patients are due to hepatitis [29]. EBV infection, either preoperatively or postoperatively (usually from donor tissue), puts the patient at risk for post-transplant lymphoproliferative disease (PTLD). Patients must be vaccinated against measles, mumps, rubella, *Hemophilus influenzae*, VZV, pneumococcus, and hepatitis A and B prior to transplantation.

## Other Organ Systems

Severe and irreversible end-organ damage, including kidney and liver failure, are usually considered contraindications to single orthotopic HTx. Multisystem organ failure carries a 1-year post-transplant mortality of 16.6% in children [3]. Requiring dialysis prior to transplantation is the second worst risk factor for 1-year mortality [3]. Given that immunosuppressive agents are highly nephrotoxic, children with moderate to severe renal impairment should be considered for combined heart-kidney transplantation [30]. End-stage liver failure or cirrhosis is most often seen in patients with single ventricle physiology who have undergone the Fontan procedure. These patients may require combined heart-liver transplantation. This procedure has been rare in the pediatric population, with 1, 3, and 5-year survivals of 93, 93, and 93% [31]. Diabetes mellitus is rarer in the pediatric population and is not considered an absolute contraindication. At present, there is no data supporting worse outcomes based on increased BMI. There was data that demonstrated increased wait times on the list for patients with increased BMI [32]. A review of the PHTS database showed few children were listed for transplantation when their BMI was more than 2 standard deviations above normal [33]. As patients on the waitlist for HTx may have difficulty with exercising, a trained nutritionist is an essential member of the HTx team.

## Psychosocial Factors

Family support is paramount to successful transplantation and long-term survival. A full assessment of the psychosocial state of the family and potential caretakers should be made. The goal is to include the child's well-being and ensure the long-term success of the transplant. A supportive family environment is essential as the care can be demanding. Compliance with care is essential. Financial resources, including insurance that will cover the hospital costs and long-term costs of medications, are necessary. It is important to consider the ability to pay for housing, food, and sundries. Access to reliable transportation is paramount. The follow-up will consist of frequent clinic appointments, procedures, and lab visits.

## Donor Selection

The number and quality of donor hearts remain significant limiting factors in pediatric HTx. An ISHLT consensus statement noted that potential HTx recipients outnumber the number of donors, and there continues to be significant waitlist mortality. In spite of this, approximately 40% of organ offers are turned down [34]. Common reasons for declining an organ included the prolonged use of cardiopulmonary resuscitation (CPR), the use of high-dose inotropes, blunt trauma to the chest wall, and prolonged ischemia time [35]. Also, donor size, donor age, cause of death, need for high-dose inotropes, and infection were reasons for declining a potential donor organ [34]. The lack of studies means clinicians rely on experience or data from the adult population. As a result, the donor pool may be unnecessarily narrow. Until recently, vital organ donation from children could only occur after a diagnosis of brain death has been established. There are also additional criteria that vary according to age [36]. In addition, an interval of between 12 and 48 h between two evaluations is required [36]. More recently, in response to a shortage of suitable donors, DCD has become an option for more centers. A review of the UNOS registry from June 2004 to June 2022 demonstrated seven children (<18 y.o.) who underwent HTx from a DCD donor [37]. Donor evaluation should include gender, age, weight, height, the cause of death, a review of any chest trauma, inotrope use, and hemodynamic status. Donor hearts have been declined in the past because of CPR use, but it has been shown to have no impact on outcomes [38]. Survival outcomes were not impacted by factors such as donor cause of death, need for CPR or inotropes [39]. Allograft ischemic time is a risk factor for survival in older children, particularly those 11–17 years old, and has almost no impact on the survival of infants < 1 year old. Longer ischemic times did not have an effect on overall recipient survival however it did negatively impact one year survival [39]. An echocardiogram should be done to exclude structural and functional abnormalities. Several adult and pediatric studies have shown a decreased utilization of the donor heart when the left ventricular (LV) ejection fraction was < 50%. This also included segmental wall abnormalities. Current ISHLT guidelines recommend refusal of donor hearts when the LV ejection fraction is less than 40% [34]. The donor echocardiogram is an important part of the decision-making process. The ECG normally shows non-specific changes that are due to hemostatic disturbances resulting from brain death. The donor to recipient weight ratio is used for size matching. An undersized donor with a ratio below 0.6 is associated with worse outcomes and most centers avoid going below 0.75 [40]. This is especially the case if the recipient suffers from pulmonary hypertension. Oversizing the donor can be done safely up to a weight ratio of 3 [41]. Donors should have serological screening for infectious agents, including, HIV, hepatitis, human T-cell lymphotropic virus (HTLV), CMV, EBV, syphilis and *Toxoplasma gondii*. A positive result for HIV, HTLV, hepatitis B or hepatitis C precludes organ use. Finding antibodies for *T. gondii*, CMV or EBV do not contraindicate transplantation but guide post-operative management. Experienced donor support is important for organ preservation. Invasive monitoring is crucial to provide hemodynamic monitoring. Brain death is usually followed by autonomic and inflammatory changes. Initially there is a catecholamine surge and subsequently a period of hypotension secondary to vasoplegia and loss of vascular tone. Hypovolemia can be seen secondary to the onset of diabetes insipidus. Management of these derangements can include inotropic and/or vasopressor support, volume repletion as well as hormonal replacement therapy [34].

## Wait List Management

The evaluation of a candidate being considered for HTx requires a multidisciplinary approach. The majority of centers meet in order to present the candidate to a multidisciplinary team consisting of the evaluating team members and the remainder team members. Many of these teams now incorporate an ethicist as well. The decision is made on suitability for transplant and urgency of listing. It is also important to note that patient life expectancy in pediatrics exceeds the current expected graft survival so re-transplantation would be necessary. Although as a group, children awaiting HTx have the worst survival of all solid organ wait lists, [42] when stratified, subgroups show large variabilities in mortality. Recent data demonstrates a mortality on the waiting list of 13% in children and 25% in infants [43]. Multiple studies have assessed risk factors for mortality or delisting. Factors demonstrating an association with death or delisting include: age, gender, insurance, race, blood type, diagnosis, weight, VAD use, inotrope use, ventilator use, defibrillator use, ECMO use, dialysis use, comorbid cancer, creatinine, and UNOS region [44]. Interestingly, hemodynamic support more reliably predicts wait list mortality than UNOS listing status [45]. The UNOS allocation policy for pediatrics was last revised in 2016. The changes resulted in a small decrease in the number of patients listed at the highest urgency status. The Organ Procurement and Transplantation Network (OPTN) considers it a priority to allocate donor hearts to those of the highest urgency. Donor allocation is determined by medical urgency, blood type and distance between the recipient and donor hospital. The changes enacted in 2016 included (1) reduced priority for candidates with cardiomyopathy, (2) requirement for hospital admission of candidates with "significant" congenital heart disease on high-dose inotropes to qualify for status 1A listing, and (3) removal of in utero listing mechanisms [46].

## Bridge to Transplant

Progression of heart failure despite maximal medical therapy is an indication for mechanical circulatory support with either ECMO or a VAD. The first VAD placed in a pediatric patient was performed in the 1960's by Dr. Michael DeBakey [47]. Children, and especially infants, were once limited in their treatment options for bridging to transplant due to a lack of VADs secondary to size limitations. The smallest patient to date who had an adult device placed had a body surface area of 0.78 $m^2$ [48]. A review of data from the PHTS of patients < 18 years over a 22-year period ending on December 31, 2015 demonstrated that of 7135 patients listed for HTx 995 (19.3%) were supported by VADs. The majority of patients placed on a VAD were older most likely due to device availability. The current limited availability of VADs due to patient size and anatomy has an impact on their use. Currently the Berlin Heart EXCOR®, the pedi- and centrimag as well as the HeartMate 3 are available for use. This has led to innovative methods to bridge the smaller patients with the available technology. Since the introduction of VADs aimed at children, its use has significantly increased, with 29% of children receiving VADs or total artificial hearts (TAH) [49, 50]. ECMO use has dropped to 5% in all children but is still 30% in the infant age group [3]. Biventricular VAD use now exceeds ECMO use [3]. Transplantation or recovery occurred in 75% of children with the EXCOR®. Mortality was 25% and the leading cause of death was thromboembolic stroke [51]. Decreased renal function, smaller patient size and elevated total bilirubin were additional risk factors for death when on EXOR® VAD therapy [51].

## Post-operative Management and Complications

### Cardiovascular System

Maintaining cardiac output (CO) post-operatively is the most significant management objective. The donor heart will have suffered a variable degree of ischemic injury during transplantation. Notably, greater than 4 h of ischemic time is associated with higher mortality in the first 30 days after transplantation due to primary graft failure [52]. Added to this are the effects of denervation, the lack of sympathetic control over the donor heart, and depleted catecholamine reserve. Support with inotropes is recommended for the first few days with a gradual wean guided by the recipients clinical status. During low cardiac output state and in the presence of systemic or pulmonary hypertension, milrinone, which has both positive inotropic, lusitropic, and vasodilator effects, can be especially beneficial. Vasopressin is typically used in vasodilatory shock in concert with other agents depending on the significance of hemodynamic instability. In infants who received an oversized heart, delayed closure can assist in supporting CO. If the CO cannot be maintained despite continuous infusion of inotropes, or if the patient was not able to be weaned off cardiopulmonary bypass intraoperatively and required ECMO, then primary graft dysfunction (PGD) should be suspected. The ISHLT guidelines recommend ECMO as the first choice for support for PGD [53]. Atrial pacing (or AV pacing if there is concern for conduction defects) via temporary pacing wires placed intraoperatively can be used to augment cardiac output while awaiting sinus node recovery. Sinus tachycardia is also common due to impaired vagal input in the denervated heart. Ventricular arrhythmias, especially ventricular ectopic beats and non-sustained ventricular tachycardia are seen in the early post-operatively period and usually do not require any treatment other than replacement of serum potassium and magnesium for subtherapeutic levels. Hypertension is a common complication owing to several contributory factors. Changes to the systemic vasculature in heart failure, initiation of corticosteroids and calcineurin inhibitors, and an oversized donor can all cause systemic hypertension.

## Respiratory System

Early extubation should be attempted where possible. Some recipients may have had mechanical ventilation for a prolonged period of time prior to transplantation. These patients need to retrain their respiratory muscles and will require additional support. Pulmonary hypertension was once regarded as a contraindication to early extubation but now appears safe in children who have undergone cardiac surgery [54]. The details of pulmonary hypertension as it pertains to the pediatric HTx population is discussed in detail earlier in the chapter. The right ventricle must be supported with catecholamines in addition to the usual post-operative regimen of positive inotropes. This allows time for the donor heart to adapt to the higher pressures. Post-operatively, inhaled nitric oxide may be continued to aid in extubation and weaning of respiratory support. For patients with single ventricle physiology and elevated PVRi prior to transplantation, and those already on PH therapy—pulmonary vasodilators may be continued until there is objective clinical and echocardiographic or hemodynamic data from catheterization that demonstrates a normalizing PVRi [55].

## Renal Function

Deranged renal function is a common complication. The kidney is susceptible to damage from underperfusion that can occur in heart failure, cardiopulmonary bypass, post-operative hypotension and low cardiac output syndrome, and with initiation of post-transplant immunosuppressants that are nephrotoxic, specifically calcineurin inhibitors (CNIs) like tacrolimus and cyclosporine. Although there is some degree of oliguria in the post-operative period, outright renal failure is rare early after transplantation.

## Gastrointestinal System

A variety of gastrointestinal (GI) problems can occur early and late after HTx in children. Stress ulcers are a concern in the post-operative period and as such patients should be given a type-2 histamine receptor antagonist prophylactically. Patients on corticosteroids or azathioprine are at increased risk of pancreatitis. Abdominal pain reported by these children warrants investigational follow-up. Enteral nutrition should be initiated early with cautious up titration of the feeding regimen. Infants, particularly those who have never fed orally, may require a nasogastric tube (NGT) for enteral feeding for a prolonged period. Some may require a percutaneous gastrostomy tube placement or a surgical gastrostomy tube if they are unable to wean off NGT feeding in the setting of oral aversion or poor PO tolerance.

## Immunosuppression

Immunosuppression in pediatric HTx recipients has been largely guided by protocols in the adult population and clinical experience. Review of the PHTS database demonstrates that while the use of induction therapy results in decreased episodes of graft rejection, the overall survival in both the low and high-risk groups is unchanged. After transplantation, it is becoming increasingly common for induction therapy to be the starting point for immunosuppression followed by maintenance therapy. The evidence on induction therapy remains equivocal. There is reportedly no difference in survival 14 days post-transplant [3]. Review of the PHTS data from 2001 to 2014 demonstrated 73% of newly transplanted patients received induction therapy. Of the group 48% were given ATG (from rabbits or horses) while the remaining 25% were given interleukin 2 receptor blockers (basiliximab) [56, 57]. Induction therapy is useful for children with a low urine-output post-operatively to delay commencement of nephrotoxic calcineurin inhibitors. Maintenance regimens are normally based on a CNI such as tacrolimus or cyclosporine. The antiproliferative drug mycophenolate mofetil (MMF) can be used in combination and has been shown to have superiority over azathioprine in adults [58]. Also in certain cases mTor inhibitors such as sirolimus or everolimus can be used in combination with a CNI. Early studies have suggested an increased time to cardiac allograft vasculopathy [56]. There is evidence to suggest that steroid-avoidance regimens can achieve equally good outcomes with fewer side effects in children who are not sensitized [59]. The side effects of these medications also play a role in guiding the immunosuppression regimen. CNIs are known to be nephrotoxic. For this reason, renal function is closely monitored. At a certain point, it may be necessary to move to a renal-sparing protocol. This may include MMF and mTor inhibitors, which are both hepatically cleared. MMF is more commonly known for its GI side effects, so an enteric-coated form can be utilized. Compliance must be reiterated, especially as the patient becomes older and more independent.

## Infection

Taking precautions to prevent infection is an essential part of the post-operative management plan. Infection is a leading cause of mortality early on after transplantation. The usual sources of infection for the surgical patient—lines, drains, and catheters—are replaced in the operating room and should be removed as soon as possible after transplantation. The most common pathogens in the postoperative period are coagulase-negative staphylococci as well as staph aureus (MSSA or MRSA) [60]. A prophylactic, short course of intravenous antibiotics is given in the immediate postoperative period. This is typically a first-generation and/or vancomycin. Patients who require prolonged intensive care or patients already colonized with MRSA require coverage with vancomycin. Prophylaxis for *Pneumocystis jirovecii* is initiated in all patients. The risk for this is highest in the first 6 months post-transplant. Patients previously on MCS therapy are at increased risk of fungal infections (particularly *Candida* and *Aspergillus*). Although fluconazole can be administered prophylactically, caution is needed because of the interaction with CNIs. Fluconazole inhibits the cytochrome P450 system that is required for CNI metabolism. Therefore, an appropriate dose reduction is required for tacrolimus. The serologic status for CMV of both the donor and recipient is central in determining the risk for the recipient. It is strongly recommended to use prophylactic therapy when there is a mismatch, especially with donor (D)+/recipient

(R)−. Prophylaxis is still recommended in cases of R+/D− however, the duration of therapy may vary. The data for prophylaxis for EBV is inconsistent [60]. While the current prophylaxis may prevent the onset of EBV viremia, frequent monitoring is paramount.

### Rejection Surveillance

Despite significant advances in the field of pediatric HTx, acute and chronic rejection remain important causes of morbidity and mortality. Endomyocardial biopsy (EMB) is the current gold standard for diagnosing allograft rejection. Children are monitored closely in the days following transplantation for symptoms and signs of early rejection. Any abdominal pain, tachycardia, new arrhythmias, and oliguria should be investigated further with an ECG and possibly EMB to exclude rejection. However, there is no consensus on the optimal surveillance protocols, and there remain significant differences across institutions in the use of routine surveillance biopsies to detect asymptomatic rejection [61]. Traditional cardio-diagnostic modalities, including echocardiography, electrocardiography, and CMR, are regaining their popularity in rejection surveillance, along with serum biomarkers such as BNP (or NT-proBNP) and donor-specific antibodies (DSAs). Furthermore, novel non-invasive methods for detecting asymptomatic rejection, such as immune cell function assay [62], gene expression profiling [63, 64], and circulating donor-derived cell-free DNA (dd cf-DNA), [65] have similarly emerged as suitable alternatives to routine surveillance biopsies.

### Rejection

Allograft rejection is generally categorized temporally and subcategorized based on type. For example, hyperacute rejection occurs intraoperatively or within hours of transplantation. Acute rejection occurs within the first week to 1-month post-transplantation. Chronic or late rejection occurs > 1 year post-transplantation. While the risk of rejection is the highest in the first year post-transplantation, reported data from two large registries, including PHTS and ISHLT, have shown a decline in rejection in the first year post-transplantation, as well as an overall decline in rejection over time [8, 66]. Allograft rejection is also characterized based on the type of rejection noted on EMB. Specifically, cellular or antibody-mediated. Cellular rejection is mediated by cytotoxic T-cells, while B-cells are implicated in antibody-mediated rejection. There are also benign findings in the form of non-specific inflammation called Quilty lesions that may be found on routine surveillance biopsies, which has only been observed in the CNI era [67]. Treatment for acute rejection is multifaceted and depends on various factors, including but limited to time post-transplant, type and grade of rejection based on EMB, clinical presentation, hemodynamic effect, co-morbidities, and confounding co-factors such as infection or non-adherence to maintenance immunosuppression. Typical treatment is with intravenous corticosteroids and may involve IVIG, plasmapheresis, adjustment of immunosuppression depending on the etiology, and initiation of novel monoclonal antibody treatment protocols.

## Long-Term Complications

### Cardiac Allograft Vasculopathy

Long-term or late complications beyond 1-year post-transplantation continue to decline over time. However, with improvements in survival, the development of cardiac allograft vasculopathy (CAV) and chronic rejection are of increasing concern. In children who survive to three years post-transplantation, CAV is a leading cause of death after graft failure [3, 8] (Fig. 24.7). Risk factors for long-term or late rejection include early rejection, presence of anti-HLA antibodies, older age, African American race, and non-adherence [68]. Specific risk factors for the development of CAV include older recipient age, older donor age, recipient black race, transplant era, no

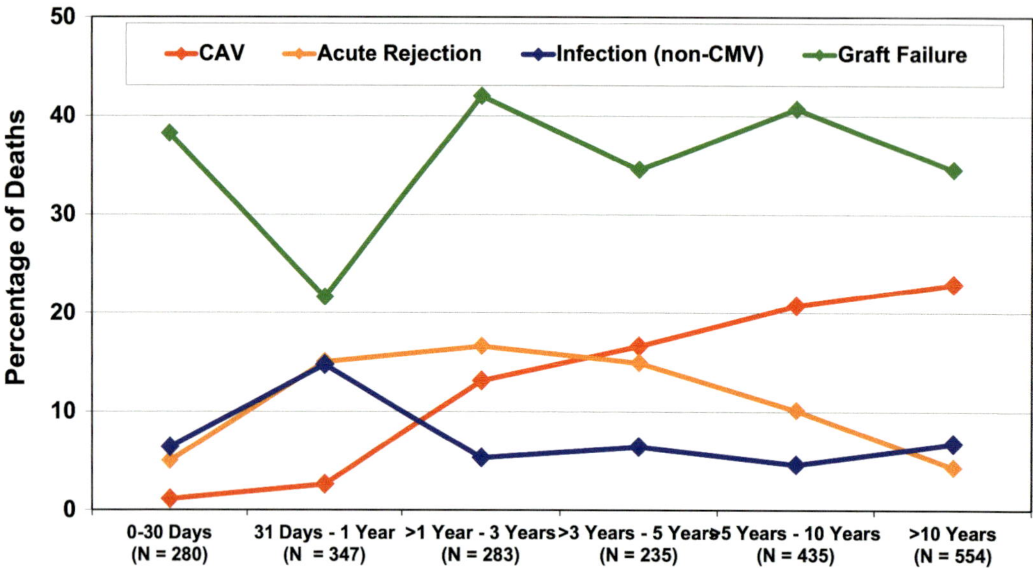


**Fig. 24.7** Relative incidence of leading cause of death in pediatric heart transplants (December 2005–June 2018). *Source* Pediatric Heart Transplantation Statistics-2019 slides, JHLT. 2019 Oct; 38(10): 1015–1066, publicly available at: https://ishltregistries.org/downloadables/slides/2019/heart_pediatric.pptx

induction therapy, early and recurrent episodes of rejection, and re-transplantation [69, 70]. From a symptoms standpoint, it is important to note that children with CAV often lack ischemic chest pain but may experience abdominal discomfort instead due to compromised end-organ perfusion to the gut. It is common for syncope or sudden death to be the first clinical manifestation of CAV in children. As such, surveillance coronary angiograms are frequently part of the long-term management plan and remain the current gold standard for diagnosing CAV. The degree of CAV is classified on a standardized ISHLT-graded system that additionally takes into account echocardiographic parameters. Other modalities, including intravascular ultrasound, cardiac MRI, and optical coherence tomography, have been previously proposed as complementary or alternative tools for the diagnosis of CAV. Although intravascular ultrasound has shown to be more sensitive for detecting CAV in adults, this has yet to be proven in children. Consequently, its use varies by institution and is limited to older children due to the size of the available catheters. From a pathophysiologic standpoint, CAV results in diastolic dysfunction due to microvascular disease. This eventually progresses to systolic dysfunction and carries a poor survival rate. While there are no definitive treatment options currently available, statins have been shown to slow the development and progression of CAV in adult studies. Many maintenance protocols for the management of pediatric HTx recipients employ statin therapy. Although beta-blockers may also provide benefits owing to their anti-ischemic effects, they are rarely used in this setting. As with adults, interventional techniques, such as stenting, do not improve outcomes, highlighted by the 52% graft loss at one-year post-procedure [71]. Retransplantation remains the only effective treatment once systolic failure ensues.

## Infection and Malignancy

The lifelong immunosuppression endured by children puts them at risk of infection from a broad spectrum of pathogens. Most infections are successfully treated; however, infection remains the second most common cause of death in the first month after transplantation and the most common reason for re-hospitalization in the first year post-transplantation [3]. Both opportunistic pathogens and ordinary pathogens afflict immunosuppressed children. Bacterial infections, specifically in the blood and lungs, predominate in the first month, while viral infections peak at two months [72]. Any signs of infection after transplantation should be treated empirically and immediately with broad-spectrum antibiotics until the causative pathogen is identified. A blood culture and/or endotracheal culture, if the patient is intubated, should be obtained to identify a source, and antibiotics should be appropriately tailored once the culture has been speciated and sensitivities have resulted. Antifungal coverage may be indicated on occasion. A full infection screen should be done, and the chest radiograph should be examined for evidence of pneumonia. Serum biomarkers of inflammation, including white blood cell count with a differential, C-reactive protein, and procalcitonin, should be obtained and trended. CMV infection remains a concern in this patient population. It predominantly affects the lungs and gastrointestinal tract, typically causing viral pneumonia requiring varying degrees of respiratory support based on its severity and diarrhea resulting in malabsorption, poor weight, and abdominal pain, respectively. Although it is common for CMV prophylaxis to be used in recipients who receive hearts from CMV-positive donors, its use has been shown to have no impact on the long-term complications of transplantation, such as the development of CAV or mortality [73]. Infection from CMV is detected with either PCR or pp65 antigen testing. Early detection usually results in successful treatment with ganciclovir or valganciclovir. EBV is similarly an important pathogen in the transplant recipient. Children are more susceptible than adults to EBV-induced PTLD. This is because immunity to EBV is typically acquired in adulthood. EBV infection can be difficult to identify as, even in the immunosuppressed patient, it can be asymptomatic or present with mild, non-specific symptoms. However, children with positive serology for EBV pre-transplant are still at risk. In addition to the disease itself, PTLD is a concern because the treatment—typically involving reduction of immunosuppression, can cause rebound rejection and lead to graft failure. This, in fact, accounts for half of deaths in children diagnosed with PTLD.

## Survival and Outcomes

Survival in pediatric HTx has shown considerable improvements over the last decade. Long-term survival in children now surpasses that of adults. Post-transplant survival was impacted by the era during which the transplant was performed. The 1-year post-transplant survival improved to 92% between 2012 and 2017. This improved survival across all age groups. One-year survival in recipients < 1 year of age is 89%, 92% in recipients between 1 and 10 years of age, and 94% in recipients 10–17 years of age. Differences in 1-year survivals were also noted between different diagnoses; however, they were improved over the prior era. Survival among recipients with the diagnosis of dilated cardiomyopathy, congenital heart disease, and retransplantation were 95, 88, and 91%, respectively (Fig. 24.8). 5-year conditional survival was 91.2% in infants less than one year, 92.3% in recipients between 1 and 10 years, and 88% in children 11–17 years (Fig. 24.9). The decrease in survival in the older age group may be impacted by compliance issues [74]. In evaluation of the different eras, there is a significant difference in freedom from CAV (Fig. 24.10). Data from the ISHLT shows that ten-year survival is 12% less for congenital heart disease patients than for cardiomyopathy patients.

## Equity

Children of minority race or ethnicity have been shown to have worse outcomes [75]. Children of black race are sicker at the time of listing. This leads to increased use of a VAD as a bridge to transplant. Early post-VAD outcomes are equal between white and non-white recipients [75]. Of note is the increase in graft loss after 1 year for

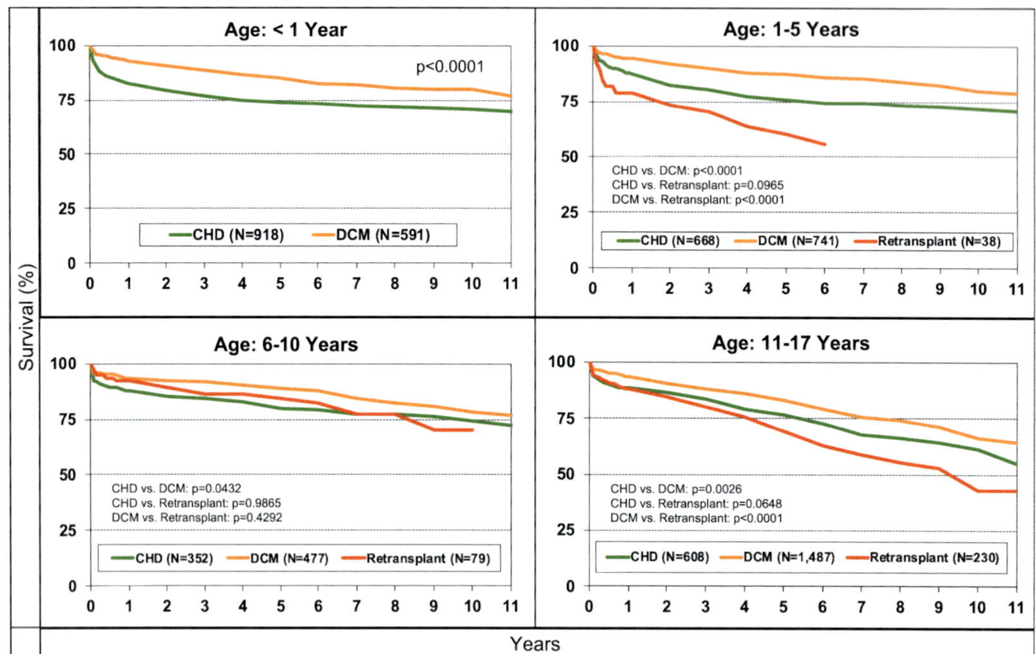


**Fig. 24.8** Kaplan–Meier survival in pediatric heart transplants by recipient age group and diagnosis (January 2005–June 2017). *Source* Pediatric Heart Transplantation Statistics-2019 slides, JHLT. 2019 Oct; 38(10): 1015–1066, publicly available at: https://ishltregistries.org/downloadables/slides/2019/heart_pediatric.pptx

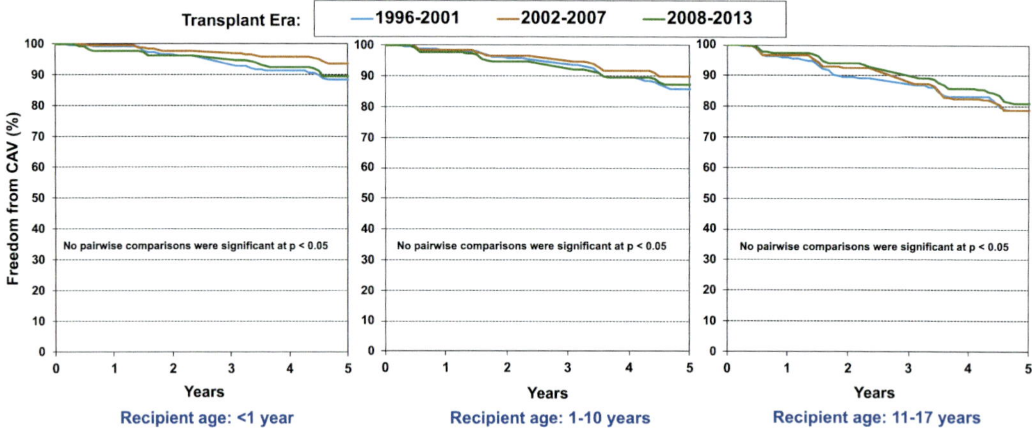


**Fig. 24.9** Freedom from CAV conditional on survival to discharge in pediatric heart transplants by recipient age and era (January 1996–June 2013). *Source* Pediatric Heart Transplantation Focus Theme, JHLT. 2021 Oct; 40(10): 1023–1072, Publicly available at: https://ishltregistries.org/downloadables/slides/2021/Pediatric_Heart_Transplantation_Focus_Theme.pptx

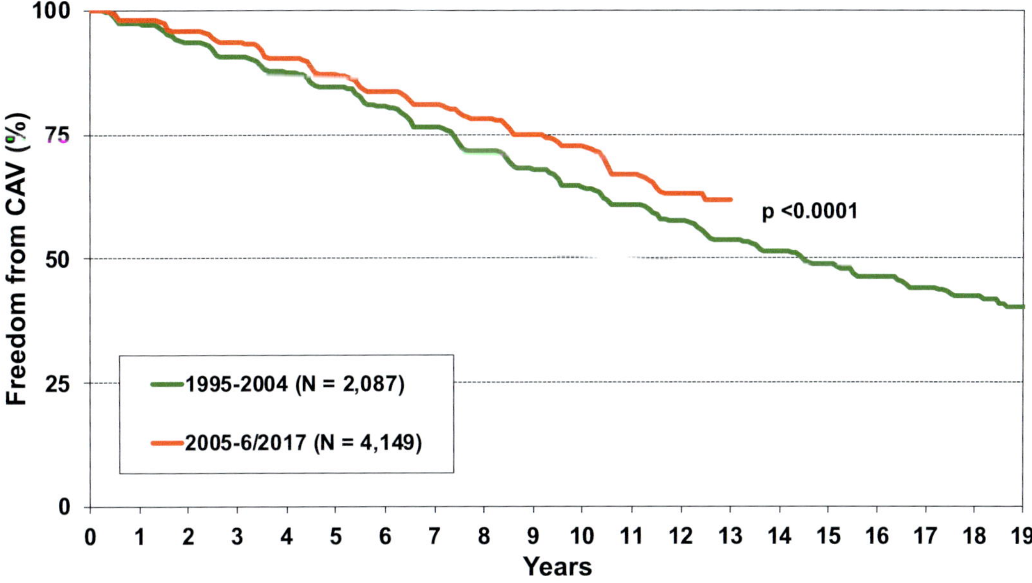


**Fig. 24.10** Freedom from CAV by era in pediatric heart transplants (January 1995–June 2017). *Source* Pediatric Heart Transplantation Statistics-2019 slides, JHLT. 2019 Oct; 38(10): 1015–1066, publicly available at: https://ishltregistries.org/downloadables/slides/2019/heart_pediatric.pptx

black patients as well as those of lower socioeconomic status [76]. At the time of listing, black children are older and sicker. They also face an increased waitlist mortality [77]. This was independent of patients receiving induction therapy as well as the incidence of treated rejection. A survey of clinicians from the Pediatric Heart Transplant Society demonstrated an implicit preference for individuals who are white and of higher socioeconomic status, as well as an explicit bias for educated people [78]. This warrants further investigation into how these biases impact clinician behavior.

## Summary

Since 1967, when Adrian Kantrowitz became the first pediatric patient to undergo a HTx, there have been major advances in the field. Survivals have improved on both the pre-and post-transplant sides. Waitlist survival has improved due to improved algorithms for the treatment of heart failure, aggressive donor utilization strategies, and improved access to suitable VAD, especially in the infant population. Post-transplant survivals continue to improve with improved regimens of immunosuppression and invasive and non-invasive techniques for monitoring rejection. The expertise of the congenital heart surgeons, pediatric transplant cardiologists, and multidisciplinary team members has resulted in improved survival and a positive quality of life.

## References

1. Kantrowitz A, Haller JD, Joos H, Cerruti MM, Carstensen HE. Transplantation of the heart in an infant and an adult. Am J Cardiol. 1968;22(6):782–90.
2. Bailey LL, Nehlsen-Cannarella SL, Concepcion W, Jolley WB. Baboon-to-human cardiac xenotransplantation in a neonate. JAMA. 1985;254(23):3321–9.
3. Dipchand AI, Rossano JW, Edwards LB, Kucheryavaya AY, Benden C, Goldfarb S, et al. The registry of the International Society for Heart and Lung Transplantation: eighteenth official pediatric heart transplantation report–2015; focus theme: early graft failure. J Heart Lung Transplant. 2015;34(10):1233–43.
4. Rossano JW, Singh TP, Cherikh WS, Chambers DC, Harhay MO, Hayes D Jr, et al. The

International Thoracic Organ Transplant registry of the International Society for Heart and Lung Transplantation: twenty-second pediatric heart transplantation report - 2019; focus theme: donor and recipient size match. J Heart Lung Transplant. 2019;38(10):1028–41.
5. Denfield SW, Azeka E, Das B, Garcia-Guereta L, Irving C, Kemna M, et al. Pediatric cardiac wait-list mortality-Still too high. Pediatr Transplant. 2020;24(3):e13671.
6. Taylor DO, Edwards LB, Boucek MM, Trulock EP, Deng MC, Keck BM, et al. Registry of the International Society for Heart and Lung Transplantation: twenty-second official adult heart transplant report–2005. J Heart Lung Transplant. 2005;24(8):945–55.
7. Rossano JW, Dipchand AI, Edwards LB, Goldfarb S, Kucheryavaya AY, Levvey Rn BJ, et al. The registry of the International Society for Heart and Lung Transplantation: nineteenth pediatric heart transplantation report-2016; focus theme: primary diagnostic indications for transplant. J Heart Lung Transplant. 2016;35(10):1185–95.
8. Dipchand AI. Current state of pediatric cardiac transplantation. Ann Cardiothorac Surg. 2018;7(1):31–55.
9. Fricker FJ, Addonizio L, Bernstein D, Boucek M, Boucek R, Canter C, et al. Heart transplantation in children: indications. Report of the Ad Hoc Subcommittee of the Pediatric Committee of the American Society of Transplantation (AST). Pediatr Transplant. 1999;3(4):333–42.
10. Canter CE, Shaddy RE, Bernstein D, Hsu DT, Chrisant MR, Kirklin JK, et al. Indications for heart transplantation in pediatric heart disease: a scientific statement from the American Heart Association Council on Cardiovascular Disease in the Young; the Councils on Clinical Cardiology, Cardiovascular Nursing, and Cardiovascular Surgery and Anesthesia; and the Quality of Care and Outcomes Research Interdisciplinary Working Group. Circulation. 2007;115(5):658–76.
11. Singh TP, Cherikh WS, Hsich E, Harhay MO, Hayes D Jr, Perch M, et al. The International thoracic organ transplant registry of the international society for heart and lung transplantation: twenty-fifth pediatric heart transplantation report-2022; focus on infant heart transplantation. J Heart Lung Transplant. 2022;41(10):1357–65.
12. Chiu P, Schaffer JM, Sheikh AY, Ha R, Reinhartz O, Mainwaring R, et al. Elevated pretransplant pulmonary vascular resistance index does not predict mortality after isolated orthotopic heart transplantation in children: a retrospective analysis of the UNOS database. Pediatr Transplant. 2015;19(6):623–33.
13. Chiu P, Russo MJ, Davies RR, Addonizio LJ, Richmond ME, Chen JM. What is high risk? Redefining elevated pulmonary vascular resistance index in pediatric heart transplantation. J Heart Lung Transplant. 2012;31(1):61–6.
14. West LJ, Pollock-Barziv SM, Dipchand AI, Lee KJ, Cardella CJ, Benson LN, et al. ABO-incompatible heart transplantation in infants. N Engl J Med. 2001;344(11):793–800.
15. Urschel S, Larsen IM, Kirk R, Flett J, Burch M, Shaw N, et al. ABO-incompatible heart transplantation in early childhood: an international multicenter study of clinical experiences and limits. J Heart Lung Transplant. 2013;32(3):285–92.
16. Chen CY, Warner P, Albers EL, Kemna MS, Delaney M, Hong BJ, et al. Donor-specific anti-HLA antibody production following pediatric ABO-incompatible heart transplantation. Pediatr Transplant. 2019;23(2):e13332.
17. Urschel S, Campbell PM, Meyer SR, Larsen IM, Nuebel J, Birnbaum J, et al. Absence of donor-specific anti-HLA antibodies after ABO-incompatible heart transplantation in infancy: altered immunity or age? Am J Transplant. 2010;10(1):149–56.
18. Chauhan D, Orlandi V, Rajab TK, Bedeir K, Volfovsky A, Mokashi S. Postoperative outcomes in infants undergoing ABO-incompatible heart transplantation in the United States. Ann Thorac Surg. 2022;114(5):1746–52.
19. Rao JN, Hasan A, Hamilton JR, Bolton D, Haynes S, Smith JH, et al. Abo-incompatible heart transplantation in infants: the Freeman Hospital experience. Transplantation. 2004;77(9):1389–94.
20. Mahle WT, Tresler MA, Edens RE, Rusconi P, George JF, Naftel DC, et al. Allosensitization and outcomes in pediatric heart transplantation. J Heart Lung Transplant. 2011;30(11):1221–7.
21. Laing BJ, Ross DB, Meyer SR, Campbell P, Halpin AM, West LJ, et al. Glutaraldehyde treatment of allograft tissue decreases allosensitization after the Norwood procedure. J Thorac Cardiovasc Surg. 2010;139(6):1402–8.
22. Gonzalez-Stawinski GV, Atik FA, McCarthy PM, Roselli EE, Hoercher K, Navia JL, et al. Early and late rejection and HLA sensitization at the time of heart transplantation in patients bridged with left ventricular assist devices. Transplant Proc. 2005;37(2):1349–51.
23. Webber S, Zeevi A, Mason K, Addonizio L, Blume E, Dipchand A, et al. Pediatric heart transplantation across a positive crossmatch: first year results from the CTOTC-04 multi-institutional study. Am J Transplant. 2018;18(9):2148–62.
24. Lytrivi ID, Koehl D, Esteso P, Frandsen EL, Gibbons MK, Kirklin JK, et al. Contemporary outcomes of pediatric cardiac transplantation with a positive retrospective crossmatch. Pediatr Transplant. 2023;27(7):e14593.
25. Kirklin JK, Pearce FB, Dabal RJ, Carlo WF Jr, Mauchley DC. Challenges of cardiac transplantation following the Fontan procedure. Los Angeles, CA: SAGE Publications Sage CA; 2017.
26. Atay G, Demirkol D. Therapeutic plasma exchange application in children requires individual decision. J Pediatr Intens Care. 2021;10(02):106–9.

27. Porter K, Babiker A, Bhaskaran K, Darbyshire J, Pezzotti P, Porter K, et al. Determinants of survival following HIV-1 seroconversion after the introduction of HAART. Lancet. 2003;362(9392):1267–74.
28. Uriel N, Jorde UP, Cotarlan V, Colombo PC, Farr M, Restaino SW, et al. Heart transplantation in human immunodeficiency virus-positive patients. J Heart Lung Transplant. 2009;28(7):667–9.
29. Hosenpud JD, Pamidi SR, Fiol BS, Cinquegrani MP, Keck BM. Outcomes in patients who are hepatitis B surface antigen-positive before transplantation: an analysis and study using the joint ISHLT/UNOS thoracic registry. J Heart Lung Transplant. 2000;19(8):781–5.
30. Leeser DB, Jeevanandam V, Furukawa S, Eisen H, Mather P, Silva P, et al. Simultaneous heart and kidney transplantation in patients with end-stage heart and renal failure. Am J Transplant. 2001;1(1):89–92.
31. Choudhry S, Dreyer WJ, Hope KD, Wang Y, Spinner JA, Tunuguntla HP, et al. Pediatric heart-liver transplant outcomes in the United States: A 25-year National Cohort Study. Pediatr Transplant. 2021;25(7):e14066.
32. Berkman E, Wightman A, Friedland-Little JM, Albers EL, Diekema D, Lewis-Newby M. An ethical analysis of obesity as a determinant of pediatric heart transplant candidacy. Pediatr Transplant. 2021;25(3):e13913.
33. Ibrahim J CC, Chinnock RE, Kirklin JK, Naftel DC, Basile S, West L, Pediatric Heart Transplant Study Group. Linear and somatic growth following pediatric heart transplantation. J Heart Lung Transplant. 2002;21(1):63.
34. Kirk R, Dipchand AI, Davies RR, Miera O, Chapman G, Conway J, et al. ISHLT consensus statement on donor organ acceptability and management in pediatric heart transplantation. J Heart Lung Transplant. 2020;39(4):331–41.
35. Bailey LL, Razzouk AJ, Hasaniya NW, Chinnock RE. Pediatric transplantation using hearts refused on the basis of donor quality. Ann Thorac Surg. 2009;87(6):1902–8; discussion 8–9.
36. Wijdicks EF. The diagnosis of brain death. N Engl J Med. 2001;344(16):1215–21.
37. Ahmed HF, Guzman-Gomez A, Kulshrestha K, Kantemneni EC, Chin C, Ashfaq A, et al. The reality of DCD donor use in pediatric thoracic transplantation in the United States. J Heart Lung Transplant. 2023.
38. L'Ecuyer T, Sloan K, Tang L. Impact of donor cardiopulmonary resuscitation on pediatric heart transplant outcome. Pediatr Transplant. 2011;15(7):742–5.
39. Conway J, Chin C, Kemna M, Burch M, Barnes A, Tresler M, et al. Donors' characteristics and impact on outcomes in pediatric heart transplant recipients. Pediatr Transplant. 2013;17(8):774–81.
40. Tang L, Du W, Delius RE, L'Ecuyer TJ, Zilberman MV. Low donor-to-recipient weight ratio does not negatively impact survival of pediatric heart transplant patients. Pediatr Transplant. 2010;14(6):741–5.
41. Kanani M, Hoskote A, Carter C, Burch M, Tsang V, Kostolny M. Increasing donor-recipient weight mismatch in pediatric orthotopic heart transplantation does not adversely affect outcome. Eur J Cardiothorac Surg. 2012;41(2):427–34.
42. Dani A, Heidel JS, Qiu T, Zhang Y, Ni Y, Hossain MM, et al. External validation and comparison of risk score models in pediatric heart transplants. Pediatr Transplant. 2022;26(3):e14204.
43. Hollander SA, Nandi D, Bansal N, Godown J, Zafar F, Rosenthal DN, et al. A coordinated approach to improving pediatric heart transplant waitlist outcomes: a summary of the ACTION November 2019 waitlist outcomes committee meeting. Pediatr Transplant. 2020;24(7):e13862.
44. Raymundo S, Wilhalme H, Chaudhary A, Karunungan K, Alejos J, Srivastava N. Pediatric risk to orthotopic heart transplant (PRO) score: Insights from United Network for Organ Sharing (UNOS) waitlist mortality findings. Pediatr Transplant. 2023;27(6):e14525.
45. Almond CSD, Thiagarajan RR, Piercey GE, Gauvreau K, Blume ED, Bastardi HJ, et al. Waiting list mortality among children listed for heart transplantation in the United States. Circulation. 2009;119(5):717–27.
46. Williams RJ, Lu M, Sleeper LA, Blume ED, Esteso P, Fynn-Thompson F, et al. Pediatric heart transplant waiting times in the United States since the 2016 allocation policy change. Am J Transplant. 2022;22(3):833–42.
47. Tume SC, Conway J, Ryan KR, Philip J, Fortkiewicz JM, Murray J. Developments in pediatric ventricular assist device support. World J Pediatr Congenit Heart Surg. 2019;10(6):759–68.
48. O'Connor MJ, Lorts A, Davies RR, Fynn-Thompson F, Joong A, Maeda K, et al. Early experience with the HeartMate 3 continuous-flow ventricular assist device in pediatric patients and patients with congenital heart disease: a multicenter registry analysis. J Heart Lung Transplant. 2020;39(6):573–9.
49. Ziegler LA, Sainathan S, Morell VO, Sharma MS. Total artificial heart as rescue therapy for primary graft failure in an infant. Ann Thorac Surg. 2018;105(4):e151–3.
50. Dipchand AI, Kirk R, Naftel DC, Pruitt E, Blume ED, Morrow R, et al. Ventricular assist device support as a bridge to transplantation in pediatric patients. J Am Coll Cardiol. 2018;72(4):402–15.
51. Zafar F, Castleberry C, Khan MS, Mehta V, Bryant R 3rd, Lorts A, et al. Pediatric heart transplant waiting list mortality in the era of ventricular assist devices. J Heart Lung Transplant. 2015;34(1):82–8.
52. Rossano JW, Cherikh WS, Chambers DC, Goldfarb S, Khush K, Kucheryavaya AY, et al. The registry of the International Society for Heart and Lung Transplantation: twentieth pediatric heart

transplantation report-2017; focus theme: allograft ischemic time. J Heart Lung Transplant. 2017;36(10):1060–9.

53. Costanzo MR, Dipchand A, Starling R, Anderson A, Chan M, Desai S, et al. The International Society of Heart and Lung Transplantation guidelines for the care of heart transplant recipients. J Heart Lung Transplant. 2010;29(8):914–56.
54. Vida VL, Leon-Wyss J, Rojas M, Mack R, Barnoya J, Castaneda AR. Pulmonary artery hypertension: is it really a contraindicating factor for early extubation in children after cardiac surgery? Ann Thorac Surg. 2006;81(4):1460–5.
55. Daftari B, Alejos JC, Perens G. Initial experience with sildenafil, bosentan, and nitric oxide for pediatric cardiomyopathy patients with elevated pulmonary vascular resistance before and after orthotopic heart transplantation. J Transplant. 2010;2010:656984.
56. Rossano JW, Jefferies JL, Pahl E, Naftel DC, Pruitt E, Lupton K, et al. Use of sirolimus in pediatric heart transplant patients: a multi-institutional study from the Pediatric Heart Transplant Study Group. J Heart Lung Transplant. 2017;36(4):427–33.
57. Castleberry C, Pruitt E, Ameduri R, Schowengerdt K, Edens E, Hagin N, et al. Risk stratification to determine the impact of induction therapy on survival, rejection and adverse events after pediatric heart transplant: a multi-institutional study. J Heart Lung Transplant. 2018;37(4):458–66.
58. Eisen HJ, Kobashigawa J, Keogh A, Bourge R, Renlund D, Mentzer R, et al. Three-year results of a randomized, double-blind, controlled trial of mycophenolate mofetil versus azathioprine in cardiac transplant recipients. J Heart Lung Transplant. 2005;24(5):517–25.
59. Singh TP, Faber C, Blume ED, Worley S, Almond CS, Smoot LB, et al. Safety and early outcomes using a corticosteroid-avoidance immunosuppression protocol in pediatric heart transplant recipients. J Heart Lung Transplant. 2010;29(5):517–22.
60. Velleca A, Shullo MA, Dhital K, Azeka E, Colvin M, DePasquale E, et al. The International Society for Heart and Lung Transplantation (ISHLT) guidelines for the care of heart transplant recipients. J Heart Lung Transplant. 2023;42(5):e1–141.
61. Godown J, Harris MT, Burger J, Dodd DA. Variation in the use of surveillance endomyocardial biopsy among pediatric heart transplant centers over time. Pediatr Transplant. 2015;19(6):612–7.
62. Chen JK, Salerno DM, Corbo H, Mantell BS, Richmond M, Rothkopf A, et al. Immune cell function assay and T lymphocyte counts lack association with rejection or infection in pediatric heart transplant recipients. Clin Transplant. 2023;37(2):e14858.
63. Knecht KR, MacLeod SL, Hobbs CA, Li M, Morrow WR. Gene expression profiling in pediatric heart transplant rejection. Int J Cardiol. 2013;168(5):5052–3.
64. Das BB, Chan KC, Winchester RW, Zakrzewski M, Niu J. Correlation of gene expression profiling score, cardiac hemodynamics and echocardiographic parameters in asymptomatic, rejection-free pediatric heart transplant recipients. Pediatr Transplant. 2020;24(3):e13673.
65. Feingold B, Rose-Felker K, West SC, Zinn MD, Berman P, Moninger A, et al. Early findings after integration of donor-derived cell-free DNA into clinical care following pediatric heart transplantation. Pediatr Transplant. 2022;26(1):e14124.
66. Gossett JG, Canter CE, Zheng J, Schechtman K, Blume ED, Rodgers S, et al. Decline in rejection in the first year after pediatric cardiac transplantation: a multi-institutional study. J Heart Lung Transplant. 2010;29(6):625–32.
67. Frank R, Dean SA, Molina MR, Kamoun M, Lal P. Correlations of lymphocyte subset infiltrates with donor-specific antibodies and acute antibody-mediated rejection in endomyocardial biopsies. Cardiovasc Pathol. 2015;24(3):168–72.
68. Everitt MD, Pahl E, Schechtman KB, Zheng J, Ringewald JM, L'Ecuyer T, et al. Rejection with hemodynamic compromise in the current era of pediatric heart transplantation: a multi-institutional study. J Heart Lung Transplant. 2011;30(3):282–8.
69. Chambers DC, Yusen RD, Cherikh WS, Goldfarb SB, Kucheryavaya AY, Khusch K, et al. The registry of the International Society for Heart and Lung Transplantation: thirty-fourth adult lung and heart-lung transplantation report-2017; focus theme: allograft ischemic time. J Heart Lung Transplant. 2017;36(10):1047–59.
70. Kobayashi D, Du W, L'Ecuyer TJ. Predictors of cardiac allograft vasculopathy in pediatric heart transplant recipients. Pediatr Transplant. 2013;17(5):436–40.
71. Jeewa A, Chin C, Pahl E, Atz AM, Carboni MP, Pruitt E, et al. Outcomes after percutaneous coronary artery revascularization procedures for cardiac allograft vasculopathy in pediatric heart transplant recipients: a multi-institutional study. J Heart Lung Transplant. 2015;34(9):1163–8.
72. Schowengerdt KO, Naftel DC, Seib PM, Pearce FB, Addonizio LJ, Kirklin JK, et al. Infection after pediatric heart transplantation: results of a multiinstitutional study. The Pediatric Heart Transplant Study Group. J Heart Lung Transplant. 1997;16(12):1207–16.
73. Dipchand AI, Kirk R, Mahle WT, Tresler MA, Naftel DC, Pahl E, et al. Ten yr of pediatric heart transplantation: a report from the Pediatric Heart Transplant Study. Pediatr Transplant. 2013;17(2):99–111.
74. Hayes D Jr, Harhay MO, Cherikh WS, Chambers DC, Perch M, Khush KK, et al. The International Thoracic Organ Transplant Registry of the International Society for Heart and Lung Transplantation: twenty-fourth pediatric lung transplantation report - 2021; focus on recipient characteristics. J Heart Lung Transplant. 2021;40(10):1023–34.

75. Greenberg JW, Bryant R 3rd, Villa C, Fields K, Fynn-Thompson F, Zafar F, et al. Racial disparity exists in the utilization and post-transplant survival benefit of ventricular assist device support in children. J Heart Lung Transplant. 2023;42(5):585–92.
76. Carlo WF, Padilla LA, Xu W, Carboni MP, Kleinmahon JA, Sparks JP, et al. Racial and socioeconomic disparities in pediatric heart transplant outcomes in the era of anti-thymocyte globulin induction. J Heart Lung Transplant. 2022;41(12):1773–80.
77. Bansal N, Lal AK, Koehl D, Cantor RS, Kirklin JK, Ravekes WJ, et al. Impact of race and health coverage on listing and waitlist mortality in pediatric cardiac transplantation. J Heart Lung Transplant. 2023;42(6):754–64.
78. Amdani S, Conway J, Kleinmahon J, Auerbach S, Hsu D, Cousino MK, et al. Race and Socioeconomic Bias in Pediatric Cardiac Transplantation. JACC Heart Fail. 2023;11(1):19–26.

# 25 Adult Congenital Heart Disease—Special Considerations

Rose Tompkins

**Abstract**

The remarkable success of congenital heart disease management in childhood has resulted in unprecedented survival to adulthood. However, survival to adulthood does not equate to normal life expectancy, with heart failure (HF) emerging as the leading cause of mortality among the adult congenital heart disease (ACHD) population. The long-term management of this highly heterogeneous patient population represents uncharted territory, resulting in a field that is persistently evolving as experience increases. The field remains nascent in the optimal strategies of ACHD-HF prevention and management, including advanced therapies and transplantation. In this chapter, we present the current state of the field and some of the current challenges unique to ACHD patients while promoting collaboration with ACHD experts to continue to inform best practices and improve patient outcomes.

**Keywords**

Congenital defects · Heart transplantation · Adult congenital heart disease

## Clinical Pearls

- Heart failure is the leading cause of mortality among contemporary cohorts of adult congenital heart disease patients.
- Early identification of advancing heart failure, optimal patient selection, and timing of transplant referral are major challenges for clinicians managing adult congenital heart disease patients.
- Given the complexity and unique characteristics of adult congenital heart disease patients, multidisciplinary collaboration is key while comprehensively evaluating these patients for transplant.
- Adult congenital heart disease patients undergoing heart transplantation are at higher surgical risk due to multiple sternotomies, complexity of anatomy, and need for vascular reconstructions, additional repairs at time of transplantation among other complications.
- Pre-transplant sensitization occurs at a higher rate among adult congenital heart disease patients secondary to their exposure to multiple blood transfusions and the use of

R. Tompkins (✉)
Cedars-Sinai Medical Center, Guerin Congenital Heart Program, Smidt Heart Institute, Los Angeles, CA, USA
e-mail: rose.tompkins@cshs.org



J. Kobashigawa (ed.), *Clinical Guide to Heart Transplantation*, https://doi.org/10.1007/978-3-031-88290-6_25

homograft and tissue allografts at the time of surgical repairs.
- Challenges to mechanical circulatory support utilization in this population include anatomic complexities to device placement, multiple prior sternotomies, persistent shunts, malnutrition from protein-losing enteropathy or cirrhosis from chronic right-sided congestion.
- Patients with adult congenital heart disease undergoing heart transplantation have consistently been shown to have higher post-operative, one-year, and ten-year mortality relative to those without congenital heart disease. However, overall survival is improving among contemporary cohorts and long-term survival is superior to non-congenital heart disease patients.
- ACHD patients, particularly single-ventricle Fontan patients, are at increased risk of severe liver dysfunction (cirrhosis) when there is underlying chronic elevation in systemic venous pressure, and may require evaluation for combined heart-liver transplantation.

## Introduction

Congenital heart defects are the most common type of birth defect, occurring in approximately 1% of live births [1]. With major advancements in medical and surgical management, the life expectancy of neonates born with congenital heart disease (CHD) has improved dramatically over the past 70 years, from a 10% survival rate before the era of cardiac surgery to now>90% surviving to adulthood [2, 3]. Due to this unprecedented survival, the number of adults living with CHD surpassed the number of children for the first time in the early 2000s, with more than an estimated 1.4 million adults (and counting) in the United States alone, with no indication of slowing for the foreseeable future [4–6]. The population growth of adult congenital heart disease (ACHD) patients is driven in large part by the improved survival of patients with the most complex congenital heart lesions [7]. However, survival to adulthood does not equate to normal life expectancy. Congenital heart repairs are palliative and not curative, with residual cardiac lesions and late sequela being the rule rather than the exception [8, 9]. ACHD patients are at an inherently higher risk for progressive heart failure (HF) due to a variety of factors, including palliated cardiac anatomy, maladaptive remodeling from persistent hemodynamic abnormalities, and limited medical therapy with proven efficacy to mitigate myocardial dysfunction [10, 11]. ACHD-HF-related hospitalizations are on the rise and will continue to increase as the growing ACHD population ages [12, 13]. Consequently, ACHD-HF has emerged as the leading cause of mortality among contemporary cohorts of ACHD patients [14–17]. With limited evidence-based guidance for ACHD-HF management and a lack of consensus on indications and timing of advanced therapies and heart transplantation (HTx) [18], many ACHD patients are referred for transplant evaluation late and denied listing as they are deemed too sick [19]. Historically, those who are accepted for transplantation, are listed at a lower status and have longer wait times relative to non-ACHD patients [20, 21], with some improvement in wait times following the UNOS change in allocation policy in 2018 [22]. While post-transplant outcomes have been improving [23, 24], the number of ACHD patients receiving HTx remains small at the present time, with only 3% of total adult HTx performed in CHD within the United States [25], an even smaller proportion thought to be for single ventricle patients with Fontan palliation. However, with the ACHD population growth, advancing age, and increasing awareness of ACHD-HF, HTx specialists will play an increasingly important role in addressing these challenges in the decades ahead.

## Challenges in Identifying Advancing ACHD-HF

Despite advances in care that have improved survivorship, the median age of death among the ACHD population ranges from 47 to 51 years of age, significantly lower than the general population. The majority of these deaths are cardiovascular, with HF being the leading cause, especially among those with more complex

CHD such as systemic right ventricle, single ventricle palliated to Fontan circulation, and unrepaired cyanotic CHD with Eisenmenger physiology [14–17]. An analysis published by a large ACHD center in Sydney, Australia, found that the median age of death for a cohort of 1043 patients with moderate CHD was 51 years old. This is in stark contrast to 552 patients with complex CHD, where the median age of death was much younger at 34 years old, with the majority of deaths attributed to HF or sudden cardiac death (SCD) [26]. Thus, highlighting that long-term survival remains adversely impacted by HF, especially among patients with more complex CHD. However, identification of advancing HF, optimal patient selection, and timing of transplant referral are major challenges for clinicians managing ACHD patients. The course and progression of ACHD-HF varies significantly from that of acquired heart disease and subsequent HF. CHD is a lifelong disease that begins in utero as a result of structural and hemodynamic abnormalities from the onset of cardiac development. There is a slow and often unpredictable progression of myocardial dysfunction that can occur over decades with additional effects of recurrent cardiac interventions, electrophysiological abnormalities, and subsequent adaptive mechanisms that limit the applicability and prognostic accuracy of traditional markers of advancing HF in use for the adult population at large (Fig. 25.1) [27–29]. Symptoms and utilization of the New York Heart Association Functional Class are hallmarks for the determination of HF severity in the general population; however, they are unreliable and under-reported for the ACHD population. Studies have consistently demonstrated that subjective symptoms and functional class correlate poorly with objective measured peak oxygen consumption (VO2) among ACHD patients, with peak VO2 often significantly reduced, even in asymptomatic patients [30–32]. This is not unexpected given that many ACHD patients have acclimated to a lifetime of reduced exercise capacity and exertional shortness of breath and, therefore, would not consider these symptoms abnormal. Unlike in acquired heart disease, ACHD patients often do not have a period of "normal" exercise capacity in which to compare their symptoms. Therefore, they may not be aware of worsening limitations until a significant change in symptomatology has occurred, particularly if they are sedentary.

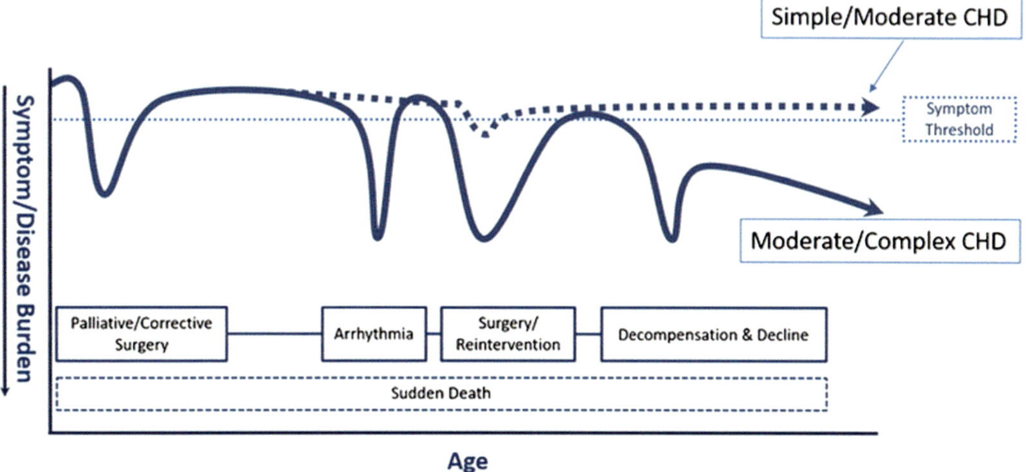


**Fig. 25.1** Schematic representation of the pattern of heart failure presentation in simple and more complex forms of congenital heart. Possible causes of acute and chronic deterioration are listed in boxes below. Sudden death is a persistent, if low-level, risk throughout the lifespan. Reused with permission from Laith I. Alshawabkeh et al., Burden of Heart Failure in Adults with Congenital Heart Disease, Current Heart Failure Reports, 13,247–254, 2016, Springer Nature. https://doi.org/10.1007/s11897-016-0301-0

However, when an ACHD patient does report a change in symptoms relative to their baseline, this often correlates with a change in NYHA class, which has then been associated with adverse HF outcomes [33]. While multiple factors have been examined in association with advancing HF among the ACHD cohort (Table 25.1), at present, no single test or risk score has been developed that adequately prognosticates HF severity for an individual ACHD patient. Ultimately, serial surveillance testing using objective data is a critical aspect of the life-long management of ACHD patients. Cardiopulmonary exercise testing remains an important tool for objective determination of functional capacity, although the majority of ACHD patients will not have a normal peak oxygen consumption (VO2) [31, 32], likely from multifactorial reasons including deconditioning from inherent limitations in cardiac reserve, exercise restrictions that had been placed on them by physicians and caregivers since childhood, and associated anxiety on part of the patient and potential unfamiliarity with what are acceptable exercise symptoms and target intensity levels. Thus, one-time measurements are less clinically predictive for an individual ACHD patient, and serial measurements over time may be more indicative of advancing disease, although robust clinical outcome data remains limited [34]. Unlike in acquired HF, there currently is no defined threshold of peak oxygen consumption (VO2) or other exercise-based parameters that reliably prognosticate when a patient should be referred for advanced therapies or HTx, and therefore should not be used alone as a determinant for appropriateness of such therapy [34]. Biomarkers, including BNP and NT-proBNP, are well established in prognostication for acquired HF; however, they are less so in ACHD-HF. BNP and NT-proBNP levels are often elevated at baseline among asymptomatic ACHD patients regardless of the underlying complexity of CHD [35]. Not unexpectedly, the more complex the CHD, the higher the baseline level. Regardless, studies have shown a higher incidence of HF events and SCD among ACHD patients with a baseline NT-proBNP level > 282 pt/mL relative to those with a level < 58 pg/mL [36]. Additionally, fewer HF events were observed over time when the NT-proBNP level remained stable. Similarly, a higher incidence of HF-related mortality was seen among ACHD patients with elevated BNP levels compared to those with lower values [33, 37, 38]. Thus, despite potentially elevated levels at baseline, BNP and NT-proBNP are still thought to be useful adjuvant measures to follow in helping to determine advancing ACHD-HF over time.

## Evaluation of the ACHD Patient Referred for Transplant Listing

### Indications for Referral and Evaluation

At present, there is no consensus on absolute indications for HTx in ACHD [18]. The decision to consider transplantation evaluation often remains empiric, driven by patient-specific factors, and when attempts at either medical or interventional optimization have failed. Additionally, difficult decisions may arise regarding whether or not a transplant should be pursued before attempt at primary or additional surgical repair and whether certain congenital lesions or conditions benefit more from transplantation. Additionally, patients may be considered stable by conventional criteria, and by the time they have further clinical decompensation, they may progress quickly to multi-organ failure, precluding transplant or requiring a multi-organ transplant. Given the complexity and unpredictability of the ACHD-HF course, early referral to a center with expertise in ACHD and HTx is strongly recommended. Unfortunately, barriers may be present that preclude patients from getting to an appropriate transplant center in a timely manner, such as geographical, social, or financial limitations. Studies have consistently shown many ACHD patients who are evaluated for transplant are denied listing as they are considered too sick, further highlighting the challenge in identifying advancing HF and appropriate timing of referral [19, 53]. Thus, erring on the side of earlier

**Table 25.1** Factors that may Indicate Advancing HF in an ACHD Patient

| Factor | Key points | First author (Ref #) |
|---|---|---|
| Functional classification | • NYHA FC I patients may under-appreciate objective functional limitation, but worsening reported NYHA FC correlates with declining pVO2 and predicted decompensating HF | Bredy et al. [39], Wang et al. [33] |
| | • 2.5× and 8.7× increased risk of mortality for NYHA FC II and III relative to NYHA FC I, respectively | |
| Cardiopulmonary exercise testing | • Baseline pVO2 is reduced in asymptomatic ACHD patients relative to age-matched controls | Diller et al. [31], Kempny et al. [32] |
| | • Increasingly complex CHD lesions have lower baseline peak VO2 | |
| | • ↓ peak VO2 (<64% pred), ↓ HRR (<1 bpm), ↑ Ve/VCO2 (>39) correlated with worse survival | Inuzuka et al. [40] |
| | • Single peak VO2 measurement not reliable sole marker for determining ACHD-HF severity | Menachem et al. [34], Wang et al. [33] |
| HF hospitalization | • ACHD-HF admission associated with a 5× increase risk of death | Zomer et al. [41] |
| | • ↑ risk of ACHD-HF hospitalization with increasing CHD lesion complexity, advancing age, pacemaker implantation, atrial arrhythmia, renal dysfunction, and PAH | Moussa et al. [42] |
| Electrophysiological | • Atrial arrhythmia and need for pacemaker ↑ risk of ACHD-HF and hospitalization | Arnaert et al. [43] |
| | • Need for pacemaker linked with reduced survival in Fontans | Poh et al. [44] |
| | • SCD is the second leading cause of ACHD mortality | Zomer et al. [17], Diller et al. [14], Engelings et al. [16] |
| | • Atrial arrhythmia a/w SCD in D-TGA s/p atrial switch | Kammeraad et al. [45] |
| Biomarkers | | |
| Anemia | • Anemia associated with 3× higher mortality risk relative to non-anemic patients | Dimopoulous et al. [46] |
| Natriuretic peptides | • Elevated BNP level correlates with increased risk of mortality | Giannakoulas et al. [37], Van De Bruaene et al. [38], Wang et al. [33] |
| | • Baseline NT-proBNP levels vary by CHD lesion and increasing levels correlate with declining NYHA FC and exercise capacity | Eindhoven et al. [35, 47] |
| | • Low NT-proBNP correlates with low risk of death and HF over median 3.5 years of f/u | Baggen et al. [36] |
| hsCRP | • Increasing hsCRP levels associated with worse NYHA FC and peak VO2 and ↑ risk of hospitalization or death | Opotowsky et al. [48] |
| Red cell distribution | • Higher RDW levels may be useful in identifying patients at increased risk for CV events including death, non-elective hospitalization, HF, arrhythmia, thromboembolic event, or cardiac intervention | Alshawabkeh et al. [49], Baggen et al. [50] |

(continued)

**Table 25.1** (continued)

| Factor | Key points | First author (Ref #) |
|---|---|---|
| Serum sodium | • Serum Na < 136 mmol/L associated with worse ACHD-HF outcomes | Van De Bruaene et al. [38] |
| Sarcopenia | • Sacropenia as measued by the volume of the psoas major muscle on CT predicted HF in Fontans | Shiina et al. [51] |
| Renal function | • CKD (EGFR < 60 mL/min/1.73 m$^2$) associated 3× risk of death, transplant, or VAD following ACHD-HF hospitalization | Krishnathasan et al. [52] |

referral is better. Not unlike patients without CHD, it is reasonable to evaluate patients who have significant symptoms limiting quality of life and/or refractory ventricular arrhythmia despite maximally tolerated medical therapy and no further options for interventional or electrophysiological optimization [18].

## Multi-disciplinary Evaluation

The number of HTx performed for ACHD has been steadily increasing [22, 25]. While early post-operative mortality remains higher among ACHD patients relative to non-ACHD patients, this has been improving in recent years, and long-term survival is comparable, if not superior [24, 54]. Notably, ACHD patients listed for transplant at centers with expertise in ACHD care have better outcomes, and there is improved post-transplant survival when performed at higher volume regional centers [55]. Multi-disciplinary collaboration is key as there are considerations that are unique to ACHD patient as part of the comprehensive transplant evaluation (Table 25.2).

## Role of the ACHD Cardiologist

The adult congenital cardiologist plays a vital role in the evaluation of the patient by determining if there are further options for interventional, electrophysiological, or pharmacological optimization in tandem with the advanced HF cardiologist [56]. This includes a thorough investigation for any residual structural lesions that are creating a hemodynamic burden that could potentially be intervened upon and stabilize/improve the patient's clinical status. These residual lesions may include valvular dysfunction, inflow or outflow obstruction, shunting, or conduit dysfunction. Evaluation by a cardiologist with expertise in ACHD is advised by guidelines as an understanding of the underlying native CHD, subsequent palliative repairs/interventions, resulting anatomy and physiology, and associated common late sequela is invaluable to help better guide the initial evaluation. Additionally, over the past decade, there have been significant advances in the field of transcatheter interventions (such as an increasing number of devices for transcatheter pulmonary valve replacements) for ACHD patients that allow more options for optimization, even for those that may have otherwise been considered a prohibitive risk for conventional open-heart surgery, especially when the patient may already have had multiple prior sternotomies. Electrophysiologic issues are also common among the ACHD population and increase with age, including atrial and ventricular arrhythmia and conduction disease that could contribute to hemodynamic deterioration if not adequately addressed. Table 25.3 includes a more detailed CHD lesion-specific approach for the evaluation of common late sequela among select moderate and severely complex CHD.

Notably, intervention may not necessarily be appropriate for all higher-risk patients. For example, while pulmonary valve replacement in a tetralogy of Fallot patient with severe pulmonary valve regurgitation or coarctation stenting

**Table 25.2** Multi-disciplinary team for the ACHD patient undergoing heart transplant evaluation

| Specialty | Expertise considerations |
|---|---|
| Cardiomyopathy/Transplant cardiology | HF optimization, including consideration of inotropes/MCS |
| | Management of post-OHT immunosuppression and surveillance for rejection |
| Adult congenital cardiology | Review CHD diagnosis, anatomy, prior surgeries/interventions, physiology |
| | Evaluation for any modifiable or treatable late sequela |
| Congenital interventional cardiology | Perform invasive hemodynamic assessment including evaluation of pulmonary pressures and PVR given higher incidence of PAH |
| | Coil embolization of collateral vessels in the chest to reduce bleeding with transplant |
| | Review vascular anatomy (abnormal venous connections that affect vascular access, peripheral venous or arterial stenosis/occlusion from prior interventions) |
| Congenital/Transplant surgery | Determine technical feasibility of transplantation: |
| | Sternal re-entry |
| | Vascular reconstruction |
| | Complex anatomy (dextrocardia, heterotaxy) |
| Immunogenetics | Evaluate antibody profiles. Increased risk of allosensitization. May require desentization |
| Transplant psychiatry | Screen and treat mood disorders. Increased incidence of depression and anxiety |
| Transplant social work | Assess social support and adherence |
| Transplant infectious disease | Treat and prevent opportunistic infections |
| Pulmonary hypertension | Evaluate pre-OHT lung function. PAH specialist may be required for evaluation of PAH |
| Nephrology | Evaluate pre-OHT renal function and need for kidney transplant, manage CKD, potential management of peri-operative dialysis for volume management |
| Hepatology | Evaluate for concurrent advanced liver disease and need for liver transplant, especially in the Fontan population |
| Liver transplant | Evaluate for liver transplant feasiblity if determined necessary |
| Lung transplant | Evaluate for lung transplant feasibility if determined necessary (for example prohibitive PAH for heart-only transplant in an Eisenmenger patient) |

in a patient with re-coarctation are generally preferable to transplantation, a high-risk surgical reoperation for a Fontan conversion in an older failing atriopulmonary Fontan may not be as appropriate. Rather, that patient may benefit more from a transplant evaluation as conventional surgery could further increase their transplant risk from the perspective of an additional sternotomy and increased sensitization from blood products with minimal long-term benefit gained. Therefore, early collaborative care with the multi-disciplinary team regarding decisions on approach and timing of possible intervention is of significant benefit for this heterogeneous, complex group of patients.

## HF Pharmacotherapy

While pharmacotherapy is a cornerstone of HF management in acquired heart disease, there is limited evidence of significant benefit in HF

**Table 25.3** Common residual structural abnormalities and resulting interventions among a selected group of moderate and severely complex CHD diagnoses

| Congenital heart lesion | Common late sequela in adulthood | Common invasive interventions |
|---|---|---|
| Tetralogy of fallot | • Pulmonary regurgitation (native or prosthetic)<br>• RV dilation and dysfunction (secondary to PR)<br>• Pulmonary stenosis (native or prosthetic)<br>• RVOT, conduit, or branch PA stenosis<br>• Aortic regurgitation ± aortic root dilation<br>• Atrial arrhythmia<br>• VT and SCD | • Transcatheter pulmonary valve replacement or conduit stenting<br>• Surgical pulmonary valve replacement or conduit replacement<br>• Surgical arterioplasty or transcatheter stenting of branch PA<br>• Surgical aortic valve replacement ± aortic root replacement<br>• VT ablation, ICD implantation |
| D-TGA atrial switch (mustard/senning) | • Interatrial baffle leak<br>• Interatrial baffle obstruction<br>• Subpulmonic LV dilation and dysfunction from baffle leak<br>• Paradoxical embolization from baffle leak<br>• Systemic RV failure ± tricuspid regurgitation<br>• Atrial arrhythmia (IART)<br>• Risk of atrial arrhythmia degenerating into VT<br>• Sinus node dysfunction | • Transcatheter intervention (baffle leak closure or stenting of baffle stenosis)<br>• Catheter ablation of atrial arrhythmia<br>• Pacemaker implantation, ICD implantation |
| D-TGA arterial switch | • Aortic root dilation ± aortic regurgitation<br>• Branch PA stenosis<br>• Ostial coronary artery stenosis | • Surgical aortic root replacement ± aortic valve replacement<br>• Transcatheter stenting of branch pulmonary artery stenosis<br>• Surgical pulmonary angioplasty<br>• Coronary intervention (PCI, CABG) |
| CC-TGA | • Systemic RV dilation and dysfunction with worsening tricuspid regurgitation<br>• Complete heart block | • Surgical tricuspid valve replacement<br>• Pacemaker implantation |
| Ebstein anomaly | • Tricuspid regurgitation with progressive RV failure<br>• Atrial arrhythmia, WPW<br>• Desaturation from commonly associated ASD or PFO | • Surgical tricuspid valve replacement<br>• Transcatheter or surgical ASD/PFO closure<br>• Catheter ablation<br>• Pacemaker implantation |
| Aortic coarctation | • Re-coarctation<br>• Aortic aneurysm at site of prior repair<br>• Ascending aortic aneurysm (esp with BAV)<br>• Persistent systemic HTN<br>• Early CAD/CVA | • Transcatheter re-coarctation balloon dilation and stenting<br>• Transcatheter covered stent implantation for aneurysm exclusion<br>• Surgical re-coarctation or aneurysm repair |
| SV Fontan | • Fontan failure<br>• Residual fenestration or venovenous collaterals → R to L shunting → desaturation → Increased fontan pressure<br>• Aortopulmonary collaterals → hemoptysis<br>• Fontan pathway obstruction<br>• Pulmonary artery stenosis<br>• Atrial arrhythmia<br>• Sinus node dysfunction, chronotropic incompetence<br>• Co-morbidities: FALD, renal dysfunction, PLE | • Transcatheter fenestration closure<br>• Transcatheter coiling of venovenous or aortopulmonary collaterals<br>• Transcatheter stenting of fontan pathway obstruction<br>• Transcatheter balloon dilation and stenting of PA stenosis<br>• Catheter ablation<br>• Epicardial pacemaker implantation<br>• Surgical fontan conversion with MAZE (older generation atriopulmonary Fontans) |

RV, right ventricle; PR, pulmonary regurgitation; RVOT, right ventricular outflow tract; PA, pulmonary artery; VT, ventricular tachycardia; SCD, sudden cardiac death; ICD, implantable cardioverter-defibrillator; D-TGA, dextro-transposition of the great arteries; LV, left ventricle; IART, intraatrial re-entrant tachycardia; PCI, percutaneous coronary intervention; CABG, coronary artery bypass grafting; CC-TGA, congenitally corrected transposition of the great arteries; WPW, Wolff-Parkinson-White syndrome; ASD, atrial septal defect; PFO, patent foramen ovale; BAV, bicuspid aortic valve; HTN, hypertension; CAD, coronary artery disease; CVA, cerebral vascular accident; R, right; L, left; FALD, Fontan associated liver disease; PLE, protein losing enteropathy

and mortality outcomes among ACHD-HF [27]. When extrapolating to the ACHD population, it stands to reason to manage patients with a similar clinical phenotype to that of patients in HF pharmacotherapy clinical trials, specifically left ventricular dysfunction in a two-ventricle circulation where the morphological left ventricle is in the systemic position. At present, benefits are less clear among those patients with a failing sub pulmonary ventricle, a two-ventricle circulation with the morphological right ventricle in the systemic position, or single ventricle circulation with or without Fontan palliation. Therefore, guideline-directed pharmacotherapy must be used cautiously in such patients and generally considered once any important residual hemodynamic lesion, if present, is addressed [27]. Ultimately, this is an evolving area of research, especially with the addition of a newer class of medications to the HF management armamentarium, like sodium-glucose transport protein 2 (SGLT2) inhibitors, and what, if any, the long-term impact remains to be seen.

## Special Considerations for the ACHD Patient

### Pre-transplant Hemodynamic and Vascular Assessment

Pre-transplant invasive hemodynamic assessment is part of the comprehensive transplant evaluation and should ideally be performed by a congenital interventional cardiologist given their knowledge of the complex cardiac congenital anatomy both for the technical aspects of performing the procedure, in addition to the interpretation of the data and potential to perform any transcatheter interventional procedures that could optimize or stabilize the patient's clinical status. Obtaining hemodynamic data may not be straightforward. For example, in a single ventricle patient with a Fontan palliation, they have total cavopulmonary anastomosis such that the superior and inferior vena cava are connected directly to the pulmonary arteries. Therefore, these patients will have non-pulsatile systemic venous and pulmonary artery pressure waveforms, and the central venous pressure should equal their mean pulmonary artery pressure. For this reason, maintaining a pulmonary artery catheter is not necessary and discouraged as central venous pressure will provide a mean pulmonary artery pressure, and an indwelling catheter in the low-flow pulmonary artery could expose the patient to potentially life-threatening pulmonary arterial thrombus. The accuracy of cardiac output and pulmonary vascular resistance calculations is affected by the non-pulsatile Fontan circulation. True pulmonary vascular resistance may be underappreciated as Fontan patients post-transplant have been shown to have higher calculated pulmonary vasculature resistance post-transplant once pulsatile pulmonary circulation has been restored [57]. Other challenges in the accurate calculation of hemodynamic data are encountered in patients with shunts or multiple sources of pulmonary blood flow, all further highlighting the importance of congenital expertise when performing these procedures. A careful review of the vascular anatomy is essential to identify both any important collateral vessels that could cause significant intraoperative bleeding and any abnormal venous connections and/or peripheral venous or arterial stenoses/occlusion that could impact vascular access [18]. ACHD patients have a propensity to develop venovenous (VV) collaterals, aortopulmonary (AP) collaterals, and pulmonary arteriovenous malformations. VV collaterals arise between systemic veins (e.g., superior vena cava, inferior vena cava, subclavian vein, abdominal veins) and the pulmonary veins in response to increased systemic venous pressure. While any patient with chronically elevated systemic venous pressure may develop VV collaterals, these are especially prevalent among Fontan patients. AP collaterals form between the aorta or its branches and the pulmonary arteries; these collaterals are usually associated with inadequate antegrade blood flow through the pulmonary artery (e.g., pulmonary atresia) or chronic cyanosis and serve as an additional source of pulmonary blood flow. Pulmonary AVMs shunt deoxygenated blood from the pulmonary arteries directly to the pulmonary veins, bypassing the pulmonary capillary bed and alveoli, thereby leading to cyanosis. While the development of pulmonary AVMs remains poorly understood, they often occur when the pulmonary circulation does not receive hepatic blood flow, suggesting that 'hepatic factor' is an important inhibitor of pulmonary AVM development [58]. This is further supported by the observation that when hepatic blood flow is restored to the pulmonary circulation, there is regression of pulmonary AVMs [59]. Major VV and AP collaterals can lead to catastrophic intraoperative bleeding, and targeted coil/device embolization at time of transplant may be considered to optimize surgical risk. However, this should be approached cautiously as collaterals may be a response to significant hemodynamic derangements for which occlusion can result in further hemodynamic deterioration (for example, single ventricle Fontan with markedly elevated Fontan pressures may have venovenous collaterals as a "pop-off" for significant central venous hypertension and acute closure could result in a sudden decrease in cardiac output). The congenital interventional cardiologist may also evaluate for venous or arterial stenoses—specifically the inferior vena cava, superior vena cava, or pulmonary arteries. However, intervention with stenting should only be performed after discussion with the transplanting surgeon as presence of stents at anastomotic sites of the new graft will add additional complexity to the transplant surgery.

## Transplant Surgical Evaluation

While there is no specific CHD sub-group or prior palliative repair that is an absolute contraindication to HTx, an ACHD patient poses an inherently higher surgical risk for a multitude of reasons including but not limited to multiple sternotomies, complexity of anatomy, and need for vascular reconstructions or additional repairs at time of transplantation. An increasing number of prior sternotomies, higher surgical complexity, and need for vascular reconstruction are associated with increased bleeding and cardiopulmonary bypass times, which results in longer graft ischemic times, a predictor of post-operative mortality [2]. Up to 30% of ACHD patients require an additional procedure at time of transplant, including reconstruction of the pulmonary arteries, systemic veins, and great vessels [10]. A majority of Fontan patients will require pulmonary artery reconstruction at time of transplant [60]. Transposition patients' status post Mustard/Senning atrial switch procedures often have calcified baffles and previously placed stents that need to be removed, leaving less tissue for atrial anastomosis. For those patients with Heterotaxy or situs inversus, baffle techniques may be necessary to direct the left-sided caval return of the donor to the right atrium of the recipient's heart. For many of these reconstructions to occur, extended harvesting of donor graft pulmonary arteries or systemic veins may be necessary, which will increase graft ischemic time. Extended harvesting may not be possible, especially of the pulmonary arteries, if the donor's lungs are to be retrieved from a separate recipient, which either limits the donor pool for a given patient or results in a further increase of the graft ischemic time with increasing complexity of the vascular reconstruction that must be taken into consideration as part of the surgical risk assessment. Therefore, evaluation by a surgeon or a surgical team with expertise in both CHD and HTx is beneficial in determination of these risks and the performance of the operation.

## Pulmonary Hypertension

Pulmonary hypertension (PH) and elevated pulmonary vascular resistance (PVR) are associated with reduced post-transplant survival secondary to right ventricle failure and progressive graft dysfunction [10, 61]. PH is common among adults with CHD, affecting up to 5–10% of patients [62]. The etiology of PH-ACHD is diverse and impacts management decisions, including eligibility for heart alone versus the need for combined heart–lung transplantation. A full review of PH-ACHD is beyond the scope of this chapter, however, the evaluation of pulmonary pressure and PVR with a hemodynamic cardiac catheterization is essential to any transplant evaluation. While fixed irreversible PH is an absolute contraindication to heart-only transplant, the threshold of PVR varies between centers, with some accepting up to 6 Woods units. Importantly, there are some instances where accurate assessment of PVR will not be possible, and that includes ACHD patients with Fontan circulation, palliative shunts, significant burden of collateral vessels, and/or multiple sources of pulmonary blood flow [62].

Eisenmenger syndrome (ES) represents the most severe form of PH-ACHD and is characterized by an unrepaired large, non-restrictive left-to-right shunt (typically a post-tricuspid shunt, meaning a ventricular septal defect, aortopulmonary window, or patent ductus arteriosus and less commonly a pre-tricuspid shunt such as atrial septal defect or partial anomalous pulmonary venous return) that leads to pulmonary vasculature remodeling, elevation in pulmonary vascular resistance (PVR), and eventual development of systemic pulmonary pressures with reversal of the shunt to right-to-left causing marked cyanosis. There may be some improvement with pulmonary vasodilatory therapy, however, evaluation for heart–lung transplantation may be indicated for those with clinical deterioration despite medical optimization. The timing of heart–lung transplant remains controversial as some well-compensated ES patients may have a better prognosis relative to the limited life expectancy post-heart–lung transplant [63]. However, their clinical course and anticipation of decline may be difficult to predict. Bilateral lung transplant with intracardiac repair has been considered as an alternative to heart–lung transplant, however, current data suggests that ES patients with pre-tricuspid shunts fare better with this strategy versus post-tricuspid shunts who had better outcomes with heart–lung transplant [64]. More studies are necessary before more definitive recommendations can be advised.

Other forms of PH-ACHD include but are not limited to: elevation in pulmonary vascular resistance from persistent left-to-right shunts, coincidental CHD when the degree of PVR elevation is out of proportion to the size and type of shunt, post-interventional PH that persists after a shunt closure or develops late (months to years) post-closure, hypoplastic or stenotic pulmonary arteries or veins causing segmental PH, or "left-heart" disease [62]. If PH-ACHD is identified, a thorough evaluation of etiology and discussion of management among the multi-disciplinary team, including physicians with expertise in ACHD and PH, is advised. Depending on the situation, if PVR is considered not to be irreversible, strategies may be employed to reduce PVR, including pulmonary vasodilatory therapy or mechanical circulatory support (MCS), where appropriate. If unsuccessful, then heart–lung transplantation can be considered.

## Cyanosis

Chronic cyanosis that may or may not be associated with pulmonary hypertension can impose additional surgical risks that should be considered. This includes advancing renal insufficiency and limited renal reserve that may not be fully unmasked until the post-operative period, requiring hemodialysis [65]. Chronic cyanosis is also associated with a higher infection risk that could complicate the early post-transplant period and the need for immunosuppression. Another significant concern is the risk of intra-operative hemorrhage from several factors, including baseline hematological abnormalities and platelet dysfunction, presence of aortopulmonary collaterals, which are often multiple and diffuse, and pulmonary arteriovenous malformations (AVMs). Pulmonary AVMs can be seen in complex heterotaxy syndromes or in patients that have undergone partial superior caval-pulmonary anastomosis with a "classic" Glenn shunt and creation of discontinuous pulmonary arteries. The pulmonary AVMs are almost exclusively in the lung that receives systemic venous return from the superior vena cava only, resulting in a lack of hepatic factor from the liver. While larger AVMs can be coil occluded, there are often innumerable microscopic AVMs present, which precludes any pre-operative interventional options. Post-transplant, with the restoration of normal systemic venous return and hepatic factor once again being received by both lungs, the AVMs may regress with time. However, there will be persistent cyanosis in the early postoperative period that increases morbidity and mortality, necessitating consideration of heart–lung transplantation in some instances [66].

## Sensitization

Panel-reactive antibody (PRA) screen is a routine part of the transplant evaluation to determine the presence of circulating antibodies to a panel of donor lymphocytes and is used to quantify the degree of sensitization of the recipient. Elevated PRA level indicates a higher degree of sensitization, with > 25% associated with worse post-transplant outcomes [67]. Sensitization occurs at a higher rate among ACHD patients secondary to their exposure to multiple blood transfusions and the use of homograft and tissue allografts at the time of surgical repairs [68]. Highly sensitized ACHD patients present a challenge as they are more likely to experience acute cellular rejection and graft failure, as well as, late antibody-mediated rejection and coronary allograft vasculopathy, which are known to be an important cause of late mortality among HTx recipients [69–71]. Thus, increased sensitization can significantly limit the donor pool and availability of a suitable graft, which can further prolong waitlist times for ACHD patients [72]. Desensitization strategies are used with variable success and dependent on center expertise.

## Liver Disease

Pre-transplant liver dysfunction is a known risk factor for early postoperative mortality and increases the risk of intra-operative bleeding and subsequent post-operative vasoplegia, which are associated with a higher risk of respiratory, cardiac, and renal complications [73]. ACHD patients, particularly single ventricle Fontan patients, are at increased risk of liver dysfunction when there is underlying chronic elevation in systemic venous pressure, dysfunction of "right-sided" ventricle, and/or "right-sided" valvular heart disease [74]. Additionally, Hepatitis C is more prevalent among ACHD patients who underwent cardiac surgical repairs prior to screening in 1992 [75]. For such patients, hepatic evaluation should be included as part of the OHT work-up to ensure that there is no evidence of significant liver disease such as cirrhosis, portal hypertension, or hepatocellular carcinoma that may negatively impact candidacy for transplantation or heart-only transplantation leading to consideration of combined heart-liver transplantation [18]. Adult single ventricle Fontan patients represent a unique subset of ACHD patients as the incidence of Fontan Associated Liver Disease (FALD) is ubiquitous [76].

## Management of ACHD Patient Listed for Transplant

Once an ACHD patient is listed, programs may benefit from a multi-disciplinary surgical planning meeting with the involved medical, surgical, intensive care unit, and anesthesiology teams for the creation of a written care plan that should account for and ensure adequate time for induction of anesthesia, safe chest entry, control of bleeding, and explant of the recipient heart, as well as, thoughtful consideration of the geographic range of donors to allow for optimization of the donor pool while balancing excessive donor ischemic time. Donor height/weight parameters should be reviewed and adjusted to ensure optimal patient size matching. For those patients undergoing multi-organ transplantation, a coordinated surgical plan should be in place with the respective surgical teams, in addition to, a strategy for induction immunosuppression [77]. Patients on the transplant waitlist remain vulnerable to clinical deterioration. Historically, ACHD patients are known to have longer waitlist times and higher waitlist mortality relative to non-ACHD patients [18]. Therefore, once a patient is listed, frequent monitoring and re-assessment, including clinical evaluation, psychosocial support, and need for mechanical circulatory support as a bridge to transplant, is necessary. Additionally, focus should be placed on maintaining or optimizing physiological status, including medication adjustments, nutritional support, and encouragement of physical activity if feasible. Ensuring no new co-morbidities have developed that would preclude transplantation is also an important aspect of clinical follow-up during this critical time period. Despite careful outpatient monitoring, an inpatient admission may be necessary to achieve adequate stabilization and allow optimization with intervention such as continuous inotrope infusion to improve end-organ perfusion, careful diuretic titration to maintain euvolemia, as well as more aggressive nutrition support to reduce sarcopenia and frailty to hopefully mitigate additional risk at the time of transplant.

## Mechanical Circulatory Support

While mechanical circulatory support (MCS) is increasingly utilized as a bridge to transplant for decompensating patients on the waitlist, use remains limited among ACHD patients, with < 1% of these devices being implanted in this population within the United States [78]. Of 159 participating centers in the INTERMACS registry, only 59 implanted a device into an ACHD patient, with the majority implanting (>70%) only 1 or 2 patients over a 9.5-year period (6/2006–12/2015). The six highest volume centers implanted devices into just 5 or 6 patients [78]. Challenges to MCS utilization for this population include anatomic complexities to device placement (dextrocardia, heterotaxy, systemic right ventricle, Fontan), multiple prior sternotomies, persistent shunts, malnutrition from PLE or cirrhosis from chronic right-sided congestion. MCS use has been associated with high morbidity and uncertain long-term outcomes [18]. However, more recent studies have shown similar survival among ACHD patients versus non-ACHD patients with left ventricular assist devices, as well as similar improvements in functional status and quality of life [78, 79]. ACHD patients did have a higher proportion receiving biventricular assist devices or total artificial heart, with this particular subgroup more likely to have an INTERMACS score of 1 or 2 and having worse survival relative to non-ACHD patients, which could suggest earlier implantation could have mitigated some of this risk [78]. When exploring MCS use among specific CHD diagnoses, there are multiple small case series supporting reasonable outcomes with use among dextro- transposition of the great arteries status-post Mustard or Senning atrial switch procedure or congenitally-corrected transposition of the great arteries with special attention to device implantation into the systemic morphological right ventricle [18, 80]. At present, there is very little experience of utilizing MCS in failing adult Fontan patients, but with careful patient selection, there has been a report of anecdotal success, although MCS use has not yet been widely adopted among the adult Fontan cohort [81, 82]. Given the evolving nature of the MCS field and the complexity and heterogeneity of the ACHD population, these patients benefit from a multi-disciplinary team to guide them in making these challenging decisions.

## ACHD Transplant Outcomes

On October 18, 2018, the United States adult heart allocation policy was changed from a three-tier to a six-tier system, resulting in most ACHD patients being initially listed as status 4, with status 1 being the highest priority [22]. In the current allocation system, status 4 ACHD patients have the same priority as those patients who are stable with durable ventricular assist devices (VAD) or on outpatient inotropic support. Analysis of the first 16–18 months following this policy change has shown that waitlist time has significantly decreased among ACHD patients and is now comparable to that of non-ACHD patients [22, 83, 84]. Remains to be seen if waitlist mortality will be significantly reduced. Notably, the majority of ACHD patients transplanted post-policy change were granted exceptions and listed at a status higher than 4 at the time of transplantation with increased utilization of aortic balloon pumps and ECMO [22]. However, one-year post-transplant survival has remained similar. ACHD patients have consistently been shown to have higher post-operative, one-year, and ten-year mortality relative to non-ACHD patients undergoing heart-only transplantation [18]. However, long-term survival is superior for ACHD patients relative to non-ACHD [23]. A review of UNOS data of 1,159 ACHD patients undergoing HTx between 2000 and 2019 found that long-term survival was better among the ACHD cohort compared to a non-ACHD cohort matched for age, gender, height, weight, year of transplant, and status at time of transplant, effectively excluding the concept that younger age at time of transplant accounts for the superior long-term survival of ACHD patients [24]. While one-year post-transplant mortality is higher among ACHD patients, there has been steady improvement relative to earlier decades [54]. Additionally, higher-volume transplant centers with ACHD expertise have better waitlist survival and one-year post-transplant mortality rates compared to low-volume centers or those without available ACHD collaboration (55). As experience continues to grow in the transplantation of ACHD patients and more data is available to better inform candidate selection and timing of transplant, the expectation is that post-transplant survival should continue to improve. A significant limitation in understanding outcome trends among ACHD patients from a population level, especially in the United States, is that UNOS does not provide more granular data regarding type of congenital heart diagnosis, rather the heterogenous population of ACHD patients are recorded in the same broad category of "Congenital Heart Disease" without further characterization of important anatomical variables that could impact selection and post-transplant outcomes including but not limited to biventricular versus univentricular circulations or those with a morphological right ventricle in the systemic position. Therefore, some caution needs to be exercised when reviewing and applying transplant outcomes when considering an individual ACHD patient. At present, much of our understanding of transplant outcomes for specific CHD subsets, such as adult single ventricle Fontan patients, is derived from single-center or limited multi-institutional large referral centers, which will carry inherent selection and referral bias limitations.

In Conclusion: The remarkable success of CHD management in childhood has resulted in unprecedented survival to adulthood, leading to an entirely new adult cardiac subspeciality of ACHD. However, survival to adulthood does not equate to normal life expectancy, with HF emerging as the leading cause of mortality among the ACHD population. The long-term management of this highly heterogeneous patient population represents uncharted territory, resulting in a field that is persistently evolving as experience increases. The field remains nascent in the optimal strategies of ACHD-HF prevention and management, including advanced therapies and transplantation. In this chapter, we presented the current state of the field and some of the current challenges unique to ACHD patients while promoting collaboration with ACHD experts to continue to inform best practices and improve patient outcomes.

## References

1. Hoffman JI, Kaplan S. The incidence of congenital heart disease. J Am Coll Cardiol. 2002;39(12):1890–900.
2. Warnes CA, Liberthson R, Danielson GK, Dore A, Harris L, Hoffman JI, et al. Task force 1: the changing profile of congenital heart disease in adult life. J Am Coll Cardiol. 2001;37(5):1170–5.
3. Moons P, Bovijn L, Budts W, Belmans A, Gewillig M. Temporal trends in survival to adulthood among patients born with congenital heart disease from 1970 to 1992 in Belgium. Circulation. 2010;122(22):2264–72.
4. Williams RG, Pearson GD, Barst RJ, Child JS, del Nido P, Gersony WM, et al. Report of the National

Heart, Lung, and Blood Institute Working Group on research in adult congenital heart disease. J Am Coll Cardiol. 2006;47(4):701–7.
5. Gilboa SM, Devine OJ, Kucik JE, Oster ME, Riehle-Colarusso T, Nembhard WN, et al. Congenital heart defects in the United States: estimating the magnitude of the affected population in 2010. Circulation. 2016;134(2):101–9.
6. Benziger CP, Stout K, Zaragoza-Macias E, Bertozzi-Villa A, Flaxman AD. Projected growth of the adult congenital heart disease population in the United States to 2050: an integrative systems modeling approach. Popul Health Metr. 2015;13:29.
7. Marelli AJ, Ionescu-Ittu R, Mackie AS, Guo L, Dendukuri N, Kaouache M. Lifetime prevalence of congenital heart disease in the general population from 2000 to 2010. Circulation. 2014;130(9):749–56.
8. Warnes CA. The adult with congenital heart disease: born to be bad? J Am Coll Cardiol. 2005;46(1):1–8.
9. Bouma BJ, Mulder BJ. Changing landscape of congenital heart disease. Circ Res. 2017;120(6):908–22.
10. Irving C, Parry G, O'Sullivan J, Dark JH, Kirk R, Crossland DS, et al. Cardiac transplantation in adults with congenital heart disease. Heart. 2010;96(15):1217–22.
11. Lewis M, Rosenbaum M. When should adult congenital heart disease patients be considered for transplant and deciding which organs to transplant. Prog Cardiovasc Dis. 2018;61(3–4):377–81.
12. Burchill LJ, Gao L, Kovacs AH, Opotowsky AR, Maxwell BG, Minnier J, et al. Hospitalization trends and health resource use for adult congenital heart disease-related heart failure. J Am Heart Assoc. 2018;7(15):e008775.
13. Agasthi P, Van Houten HK, Yao X, Jain CC, Egbe A, Warnes CA, et al. Mortality and morbidity of heart failure hospitalization in adult patients with congenital heart disease. J Am Heart Assoc. 2023;12(23):e030649.
14. Diller GP, Kempny A, Alonso-Gonzalez R, Swan L, Uebing A, Li W, et al. Survival prospects and circumstances of death in contemporary adult congenital heart disease patients under follow-up at a large tertiary centre. Circulation. 2015;132(22):2118–25.
15. Verheugt CL, Uiterwaal CS, van der Velde ET, Meijboom FJ, Pieper PG, van Dijk AP, et al. Mortality in adult congenital heart disease. Eur Heart J. 2010;31(10):1220–9.
16. Engelings CC, Helm PC, Abdul-Khaliq H, Asfour B, Bauer UM, Baumgartner H, et al. Cause of death in adults with congenital heart disease - an analysis of the German national register for congenital heart defects. Int J Cardiol. 2016;211:31–6.
17. Zomer AC, Vaartjes I, Uiterwaal CS, van der Velde ET, van den Merkhof LF, Baur LH, et al. Circumstances of death in adult congenital heart disease. Int J Cardiol. 2012;154(2):168–72.
18. Ross HJ, Law Y, Book WM, Broberg CS, Burchill L, Cecchin F, et al. Transplantation and mechanical circulatory support in congenital heart disease: a scientific statement from the American Heart Association. Circulation. 2016;133(8):802–20.
19. Meras P, Riesgo-Gil F, Rybicka J, Barradas-Pires A, Smith J, Kempny A, et al. Heart transplantation at a single tertiary adult congenital heart disease centre: too little, too late? Int J Cardiol. 2021;322:107–13.
20. Everitt MD, Donaldson AE, Stehlik J, Kaza AK, Budge D, Alharethi R, et al. Would access to device therapies improve transplant outcomes for adults with congenital heart disease? Analysis of the United Network for Organ Sharing (UNOS). J Heart Lung Transplant. 2011;30(4):395–401.
21. Goldberg SW, Fisher SA, Wehman B, Mehra MR. Adults with congenital heart disease and heart transplantation: optimizing outcomes. J Heart Lung Transplant. 2014;33(9):873–7.
22. Ashraf SF, Hess N, Seese L, Kavarana MN, Tedford RJ, Rajab TK, et al. Impact of the 2018 change in US allocation policy on adults with congenital heart disease. J Heart Lung Transplant. 2022;41(3):373–81.
23. Burchill LJ, Edwards LB, Dipchand AI, Stehlik J, Ross HJ. Impact of adult congenital heart disease on survival and mortality after heart transplantation. J Heart Lung Transplant. 2014;33(11):1157–63.
24. Dolgner SJ, Nguyen VP, Krieger EV, Stempien-Otero A, Dardas TF. Long-term adult congenital heart disease survival after heart transplantation: a restricted mean survival time analysis. J Heart Lung Transplant. 2021;40(7):698–706.
25. Khush KK, Cherikh WS, Chambers DC, Goldfarb S, Hayes D Jr, Kucheryavaya AY, et al. The International Thoracic Organ Transplant registry of the International Society for Heart and Lung Transplantation: thirty-fifth adult heart transplantation report-2018; focus theme: multiorgan transplantation. J Heart Lung Transplant. 2018;37(10):1155–68.
26. Yu C, Moore BM, Kotchetkova I, Cordina RL, Celermajer DS. Causes of death in a contemporary adult congenital heart disease cohort. Heart. 2018;104(20):1678–82.
27. Stout KK, Broberg CS, Book WM, Cecchin F, Chen JM, Dimopoulos K, et al. Chronic heart failure in congenital heart disease: a scientific statement from the American Heart Association. Circulation. 2016;133(8):770–801.
28. Alshawabkeh LI, Opotowsky AR. Burden of heart failure in adults with congenital heart disease. Curr Heart Fail Rep. 2016;13(5):247–54.
29. Bolger AP, Coats AJ, Gatzoulis MA. Congenital heart disease: the original heart failure syndrome. Eur Heart J. 2003;24(10):970–6.
30. Fredriksen PM, Veldtman G, Hechter S, Therrien J, Chen A, Warsi MA, et al. Aerobic capacity in

adults with various congenital heart diseases. Am J Cardiol. 2001;87(3):310–4.
31. Diller GP, Dimopoulos K, Okonko D, Li W, Babu-Narayan SV, Broberg CS, et al. Exercise intolerance in adult congenital heart disease: comparative severity, correlates, and prognostic implication. Circulation. 2005;112(6):828–35.
32. Kempny A, Dimopoulos K, Uebing A, Moceri P, Swan L, Gatzoulis MA, et al. Reference values for exercise limitations among adults with congenital heart disease. Relation to activities of daily life--single centre experience and review of published data. Eur Heart J. 2012;33(11):1386–96.
33. Wang F, Harel-Sterling L, Cohen S, Liu A, Brophy JM, Paradis G, et al. Heart failure risk predictions in adult patients with congenital heart disease: a systematic review. Heart. 2019;105(21):1661–9.
34. Menachem JN, Reza N, Mazurek JA, Burstein D, Birati EY, Fox A, et al. Cardiopulmonary exercise testing-A valuable tool, not gatekeeper when referring patients with adult congenital heart disease for transplant evaluation. World J Pediatr Congenit Heart Surg. 2019;10(3):286–91.
35. Eindhoven JA, van den Bosch AE, Boersma E, Roos-Hesselink JW. The usefulness of brain natriuretic peptide in simple congenital heart disease - a systematic review. Cardiol Young. 2013;23(3):315–24.
36. Baggen VJ, van den Bosch AE, Eindhoven JA, Schut AW, Cuypers JA, Witsenburg M, et al. Prognostic value of N-terminal pro-B-type natriuretic peptide, troponin-T, and growth-differentiation factor 15 in adult congenital heart disease. Circulation. 2017;135(3):264–79.
37. Giannakoulas G, Dimopoulos K, Bolger AP, Tay EL, Inuzuka R, Bedard E, et al. Usefulness of natriuretic peptide levels to predict mortality in adults with congenital heart disease. Am J Cardiol. 2010;105(6):869–73.
38. Van De Bruaene A, Hickey EJ, Kovacs AH, Crean AM, Wald RM, Silversides CK, et al. Phenotype, management and predictors of outcome in a large cohort of adult congenital heart disease patients with heart failure. Int J Cardiol. 2018;252:80–7.
39. Bredy C, Ministeri M, Kempny A, Alonso-Gonzalez R, Swan L, Uebing A, et al. New York Heart Association (NYHA) classification in adults with congenital heart disease: relation to objective measures of exercise and outcome. Eur Heart J Qual Care Clin Outcomes. 2018;4(1):51–8.
40. Inuzuka R, Diller GP, Borgia F, Benson L, Tay EL, Alonso-Gonzalez R, et al. Comprehensive use of cardiopulmonary exercise testing identifies adults with congenital heart disease at increased mortality risk in the medium term. Circulation. 2012;125(2):250–9.
41. Zomer AC, Vaartjes I, van der Velde ET, de Jong HM, Konings TC, Wagenaar LJ, et al. Heart failure admissions in adults with congenital heart disease; risk factors and prognosis. Int J Cardiol. 2013;168(3):2487–93.
42. Moussa NB, Karsenty C, Pontnau F, Malekzadeh-Milani S, Boudjemline Y, Legendre A, et al. Characteristics and outcomes of heart failure-related hospitalization in adults with congenital heart disease. Arch Cardiovasc Dis. 2017;110(5):283–91.
43. Arnaert S, De Meester P, Troost E, Droogne W, Van Aelst L, Van Cleemput J, et al. Heart failure related to adult congenital heart disease: prevalence, outcome and risk factors. ESC Heart Fail. 2021;8(4):2940–50.
44. Poh CL, d'Udekem Y. Life after surviving Fontan surgery: a meta-analysis of the Incidence and predictors of late death. Heart Lung Circ. 2018;27(5):552–9.
45. Kammeraad JA, van Deurzen CH, Sreeram N, Bink-Boelkens MT, Ottenkamp J, Helbing WA, et al. Predictors of sudden cardiac death after mustard or senning repair for transposition of the great arteries. J Am Coll Cardiol. 2004;44(5):1095–102.
46. Dimopoulos K, Diller GP, Giannakoulas G, Petraco R, Chamaidi A, Karaoli E, et al. Anemia in adults with congenital heart disease relates to adverse outcome. J Am Coll Cardiol. 2009;54(22):2093–100.
47. Eindhoven JA, van den Bosch AE, Ruys TP, Opic P, Cuypers JA, McGhie JS, et al. N-terminal pro-B-type natriuretic peptide and its relationship with cardiac function in adults with congenital heart disease. J Am Coll Cardiol. 2013;62(13):1203–12.
48. Opotowsky AR, Valente AM, Alshawabkeh L, Cheng S, Bradley A, Rimm EB, et al. Prospective cohort study of C-reactive protein as a predictor of clinical events in adults with congenital heart disease: results of the Boston adult congenital heart disease biobank. Eur Heart J. 2018;39(34):3253–61.
49. Alshawabkeh L, Rajpal S, Landzberg MJ, Emani S, Ephrem G, Gray C, et al. Relationship of red cell distribution width to adverse outcomes in adults with congenital heart disease (from the Boston adult congenital heart biobank). Am J Cardiol. 2018;122(9):1557–64.
50. Baggen VJM, van den Bosch AE, van Kimmenade RR, Eindhoven JA, Witsenburg M, Cuypers J, et al. Red cell distribution width in adults with congenital heart disease: a worldwide available and low-cost predictor of cardiovascular events. Int J Cardiol. 2018;260:60–5.
51. Shiina Y, Nagao M, Shimomiya Y, Inai K. Secondary sarcopenia assessed by computed tomography can predict hospitalization for heart failure in adults with Fontan circulation. J Cardiol. 2021;77(1):10–6.
52. Krishnathasan K, Dimopoulos K, Duncan N, Ricci P, Kempny A, Rafiq I, et al. Advanced heart failure in adult congenital heart disease: the role of renal dysfunction in management and outcomes. Eur J Prev Cardiol. 2023;30(13):1335–42.
53. Crossland DS, Van De Bruaene A, Silversides CK, Hickey EJ, Roche SL. Heart failure in

adult congenital heart disease: from advanced therapies to end-of-life care. Can J Cardiol. 2019;35(12):1723–39.

54. Riggs KW, Zafar F, Radzi Y, Yu PJ, Bryant R 3rd, Morales DLS. Adult Congenital Heart Disease: Current Early Expectations After Cardiac Transplantation. Ann Thorac Surg. 2020;109(2):480–6.
55. Nguyen VP, Dolgner SJ, Dardas TF, Verrier ED, McMullan DM, Krieger EV. Improved outcomes of heart transplantation in adults with congenital heart disease receiving regionalized care. J Am Coll Cardiol. 2019;74(23):2908–18.
56. Tompkins R, Romfh A. General principles of heart failure management in adult congenital heart disease. Heart Fail Rev. 2020;25(4):555–67.
57. Mitchell MB, Campbell DN, Ivy D, Boucek MM, Sondheimer HM, Pietra B, et al. Evidence of pulmonary vascular disease after heart transplantation for Fontan circulation failure. J Thorac Cardiovasc Surg. 2004;128(5):693–702.
58. Rajagopal SK, Fineman JR. Pulmonary arteriovenous malformations and the hepatic "black box": are we emerging from the darkness? JACC Basic Transl Sci. 2021;6(3):236–8.
59. Pike NA, Vricella LA, Feinstein JA, Black MD, Reitz BA. Regression of severe pulmonary arteriovenous malformations after Fontan revision and "hepatic factor" rerouting. Ann Thorac Surg. 2004;78(2):697–9.
60. Shi WY, Saxena P, Yong MS, Marasco SF, McGiffin DC, Shipp A, et al. Increasing complexity of heart transplantation in patients with congenital heart disease. Semin Thorac Cardiovasc Surg. 2016;28(2):487–97.
61. Burchill LJ. Heart transplantation in adult congenital heart disease. Heart. 2016;102(23):1871–7.
62. Goldstein SA, Krasuski RA. Pulmonary hypertension in adults with congenital heart disease. Cardiol Clin. 2022;40(1):55–67.
63. Arvanitaki A, Gatzoulis MA, Opotowsky AR, Khairy P, Dimopoulos K, Diller GP, et al. Eisenmenger syndrome: JACC state-of-the-art review. J Am Coll Cardiol. 2022;79(12):1183–98.
64. Sertic F, Han J, Diagne D, Richards T, Chavez L, Berg A, et al. Not all septal defects are equal: outcomes of bilateral lung transplant with cardiac defect repair vs combined heart-lung transplant in patients with Eisenmenger syndrome in the United States. Chest. 2020;158(5):2097–106.
65. Dimopoulos K, Diller GP, Koltsida E, Pijuan-Domenech A, Papadopoulou SA, Babu-Narayan SV, et al. Prevalence, predictors, and prognostic value of renal dysfunction in adults with congenital heart disease. Circulation. 2008;117(18):2320–8.
66. Houyel L, To-Dumortier NT, Lepers Y, Petit J, Roussin R, Ly M, et al. Heart transplantation in adults with congenital heart disease. Arch Cardiovasc Dis. 2017;110(5):346–53.
67. Nwakanma LU, Williams JA, Weiss ES, Russell SD, Baumgartner WA, Conte JV. Influence of pretransplant panel-reactive antibody on outcomes in 8,160 heart transplant recipients in recent era. Ann Thorac Surg. 2007;84(5):1556–62; discussion 62–3.
68. Kaufman BD, Shaddy RE. Immunologic considerations in heart transplantation for congenital heart disease. Curr Cardiol Rev. 2011;7(2):67–71.
69. Kfoury AG, Stehlik J, Renlund DG, Snow G, Seaman JT, Gilbert EM, et al. Impact of repetitive episodes of antibody-mediated or cellular rejection on cardiovascular mortality in cardiac transplant recipients: defining rejection patterns. J Heart Lung Transplant. 2006;25(11):1277–82.
70. Wu GW, Kobashigawa JA, Fishbein MC, Patel JK, Kittleson MM, Reed EF, et al. Asymptomatic antibody-mediated rejection after heart transplantation predicts poor outcomes. J Heart Lung Transplant. 2009;28(5):417–22.
71. Smith JD, Banner NR, Hamour IM, Ozawa M, Goh A, Robinson D, et al. De novo donor HLA-specific antibodies after heart transplantation are an independent predictor of poor patient survival. Am J Transplant. 2011;11(2):312–9.
72. Patel ND, Weiss ES, Allen szszJG, Russell SD, Shah AS, Vricella LA, et al. Heart transplantation for adults with congenital heart disease: analysis of the United network for organ sharing database. Ann Thorac Surg. 2009;88(3):814–21; discussion 21–2.
73. Hsu RB, Chang CI, Lin FY, Chou NK, Chi NH, Wang SS, et al. Heart transplantation in patients with liver cirrhosis. Eur J Cardiothorac Surg. 2008;34(2):307–12.
74. Reiter FP, Hadjamu NJ, Nagdyman N, Zachoval R, Mayerle J, De Toni EN, et al. Congenital heart disease-associated liver disease: a narrative review. Cardiovasc Diagn Ther. 2021;11(2):577–90.
75. Wang A, Book WM, McConnell M, Lyle T, Rodby K, Mahle WT. Prevalence of hepatitis C infection in adult patients who underwent congenital heart surgery prior to screening in 1992. Am J Cardiol. 2007;100(8):1307–9.
76. Emamaullee J, Zaidi AN, Schiano T, Kahn J, Valentino PL, Hofer RE, et al. Fontan-associated liver disease: screening, management, and transplant considerations. Circulation. 2020;142(6):591–604.
77. Reardon L, Lin J. Advanced heart failure and transplant in congenital heart disease. Heart. 2021;107(3):245–53.
78. VanderPluym CJ, Cedars A, Eghtesady P, Maxwell BG, Gelow JM, Burchill LJ, et al. Outcomes following implantation of mechanical circulatory support in adults with congenital heart disease: An analysis of the Interagency Registry for Mechanically Assisted Circulatory Support (INTERMACS). J Heart Lung Transplant. 2018;37(1):89–99.
79. Cedars A, Vanderpluym C, Koehl D, Cantor R, Kutty S, Kirklin JK. An Interagency Registry for Mechanically Assisted Circulatory Support

(INTERMACS) analysis of hospitalization, functional status, and mortality after mechanical circulatory support in adults with congenital heart disease. J Heart Lung Transplant. 2018;37(5):619–30.
80. Gyoten T, Rojas SV, Fox H, Schramm R, Hakim-Meibodi K, Ruiz-Cano M, et al. Mechanical circulatory support as a bridge to candidacy in adults with transposition of the great arteries and a systemic right ventricle. Eur J Cardiothorac Surg. 2020.
81. Steiner JM, Krieger EV, Stout KK, Stempien-Otero A, Mahr C, Mokadam NA, et al. Durable mechanical circulatory support in teenagers and adults with congenital heart disease: a systematic review. Int J Cardiol. 2017;245:135–40.
82. Carlo WF, Villa CR, Lal AK, Morales DL. Ventricular assist device use in single ventricle congenital heart disease. Pediatr Transplant. 2017;21(7).
83. Kainuma A, Ning Y, Kurlansky PA, Wang AS, Axom K, Farr M, et al. Changes in waitlist and posttransplant outcomes in patients with adult congenital heart disease after the new heart transplant allocation system. Clin Transplant. 2021;35(11):e14458.
84. Bravo-Jaimes K, Axsom K, Menachem J, Danford D, Kutty S, Cedars A. Impact of the new UNOS donor heart allocation system on waitlist outcomes and early posttransplant mortality among adults with congenital heart disease. Am J Transplant. 2022;22(4):1123–32.

# 26 Combined Heart and Other Organ Transplants

Jon Kobashigawa and Yosef Manla

**Abstract**

Advances in immunosuppressive therapies and surgical and organ preservation techniques have significantly improved transplant patient outcomes. Inevitably, multiorgan transplants involving heart transplantation (HTx) have steadily increased in the United States. Given the scarcity of organ donors, appropriate allocation of these resources is essential. The approach to HTx candidates with concomitant organ dysfunction necessitates multidisciplinary collaboration between subspecialties and transplantation surgeons. This chapter will cover the clinical aspects, indications, donor-recipient considerations, and management of combined HTx organ transplants.

**Keywords**

Heart · Lung · Kidney · Solid organ transplantation · Combined heart transplant · Multidisciplinary team

J. Kobashigawa (✉) · Y. Manla
Cedars-Sinai Smidt Heart Institute, Los Angeles, CA, USA
e-mail: Jon.Kobashigawa@cshs.org

Y. Manla
e-mail: Yosef.manla@cshs.org; Yosef.manla1@gmail.com

## Clinical Pearls

- Patients with severe heart disease frequently have concomitant kidney, liver, or lung disease. Dual heart and other organ transplantation has been demonstrated to have outcomes benefit not only in survival but in reduction of cardiac rejection.
- To qualify for evaluation for simultaneous heart-kidney transplant (sHKT), patients need to have established chronic kidney disease (CKD) defined as GFR ≤ 60 ml/min/1.73 m$^2$ measured 90 days apart. Thereafter, these patients must have established GFR < 30 ml/min/1.73 m$^2$ to qualify for sHKT.
- For pre-HTx patients who do not undergo sHKT but HTx alone, a safety net policy for after HTx (modified from liver-kidney policy) is in place. This safety net policy provides that HTx patients on chronic dialysis or with persistent GFR ≤ 20 ml/min/1.73 m$^2$ for 6 weeks during day 30 to day 365 post-transplant, should be given priority for kidney transplantation (donors with KDPI > 20%).
- Induction therapy for sHKT will be left to the discretion of the transplant program. If ATG is used for induction, a delay in initiation of calcineurin inhibitor of 1–3 days is considered safe, especially if kidney function appears impaired post-operatively.
- It is safe for corticosteroids to be weaned in select (low immunologic risk) sHKT



J. Kobashigawa (ed.), *Clinical Guide to Heart Transplantation*, https://doi.org/10.1007/978-3-031-88290-6_26

recipients after carefully weighing risks versus benefits.

- Liver transplant evaluation should be performed in heart transplant (HTx) candidates if there is concern for co-existing liver disease based on clinical/laboratory findings or if the liver appears nodular on imaging.
- In patients being considered for combined heart-liver transplantation (CHLT), a liver biopsy is highly encouraged when technically feasible and acceptably safe.
- Biopsy-proven cirrhosis, regardless of portal hypertension, is an indication of CHLT. Biopsy-proven fibrosis of any stage with clinical evidence of portal hypertension (hepatic ascites and portosystemic collaterals) should be a consideration for CHLT.
- Biopsy-proven stage 3 fibrosis (F3 disease) without clinical evidence for portal hypertension may not require CHLT.
- Adult patients with Fontan physiology may have more tendency toward CHLT due to chronically elevated central venous pressure that results in Fontan-associated liver disease
- Induction therapy for CHLT should be used on an individualized basis based on factors including antibody sensitization, renal function, risk of infection, and risk of bleeding. In low-risk patients, prednisone can be weaned off in the setting of CHLT.
- Less frequent acute and chronic rejection surveillance for the HTx is needed for low risk CHLT patients due to immune protective effect of the liver transplant.
- Heart–lung transplantation (HLT) is an effective and definitive treatment option for patients with advanced cardiopulmonary failure with pulmonary arterial hypertension and cystic fibrosis as leading indications for HLT.
- Advanced donor age, recipient male sex, recipient ECMO support, and HLT performed in low- and medium-volume centers as independent predictors of death or retransplant post-HLT.
- The day-to-day management of the HLT patient is primarily done by the lung transplant team due to most post-transplant complication occurring in that organ.
- In sHKT, CHLT and HLT, the immunosuppression protocols should involve multidisciplinary collaboration between HTx and other organ transplant specialists balancing the risk of infection and rejection.

## Introduction

Advances in immunosuppressive therapies and surgical and organ preservation techniques have significantly improved transplant patient outcomes [1]. In the case of heart transplantation (HTx), the presence of other concomitant comorbidities, including renal, hepatic, or respiratory failure, may limit isolated HTx [2]. Multiorgan transplants involving HTx have steadily increased in the United States. According to the 2022 Organ Procurement and Transplantation Network (OPTN) and Scientific Registry of Transplant Recipients (SRTR) report, 14% of HTx were combined with transplant of other organs in 2021 versus 5.7% in 2011 in the US, with simultaneous heart-kidney transplant (sHKT) recording an increase of 442.3% (71–385 transplants) over the years 2011–2021. Similarly, combined heart-liver transplant (CHLT) increased by 393.3% (from 15 to 74), and heart–lung transplants (HLT) increased by 87.5% (from 24 to 45) (Fig. 26.1) [3]. Dual heart and other organ transplantation has been demonstrated to have outcomes benefit not only in survival but also in reduction of cardiac rejection [4]. The more vascularized organ provides immune protection for the less vascularized organ, this being the heart in sHKT, CHLT, and HLT. Given the scarcity of organ donors, appropriate allocation of these resources is essential. The approach to HTx candidates with concomitant organ dysfunction necessitates multidisciplinary collaboration between subspecialties and transplantation surgeons. This chapter will cover the clinical aspects, indications, donor-recipient considerations, and management of multi-organ Tx, including sHKT, CHLT, and HLT, from a cardiologist's perspective.

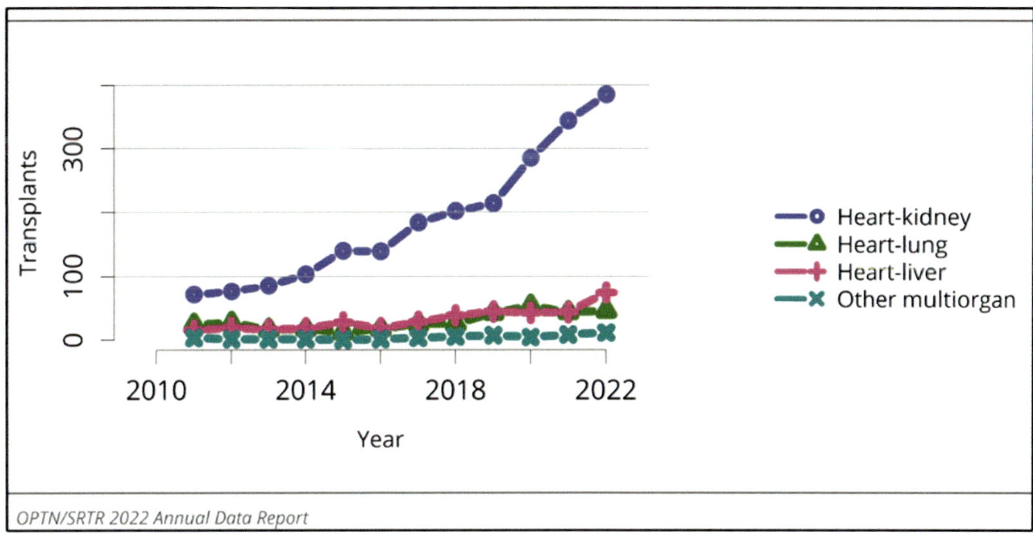


**Fig. 26.1** Adult heart transplant by multiorgan transplant type (2011–2022). *Source* OPTN/SRTR 2022 Annual Data Report. HHS/HRSA; 2024. Accessed [October 1st 2024]., not copyrighted. https://srtr.transplant.hrsa.gov/ADR/Chapter?name=Heart&year=2022

## The Ethics of Dual Organ Transplantation: Evaluating Fairness in Organ Allocation

Organ Procurement and Transplantation Network's (OPTN) policies for organ allocation make an implicit distinction between life-saving organs (heart, lung and liver) and those that are life-prolonging, or that improve the quality of life for recipients (kidney and pancreas). The most recent UNOS policy states: "When multi-organ candidates are registered on the heart, lung, or liver waiting list, the second required organ will be allocated to the multi-organ candidate from the same donor if the candidate is qualified for dual organ transplant. In practice, this means that a recipient listed for sHKT or simultaneous liver/kidney (a) will have the primary life-saving organ allocated on the basis of the acuity of need and (b) will then receive the second, life-prolonging organ based on qualification of need for that organ. Another ethically distinctive feature of simultaneous multi-organ transplantation (sMOT) is that this ethical reasoning based on life-saving and life-prolonging views support bypassing other potential recipients who may be on the waiting list for a life-prolonging organ, whereas the sMOT recipient may have a more immediate need for that organ. Preemptive KT for patients requiring another life-saving solid organ is a rare instance when a future event is considered in the evaluation and allocation of an organ.

**Is an immediate or proven need more ethically justified than an anticipated or potential need?** In this sense, eligible patients are not unfairly disadvantaged because they have a life-sustaining alternative (dialysis) until an organ becomes available and because the allocation of both a life-saving organ and a life-prolonging organ is well-supported by both beneficence and utility. The most obvious issue with utility in a sMOT is the single recipient. Rather than helping two or three people, only one person benefits. Typically, utility beyond the individual has not been considered in either candidate consideration or allocation policies. The methods for determining social utility are imperfect, and they are not generally considered in transplantation decisions. In the setting of sMOT, however, when there are multiple waiting lists of competing recipients for several organs, some consideration of utility might help determine which patient would be the most appropriate candidate for sMOT. The usual criteria for determining transplant outcomes are affected by other considerations such as quality of life and potential alternative treatments, namely dialysis. These and other issues around fairness and distribution of organs across waitlists and different types of candidates warrant ongoing discussion and consensus in order to move toward sensible policy.

## Heart-Kidney Transplantation

These patients with kidney disease who undergo alone have reduced survival. Kidney failure is a predictor of morbidity and mortality in post-patients [5, 6]. sHKT has enabled the successful transplantation of patients with end-stage heart disease and concomitant kidney disease, with increasing numbers since 2010. The rise of sHKs has raised concerns due to the incremental benefit attributable to the kidney in the sHKT recipient is difficult to assess, proper candidate selection remains debated, and sHKT diverts deceased donor kidneys away from candidates for kidney transplant alone. The decision for sHKT transplantation is further challenged by difficulties in differentiating those patients with a reversible kidney injury due to cardiorenal syndrome who may recover kidney function after HTx, from those with intrinsic advanced kidney disease who would benefit most from sHKT.

## The Pathophysiology of Cardiorenal Disease Leading to End Organ Failure

Heart failure and kidney failure share complex pathophysiological pathways that affect myocardial and vascular remodeling, endothelial dysfunction, as well as systemic neurohormonal activation, inflammation and oxidative stress [7, 8]. Hemodynamic factors in myocardial dysfunction leading to kidney failure include not only impaired cardiac output and arterial underfilling, but also venous congestion leading to kidney congestion. All this leads to reduced glomerular filtration and rise in serum creatinine which we call cardiorenal syndrome [9–11]. In the acute setting, restoration of cardiac performance often results in improvement of kidney function.

Kidney disease can also affect the heart. Progressive kidney failure triggers metabolic disorders that can accelerate atherosclerosis, as well as precipitate uremic cardiomyopathy. Concomitant anemia from kidney failure, as well as the presence of an arteriovenous fistula, can create a state of "high performance" volume overload that may be reversible after restoration of cardiac function [12, 13]. It is important to emphasize that the ongoing findings of traditional biomarkers of kidney function such as creatinine and proteinuria may not reflect the spectrum of kidney dysfunction seen in heart failure and kidney disease. Specifically, the frequent occurrence of electrolyte imbalances, metabolic disturbances, and persistent volume overload may further exacerbate cardiorenal syndrome [14].

## Evaluation for Combined Heart-Kidney Transplantation

CKD is defined as having documentation of GFR $<$ 60 ml/min/1.73 m$^2$ on at least 2 occasions 90 days apart. In addition, any history of kidney disease or kidney disease risk factors, such as diabetes or hypertension, will be helpful. In addition, kidney ultrasound to assess for kidney size asymmetry, shrinkage or cortical thinning can indicate the diagnosis of CKD [15]. Native kidney biopsies are not always feasible and can carry significant risk but may be valuable in select clinical circumstances. Some patients with normal kidney function who develop sudden decompensated heart failure or cardiogenic shock may experience an acute rise in serum creatinine and, in some cases, temporary dialysis may even be necessary. These patients will have predominantly cardiorenal syndrome and/or acute tubular injury and will typically recover kidney function with HTx alone.

There remains some uncertainty as to what lower GFR threshold should warrant evaluation of a pre-HTx patient for sHKT. Large registry studies on pre-HTx patients have demonstrated post-HTx mortality and complication risks for various baseline levels of GFR. A large review of the UNOS database assessed pre-HTx GFR in patients aged $\geq$ 18 years who underwent HTx between 1988 and 2013 [16]. In this study, patients were stratified into 5 different GFR categories ($\geq$ 90, 60–89, 45–59, 30–44 and < 30 ml/min/1.73 m$^2$). A total of 30,090 patients were included in the study; of these, 46.1% and 39.9% had an GFR < 60 ml/min/1.73 m$^2$ by Modification of Diet in Renal Disease (MDRD) and Chronic Kidney Disease Epidemiology Collaboration (CKD-EPI), respectively. Compared with GFR $\geq$ 90 ml/min/1.73 m$^2$, the adjusted hazard ratio of mortality was 1.09 (95% confidence interval [CI] 1.02–1.26) for GFR 45–59 ml/min/1.73 m$^2$, 1.22 (95% CI −1.23 to 1.31) for GFR 30–44 ml/min/1.73 m$^2$ and 1.55 (95% CI 1.41–1.70) for GFR < 30 ml/min/1.73 m$^2$ by MDRD. There was no advantage for CKD-EPI over MDRD in determining post-HTx mortality. Pre-HTx GFR by either equation was predictive of post-HTx end-stage kidney disease and the need for KT, with the highest risk in those with pre-HTx GFR < 30 ml/min/1.73 m$^2$ by either equation.

In other studies, pre-HTx GFR < 60 mL/min/1.73 m$^2$ was similarly associated with increased mortality after HTx. Thus, lower GFR portended higher mortality after isolated HTx but there was no indication that all patients with GFR < 60 mL/min/1.73 m$^2$ would require sHKT [5, 6].

As noted, sHKT improves survival in patients with a recent International Society for Heart and Lung Transplant registry analysis, demonstrating that multiorgan transplantation is associated with a survival advantage in comparison with HTx alone [17]. In addition, recent data show that heart-kidney and heart-liver transplantation provide immune-protection to the cardiac allograft showing less rejection [18]. A recent intravascular ultrasound (IVUS) study has demonstrated less first-year allograft vasculopathy in sHKT recipients when compared with HTx alone [19].

## Medical Eligibility Criteria for Heart-Kidney Allocation

As of September 2023, UNOS made formal guidelines for the criteria for when to proceed with sHKT. To qualify for sHKT evaluation the following must occur.

If the candidate's transplant nephrologist confirms a diagnosis of: CKD with a measured or estimated GFR less than or equal to 60 mL/min/1.73 m$^2$ for greater than 90 consecutive days.

Then the transplant program must report to the OPTN and document in the candidate's medical record at least one of the following:

- That the candidate has begun regularly administered dialysis as an end-stage renal disease (ESRD) patient in a hospital based, independent non-hospital based, or home setting.
- At the time of registration on the kidney waiting list, that the candidate's most recent measured or estimated creatinine clearance (CrCl) or GFR is less than or equal to 30 mL/min/1.73 m$^2$
- On a date after registration on the kidney waiting list, that the candidate's measured or estimated CrCl or GFR is less than or equal to 30 mL/min/1.73 m$^2$.

If the candidate's transplant nephrologist confirms a diagnosis of: Sustained acute kidney injury at least one of the following, or a combination of both of the following, for the last 6 weeks:

- That the candidate has been on dialysis at least once every 7 days.
- That the candidate has a measured or estimated CrCl or GFR less than or equal to 25 mL/min/1.73 m$^2$ at least once every 7 days.

If the candidate's eligibility is not confirmed at least once every seven days for the last 6 weeks, the candidate is not eligible to receive a heart and a kidney from the same donor.

## Safety Net

To reduce unnecessary KTs a safety net policy for HTx patients was initiated (September 2023) for those patients who do not undergo sHKT, a policy currently applied to kidney after liver transplantation [20]. For pre-HTx patients who do not undergo sHKT but HTx alone, a safety net policy for after HTx (modified from liver-kidney policy) is in place. This safety net policy provides that HTx patients on chronic dialysis or with persistent GFR ≤ 20 ml/min/1.73 m$^2$ for 6 weeks during day 30 to day 365 post-transplant, should be given priority for kidney transplantation (donors with kidney donor profile index, KDPI, >20%). The safety net thus alleviates the burden of "guessing incorrectly," and incentivizes isolated HTx when there remains potential for kidney recovery.

## Outcomes of Heart-Kidney Transplantation

Patients who undergo sHKT may have improved survival, less rejection, and less cardiac allograft vasculopathy than patients undergoing HTx alone. Nonetheless, sHKT does not fully mitigate the risk of adverse renal disease after HTx. Recipients of sHKT experience a higher rate of severe AKI after transplantation due to adverse effect of medications and abnormal cardiac hemodynamics, with 26–37% of sHKT recipients needing dialysis in the early post transplantation period compared with recipients of HTx alone (7–22%) [21]. Furthermore, similar to patients undergoing HTx, progressive renal dysfunction may still develop over time after sHKT in part due to chronic immunosuppression medications.

## Management of the sHKT Patient

There is a lack of specific evidence on the benefit of induction therapy and an absence of consensus among centers performing induction therapy for sHKT. If induction is to be used, the choice of agent for induction therapy needs to be personalized based on recipient's risk factors for infection, presence or absence of delayed graft function and recipient's immunologic profile [22]. For sensitized recipients and patients with delayed graft function, anti-thymocyte globulin (ATG) induction can be considered [23]. For recipients with lower immunologic risk or at risk for infection, basiliximab induction can be considered. Although it is believed that calcineurin inhibitor (CNI) delay is not necessary for kidney protection, if ATG is used for induction, a delay in initiation of CNI of 1–2 days was considered safe, especially if kidney function appears impaired post-operatively [24]. There was no consensus on a specific goal level for CNI in the case of delayed kidney graft function, but CNI can be safely continued through kidney dysfunction. If basiliximab is used for induction, CNI introduction should not be delayed and preferably given within 24 h of sHKT. Lastly, it is believed that corticosteroids can be weaned in select (low immunologic risk) sHKT recipients carefully weighing the risks versus benefits. Low risk is understood as no treated rejection episodes, no donor-specific antibodies and normal heart/kidney function. For those sHKT patients not weaned off steroids, they may be maintained on 5 mg Prednisone per day which is standard for alone patients.

## Heart-Liver Transplantation

Patients with severe heart disease may have co-existing liver disease from various causes. The incidence of combined heart-liver transplant (CHLT) is increasing as more patients with congenital heart disease are surviving to adulthood. However, these patients over time may develop advanced heart failure with associated liver disease from chronic right-sided heart or Fontan failure. Patients with advanced heart failure and chronic liver disease who undergo alone have reduced survival compared to those without liver disease. In recent years, approximately 40–50 CHLT surgeries have been performed annually in 25 centers in the United States with comparable 1-year survival outcomes to heart alone [25]. However, the decision of when liver transplantation is warranted in a patient with advanced HF and compensated chronic liver disease is challenged by difficulties in differentiating those patients with moderate hepatic fibrosis (which may be reversible) from those with advanced fibrosis and/or cirrhosis who could benefit from this intervention. This can be particularly challenging given the overlap in clinical symptoms in advanced cardiac and liver disease.

## Indications and the Standard Liver-Related Workup of the CHLT Patient

The most common indications for liver transplant in CHLT include cardiomyopathy with non-cardiac cirrhosis (e.g., hepatitis C virus (HCV), alcohol-associated cirrhosis), congenital heart disease (CHD) with congestive hepatopathy and transthyretin cardiac amyloidosis (though less common in the current era due to the advent of effective disease-directed therapies).

All candidates should undergo liver-related assessment, with those patients who are found to have abnormal findings referred to transplant hepatology for further testing (Fig. 26.2) [26]. An example protocol has been suggested (Fig. 26.3) [27]. Dedicated liver imaging should be performed for candidates with presence or prior history of liver disease or greater than 10 years of cardiac disease. If the liver has nodularity on imaging, suggestive of cirrhosis, then liver transplant evaluation should be pursued. In these cases, a liver biopsy should be performed when technically feasible and safe.

A liver biopsy may not be required if there are clinical signs of portal hypertension (e.g., varices, *ascites*) [28]. Isolated hepatic venous pressure gradient (HVPG) should not be used to rule in or rule out portal hypertension especially in patients with Fontan-associated liver disease (FALD) as it may not be reliable. If cross-sectional imaging reveals portosystemic collaterals, upper endoscopy should be performed for variceal screening. In lower-risk patients (those with compensated HF), a normal elastography result can be used to exclude advanced liver disease.

## Concerns for CHD Patients, Particularly the Fontan Population Who Require CHLT

Many survivors of specific CHD had undergone the Fontan procedure, with an estimated global population of 70,000 by the mid-2020s, which creates the potential for chronic FALD warranting CHLT. Survival has been shown to be comparable between the CHD-Heart transplant alone and CHD-CHLT groups [29]. Therefore, it is important that chronic CHD patients with disease of several years undergo liver assessment to exclude the need for CHLT [30].

There are numerous considerations for Fontan patients undergoing including anatomical complexity and surgical reconstruction (may result in longer bypass, ischemic time, and prolonged bleeding). Fontan patients are generally not candidates for temporary or durable mechanical circulatory support (MCS) due to anatomical considerations. Therefore these patients may qualify for prioritization at Status 1–3 only by seeking exceptions. CHD specific conditions such as hepatocellular cancer (HCC), cyanosis, protein losing enteropathy, plastic bronchitis, unsuitability for inotropic support or MCS may be considered for exception status [31].

Liver cirrhosis identified by computed tomography (CT) imaging may not be an absolute contraindication to alone in the Fontan population [32]. In one study, 41% of Fontan patients evaluated for had cirrhosis suggested by imaging, however, one-year mortality and post-transplant liver function was comparable between alone and CHLT.

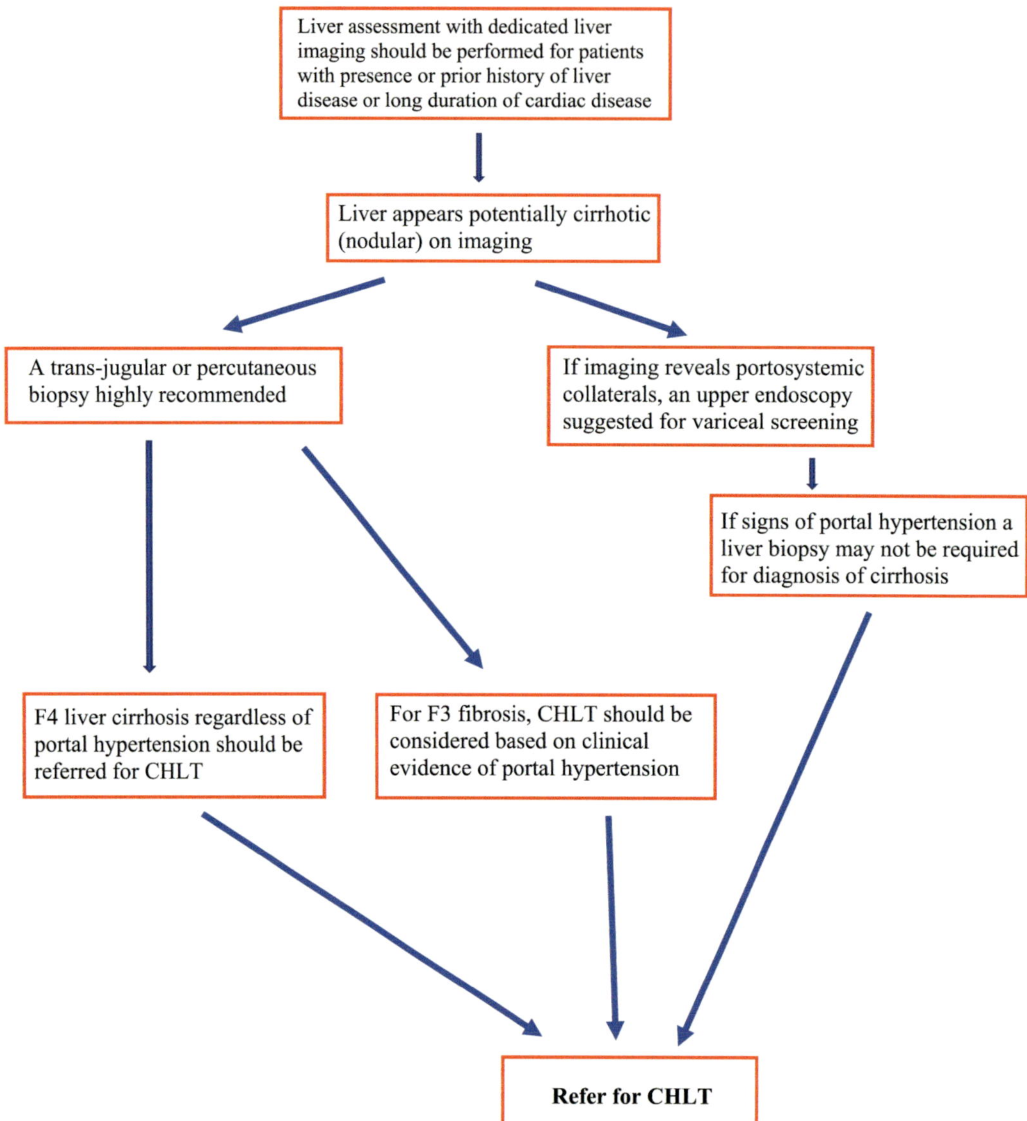


**Fig. 26.2** Workflow for liver-related assessment in non-congenital combined heart-liver transplant. Reused with permission from American Journal of Transplantation, 24(3), Kobashigawa, Jon, Lisa B. VanWagner, Shelley Hall, Juliet Emamaullee, John W. Entwistle, Daniel Ganger, Howard Gebel et al., Summary of a consensus conference on heart-liver transplantation, 380–390, Copyright Elsevier (2024)

## Criteria to Proceed with CHLT

Biopsy-proven cirrhosis, regardless of the presence of portal hypertension, is generally considered an indication for CHLT. Biopsy-proven stage 3 fibrosis (F3) and/or clinical evidence of portal hypertension should be a consideration for CHLT. In patients with F3 fibrosis, consideration for CHLT may also depend on recipient's age, the chronicity of right-sided heart or Fontan failure, and presence of clinical signs of portal hypertension. In patients with biopsy proven F3 fibrosis, F4 fibrosis (cirrhosis) is likely imminent due to the natural history of congestive

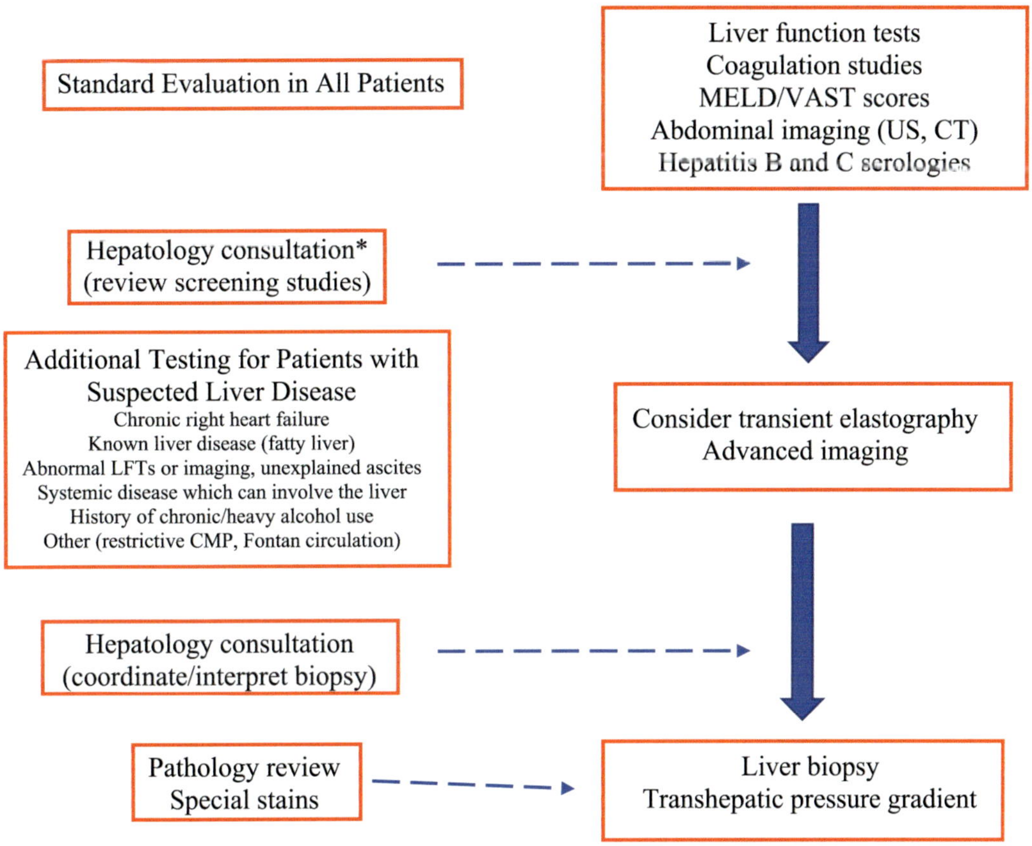

Standard Evaluation in All Patients

Liver function tests
Coagulation studies
MELD/VAST scores
Abdominal imaging (US, CT)
Hepatitis B and C serologies

Hepatology consultation*
(review screening studies)

Additional Testing for Patients with Suspected Liver Disease
Chronic right heart failure
Known liver disease (fatty liver)
Abnormal LFTs or imaging, unexplained ascites
Systemic disease which can involve the liver
History of chronic/heavy alcohol use
Other (restrictive CMP, Fontan circulation)

Consider transient elastography
Advanced imaging

Hepatology consultation
(coordinate/interpret biopsy)

Pathology review
Special stains

Liver biopsy
Transhepatic pressure gradient

**Fig. 26.3** Proposed algorithm for evaluation of liver disease in potential heart transplant candidates. *An early hepatology consultation may result in a clear recommendation for liver biopsy (e.g., in a patient with a history or imaging suggestive of cirrhosis, but no prior tissue diagnosis), thereby obviating the need for additional testing. CMP, cardiomyopathy; CT, computed tomography; HCV, hepatitis C virus; LFTs, liver function tests; MELD, model for end-stage liver disease; US, ultrasound. Reused with permission from American Journal of Transplantation, 24(3), Kobashigawa, Jon, Lisa B. VanWagner, Shelley Hall, Juliet Emamaullee, John W. Entwistle, Daniel Ganger, Howard Gebel et al., mary of a consensus conference on heart-liver transplantation, 380–390, Copyright Elsevier (2024)

hepatopathy or under-staging due to sampling error [28]. In contrast, patients with F3 fibrosis may also have regression of fibrosis as has been observed in patients with nonalcoholic steatohepatitis (NASH) post bariatric surgery and in those with HCV post curative antiviral treatment [33, 34]. In rare circumstances patients with F3 fibrosis who are highly sensitized have been considered for CHLT due to reported superior heart outcomes, where the donor liver is known to absorb circulating antibodies [35]. Regarding contraindications, although some programs reported an upper age limit for CHLT of 60 years, one should consider a physiological age rather than chronological age for older patients being evaluated for CHLT.

Liver biopsy may play a smaller role in the evaluation of FALD, owing to low inter-rater reliability among pathologists for qualitative interpretation of degree of fibrosis in FALD. Information from imaging and biomarkers may be sufficient to determine need for CHLT. However, in certain patients biopsy may be helpful where there is ambiguity about the severity of liver disease. Workup of patients with FALD should be based on multiple assessment modalities to include staging of liver fibrosis (if biopsy done), portal hypertension assessment and HCC screening imaging. From previous studies, it is expected that most Fontan patients will have some degree of liver disease due to chronic congestive hepatopathy [36].

## Surgical Approach and CHLT for Highly Sensitized Patients

Surgical approaches of CHLT include heart-first approach, en-bloc technique, or liver-first approach [37]. The heart-first approach is most used and provides maximal technical flexibility and less procurement risk. It also allows rapid cardiac implantation and cardiac recovery prior to liver reperfusion. However, there are advantages to the other methods. The en-bloc CHLT technique reduces surgery time and shortens liver cold ischemic time but increases the risk for phrenic nerve injury [38]. There is no clear indication for the liver-first approach except possibly in the highly sensitized patient. The liver-first approach may be applicable in experienced centers for the highly sensitized patient where it has been demonstrated to provide a protective effect on the donor heart by absorption of circulating antibodies [39]. For all approaches, a comprehensive team approach is critical to optimize care for patients.

Performing CHLT solely for the purpose of sensitization (no F3/F4 on liver biopsy) may not be appropriate because of significant surgical risk, ethical issues (i.e., the liver doesn't go to the patient who is highest on the list) and the current effective strategies for managing desensitization.

## Recommendations for Post-CHLT Management

The use of induction therapy in CHLT has not been established. It is usually administered to patients at higher risk for rejection and to allow delayed initiation of nephrotoxic immunosuppressive drugs in patients with compromised renal function (i.e., anti-thymocyte globulin or IL-2 receptor monoclonal antibody, basiliximab). According to the UNOS registry queried January 2000 to June 2018, 135 of 260 CHLT recipients (52%) were administered induction therapy with no difference in survival with induction versus no induction [40].

Surveillance protocols for acute rejection in both heart and liver transplant recipients vary across respective programs. Because CHLT recipients have a lower risk of acute rejection than heart-alone recipients, less frequent rejection surveillance may be feasible [41]. The role of noninvasive methods of rejection surveillance such as gene expression profiling and donor-derived cell-free DNA (dd-cfDNA) is uncertain given the lack of validation in heart-liver transplant recipients.

In addition, CHLT recipients have a reported lower risk of CAV than recipients of alone [41]. Therefore, routine surveillance with annual coronary angiography is also less frequent. Non-invasive measures of surveillance for CAV are currently being utilized in place of these angiograms [42].

In low-risk patients, prednisone could be weaned off in the setting of CHLT given the immunologically privileged status of CHLT. However, pre-transplant conditions may support ongoing steroid maintenance, such as autoimmune hepatitis and sarcoidosis. Proliferation signal inhibitors (PSI) should be avoided early given the risk for early renal insufficiency (potentiating CNI nephrotoxicity) and delayed wound healing as well as the box warning for increased risk of hepatic artery thrombosis in the first 30 days post-transplant. Using PSIs later after CHLT should be considered for renal sparing in liver transplant and possible benefits regarding HCC [43]. The immunosuppression protocols in CHLT recipients should involve multidisciplinary collaboration between and liver transplant specialists balancing the risk of infection and rejection.

## Heart–Lung Transplantation

Combined HLT is an effective and definitive treatment option for patients with advanced cardiopulmonary failure [44]. In a historical course like that of HTx alone, HLT in humans was first attempted in the late 1960s. Still, it was not a viable procedure for favorable long-term outcomes until the early 1980s, with the first successful HLT in 1981 by Reitz [45]. By 2018, 4,128 adult HLT were performed worldwide [46].

## Indications for Heart–Lung Transplantation

In an analysis of the 2019 International Heart and Lung Transplantation Registry report of more than 3000 adults undergoing HLT between 1988 and 2018, non-idiopathic pulmonary arterial hypertension (PAH) due to congenital heart disease, cardiomyopathy, or other conditions (37.7%), idiopathic PAH (28.4%), and cystic fibrosis (14.9%) were the overall leading indications [46, 47]. More recent data of 216 patients listed for HLT following an allocation system change in 2018 revealed that World Health Organization group 1 PAH accounted for two-thirds of transplants, including IPAH, representing 64% of these cases [47, 48]. In the past, HLT was far more common for primary lung diseases such as emphysema, idiopathic pulmonary fibrosis, and suppurative lung diseases. However, due to the shortage of donor hearts and increasing evidence of the non-inferiority of the double-lung transplant, there has been a decreased rate of HLT for these indications [49].

## Recipient and Donor Considerations for Heart–Lung Transplant

Regarding formal evaluation for transplant, the process is very similar to that of HTx alone, as addressed in Chap. 3. Additional factors such as the consistency of low oxygen saturation, the frequency of exacerbations, and a forced expiratory volume of below 30% of predicted have been associated with poor survival [50]. A thorough pre-operative assessment can guide listing and aid in achieving optimal management. For those with congenital heart disease and Eisenmenger's syndrome, clinical features should be evaluated in conjunction with hemodynamics, each patient's unique cardiac anatomy, and the overall health and functionality of the patient [51]. Many congenital heart disease patients present with their unique complications and pathophysiology and do not fit neatly into the standard model of single-organ failure on which current recommendations are based. Factors explaining the decreased use of HLT in patients with congenital heart disease may include HLA antibody development due to blood transfusions and size shorter height in patients with congenital heart disease. In addition to adhesions due to multiple prior surgeries, anatomical alterations, and collateral blood vessels, thereby creating technical difficulties [49, 52, 53]. In addition to the usual pre-operative assessments mentioned in Chap. 3. Detailed imaging with computed tomography should be performed in patients with primary lung disease, as well as to assess for aortopulmonary collaterals in congenital heart disease patients [51]. As with HTx, patients should be constantly monitored and reassessed as to whether they remain eligible for dual HLT. A failure to delist when patients deteriorate while on the waiting list may result in worse outcomes [49]. Shudo et al. studied 997 patients who underwent HLT between 1987 and 2017 [44] and analyzed 25 donor and 26 recipient characteristics. Among significant recipient characteristics significantly predicting worse outcomes, they identified advanced donor age, recipient male sex, earlier transplant year, recipient ECMO support, and HLT performed in low- and medium-volume centers as independent predictors of death or retransplant. Importantly, they found donor LVEF, donor or recipient history of cigarette usage, recipient lung allocation score, and allograft ischemic time, did not impact post-HLT outcomes. Additionally, Weingarten et al. recently found in their study of HLT that those receiving extended criteria donor (ECD) hearts and lungs did not experience worse mortality compared to recipients of ECD lung only, ECD heart only, or standard donor criteria organs. However, advanced donor age and the ratio of arterial oxygen partial pressure to the fraction of inspired oxygen (P/F ratio) were significant predictors of mortality overall in this study [54].

## Management and Complications of Heart Lung Transplant Recipients:

Overall, the post-operative management guidelines outlined in Chap. 11 still hold true for dual HLT, and as detailed in Chaps. 12 and 13, the immunosuppression and infection protocols used in HTx are also applicable to patients undergoing HLT. However, the day-to-day management of the HLT patient is primarily done by the lung transplant team due to most complications occurring in that organ. The use of induction therapy after dual HLT is center-dependent and usually follows the protocols used for lung transplantation alone [46, 55, 56]. Acute cellular rejection of either the heart or lung allografts is less common than after isolated heart or lung transplantation, and most of the common complications are infections arising from the lung allograft [46].

## Survival After Heart–Lung Transplantation

HLT recipients continue to have lower survival than isolated HTx or other combined HTx [3]. In a long-term analysis of 1,294 HLT recipients from the UNOS database. Kaplan–Meier Survival Curve showed 1, 3, 5, and 10-year survival outcomes of 68.5, 53.1, 44.7, and 29.8%, respectively [52]. During the first month after HLT, graft failure, technical complications, and infection remain the leading causes of death, whereas bronchiolitis obliterans syndrome and chronic lung allograft dysfunction cause the most deaths beyond the first year [57]. High-volume centers have been found to have better HLT outcomes, which could be due to an interdisciplinary approach to HLT workup, optimal pre-transplant assessment before transplant, well-tailored protocols for donor selection, improving procurement and preservation, and surgical techniques [44]. Furthermore, the US 2018 allocation policy change has been associated with improvements in waitlist outcomes of HLT candidates, including increased likelihood of and decreased waitlist mortality. Despite increased ischemic times and the use of ECMO after the policy change, early post-transplant survival was comparable to HLT recipients in the pre-policy change [48].

## References


1. Jou S, Mendez SR, Feinman J, Mitrani LR, Fuster V, Mangiola M, et al. Heart transplantation: advances in expanding the donor pool and xenotransplantation. Nat Rev Cardiol. 2024;21(1):25–36.
2. Kittleson MM, Sharma K, Brennan DC, Cheng XS, Chow SL, Colvin M, et al. Dual-organ transplantation: indications, evaluation, and outcomes for heart-kidney and heart-liver transplantation: a scientific statement from the American Heart Association. Circulation. 2023;148(7):622–36.
3. Colvin MM, Smith JM, Ahn YS, Handarova DK, Martinez AC, Lindblad KA, et al. OPTN/SRTR 2022 annual data report: Heart. Am J Transplant. 2024;24(2):S305-93.
4. Rana A, Robles S, Russo MJ, Halazun KJ, Woodland DC, Witkowski P, et al. The combined organ effect: protection against rejection? Ann Surg. 2008;248(5):871–9.
5. Grupper A, Grupper A, Daly RC, Pereira NL, Hathcock MA, Kremers WK, et al. Renal allograft outcome after simultaneous heart and kidney transplantation. Am J Cardiol. 2017;120(3):494–9.
6. Karamlou T, Welke KF, McMullan DM, Cohen GA, Gelow J, Tibayan FA, et al. Combined heart-kidney transplant improves post-transplant survival compared with isolated heart transplant in recipients with reduced glomerular filtration rate: analysis of 593 combined heart-kidney transplants from the United Network Organ Sharing Database. J Thorac Cardiovasc Surg. 2014;147(1):456–61.
7. Mentz RJ, O'connor CM. Pathophysiology and clinical evaluation of acute heart failure. Nat Rev Cardiol. 2016;13(1):28–35.
8. Liu S. Heart-kidney interactions: mechanistic insights from animal models. Am J Physiol-Renal Physiol. 2019;316(5):F974-85.

9. Mullens W, Abrahams Z, Francis GS, Sokos G, Taylor DO, Starling RC, et al. Importance of venous congestion for worsening of renal function in advanced decompensated heart failure. J Am Coll Cardiol. 2009;53(7):589–96.
10. Nijst P, Verbrugge FH, Martens P, Dupont M, Tang WHW, Mullens W. Renal response to intravascular volume expansion in euvolemic heart failure patients with reduced ejection fraction: Mechanistic insights and clinical implications. Int J Cardiol. 2017;243:318–25.
11. Tang WHW, Mullens W. Cardiorenal syndrome in decompensated heart failure. Heart. 2010;96(4):255–60.
12. Hawwa N, Shrestha K, Hammadah M, Yeo PSD, Fatica R, Tang WHW. Reverse remodeling and prognosis following kidney transplantation in contemporary patients with cardiac dysfunction. J Am Coll Cardiol. 2015;66(16):1779–87.
13. Rao NN, Stokes MB, Rajwani A, Ullah S, Williams K, King D, et al. Effects of arteriovenous fistula ligation on cardiac structure and function in kidney transplant recipients. Circulation. 2019;139(25):2809–18.
14. Chirakarnjanakorn S, Navaneethan SD, Francis GS, Tang WHW. Cardiovascular impact in patients undergoing maintenance hemodialysis: clinical management considerations. Int J Cardiol. 2017;232:12–23.
15. Emamian SA, Nielsen MB, Pedersen JF, Ytte L. Kidney dimensions at sonography: correlation with age, sex, and habitus in 665 adult volunteers. AJR Am J Roentgenol. 1993;160(1):83–6.
16. Habib PJ, Patel PC, Hodge D, Chimato N, Yip DS, Hosenpud JD, et al. Pre-orthotopic heart transplant estimated glomerular filtration rate predicts post-transplant mortality and renal outcomes: an analysis of the UNOS database. J Heart Lung Transplant. 2016;35(12):1471–9.
17. Khush KK, Hsich E, Potena L, Cherikh WS, Chambers DC, Harhay MO, et al. The International Thoracic Organ Transplant Registry of the International Society for Heart and Lung Transplantation: thirty-eighth adult heart transplantation report—2021; focus on recipient characteristics. J Heart Lung Transplant. 2021;40(10):1035–49.
18. Chou AS, Habertheuer A, Chin AL, Sultan I, Vallabhajosyula P. Heart-kidney and heart-liver transplantation provide immunoprotection to the cardiac allograft. Ann Thorac Surg. 2019;108(2):458–66.
19. Sato T, Cheng R, Azarbal B, Kittleson M, Patel J, Czer L, et al. Combined heart and kidney transplantation—Is there a protective effect against cardiac allograft vasculopathy using intravascular ultrasound? J Heart Lung Transplant. 2019;38(9):956–62.
20. Safety net policies for kidney-after-heart and kidney-after-lung allocation in effect June 29 - UNOS [Internet]. https://unos.org/news/policy-changes/safety-net-mot-in-effect-june-29/. Accessed 17 Oct 2024
21. Agarwal KA, Patel H, Agrawal N, Cardarelli F, Goyal N. Cardiac outcomes in isolated heart and simultaneous kidney and heart transplants in the United States. Kidney Int Rep. 2021;6(9):2340–57.
22. Awad MA, Czer LSC, Emerson D, Jordan S, De Robertis MA, Mirocha J, et al. Combined heart and kidney transplantation: clinical experience in 100 consecutive patients. J Am Heart Assoc. 2019;8(4):e010570.
23. Ariyamuthu VK, Amin AA, Drazner MH, Araj F, Mammen PPA, Ayvaci M, et al. Induction regimen and survival in simultaneous heart-kidney transplant recipients. J Heart Lung Transplant. 2018;37(5):587–95.
24. Kobashigawa J, Dadhania DM, Farr M, Tang WHW, Bhimaraj A, Czer L, et al. Consensus conference on heart-kidney transplantation. Am J Transplant. 2021;21(7):2459–67.
25. Alexopoulos SP, Wu WK, Ziogas IA, Matsuoka LK, Rauf MA, Izzy M, et al. Adult combined heart-liver transplantation: the United States experience. Transpl Int. 2022;35:10036.
26. Kobashigawa J, VanWagner LB, Hall S, Emamaullee J, Entwistle JW, Ganger D, et al. Summary of a consensus conference on heart-liver transplantation. Am J Transplant. 2024;24(3):380–90.
27. Givertz MM. Assessing the liver to predict outcomes in heart transplantation. J Heart Lung Transplant. 2015;34(7):869–72.
28. Louie CY, Pham MX, Daugherty TJ, Kambham N, Higgins JPT. The liver in heart failure: a biopsy and explant series of the histopathologic and laboratory findings with a particular focus on pre-cardiac transplant evaluation. Mod Pathol. 2015;28(7):932–43.
29. Bryant R 3rd, Rizwan R, Zafar F, Shah SA, Chin C, Tweddell JS, et al. Contemporary outcomes of combined heart-liver transplant in patients with congenital heart disease. Transplantation. 2018;102(2):e67-73.
30. Emamaullee J, Zaidi AN, Schiano T, Kahn J, Valentino PL, Hofer RE, et al. Fontan-associated liver disease: screening, management, and transplant considerations. Circulation. 2020;142(6):591–604.
31. Reardon LC, Lin JP, VanArsdell GS, Kaldas FM, Lluri G, Tan W, et al. Orthotopic heart and combined heart liver transplantation: the ultimate treatment option for failing Fontan physiology. Curr Transplant Rep. 2021;8:9–20.
32. Simpson KE, Esmaeeli A, Khanna G, White F, Turnmelle Y, Eghtesady P, et al. Liver cirrhosis in Fontan patients does not affect 1-year post-heart transplant mortality or markers of liver function. J Heart Lung Transplant. 2014;33(2):170–7.
33. Lassailly G, Caiazzo R, Ntandja-Wandji LC, Gnemmi V, Baud G, Verkindt H, et al. Bariatric

surgery provides long-term resolution of nonalcoholic steatohepatitis and regression of fibrosis. Gastroenterology. 2020;159(4):1290–301.

34. Rockey DC, Friedman SL. Fibrosis regression after eradication of hepatitis C virus: from bench to bedside. Gastroenterology. 2021;160(5):1502–20.
35. Vaikunth SS, Higgins JP, Concepcion W, Haeffele C, Wright GE, Chen S, et al. Does liver biopsy accurately measure fibrosis in Fontan-associated liver disease? A comparison of liver biopsy pre–combined heart and liver transplant and liver explant post-transplant. Clin Transplant. 2020;34(12):e14120.
36. Goldberg DJ, Surrey LF, Glatz AC, Dodds K, O'Byrne ML, Lin HC, et al. Hepatic fibrosis is universal following Fontan operation, and severity is associated with time from surgery: a liver biopsy and hemodynamic study. J Am Heart Assoc. 2017;6(5):e004809.
37. Ceulemans LJ, Strypstein S, Neyrinck A, Verleden S, Ruttens D, Monbaliu D, et al. Combined liver–thoracic transplantation: single-center experience with introduction of the 'Liver-first'principle. Transpl Int. 2016;29(6):715–26.
38. Brozzi NA, Loebe M, Souki FG, Beduschi T, Ghodzisad A, Tekin A, et al. En-bloc simultaneous heart-liver transplantation in adult patients. Ann Surg. 2021;274(6):e1284-9.
39. Daly RC, Rosenbaum AN, Dearani JA, Clavell AL, Pereira NL, Boilson BA, et al. Heart-after-liver transplantation attenuates rejection of cardiac allografts in sensitized patients. J Am Coll Cardiol. 2021;77(10):1331–40.
40. Abdulameer H. Outcomes of induction immunosuppressive therapy in combined heart-liver transplantation. J Heart Lung Transplant. 2021;40(4):S134-5.
41. Wong TW, Gandhi MJ, Daly RC, Kushwaha SS, Pereira NL, Rosen CB, et al. Liver allograft provides immunoprotection for the cardiac allograft in combined heart–liver transplantation. Am J Transplant. 2016;16(12):3522–31.
42. Nikolova AP, Kobashigawa JA. Cardiac allograft vasculopathy: the enduring enemy of cardiac transplantation. Transplantation. 2019;103(7):1338–48.
43. Cillo U, De Carlis L, Del Gaudio M, De Simone P, Fagiuoli S, Lupo F, et al. Immunosuppressive regimens for adult liver transplant recipients in real-life practice: consensus recommendations from an Italian Working Group. Hepatol Int. 2020;14:930–43.
44. Shudo Y, Wang H, Lingala B, He H, Kim FY, Hiesinger W, et al. Evaluation of risk factors for heart-lung transplant recipient outcome: an analysis of the united network for organ sharing database. Circulation. 2019;140(15):1261–72.
45. Reitz BA, Wallwork JL, Hunt SA, Pennock JL, Billingham ME, Oyer PE, et al. Heart-lung transplantation: successful therapy for patients with pulmonary vascular disease. N Engl J Med. 1982;306(10):557–64.
46. Chambers DC, Cherikh WS, Harhay MO, Hayes D, Hsich E, Khush KK, et al. The International Thoracic Organ Transplant Registry of the International Society for Heart and Lung Transplantation: thirty-sixth adult lung and heart–lung transplantation report—2019; focus theme: donor and recipient size match. J Heart Lung Transplant. 2019;38(10):1042–55.
47. Heart-lung transplantation in adults - UpToDate [Internet]. https://www.uptodate.com/contents/heart-lung-transplantation-in-adults. Accessed 16 Oct 2024
48. Shin M, Iyengar A, Helmers MR, Kelly JJ, Song C, Rekhtman D, et al. Modern outcomes of heart-lung transplantation: assessing the impact of the updated US allocation system. Eur J Cardio-Thorac Surg. 2023;63(1):ezac559.
49. Idrees JJ, Pettersson GB. State of the art of combined heart-lung transplantation for advanced cardiac and pulmonary dysfunction. Curr Cardiol Rep. 2016;18:1–9.
50. Anthonisen NR. Prognosis in chronic obstructive pulmonary disease: results from multicenter clinical trials. Am Rev Respir Dis. 1989;140(3 Pt 2):S95-9.
51. Kobashigawa J, Olymbios M, Luu M. Combined heart and other organ transplant. In: Clinical Guide to Heart Transplantation; 2017. p. 213–25.
52. Le Pavec J, Hascoët S, Fadel E. Heart-lung transplantation: current indications, prognosis and specific considerations. J Thorac Dis. 2018;10(10):5946.
53. Pasupneti S, Dhillon G, Reitz B, Khush K. Combined heart lung transplantation: an updated review of the current literature. Transplantation. 2017;101(10):2297–302.
54. Weingarten N, Iyengar A, Herbst DA, Helmers M, Meldrum D, Guevara-Plunkett S, et al. Extended criteria donor organ use for heart-lung transplantation in the modern era. Clinics. 2023;78:100205.
55. Sweet SC. Induction therapy in lung transplantation. Transpl Int. 2013;26(7):696–703.
56. Hsiao S, Khush KK. Donor selection for multiorgan transplantation. Curr Opin Organ Transplant. 2022;27(1):52–6.
57. Suryapalam M, Kashem M, Shigemura N, Toyoda Y. Combined heart-lung transplantation: UNOS data analysis for long-term survival outcome. J Heart Lung Transplant. 2021;40(4):S251.

# Pregnancy in Heart Transplant Recipients

27

Michelle M. Kittleson

**Abstract**

With improved outcomes after heart transplantation (HTx), there is a growing pool of individuals of childbearing age who may wish to consider pregnancy. Pregnancy after HTx requires anticipatory planning and guidance, careful patient risk assessment with a discussion of individualized risk, close monitoring of graft function and immunosuppression, and vigilance for optimization of comorbid conditions. With a multidisciplinary approach and team, pregnancy after HTx is feasible in selected patients. In the future, multicenter registries may provide much-needed experience to craft future guidelines and recommendations concerning pregnancy after HTx.

**Keywords**

Heart failure · Heart transplantation · Pregnancy

M. M. Kittleson (✉)
Cedars-Sinai Smidt Heart Institute, Los Angeles, CA, USA
e-mail: michelle.kittleson@cshs.org

## Clinical Pearls

- The keys to successful post-transplant pregnancy are preconception and contraceptive planning, appropriate patient risk assessment with comprehensive risk stratification, and optimization of maternal comorbidities and fetal health through careful monitoring.
- Counseling and shared decision-making should be facilitated in an experienced transplant center with a multidisciplinary expert team and should ideally include both the patient and the partner.
- Due to the teratogenicity of mycophenolate mofetil, this drug should be discontinued 6 weeks prior to conception. A transplant recipient who has been weaned off prednisone and requires lower tacrolimus target trough levels due to side effects may warrant azathioprine at 50–100 mg.
- Diabetic control improves both maternal and fetal outcomes, and the cornerstones of pharmacological measures are insulin or metformin.
- Meticulous blood pressure control is advisable; nifedipine, amlodipine, labetalol, hydralazine, and methyldopa can generally be used safely in pregnancy.
- Infections, especially those of the urinary tract and respiratory tract, can be more common in pregnancy and should be actively screened for and treated.


J. Kobashigawa (ed.), *Clinical Guide to Heart Transplantation*, https://doi.org/10.1007/978-3-031-88290-6_27

- Given the increased risk of cardiovascular events in the immediate postpartum period, postpartum care in an intensive care unit setting is recommended, and early discharge from the hospital (<72 h) should be discouraged.

## Introduction

With surgical and immunosuppressive advances in thoracic organ transplantation over the past three decades and attendant improved long-term outcomes, post-transplant pregnancy is an achievable goal for many heart transplant (HTx) recipients [1]. The keys to successful post-transplant pregnancy are preconception and contraceptive planning, appropriate patient risk assessment with comprehensive risk stratification, and optimization of maternal comorbidities and fetal health through careful monitoring [2]. This chapter will summarize the current evidence and provide guidance surrounding these issues.

## Preconception Counseling

Preconception counseling for all individuals of childbearing age encompasses pregnancy intention, contraception, timing of conception after transplant, maternal risks, including those unique to transplant recipients, fetal risks, and psychosocial support for optimal shared decision-making [3, 4]. Whenever possible, counseling and shared decision-making should be facilitated in an experienced transplant center with a multidisciplinary expert team. Unfortunately, about half of pregnancies in HTx recipients are unplanned [5, 6], demonstrating a significant opportunity for education both pre- and post-transplantation regarding contraception and transition to medications that are safe during pregnancy. Because of the potential risks involved with pregnancy after HTx, these discussions should ideally include both the patient and partner and begin during the pre-transplant evaluation. Revisiting these discussions annually throughout the post-transplant period allows recipients opportunities to reassess their decisions. Pre-pregnancy planning allows for the adjustment of medications to those with a safety profile compatible with pregnancy, time to optimize comorbidities, and the opportunity to consider genetic counseling for potentially heritable pre-transplant diagnoses. Figure 27.1 summarizes the key components of preconception counseling. Figure 27.2 provides a patient-focused summary of important concepts for patients to discuss with their treating clinicians. A major component of preconception counseling is a frank discussion of how transplant status influences maternal and fetal risks during pregnancy.

## Contraception

As any disruption to the hypothalamic-gonadal axis is usually restored within 2–6 months following transplant, effective contraception should be recommended immediately; options are summarized in Table 27.1 [7]. Intrauterine devices (copper-containing IUD and levonorgestrel-releasing IUD) offer long-term, highly effective, reversible contraception [4, 8, 9]. Immunosuppression is not a contraindication to IUD use [10, 11]. IUDs are the contraceptive method of choice [2] and are considered the only acceptable sole method of contraception in transplant recipients taking mycophenolate mofetil. IUDs are considered preferable to other forms of birth control in transplant recipients because of their low failure rate, ability to remain in place for several years, lack of required daily adherence for effectiveness, lack of drug-drug interactions, and straightforward removal to reverse contraception. Depo-medroxyprogesterone acetate administered every three months is another highly effective form of contraception, but it is associated with delayed return to fertility after cessation and decreased bone mineral density and weight gain [12], which may be significant in transplant recipients who are also exposed to long-term corticosteroid therapy [13]. Thus,

**Preconception Counseling**

- Assess graft function by echocardiogram
- Review transplant history of rejection, DSA, CAV (HT)
- Consider associated conditions such as PPCM, CHD, and heritable diseases
- Optimize other medical conditions (hypertension, diabetes)
- Perform psychosocial assessment

**Discuss risks**

- Maternal and paternal risks, including maternal survival
- Fetal risks, including heritable conditions
- Potential effects on allograft
- Obstetric risks
- Psychological morbidity

**Review Plans**

- Pre-pregnancy contraception
- Defer until at least 1 year post-transplant
- Ensure teratogenic medications are stopped and replaced, if necessary
- Multidisciplinary delivery plan
- Enhanced monitoring plan during pregnancy & following delivery
- Psychological follow-up, treatment, and support

**Fig. 27.1** Approach to preconception counseling in lung and heart transplant recipients. CAV = cardiac allograft vasculopathy, CHD = congenital heart disease, DSA = donor-specific antibodies, HT = heart transplant, PPCM = peripartum cardiomyopathy. Reprinted from The Journal of Heart and Lung Transplantation, 42(3), Kittleson, Michelle M., Ersilia M. DeFilippis, Catriona J. Bhagra, Jillian P. Casale, Matthew Cauldwell, Lisa A. Coscia, Rohan D'Souza et al., Reproductive health after thoracic transplantation: an ISHLT expert consensus statement, e1–e42, Copyright (2023), with permission from Elsevier.

EDUCATING PATIENTS ON POST-TRANSPLANT PREGNANCY

**Before transplant**

- ✓ Begin pre-conception counseling before transplant and continue post-transplant
- ✓ Avoid unplanned pregnancy, discuss contraception or other pregnancy options including surrogacy, adoption and oocyte cryopreservation
- ✓ Meet with a genetic counselor for a familial or hereditary form of heart or lung disease

**After transplant, prior to pregnancy**

- ✓ Continue contraception during childbearing years
- ✓ Wait at least 1 year after HT, 2 years after LT to become pregnant
- ✓ Discuss timing and unique risks to mother and baby prior to becoming pregnant
- ✓ Plan transition to medications safe during pregnancy
- ✓ Control high blood pressure and diabetes
- ✓ Discuss psychological, social, financial concerns

**After transplant, during pregnancy**

- ✓ Take medications which are safe in pregnancy
- ✓ Follow enhanced monitoring plan: labs, clinic, transplant-specific testing
- ✓ Monitor blood pressure
- ✓ Continue to control other medical conditions
- ✓ Discuss psychological, social, financial concerns

**After transplant, after pregnancy**

- ✓ Discuss safety of medications during breastfeeding
- ✓ Discuss contraception
- ✓ Monitor labs and other transplant testing early after delivery
- ✓ Transition back to prior, stable immunosuppression
- ✓ Discuss mental health concerns
- ✓ Discuss psychological, social, financial concerns

**Fig. 27.2** Educating patients on post-transplant pregnancy. HT = heart transplant, LT; Lung transplant. Reprinted from The Journal of Heart and Lung Transplantation, 42(3), Kittleson, Michelle M., Ersilia M. DeFilippis, Catriona J. Bhagra, Jillian P. Casale, Matthew Cauldwell, Lisa A. Coscia, Rohan D'Souza et al., Reproductive health after thoracic transplantation: an ISHLT expert consensus statement, e1–e42, Copyright (2023), with permission from Elsevier.

**Table 27.1** Summary of contraceptive options in transplant recipients

| Type of contraception | Consensus recommendations | Use in transplant recipients taking mycophenolate products | Safe in breastfeeding | Notes |
|---|---|---|---|---|
| Intrauterine devices (hormonal and non-hormonal) | Preferred method for long-term contraception | Acceptable as sole method of contraception | Yes | • Long-term, highly effective<br>• Immunosuppression is not a contraindication<br>• Lack of drug-drug interactions<br>• Straightforward removal for reversal |
| Progesterone depot injection | Not recommended for long-term (i.e., >2 years) contraception due to risk of decreased bone mineral density | Use with barrier method | Yes | • Highly effective<br>• Delayed return to fertility after cessation<br>• Decreased bone mineral density<br>• Weight gain |
| Progesterone subdermal implant | Acceptable method of long-term contraception | Use with barrier method | Yes | • Long-term, highly effective<br>• Rapid return of fertility once removed |
| Combined hormonal contraceptives (pills, vaginal ring, transdermal patch) | Not recommended as sole method of contraception given contraindications and drug interactions | Use with barrier method | May reduce milk production | • Screen for hypercoagulable states prior to the initiation of combination hormonal contraception<br>• Avoid in patient with transplant-related coronary artery disease or hypertension<br>• Contraindicated in patients with a history of stroke, increased risk of thrombosis, liver disease, and estrogen-sensitive malignancies<br>• Subject to drug interactions that may reduce contraception efficacy<br>• Due to the inhibition of the cytochrome P450 3A4 pathway seen with these drugs, monitoring blood levels of immunosuppressive medications is required after initiation<br>• Avoid early postpartum due to risk of thrombosis |
| Progestin-only pills | Not routinely recommended given effectiveness diminishes with nonadherence | Use with barrier method | Yes | • Efficacy strongly dependent on consistent timing of administration due to short half-life |
| Barrier methods (condoms, sponge, diaphragm, cervical cap with or without spermicide) | Not recommended as sole contraception | Use with another method | Yes | • Should be used in combination with non-IUD hormonal methods for prevention of pregnancy<br>• Should be used in combination with any another form of contraception for protection against sexually transmitted diseases |

Barrier methods are recommended for use with progesterone implant or depot injection based on the Mycophenolate Risk Evaluation and Mitigation Strategies (REMS) program (https://www.mycophenolaterems.com). Reprinted from The Journal of Heart and Lung Transplantation, 42(3), Kittleson, Michelle M., Ersilia M. DeFilippis, Catriona J. Bhagra, Jillian P. Casale, Matthew Cauldwell, Lisa A. Coscia, Rohan D'Souza et al., Reproductive health after thoracic transplantation: an ISHLT expert consensus statement, e1–e42, Copyright (2023), with permission from Elsevier.

depo-medroxyprogesterone acetate is not routinely recommended as a long-term contraceptive option [2, 14]. The use of combined hormonal contraceptives should be considered carefully in patients with cardiac allograft vasculopathy (CAV) or hypertension, and their use is contraindicated in patients with an increased risk of thrombosis, liver disease, or estrogen-sensitive malignancies [4]. Combined hormonal contraceptives portend increased risk in patients with prior myocardial infarction, stroke or deep venous thrombosis, hypertension, migraine with aura, and liver disease [13]. Transplant recipients should be screened for hypercoagulable states prior to the initiation of combination hormonal contraception [14]. Furthermore, due to the inhibition of the cytochrome P450 3A4 pathway with these drugs, additional monitoring of immunosuppression blood levels is required after initiation. Progestin-only pills are not routinely recommended as their efficacy is strongly dependent on consistent timing of administration due to the short half-life, and thus, the effectiveness will diminish with non-adherence. Barrier methods are not sufficient as a sole method of contraception, given their relatively high failure rates. They should be used, in combination with another reliable form of birth control, for protection against sexually transmitted infection when indicated.

## Assisted Reproductive Technology (ART)

A survey of 1090 solid organ transplant recipients in the Transplant Pregnancy Registry International (TPRI) revealed that 22% of women experienced difficulty achieving pregnancy [5]. For such patients and for those transplant recipients for whom pregnancy portends prohibitive risk and is not recommended, the options of surrogacy, adoption, and oocyte preservation may be considered. For other patients, ART may be an option. The decision to proceed with ART requires consultation between the transplant physician and the reproductive endocrinologist, considering the transplant recipient's graft function, any comorbid conditions, and the potential for success with ART. Of note, the risk of thromboembolism is low with ART, 0.6% in a large registry [15], which is reassuring when considering ART for HTx recipients without risk factors for or prior history of thromboembolism. One risk of fertility treatments is an increased incidence of multiple gestations, a known risk factor for hypertension and preeclampsia, for which transplant recipients are already at increased risk [6, 16–21]. To avoid multiple gestations, guidelines from the American Society of Reproductive Medicine recommend single embryo transfer at the blastocyst stage, allowing for high implantation rates with a lower risk of multiple pregnancies [22]. Controlled ovarian stimulation may cause increased vascular fluid shifts [23], which should be tolerated in transplant recipients with normal graft function. However, a potentially life-threatening complication of controlled ovarian stimulation is ovarian hyperstimulation syndrome (OHSS). OHSS is characterized by third-spacing fluid accumulation with increased vascular permeability and may result in ascites, hypercoagulability, and electrolyte imbalances [24]. In some cases, OHSS can lead to arrhythmias, pericardial effusion, and adult respiratory distress syndrome. It is not established that the risk of OHSS is higher in transplant recipients than in the general population undergoing controlled ovarian stimulation, and, thus, if felt to be an important component of ART, controlled ovarian stimulation may be used with close monitoring for potential complications.

## Shared Decision-Making

A critical component of transplant care is shared decision-making, a model of patient-clinician communication that promotes the integration of patient values and preferences with discussion of potential risks, benefits, and harms to inform treatment decisions [25, 26]. Shared decision-making is especially important given the unique physical and psychological complexities faced by transplant recipients and their families

[27–33]. Key components of communication in shared decision-making are trust, understanding patient values, goals, and preferences, and continued discussion of evolving choices as new situations arise [34]. Ideally, shared decision-making about contraception and risks associated with pregnancy after HTx will occur pre-transplant, regularly during post-transplant follow-up, and prior to conception. If pregnancy is unplanned or undesired, counseling on maternal and fetal risks associated with pregnancy continuation is necessary, particularly if pregnancy is medically contraindicated. Shared decision-making is a central feature of care for transplant recipients in general and specifically for individuals of reproductive age. Clinicians and patients should work toward patient-centered care that factors in individual and family values, goals, and preferences [34].

## Fatherhood After Transplantation

The reproductive health of the non-gestational parent should also be considered. Some issues are common to both the pregnant individual and the non-gestational parent, including the impact of post-transplant life expectancy on parenthood and the role of potentially inheritable conditions. A specific issue for the non-gestational parent would be the potential teratogenicity of immunosuppression. Fortunately, offspring fathered by kidney, kidney-pancreas, liver, and HTx recipients on mycophenolate at the time of conception do not have a higher incidence of adverse outcomes of pregnancy, congenital malformations, or other adverse neonatal outcomes, and thus mycophenolate avoidance is not necessary for the non-gestational parent [35–37]. Similar reassuring findings have been noted with corticosteroids, calcineurin inhibitors, and azathioprine, though sirolimus may cause lower sperm counts, dysmotility, and reduced spontaneous pregnancy rates [38].

## Risk Assessment, Management, and Outcomes of Pregnancy After Heart Transplantation

### Timing of Pregnancy

The risk of allograft rejection is highest, and the immunosuppression regimen most aggressive, in the first 6–12 months after transplantation; hence the 2023 ISHLT Consensus Statement on Reproductive Health in Thoracic Transplantation advises that pregnancy should not be attempted within the first year and recommends that HTx recipients have stable graft function with no rejection in the past 12 months, no active infection, and a stable immunosuppression regimen to maximize the chance of a favorable outcome [2].

### Patient Risk Assessment

Figure 27.3 illustrates some of the factors requiring consideration when assessing the risk of pregnancy in HTx recipients. The estimation of the risk of pregnancy for any given individual post-transplantation is complex. Due to the lack of data and unique patient factors to be considered, no risk calculator specific to transplantation currently exists. There are some conditions under which pregnancy in a HTx recipient is considered very high risk or contraindicated; these include poor graft function (LVEF < 30%), which falls into the modified World Health Organization (WHO) classification IV of maternal risk as prohibitive (LVEF 30–45% is WHO classification II-III as intermediate risk) [39], non-adherence with immunosuppression or other important medical therapy, significant CAV, active infection, and poorly controlled hypertension, diabetes or renal dysfunction (eGFR < 30 ml/min/1.73 $m^2$) [1, 14, 40]. Prior rejection is a concern. While treated acute cellular rejection more than one year prior to pregnancy may be a relative contraindication,

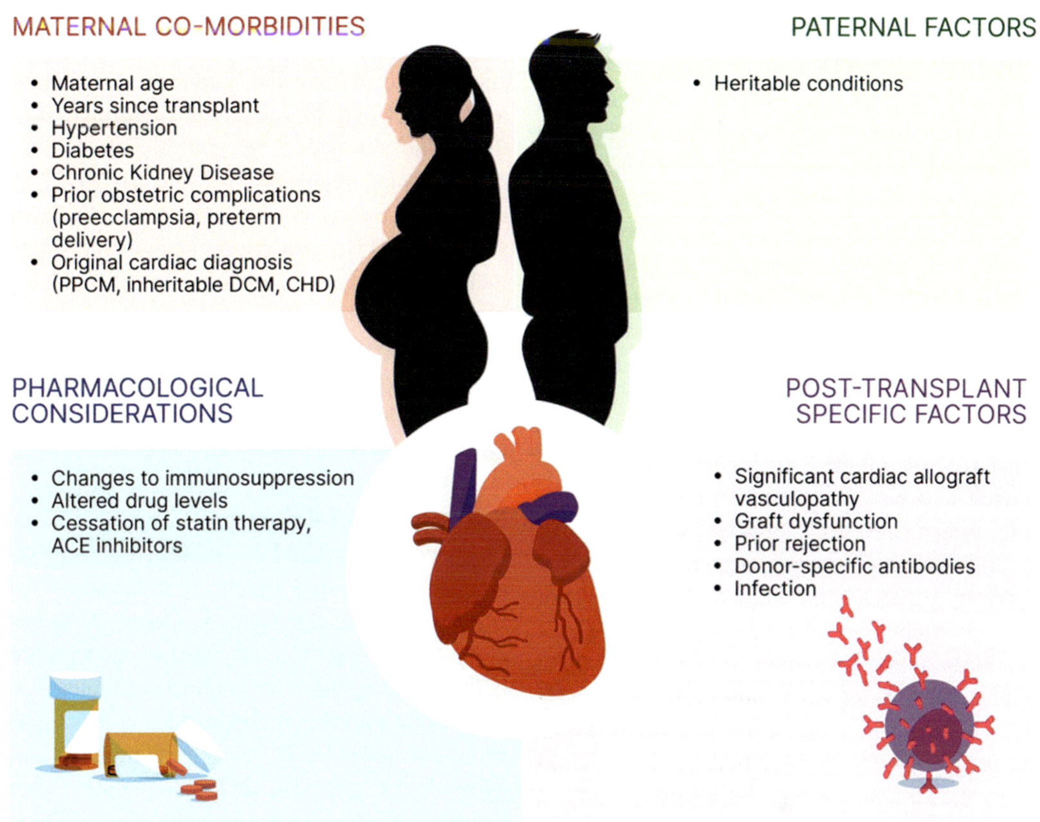


**Fig. 27.3** Factors to be considered in risk assessment for pregnancy after heart transplantation. Reprinted from The Journal of Heart and Lung Transplantation, 42(3), Kittleson, Michelle M., Ersilia M. DeFilippis, Catriona J. Bhagra, Jillian P. Casale, Matthew Cauldwell, Lisa A. Coscia, Rohan D'Souza et al., Reproductive health after thoracic transplantation: an ISHLT expert consensus statement, e1–e42, Copyright (2023), with permission from Elsevier. ACE = angiotensin-converting enzyme, CHD = congenital heart disease, CM = cardiomyopathy, PPCM = peripartum cardiomyopathy

any history of antibody-mediated rejection (AMR) or donor-specific antibodies (DSA) should also be considered a contraindication to pregnancy, given the risk of a heightened humoral response from fetal exposure. When adverse consequences to the cardiac allograft, such as left ventricular dysfunction, valvular disease, or arrhythmias, are present, the risk of long-term cardiovascular complications may be identified by using risk prediction tools such as the CARPREG II (Canadian Cardiac Disease in Pregnancy) risk score [3, 41–43]. In addition to these risks, the importance of co-morbidities must be emphasized. In an ISHLT registry analysis of women of childbearing age, the presence of DM and/or severe kidney dysfunction (sCKD) strongly impacted survival: DM versus No-DM: median survival 8.9 versus 14.7 years ($p < 0.0001$); sCKD versus no-sCKD: median survival 10.8 versus 14.5 years ($p < 0.0001$); and DM plus CKD versus none: median survival 2.5 years versus 14.9 years ($p < 0.0001$) [44].

The impact of these comorbidities on maternal survival and on the decision to proceed or not with pregnancy should be discussed with patients. Additional maternal comorbidities that may increase the risk of pregnancy from a general cardiovascular perspective include advanced maternal age, obesity, and significant prior pregnancy-related cardiac or obstetric complications. The presence of CAV negatively affects survival. Hence, even early-stage CAV requires aggressive treatment with statins and mammalian target of rapamycin (mTOR) inhibitors. However, the safety of these agents has not been established during pregnancy, and discontinuation may potentially expose the patient to the risk of further CAV progression as another possible risk of pregnancy [45]. While significant CAV (Grade 2 or higher) may be considered a contraindication to pregnancy, those with milder CAV may consider pregnancy and, in this situation, warrant ongoing therapy for CAV. In patients with known CAV, the fetal risks of potential exposure to statins and mTOR inhibitors during pregnancy should be weighed against the risks of worsening graft function. If statin and mTOR inhibitor use is continued during pregnancy, the lowest effective dose should be used to minimize fetal exposure. Finally, a discussion regarding post-transplant life expectancy may impact decisions surrounding pregnancy planning. The median survival for HTx recipients is 12.5 years, extending to 14.8 years in those surviving the first year [46]. Median survival for women is higher than for men (12.2 years vs. 11.4 respectively), and leading causes of death are graft failure (mainly related to CAV), Cytomegalovirus infection, and multi-system organ failure [46]. These considerations emphasize the complexity of preconception counseling, and a comprehensive approach is advised. Parenthood, however, is a deeply personal choice, and some may choose to try to conceive despite an individualized risk assessment.

## Surveillance

### Baseline Evaluation of Graft Function and Risk Assessment

If not completed as part of usual post-transplant surveillance within the previous six months, an echocardiogram should be performed for a diagnostic assessment of graft function with a more detailed assessment for rejection and CAV depending on the patient's history and clinical status [14, 47]. Laboratory assessment should include immunosuppression levels, complete blood count, assessment of liver and renal function, urinalysis to assess for proteinuria, and screening for infection (urinary, CMV) [47]. The list of recommended exams, with rationale and impact of results, is shown in Table 27.2 [2].

### Surveillance of Rejection

Pregnancy can proceed successfully in many HTx recipients, provided timely preconception risk assessment and management (Table 27.2) and close monitoring of graft function and comorbidities during and after pregnancy (Table 27.3). Echocardiography is recommended at least every trimester and ideally every 1–2 months until 24 weeks of gestation and then monthly until delivery. Non-invasive screening for rejection, through gene expression profiling (GEP) and donor-derived cell-free DNA (dd-cfDNA) testing, are useful tools in monitoring for acute rejection [48, 49]. However, dd-cfDNA testing will detect fetal DNA and thus, cannot be reliably used in pregnancy.

### Diagnosis and Treatment of Acute Rejection

Endomyocardial biopsy for cause should be performed when acute rejection is suspected based on findings of the clinical assessment, echocardiography, and genetic testing. An echocardiographic-guided procedure is preferred. Otherwise, fluoroscopy should be

**Table 27.2** Recommended baseline assessment of clinical status and graft function in lung transplant and heart transplant recipients desiring pregnancy

| Assessment | Impact on management or outcome | Contraindications to planned pregnancy |
|---|---|---|
| History | • Genetic condition may trigger need for genetic counseling (ARVC, HCM, CHD, familial CM); special considerations for patients with pre-transplant diagnosis of PPCM<br>• Social history | • Less than 1 year post-transplant<br>• Nonadherence |
| Clinical examination | • Arterial hypertension is associated with higher risk of preeclampsia | • Symptomatic graft dysfunction<br>• Uncontrolled hypertension |
| Laboratory assessment: comprehensive metabolic panel, Hgb A1c, urinalysis | • Pre-pregnancy DM, renal dysfunction and proteinuria are associated with higher risk of preeclampsia<br>• DM requires close monitoring to lessen risk for macrosomia and shoulder dystocia | • Poorly controlled diabetes<br>• Severe renal dysfunction (creatinine > 2.5 mg/dl, eGFR < 30 ml/min/1.73m$^2$, or dialysis)<br>• Significant proteinuria |
| Anti-HLA antibodies | • Pregnancy could trigger alloimmunization<br>• Sensitized patients have a worse long-term outcome | • Donor-specific antibodies |
| Immunosuppressive levels | • Trough levels of immunosuppression should be stable before pregnancy, to minimize the risk of rejection<br>• Close monitoring of immunosuppression levels is recommended | • Inability to maintain therapeutic levels of maintenance immunosuppression with CNI<br>• Inability to stop mycophenolate products |
| Serology and PCR for CMV | • Primary CMV infection and, to a lesser extent, CMV reactivation are associated with the risk of fetal CMV disease<br>• CMV seronegative patients should be advised to take additional precautions | • CMV infection within the past year |
| Standard assessment of graft function with echocardiogram | • Graft dysfunction is associated with high risk of complications during pregnancy and a worse long-term outcome | • Heart transplant: reduced EF (<30%), severe valvular disease (stenotic lesions) |
| In-depth assessment of the graft function (if clinically indicated) with RHC/biopsy, coronary angiogram | • Rejection may recur during pregnancy or after delivery and portends increased risk<br>• CAV portends increased risk | • Heart transplant: cellular rejection in the past year, any history of AMR, CAV grade 2 or greater<br>• Active infection |

AMR = antibody-mediated rejection; ARVC = arrhythmogenic right ventricular cardiomyopathy; CAV = cardiac allograft vasculopathy; CHD = congenital heart disease; CMV = cytomegalovirus; DM = diabetes mellitus; EF = ejection fraction; HCM = hypertrophic cardiomyopathy; PPCM = peripartum cardiomyopathy; RHC = right heart catheterization. Reprinted from The Journal of Heart and Lung Transplantation, 42(3), Kittleson, Michelle M., Ersilia M. DeFilippis, Catriona J. Bhagra, Jillian F. Casale, Matthew Cauldwell, Lisa A. Coscia, Rohan D'Souza et al., Reproductive health after thoracic transplantation: an ISHLT expert consensus statement, e1–e42, Copyright (2023), with permission from Elsevier

**Table 27.3** Timetable of periodic assessment during pregnancy in lung transplant and heart transplant recipients

| Exam | Timing | Notes |
|---|---|---|
| **Graft function and rejection** | | |
| Physical examination, vital parameters | Every 4 weeks | 24 h-monitoring of BP if hypertension is suspected |
| 12-lead EKG | Every 4 weeks | EMB (preferably echo-guided) if rejection is suspected |
| Echocardiography | At least every trimester and ideally every 1–2 months until 24$^{th}$ week and then every 4 weeks until delivery | EMB (preferably echo-guided) if rejection is suspected |
| **Hypertensive disorders** | | |
| Renal function, liver function, blood cells count | Every 4 weeks | Increase in eGFR is expected<br>Monitoring liver enzymes and platelet count if HELLP syndrome is suspected |
| Urinalysis | Every 4 weeks | Check for proteinuria |
| **Diabetes mellitus** | | |
| Fasting plasma glucose | Every 4 weeks | Additional therapy if increase in steroid dose is needed |
| Glucose challenge test | Between 24 and 28 weeks | May be performed earlier in patients at risk for diabetes |
| **Immunosuppression** | | |
| Circulating levels | Every 4 weeks until 32nd week; every 2 weeks until 36th week; weekly until delivery and the first month after delivery | Additional therapeutic drug monitoring in the first two trimesters may be suggested, following daily dose adaptation, as needed |
| HLA-specific antibodies | 1–3 months after delivery | Earlier testing of HLA-specific Ab if acute rejection during pregnancy |
| **Infections** | | |
| Complete blood count, CRP | Every 4 weeks | |
| PCR for CMV genome | Every 4 weeks | |
| Urine culture | Every 4 weeks | |
| Serology for Toxoplasma (in seronegative patients), HSV, hepatitis | Third trimester (36 0/7–37 6/7 weeks of gestation) | |
| Vaginal swab culture for Streptococci B | Third trimester (36 0/7–37 6/7 weeks of gestation) | |

(continued)

**Table 27.3** (continued)

| Exam | Timing | Notes |
|---|---|---|
| **Fetal growth** | | |
| Echo assessment of fetal well-being | Routine dating ultrasound between 8 and 9 weeks of gestation when available<br>Nuchal translucency scan between 11 and 14 weeks gestation when available<br>Early (transabdominal or transvaginal) anatomy scan between 11 and 16 weeks of gestation when available<br>Every 2 months until 24th week; every 4 weeks until delivery | In diabetic patients:<br>– consider closer monitoring of fetal growth from 28th week<br>– weekly monitoring from 32nd week |

*Abbreviations* BP = blood pression; CMV = cytomegalovirus; CNI = calcineurin-inhibitors; CRP = C-reactive protein; eGFR = estimated glomerular filtration rate; EMB = endomyocardial biopsy; HELLP = hemolysis, elevated liver enzymes, low platelets; HLA = human leukocyte antigen; HSV = herpes-simplex virus; PCR = polymerase chain reaction. Reprinted from The Journal of Heart and Lung Transplantation, 42(3), Kittleson, Michelle M., Ersilia M. DeFilippis, Catriona J. Bhagra, Jillian P. Casale, Matthew Cauldwell, Lisa A. Coscia, Rohan D'Souza et al., Reproductive health after thoracic transplantation: an ISHLT expert consensus statement, e1–e42, Copyright (2023), with permission from Elsevier

**Table 27.4** Summary of Maternal and Fetal Outcomes in Heart Transplant Recipients across contemporary published series, with > 10 reported pregnancies

| Series (year) | Punnoose et al. [6] (includes TPRI data [5]) | Macera et al. [50] | D'Souza et al. [51] | Dagher et al. [16] | Bhagra et al. [17] |
|---|---|---|---|---|---|
| Number of pregnancies (number of women) | 157 (91) | 17 (11) | 17 (16) | 18 (8) | 22 (17) |
| Unplanned pregnancies, n (%) | 59 (46) | Not reported | Not reported | 10 (56) | 18 (82) |
| Mean time from transplant (years) | 7 ± 6 | 5.6 | 7.3 ± 4 | 8.2 (2.6–24.6) | 8.2 ± 5.2 |
| Mean age at transplant (years) | 20 ± 8 | Not reported | Not reported | 16.0 (6.2–26.6) | Not reported |
| Mean age at pregnancy (years) | 27 ± 5.6 | 33 | 28 ± 5.8 | 25.5 (17.6–33.3) | 25.3 ± 5.8 |
| LVEF (%) pre-pregnancy | Not reported | All with normal graft function but no LVEF reported | All with normal graft function but LVEF not reported | 61 (55–65) | All with normal graft function, no LVEF reported |
| Maternal complications (as % of pregnancies) | | | | | |
| Hypertension, n (%) | Before pregnancy: 65 (42)<br>During pregnancy: 72 (46) | Before pregnancy: 5 (45)<br>During pregnancy: 1 (6) | – | Before pregnancy: 2 (25)<br>During pregnancy: 5 (39) | Before pregnancy: 5 (36)<br>During pregnancy: 3 (14) |
| Preeclampsia, n (%) | 27 (23) | 0 (0) | 2 (12) | 2 (15) | 13 (4) |
| Diabetes mellitus, n (%) | Before pregnancy: 7 (5)<br>During pregnancy: 11 (7) | 0 (0) | During pregnancy: 1 (6) | Before pregnancy: 1 (13)<br>During pregnancy: 2 (15) | 0 (0) |
| Renal failure, n (%) | Not reported | Not reported | 4 (24) | Not reported | Not reported |
| Infection, n (%) | 22 (14) | 0 (0) | 2 (12) | 3 (23) | Not reported |
| Graft loss (within 2 years of delivery/termination), n (%) | 2 (2) | 0 | 0 | 0 (0) | 0 |
| Rejection, n (%) | 14 (9) | 0 (0) | 2 (12) | 0 (0) | 1 (5) |

(continued)

**Table 27.4** (continued)

| Series (year) | Punnoose et al. [6] (includes TPRI data [5]) | Macera et al. [50] | D'Souza et al. [51] | Dagher et al. [16] | Bhagra et al. [17] |
|---|---|---|---|---|---|
| Maternal Death during Pregnancy, n (%) | 0 | 0 (0) | 0 (0) | 0 (0) | 1 (during immediate postpartum period from postpartum hemorrhage) |
| Maternal death, n (%) | 30 (33) | 3 (27) | 2 (12) | 3 (38) | 4 (24) |
| Mean time from pregnancy to maternal death (yrs) | 9.4 (0.5–26) | 11 | At 10 and 18 months after delivery (attributed to rejection from nonadherence with immunosuppression) | 3.9 (2.6–5.4) | Not reported |
| Obstetric and Fetal outcomes (as % of pregnancies except as noted) | | | | | |
| Live birth, n (%) | 111 (69) | 12 (71) | 14 (81) | 13 (72) | 20 (91) |
| Mean gestational age at delivery (weeks) | 36 | 36.5 | Not reported | 35 | $34 \pm 4$ |
| Fertility treatments used, n (%) | Not reported | Not reported | Not reported | Not reported | 1 (5) |
| Cesarean delivery, n (% of live births) | 45 (42) | 10 (83) | 8 (46) | 5 (39) | 11 (55) |
| Miscarriage, n (%) | 41 (25) | 3 (18) | 1 (6) | 3 (17) | 2 (9) |
| Ectopic pregnancies, n (%) | 2 (1) | Not reported | Not reported | Not reported | Not reported |
| Terminations, n (%) | 7 (4) | 2 (12) | 2 (12) | 2 (11) | 0 (0) |
| Low birth weight (<2500 g), n (%) | 41 (37) | 4 (36) | Not reported | 6 (46) | 9 (45) |
| Preterm (<37 weeks), n (%) | 45 (41) | 4 (36) | 6 (46) | 7 (54) | 9 (45) |
| Congenital malformations, n (% of live births) | 9 (8) * | Not reported | 2 (14%) ** | 1 (8) | 0 |

* Duodenal atresia, tetralogy of Fallot, laryngomalacia, facial deformities, vermian hypoplasia of the cerebellum, hypospadias, cystic hygroma, pectus excavatum, lip and tongue tie, and long QT syndrome

** Frontonasal dysplasia, bilateral radial ray anomalies with oligodactyly

*** Only fetal cardiac malformations noted; perimembranous ventricular septal defect

LVEF, left ventricular ejection fraction; TPRI, Transplant Pregnancy Registry International

**Table 27.5** Treatment of hypertension during pregnancy in transplant recipients

| Measure | Rationale | Potential side-effects | Comments |
|---|---|---|---|
| Non-pharmacological | | | |
| Low-sodium diet | To prevent RAAS-mediated sodium and water retention | None | |
| Pharmacological | | | |
| Dihydropyridine calcium-channels blockers<br>Amlodipine<br>Nifedipine | To promote peripheral vasodilation | Edema, headache, tachycardia | Safe during pregnancy and breastfeeding<br>No significant interactions with CNI |
| Methyldopa | Available data about safety in offspring up to 7 years | Sedation, dizziness, depression | Safe during pregnancy; may be avoided during breastfeeding due to association with depression |
| Beta-blockers<br>Labetalol | To lower systemic vascular resistance (α-antagonism is more pronounced than β-blocking activity)<br>Often used for hypertensive crisis (intravenous) | Postural hypotension<br>Bronchospasm (if history of asthma or COPD)<br>Fetal bradycardia, growth restriction | Beta-blockers may be less well-tolerated in heart transplant recipients due to denervation with reduced exercise tolerance; propranolol, metoprolol, and labetalol have the lowest transfer into breast milk |
| Hydralazine | Peripheral vasodilatation | May increase CNI trough levels (by decreasing their metabolism) | TID dosing may limit adherence; safe during breastfeeding |
| Diuretics<br>Loop diuretics<br>Thiazide diuretics | To treat water retention<br>Complementary treatment in severe drug-resistant hypertension and oliguria | Hypovolemia, transient electrolytes and metabolic disbalance in mother and fetus | Should be avoided in the first trimester (data about teratogenicity showed conflicting results); may reduce milk volume during breastfeeding |

*Abbreviations* CCB = calcium-channels blockers; CNI = calcineurin-inhibitors; COPD = chronic obstructive pulmonary disease; HT = heart transplantation; RAAS = renin-angiotensin aldosterone system. Reprinted from The Journal of Heart and Lung Transplantation, 42(3), Kittleson, Michelle M., Ersilia M. DeFilippis, Catriona J. Bhagra, Jillian P. Casale, Matthew Cauldwell, Lisa A. Coscia, Rohan D'Souza et al., Reproductive health after thoracic transplantation: an ISHLT expert consensus statement, e1–e42, Copyright (2023), with permission from Elsevier

**Table 27.6** Immunosuppressive agents in pregnancy

| Drug class | Safety for use in pregnancy | Risk of teratogenicity | Special instruction | Safety for use while breastfeeding |
|---|---|---|---|---|
| Corticosteroids | Relatively safe at contemporary clinical dosing | Cleft palate may occur with high doses used in the first trimester (over, 10–15 mg prednisolone daily) | Continue treatment with corticosteroids when indicated | Yes |
| Calcineurin inhibitors<br>Cyclosporine<br>Tacrolimus | Relatively safe at contemporary clinical dosing | No teratogenic potential in human registries | Frequent monitoring of levels (every 2–4 weeks) | Yes |
| mTOR inhibitors<br>Everolimus<br>Sirolimus | Insufficient data to affirm safety | Limited data in humans; potential risk from animal studies | Discontinue 6–12 weeks before planned conception; evaluate risk vs benefit on case-by-case basis in heart transplant recipients with CAV | Limited evidence |
| Mycophenolate products<br>Mycophenolate mofetil<br>Mycophenolate sodium | No | Teratogen: risk of spontaneous abortion and congenital malformations | Discontinue 6–12 weeks before planned conception or immediately if unplanned | Not recommended |
| Azathioprine | No evidence of teratogenic effect in human studies | May use in place of mycophenolate depending on patient's risk of rejection | Relatively safe at contemporary clinical dosing | No evidence of teratogenic effect in human studies |

CAV = cardiac allograft vasculopathy; mTOR = mammalian target of rapamycin. Reprinted from The Journal of Heart and Lung Transplantation, 42(3), Kittleson, Michelle M., Ersilia M. DeFilippis, Catriona J. Bhagra, Jillian P. Casale, Matthew Cauldwell, Lisa A. Coscia, Rohan D'Souza et al., Reproductive health after thoracic transplantation: an ISHLT expert consensus statement, e1–e42, Copyright (2023), with permission from Elsevier.

done with lead draping of the abdomen [14]. Recommended regimens for the treatment of acute cellular rejection during pregnancy include high-dose corticosteroids; however, due to the relative insulin resistance induced by pregnancy, closer glucose monitoring is recommended if steroids are used. The safety of other agents for the treatment of rejection, such as anti-thymocyte globulin, in pregnancy has not been established and should be used with utmost caution.

## Maternal and Fetal Outcomes

A key component of preconception counseling is explaining the maternal and fetal pregnancy outcomes. Table 27.4 provides a summary of the key maternal and fetal outcomes in HTx recipients across a review of the largest series in the literature.

### Maternal Outcomes

HTx rejection is uncommon during pregnancy but occurs more frequently after delivery. Rejection rates in the peripartum period range from 5 to 12% and episodes are most commonly low grade without significant hemodynamic compromise [5, 6, 16, 17, 50, 51]. Episodes can often be treated with adjustments to baseline immunosuppression and may be related to both activation of maternal alloreactive T-cells and subtherapeutic exposure to immunosuppressive drugs, the latter being secondary to changes in circulating blood volume, intestinal motility, and renal function [17, 50]. However, rejection in HTx recipients may also occur after delivery, noted in 7% of patients within 3 months after delivery [6]. The cause for rejection may be due to variable immunosuppressant levels due to increased blood volume.

The association between pregnancy and the development of CAV is not clear. In 157 pregnancies in 97 HTx recipients, 2 individuals developed CAV after pregnancy, leading to listing for re-transplantation, and 5 had CAV or myocardial infarction listed as the cause of death [6].

In a large series of HTx recipients, mortality during pregnancy was low at 0.5% [52]. However, the longer-term survival of HTx recipients after pregnancy warrants consideration. In one analysis, 33% of HTx recipients who experienced pregnancy died with the median time after first pregnancy to death of 8.9 years with an average survival of 9.4 years [6]. In other series, post-pregnancy mortality in HTx recipients ranges from 10.8% over 3–7 years follow-up [52] to 33% with 8.7 years of follow-up [5]. Notably, the mean age of the child at the time of maternal death was 10.8 years [5].

### Fetal Outcomes

The rate of miscarriage in HTx recipients ranges can be as high as 25% [19, 52] compared to 16% in non-transplant pregnancies [53]. However, several contemporary published series have shown that with careful intrapartum management pregnancy in HTx recipients can be successful with a reported live birth rate between 69 and 91% [5, 6, 16, 17, 50–52]. Cesarean delivery occurs commonly in HTx recipients, 39–83% [5, 19, 54]. Nonetheless, about half of the infants in the published series were delivered preterm, prior to 37 weeks gestation, and 35–40% had low birth weight (<2500 g) [5, 6, 16, 17, 50–52]. About 20% of infants born to HTx recipients are admitted to neonatal intensive care units [52] and 6.5–9% have congenital anomalies [5, 52]. Data are limited regarding detailed longer-term follow-up of offspring of HTx recipients.

## Management of Comorbid Conditions During Pregnancy

### Diabetes

Pregnancy can exacerbate pregestational diabetes and lead to gestational diabetes with significant impacts on both the fetus and pregnant individual [55]. Pregestational diabetes, both type 1 and type 2, is associated with congenital anomalies and both pregestational and gestational diabetes are associated with fetal growth abnormalities, fetal growth restriction and macrosomia, and fetal demise if glycemic control is poor [56]. Pregestational diabetes is common in HTx recipients; 21% develop diabetes within 5 years of transplant [57] and up to 11% of HTx recipients have pregestational and gestational diabetes [6, 17, 50]. This is not surprising, as pregnancy is physiologically associated with insulin resistance, mediated by progesterone, cortisol, and prolactin. Furthermore, compensatory increases in insulin production may be impaired in transplant recipients, due to predisposing factors and diabetogenic effects of calcineurin inhibitors and steroids [58]. Consistent with recommendations from the American College of Obstetrics and Gynecology (ACOG), screening for gestational DM should be performed at 24–28 weeks in pregnant HTx recipients, potentially earlier in those with an increased risk for diabetes [59, 60]. Treatment of DM during pregnancy should occur in consultation with a maternal–fetal-medicine specialist or an endocrinologist.

## Hypertension

In HTx recipients, hypertension is common, with a prevalence of 72% at 1 year and 92% at 5 years after HTx [61]. The pathophysiological mechanisms of post-transplant hypertension are related to systemic and renal vasoconstriction resulting from calcineurin inhibitors as well as cardiac denervation in HTx recipients. Cardiac denervation results in the inability to suppress the renin–angiotensin–aldosterone system (RAAS), thus leading to sodium and water retention, which may be exacerbated by corticosteroids. The expansion of circulating volume and hemodilution occurring during pregnancy can further enhance the development of hypertension [7, 62]. Physiologic pregnancy is usually associated with estrogen-promoted peripheral vasodilation and an increase in creatinine clearance, which may partially counterbalance this process [63]. However, hypertension during pregnancy is commonly diagnosed post-transplant in 25–48% of HTx recipients [5, 52]. Baseline hypertension in transplant recipients results in an increased risk of preeclampsia, observed in 17–29% of HTx recipients [5, 52], and preterm delivery [1]. To manage hypertension in these patients, one must consider the cardiovascular adaptation to hemodynamic changes related to pregnancy, as well as the pharmacological interactions between anti-hypertensive drugs and immunosuppression [14, 39, 64–66]. Meticulous control of blood pressure is advisable; generally nifedipine, amlodipine, labetalol, hydralazine, and methyldopa can be used safely in pregnancy (Table 27.5).

## Infections

Infections, especially those of the urinary tract and respiratory tract, can be more common in pregnancy and should be actively screened for and treated [7]. CMV infection is of particular concern in pregnant transplant recipients. Primary CMV infection and reactivation are common after transplantation, and during pregnancy, there are additional concerns about the risk of congenital CMV disease in the fetus, a potentially serious condition associated with intellectual disability, microcephaly, and visual or hearing loss [67]. The risk of transmission of CMV to the fetus could be as high as 40% [67, 68] during primary infection, while for reactivation, the risk is lower [69]. As CMV carries a significant risk to the fetus [70] as well as to the transplant recipient, pregnant transplant recipients should be tested monthly for CMV viremia during pregnancy. Patients who are CMV-seronegative at the time of pregnancy should be advised to adopt specific behaviors to minimize the risk of primary infection. As CMV is often transmitted through the care of young children, regular hand washing, particularly after changing diapers, is recommended to decrease the spread of infection and may reduce exposure to CMV [71]. Maternal primary infection should be treated to reduce the risk of vertical transmission, especially in the first trimester.

## Immunosuppression During Pregnancy

Given the need to maintain adequate immunosuppression during pregnancy to prevent graft rejection and loss, several important pharmacologic considerations must be considered in the management of pregnancy after HTx. The physiological changes observed during pregnancy can have a significant impact on the pharmacokinetics of immunosuppressants and other agents critical to a transplant recipient's medication regimen. The risks of fetal toxicities resulting from in utero medication exposure must be weighed against the pregnant transplant recipient's requirements. Many of these medications also transfer into human milk, and the potential for drug exposure to the infant via breastfeeding should be considered. The efficacy and safety of immunosuppression medications in pregnancy and their use in breast feeding are summarized in Table 27.6. Due to the inability to study the safety of medication use during pregnancy and lactation through robust, randomized controlled trials, data to guide clinical decision-making are limited to case reports and series. There is also no international standard for risk assessment in pregnancy and lactation in drug labeling.

The Transplant Pregnancy Registry International is a critical source of information regarding maternal and fetal outcomes of pregnant transplant recipients. As a voluntary registry, clinicians are strongly encouraged to enroll pregnant patients to contribute to this body of knowledge. Physiological changes affecting pharmacokinetics during pregnancy can have unpredictable effects on drug levels. Reduced gastrointestinal motility, nausea and vomiting, increased plasma volume and fat stores, changes in plasma binding protein concentrations, and drug metabolism can all impact immunosuppression levels [72–75]. While some studies have described no change in immunosuppression levels during pregnancy, others report the need for dosage escalation [21, 76, 77]. Due to this unpredictability, therapeutic drug monitoring every 2–4 weeks with dose adjustment as required to achieve target levels is advised during pregnancy [21, 77]. Frequent evaluation of immunosuppression levels after delivery is also essential as drug distribution and hepatic metabolism normalize in the postpartum period.

## Postpartum Management

Given the increased risk of cardiovascular events in the immediate postpartum period, postpartum care in an intensive care unit setting is recommended, and early discharge from the hospital (<72 h) should be discouraged. Postpartum thromboprophylaxis should follow local protocols. Postpartum monitoring of immunosuppression levels and for infection is critical. In the general population, breastfeeding is associated with a myriad of immunologic, emotional, and nutritional benefits. In HTx recipients, the decision to breastfeed should be based on a risk–benefit analysis of the potential for immunosuppressive medications to be excreted in the breast milk. After 1–2 weeks of breastfeeding, it is reasonable to check the infant's serum for measurable drug levels of cyclosporine or tacrolimus [78]. If significant levels are detected, the mother may be counseled to discontinue breastfeeding. Limited data are available regarding the excretion of mTOR inhibitors in breast milk. Therefore, caution must be advised regarding breastfeeding in mothers taking mTOR inhibitors. The Drugs and Lactation Database (LactMed) and e-lactancia can be helpful resources for physicians and patients when determining which medications are safe for breastfeeding mothers after HTx [79, 80].

## References

1. Mastrobattista JM, Gomez-Lobo V. Pregnancy after solid organ transplantation. Obstet Gynecol. 2008;112(4):919–32.
2. Kittleson MM, DeFilippis EM, Bhagra CJ, Casale JP, Cauldwell M, Coscia LA, et al. Reproductive health after thoracic transplantation: an ISHLT expert consensus statement. J Heart Lung Transplant. 2023;42(3):e1–42.

3. Davis MB, Arendt K, Bello NA, Brown H, Briller J, Epps K, et al. Team-based care of women with cardiovascular disease from pre-conception through pregnancy and postpartum: JACC focus seminar 1/5. J Am Coll Cardiol. 2021;77(14):1763–77.
4. Rajapreyar IN, Sinkey RG, Joly JM, Pamboukian SV, Lenneman A, Hoopes CW, et al. Management of reproductive health after cardiac transplantation. J Matern Fetal Neonatal Med. 2021;34(9):1469–78.
5. Moritz MJ, Constantinescu, S., Coscia, L.A., et al. 2019 annual report. Transplant Pregnancy Registry International (TPRI). Philadelphia, PA: Gift of Life Institute. 2019. p. 1–22.
6. Punnoose LR, Coscia LA, Armenti DP, Constantinescu S, Moritz MJ. Pregnancy outcomes in heart transplant recipients. J Heart Lung Transplant. 2020;39(5):473–80.
7. Vos R, Ruttens D, Verleden SE, Vandermeulen E, Bellon H, Vanaudenaerde BM, et al. Pregnancy after heart and lung transplantation. Best Pract Res Clin Obstet Gynaecol. 2014;28(8):1146–62.
8. Curtis KM, Jatlaoui TC, Tepper NK, Zapata LB, Horton LG, Jamieson DJ, et al. U.S. selected practice recommendations for contraceptive use. MMWR Recomm Rep. 2016;65(4):1–66.
9. Curtis KM, Tepper NK, Jatlaoui TC, Berry-Bibee E, Horton LG, Zapata LB, et al. U.S. medical eligibility criteria for contraceptive use. MMWR Recomm Rep. 2016;65(3):1–103.
10. Gordon C, Harken T. Controversies in family planning: intrauterine device placement in solid organ transplant patients. Contraception. 2019;100(3):250–2.
11. Krajewski CM, Geetha D, Gomez-Lobo V. Contraceptive options for women with a history of solid-organ transplantation. Transplantation. 2013;95(10):1183–6.
12. Sims J, Lutz E, Wallace K, Kassahun-Yimer W, Ngwudike C, Shwayder J. Depo-medroxyprogesterone acetate, weight gain and amenorrhea among obese adolescent and adult women. Eur J Contracept Reprod Health Care. 2020;25(1):54–9.
13. Estes CM, Westhoff C, editors. Contraception for the transplant patient. In: Seminars in perinatology; 2007: Elsevier.
14. Costanzo MR, Costanzo MR, Dipchand A, Starling R, Anderson A, Chan M, et al. The International Society of Heart and Lung Transplantation guidelines for the care of heart transplant recipients. J Heart Lung Transplant. 2010;29(8):914–56.
15. Grandone E, Di Micco PP, Villani M, Colaizzo D, Fernández-Capitán C, Del Toro J, et al. Venous thromboembolism in women undergoing assisted reproductive technologies: data from the RIETE registry. Thromb Haemost. 2018;118(11):1962–8.
16. Dagher O, Alami Laroussi N, Carrier M, Cecere R, Charbonneau E, De Denus S, et al. Pregnancy after heart transplantation: a well-thought-out decision? The Quebec provincial experience - a multi-centre cohort study. Transpl Int. 2018;31(9):977–87.
17. Bhagra CJ, Bhagra SK, Donado A, Butt T, Forrest L, Macgowan GA, et al. Pregnancy in cardiac transplant recipients. Clin Transplant. 2016;30(9):1059–65.
18. Bry C, Hubert D, Reynaud-Gaubert M, Dromer C, Mal H, Roux A, et al. Pregnancy after lung and heart–lung transplantation: a French multicentric retrospective study of 39 pregnancies. ERJ Open Res. 2019;5(4).
19. Daly TA, Coscia L, Nathan HM, Hasz RD, Constantinescu S, Moritz MJ. Pregnancy outcomes in 36 lung transplant recipients. Transplantation. 2020;104(S3).
20. Gadre S, Gadre SK. Pregnancy and lung transplantation. Curr Pulmonol Rep. 2021:1–9.
21. Thakrar MV, Morley K, Lordan JL, Meachery G, Fisher AJ, Parry G, et al. Pregnancy after lung and heart-lung transplantation. J Heart Lung Transplant. 2014;33(6):593–8.
22. Penzias A, Bendikson K, Butts S, Coutifaris C, Falcone T, Fossum G, et al. ASRM standard embryo transfer protocol template: a committee opinion. Fertil Steril. 2017;107(4):897–900.
23. De Pinho JC, Sauer MV. Infertility and ART after transplantation. Best Pract Res Clin Obstet Gynaecol. 2014;28(8):1235–50.
24. Prevention and treatment of moderate and severe ovarian hyperstimulation syndrome: a guideline. Fertil Steril. 2016;106(7):1634–47.
25. Dy SM, Purnell TS. Key concepts relevant to quality of complex and shared decision-making in health care: a literature review. Soc Sci Med. 2012;74(4):582–7.
26. Oshima Lee E, Emanuel EJ. Shared decision making to improve care and reduce costs. N Engl J Med. 2013;368(1):6–8.
27. Duffy J, Thompson T, Hinton L, Salinas M, McManus R, Ziebland S. What outcomes should researchers select, collect and report in pre-eclampsia research? A qualitative study exploring the views of women with lived experience of pre-eclampsia. BJOG: Int J Obstet & Gynaecol. 2019; 637–46.
28. Hinton L, Locock L, Knight M. Support for mothers and their families after life-threatening illness in pregnancy and childbirth: a qualitative study in primary care. Br J Gen Pract: R Coll Gen Pract. 2015;e563–e9.
29. Hinton L, Locock L, Knight M. Maternal critical care: what can we learn from patient experience? A qualitative study. BMJ open: BMJ Open. 2015:e006676.
30. Khan A, Pare E, Shah S. Peripartum cardiomyopathy: a review for the clinician. Curr Treat Options Cardiovasc Med. 2018;20(11):91.
31. Hinton L, Locock L, Knight M. Partner experiences of "near-miss" events in pregnancy and childbirth in the UK: a qualitative study. PLoS ONE: Public Library of Science; 2014.

32. Evangelista LS, Doering L, Dracup K. Meaning and life purpose: the perspectives of post-transplant women. Heart Lung. 2003;32(4):250–7.
33. Conway A, Schadewaldt V, Clark R, Ski C, Thompson DR, Kynoch K, et al. The effectiveness of non-pharmacological interventions in improving psychological outcomes for heart transplant recipients: a systematic review. Eur J Cardiovasc Nurs. 2014;13(2):108–15.
34. Allen LA, Stevenson LW, Grady KL, Goldstein NE, Matlock DD, Arnold RM, et al. Decision making in advanced heart failure: a scientific statement from the American Heart Association. Circulation. 2012;125(15):1928–52.
35. Coscia L, Daly T, Nathan H, Armenti D, Kliniewski D, Constantinescu S, et al. Transplant pregnancy registry international. Transplantation. 2017;101:S64.
36. Jones A, Clary MJ, McDermott E, Coscia LA, Constantinescu S, Moritz MJ, et al. Outcomes of pregnancies fathered by solid-organ transplant recipients exposed to mycophenolic acid products. Prog Transplant. 2013;23(2):153–7.
37. Midtvedt K, Bergan S, Reisæter AV, Vikse BE, Åsberg A. Exposure to mycophenolate and fatherhood. Transplantation. 2017;101(7):e214.
38. Zuber J, Anglicheau D, Elie C, Bererhi L, Timsit MO, Mamzer-Bruneel MF, et al. Sirolimus may reduce fertility in male renal transplant recipients. Am J Transplant. 2008;8(7):1471–9.
39. Regitz-Zagrosek V, Roos-Hesselink JW, Bauersachs J, Blomström-Lundqvist C, Cífková R, De Bonis M, et al. 2018 ESC guidelines for the management of cardiovascular diseases during pregnancy. Eur Heart J. 2018;39(34):3165–241.
40. DeFilippis EM, Haythe J, Farr MA, Kobashigawa J, Kittleson MM. Practice patterns surrounding pregnancy after heart transplantation. Circ Heart Fail. 2020;13(4):e006811.
41. Siu SC, Lee DS, Rashid M, Fang J, Austin PC, Silversides CK. Long-term cardiovascular outcomes after pregnancy in women with heart disease. J Am Heart Assoc. 2021;10(11):e020584.
42. Botero D, Senior J, Velasquez J, Gandara J, Zapata A, Holguin E, et al. Validation of the CARPREG II risk stratification model and the WHOm scale in pregnant women with heart disease. Eur Heart J. 2021;42(Supplement_1).
43. Silversides CK, Grewal J, Mason J, Sermer M, Kiess M, Rychel V, et al. Pregnancy outcomes in women with heart disease: the CARPREG II study. J Am Coll Cardiol. 2018;71(21):2419–30.
44. Personal communication with Josef Stehlik February 14, 2022.
45. Chih S, Chong AY, Mielniczuk LM, Bhatt DL, Beanlands RS. Allograft vasculopathy: the achilles' heel of heart transplantation. J Am Coll Cardiol. 2016;68(1):80–91.
46. Khush KK, Potena L, Cherikh WS, Chambers DC, Harhay MO, Hayes D Jr, et al. The International Thoracic Organ Transplant Registry of the International Society for Heart and Lung Transplantation: 37th adult heart transplantation report-2020; focus on deceased donor characteristics. J Heart Lung Transplant. 2020;39(10):1003–15.
47. Defilippis EM, Kittleson MM. Pregnancy after heart transplantation. J Card Fail. 2021;27(2):176–84.
48. Moayedi Y, Foroutan F, Miller RJH, Fan CS, Posada JGD, Alhussein M, et al. Risk evaluation using gene expression screening to monitor for acute cellular rejection in heart transplant recipients. J Heart Lung Transplant. 2019;38(1):51–8.
49. Khush KK, Patel J, Pinney S, Kao A, Alharethi R, DePasquale E, et al. Noninvasive detection of graft injury after heart transplant using donor-derived cell-free DNA: a prospective multicenter study. Am J Transplant. 2019;19(10):2889–99.
50. Macera F, Occhi L, Masciocco G, Varrenti M, Frigerio M. A new life: motherhood after heart transplantation. A single-center experience and review of literature. Transplantation. 2018;102(9):1538–44.
51. D'Souza R, Soete E, Silversides CK, Zaffar N, Van Mieghem T, Van Cleemput J, et al. Pregnancy outcomes following cardiac transplantation. J Obstet Gynaecol Can. 2018;40(5):566–71.
52. Acuna S, Zaffar N, Dong S, Ross H, D'Souza R. Pregnancy outcomes in women with cardiothoracic transplants: a systematic review and meta-analysis. J Heart Lung Transplant. 2020;39(2):93–102.
53. Collier AY, Molina RL. Maternal mortality in the United States: updates on trends, causes, and solutions. NeoReviews. 2019;20(10):e561–74.
54. Kallapur A, Jang C, Yin O, Mei JY, Afshar Y. Pregnancy care in solid organ transplant recipients. Int J Gynaecol Obstet. 2021.
55. Deputy NP, Kim SY, Conrey EJ, Bullard KM. Prevalence and changes in preexisting diabetes and gestational diabetes among women who had a live birth - United States, 2012–2016. MMWR Morb Mortal Wkly Rep. 2018;67(43):1201–7.
56. Kitzmiller JL, Wallerstein R, Correa A, Kwan S. Preconception care for women with diabetes and prevention of major congenital malformations. Birth Defects Res A Clin Mol Teratol. 2010;88(10):791–803.
57. Vest AR, Cherikh WS, Noreen SM, Stehlik J, Khush KK. New-onset diabetes mellitus after adult heart transplantation and the risk of renal dysfunction or mortality. Transplantation. 2022;106(1):178–87.
58. Ramlakhan KP, Johnson MR, Roos-Hesselink JW. Pregnancy and cardiovascular disease. Nat Rev Cardiol. 2020;17(11):718–31.
59. Chamberlain JJ, Johnson EL, Leal S, Rhinehart AS, Shubrook JH, Peterson L. Cardiovascular disease and risk management: review of the

American Diabetes Association standards of medical care in diabetes 2018. Ann Intern Med. 2018;168(9):640–50.
60. National Institute for Health and Care Excellence: Guidelines. Diabetes in pregnancy: management from preconception to the postnatal period. London: National Institute for Health and Care Excellence (NICE) Copyright © NICE 2020. 2020.
61. Lund LH, Edwards LB, Kucheryavaya AY, Benden C, Christie JD, Dipchand AI, et al. The registry of the International Society for Heart and Lung Transplantation: thirty-first official adult heart transplant report–2014; focus theme: retransplantation. J Heart Lung Transplant. 2014;33(10):996–1008.
62. Campbell PT, Krim SR. Hypertension in cardiac transplant recipients: tackling a new face of an old foe. Curr Opin Cardiol. 2020;35(4):368–75.
63. Mata KM, Li W, Reslan OM, Siddiqui WT, Opsasnick LA, Khalil RA. Adaptive increases in expression and vasodilator activity of estrogen receptor subtypes in a blood vessel-specific pattern during pregnancy. Am J Physiol Heart Circ Physiol. 2015;309(10):H1679-96.
64. (NICE) LNIfHaCE. Hypertension in pregnancy: diagnosis and management. : NICE Guideline, No. 133. 2019. https://www.ncbi.nlm.nih.gov/books/NBK546004/.
65. Brown MA, Magee LA, Kenny LC, Karumanchi SA, McCarthy FP, Saito S, et al. Hypertensive disorders of pregnancy: ISSHP classification, diagnosis, and management recommendations for international practice. Hypertension. 2018;72(1):24–43.
66. ACOG Practice Bulletin No. 203: Chronic Hypertension in Pregnancy. Obstet Gynecol. 2019;133(1):e26-e50.
67. Stagno S, Pass RF, Dworsky ME, Alford CA. Maternal cytomegalovirus infection and perinatal transmission. Clin Obstet Gynecol. 1982;25(3):563–76.
68. Stagno S, Pass RF, Cloud G, Britt WJ, Henderson RE, Walton PD, et al. Primary cytomegalovirus infection in pregnancy: incidence, transmission to fetus, and clinical outcome. JAMA. 1986;256(14):1904–8.
69. Fowler KB, Stagno S, Pass RF, Britt WJ, Boll TJ, Alford CA. The outcome of congenital cytomegalovirus infection in relation to maternal antibody status. N Engl J Med. 1992;326(10):663–7.
70. Rawlinson WD, Boppana SB, Fowler KB, Kimberlin DW, Lazzarotto T, Alain S, et al. Congenital cytomegalovirus infection in pregnancy and the neonate: consensus recommendations for prevention, diagnosis, and therapy. Lancet Infect Dis. 2017;17(6):e177–88.
71. Pass RF, Arav-Boger R. Maternal and fetal cytomegalovirus infection: diagnosis, management, and prevention. F1000Res. 2018;7:255.
72. Anderson GD. Pregnancy-induced changes in pharmacokinetics: a mechanistic-based approach. Clin Pharmacokinet. 2005;44(10):989–1008.
73. Casale JP, Doligalski CT. Pharmacologic considerations for solid organ transplant recipients who become pregnant. Pharmacotherapy. 2016;36(9):971–82.
74. Hebert MF, Zheng S, Hays K, Shen DD, Davis CL, Umans JG, et al. Interpreting tacrolimus concentrations during pregnancy and postpartum. Transplantation. 2013;95(7):908–15.
75. Zheng S, Easterling TR, Umans JG, Miodovnik M, Calamia JC, Thummel KE, et al. Pharmacokinetics of tacrolimus during pregnancy. Ther Drug Monit. 2012;34(6):660–70.
76. Divithotawela C, Chambers D, Hopkins P. Pregnancy after lung transplant: case report. Breathe (Sheff). 2015;11(4):291–5.
77. Gyi KM, Hodson ME, Yacoub MY. Pregnancy in cystic fibrosis lung transplant recipients: case series and review. J Cyst Fibros. 2006;5(3):171–5.
78. Thiagarajan K, Arakali SR, Mealey KJ, Cardonick EH, Gaughan WJ, Davison JM, et al. Safety considerations: breastfeeding after transplant. Prog Transplant. 2013;23(2):137–46.
79. Drugs and lactation database (LactMed) https://www-ncbi-nlm-nih-gov.mlprox.csmc.edu/books/NBK501922/?report=classic.
80. Is it compatible with breastfeeding? https://www.e-lactancia.org/.

# Part VI
# The Future of Heart Transplantation

# The Total Artificial Heart

# 28

Jaime D. Moriguchi

**Abstract**

Despite optimized heart failure (HF) medical, surgical, and device therapies, many patients may still have progressive, persistent, severe signs and symptoms of HF, thus requiring advanced HF therapies. For a very small fraction of patients with severe biventricular HF and other anatomic or rhythm issues for which durable mechanical circulatory support would not be appropriate, the total artificial (TAH) is often the only viable option as a bridge to transplant. This chapter will describe the history, clinical indications, available devices, and outcomes of TAH as utilized in the US and the world for end-stage HF.

**Keywords**

Advanced heart failure · Mechanical circulatory support · Total Artificial Heart · Heart transplantation

J. D. Moriguchi (✉)
Cedars-Sinai Smidt Heart Institute, Los Angeles, CA, USA
e-mail: MoriguchiJ@csmns.org

## Clinical Pearls

- The total artificial heart is often the only viable option as a bridge to transplantation in patients with severe biventricular failure and other anatomic or rhythm issues for which a left ventricular assist devices is not appropriate.
- Total artificial heart contraindications include non-transplant candidates, reversible cardiomyopathies, advanced age, size limitations, multisystem or irreversible organ failure, uncontrolled bleeding, diathesis or infection/sepsis, among others
- Bleeding is the most frequent early issue, and emphasis on meticulous surgical attention to hemostasis and correction of thrombocytopenia/coagulopathy prior to leaving the operative room cannot be overemphasized.
- Patients bridged to transplantation with a total artificial heart demonstrated acceptable waitlist and 1-year post-transplant survival.

## Introduction

Since the beginning of time, scientists, physicians and philosophers alike have pondered the holy grail of medicine and cardiology in search of a suitable man-made pump to replace the human heart. Although temporary percutaneous



J. Kobashigawa (ed.), *Clinical Guide to Heart Transplantation*, https://doi.org/10.1007/978-3-031-88290-6_28

mechanical support and durable left ventricular assist devices (LVAD) are now available as bridges to heart transplantation (HTx) with excellent outcomes, a permanent total mechanical heart replacement has yet to be developed.

In patients with heart failure (HF), the 'four pillars' of guideline-directed medical therapies (GDMT) including beta-blockers (BB), angiotensin receptor-neprilysin inhibitors (ARNIs)/angiotensin receptor blocker (ARB)/angiotensin-converting enzyme inhibitors (ACEIs), mineralocorticoid receptor antagonists (MRAs), and sodium-glucose co-transporter 2 inhibitors (SGLT-2i) have shown to greatly improve quality of life and prolong survival [1].

Despite optimized medical, surgical, and device therapies, many patients (0.2–2.7% of Americans) may still have progressive/persistent severe signs and symptoms of HF (New York Heart Association (NYHA) functional class IV, AHA-ACC Stage D), thus requiring more aggressive interventions: advanced HF therapies [2, 3]. If a patient is evaluated and found to be a suitable candidate for HTx, listing actively through the United Network for Organ Sharing (UNOS) is an excellent option with 1-year survival near 90%, 5-year survival of 80%, and a median survival approaching 12 years [4]. Waiting times for a suitable donor vary depending on the patient's blood type, body size, and UNOS status. For instance, a large male (body service area (BSA)>2.5), blood type O, may wait 3–4 years as a status 6 candidate in some regions. There are also many patients who become hemodynamically unstable (cardiogenic shock) and require the initiation of inotropes, intra-aortic balloon pump (IABP), or percutaneous ventricular assist devices to support them temporarily [4]. These critically ill patients may qualify for a higher priority (UNOS status 2) to improve their chances of receiving a suitable donor heart in time. Others, in severe cardiogenic shock may require venoarterial extracorporeal membrane oxygenation (VA-ECMO) (Status I) to fully support their circulation, which markedly increases morbidity, mortality, and perioperative risk. Others may qualify for a durable LVAD (HeartMate III, Abbott) for extended support as a bridge to transplant (BTT) or destination therapy with 1 and 5-year survivals approaching that of HTx recipients [5]. For a very small proportion of patients (< 5% of those who qualify for durable devices) with severe biventricular HF and other anatomic or rhythm issues for which LVADs would not be appropriate, the total artificial heart (TAH) is often the only viable option as a BTT [6]. This chapter will describe the history, clinical indications, available devices, and outcomes of TAH as utilized in the US and the world for end-stage HF.

## Historical Perspectives

In 1920, Charles Lindburgh and Alexis Carrel joined forces to promote the concept of mechanical circulatory support (MCS). Lindbergh, better known as an aviator for flying across the Atlantic, was also an inventor. Carrel, a surgeon and Nobel Laureate (for his innovative work in HTx), performed many heart surgeries and recognized the need for an MCS device in the operative room [7]. Together, they created several blood pumps that provided temporary circulatory support and supported organs removed from a donor for subsequent transplant.

In 1937, Vladimir P. Demikhov, a Russian scientist, developed a TAH consisting of two separate pumps driven by an external driver (transcutaneous drive shaft) [8]. He implanted this device into a dog that lived for 5 h on support. In 1946, Demikhov successfully transplanted a heart–lung with the aid of a cardiopulmonary bypass and also performed the first known heterotopic HTx into a dog that survived 30 days [8].

In 1939, Dr. John H. Gibbon created a heart–lung machine used for cardiopulmonary bypass (CPB) in the U.S. His early experience with children, however, was uniformly unsuccessful. Subsequently, he teamed up with the Mayo Clinic and created a successful version of CPB, the Mayo-Gibbon-type oxygenator [8].

Tetsuzu Akutsu and Willem Kolff created and successfully implanted the first TAH into an animal in 1957 at the Cleveland Clinic, and it survived for 1.5 h. Dr Domingo Liotta from Argentina later created his version of a TAH model, which allowed an animal to survive up to 13 h. He subsequently joined Dr Michael DeBakey at Baylor in 1963 and implanted the first pulsatile LVAD. On April 4, 1969, Dr. Denton Cooley implanted a TAH into a 47-year-old male, Haskell Karp, whose native heart was failing without any suitable donor hearts available. This represented the first use of a TAH in man [9]. Unfortunately, due to hemolysis and renal failure, the device only supported the patient for 64 h before an emergency transplant was performed. The patient died 32 h post-transplant of infection.

In 1982, Dr. Robert Jarvik joined Dr. Willem Kolff at the University of Utah's heart program and, together with Dr. William DeVries, successfully implanted the first permanent TAH into a 61-year-old male, Barney Clark, on December 2, 1982 [10]. The device was the Symbion Jarvik 7 TAH. Mr. Clark lived for 112 days before succumbing to pneumonia and other ailments. The second recipient of the Jarvik 7 lived 620 days. Five other patients received this device, dying of multi-system organ failure, stroke, infection, and blood loss. The Jarvik 7, a precursor to the current TAH, was powered by a very large, external pneumatic driver that essentially confined the patient to a hospital existence [10].

## SynCardia Temporary Total Artificial Heart

The Symbion Jarvik 7 TAH evolved over the past 60 years, transitioning to the CardioWest TAH in 1991. In 2010, the device assumed the name of the SynCardia t-TAH manufactured in Tucson, AZ (SynCardia Systems Inc, Tucson, AZ) (Fig. 28.1). The current t-TAH is made of t wo independent artificial ventricles and is available in two sizes—70 cc and 50 cc. Four

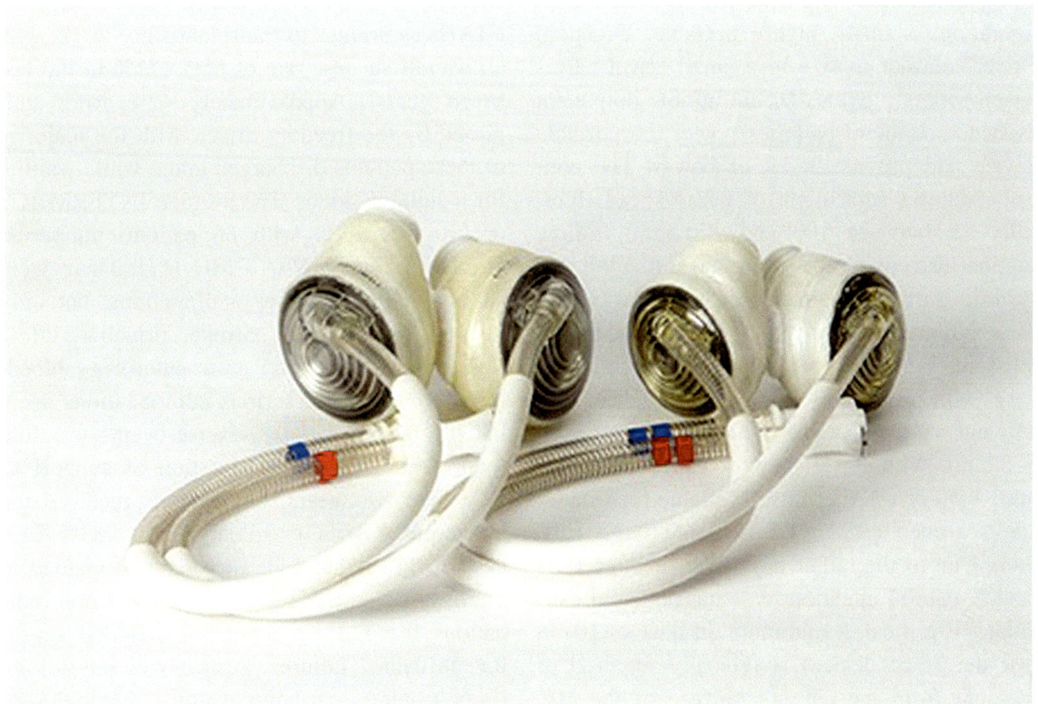

**Fig. 28.1** Syncardia TAH 70 cc (left) and 50 cc (right) devices. Reused from Villa CR, Morales DLS. The total artificial heart in end-stage congenital heart disease. Front Physiol. 2017;8:131

Medtronic-Hall valves, two (inflow & outflow) for each ventricle were utilized. After moving to Tucson, the MH valve was no longer being manufactured, and SynCardia secured the right to produce its own (Syn-Hall) valves. The two inflow cuffs were sutured to the native atria with outflow dacron grafts anastomosed from the right and left ventricles to the pulmonary artery and aorta, respectively. The ventricles are attached by Velcro to allow appropriate positioning within the mediastinum. Each ventricle has a stroke volume of 70 cc and is pneumatically driven using 5-layer polyurethane diaphragmatic membranes. Two pneumatic drivelines (1 cm diameter) are tunneled from the orthotopically positioned device to the subxiphoid or subcostal area [11]. Several modifications of the CardioWest TAH included covering the drivelines with Dacron velour and coating the diaphragm with silicone oil. The drivelines are connected to a large, external driver that weighed 350 lbs and was affectionately known as "Big Blue." Over time, the Companion II (C 2) driver, which was much smaller and more portable, replaced "Big Blue". In its current configuration, a small, highly portable "Freedom Driver" similar in size to a small travel carry-on on rollers provides a comfortable outpatient existence. Lithium batteries power the portable device and provide 3–4 h of power. The controller allows adjustment of pump speed (typically set between 100 and 120 bpm), inflow suction, drive pressure (right and left side), and systolic duration to match the vascular resistance and maintain physiologic systemic blood pressure. Pump flows for a given pump speed vary with peripheral vascular resistance, dP/dT, and suction but are typically backed with 5–8 l/min with top capability exceeding 9.5 l/min. A 50-cc t-TAH is also available for smaller adults/women (BSA $\geq$ 1.5 m$^2$) and large children. Due to the rather large size of the t-TAH device, careful attention to sizing potential candidates is critical. A minimum distance of 10 cm (for the 70 cc device) is typically required to measure from the anterior surface of the 10$^{th}$ thoracic vertebra (on chest CT) to the posterior surface of the sternum, often facilitated by 3-D reconstructed images. As a general rule, patients with a BSA of > 1.7 m$^2$ are potential candidates for the device. The surgical implantation of this device is well described elsewhere [12, 13] and will not be covered in this section.

The CardioWest TAH was implanted through clinical trial from 1983 and based on several landmark publications [14], this t-TAH was finally approved as a BTT in 2004. Specific indications included patients with irreversible, severe biventricular HF or who could not be supported with an LVAD, patients with restrictive physiology, refractory VT, and anatomic variants (massive myocardial infarction with ventricular septal defect/rupture). Since 1982, over 2080 t-TAH have been implanted worldwide with a success rate of 52.8–86.6%. Larger centers with > 10 implants appear to have better outcomes, and risk factors for poor outcomes include renal failure, advanced age, liver dysfunction, and ventilatory support. Many larger transplant centers have published favorable survival data on the Syncardia t-TAH as BTT [15, 16].

At our own institution (Cedars-Sinai Medical Center), we have implanted 101 Syncardia t-TAHs as bridges to transplant since 2012, with an overall success rate of 65% (71% in the last seven years). Approximately 42% were supported by the freedom driver, with the majority of these patients discharged home while waiting for a suitable donor. The average INTERMACS profile was 1.72, with 36 patients supported at some point by VA-ECMO [17]. There were six major device/driver malfunctions, but only resulting in 1 death. Stroke, driveline infection, renal failure, and gastroenterology bleeding were the most serious complications seen, but the rate of serious adverse events was less than 20%. The longest duration of support as BTT was two years. Six patients received the 50 cc pump with excellent results (83% successful BTT), although all patients remained in the hospital until HTx. The most common indications for TAH implantation included severe biventricular failure, restrictive physiology (hypertrophic cardiomyopathy, amyloidosis), refractory ventricular tachyarrhythmias, and congenital heart disease [18].

## Abiomed AbioCor TAH

The AbioCor TAH was the only fully implantable, self-contained artificial heart designed and developed in the Abiomed laboratories (AbioMed Danvers, MA) in the 1980–1990s [19]. It had a systemic pumping chamber and a pulmonary chamber formed from flexible membranes that were alternatively compressed by an internal pump. The blood bladders were compressed by surrounding hydraulic fluid (silicone oil) alternatively pumped by a centrifugal rotor at speeds of 4,000–8,000 rpm. This continuous rotation, as opposed to oscillating rotation, was felt to be the key to enhanced durability. This device was considered a major breakthrough from previous technologies in that it was truly and fully implantable using transcutaneous energy transmission (TET). There were no wires that exited the body, thereby eliminating the risk of percutaneous line-associated infections. In addition, instead of pusher plate technology, a gentler hydraulic fluid compression using a highly compliant diaphragm would minimize hemolysis and promote the device's durability. Because it is powered electrically, bulky pneumatic drivelines were eliminated, and a fully implantable unit, including a short-term internal battery, made for an untethered and completely silent existence (Fig. 28.2). Four tri-leaflet polyurethane valves promoted unidirectional flow but mandated systemic anticoagulation. The pump itself weighed only 2 lbs and was orthotopically implanted. A transcutaneous TET coil was also implanted along with a controller and internal battery (15–20' pump time). For the US trial, patient selection was limited to individuals > 75 years old who had end-stage biventricular failure and were not HTx candidates. The first implantation, Robert Tools, occurred at the University of Louisville by Drs. Bowman Gray and Robert Dowling in 2001 and survived for five months. Three other centers were involved, and, in all, 14 patients received the AbioCor TAH [19, 20]. Two patients were discharged home, and the second patient, Tom Christerson, survived for 17 months. For the initial seven patients, the 30-day mortality was over 70%,

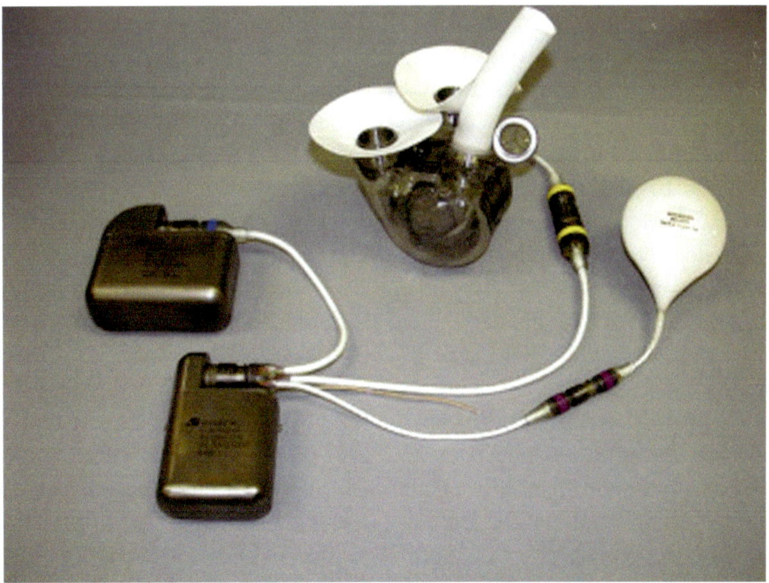

**Fig. 28.2** AbioCor® system, artificial heart system. Reprinted from Cardiovascular Pathology, (Fourth Edition), Berthiaume JM, Kirk JA, Ranek MJ, Lyon RC, Sheikh F, Jensen BC, et al., Chap. 8—Pathophysiology of Heart Failure and an Overview of Therapies, 271–339, Copyright (2016), with permission from Elsevier

including one intraoperative mortality. Four patients died on postop days 51–151. The longest survivor was ultimately able to spend time with his family at home, although his wife claimed he was not able to ambulate or enjoy a good quality of life [19, 20]. Many patients also complained of orthostatic hypotension and inadequate physiological response to activities. Acute renal failure was often a marker of poor outcomes. The AbioCor was FDA-approved in 2006 for inotrope-dependent patients with irreversible biventricular failure who were ineligible for HTx < 30 days anticipated survival. However, over time, the device fell out of favor clinically and is no longer available.

## Carmat Aeson TAH

The Carmat Aeson (France) is an electrohydraulically powered heart replacement device that was developed between 2008 and 2021. It consists of a left and right ventricle, which are housed within a single structure. Separate compartments contain the electrohydraulic actuators and control systems. There is a double-layered hybrid membrane made of polyurethrane on the hydraulic surface and a glutaraldehyde-treated bovine pericardial membrane in contact with the blood elements. The static surfaces are also covered by expanded polytetrafluoroethylene (ePTFE). There are four biological valves (two inlet, two outlet) and two rotary pumps located in the device's technical compartments. Blood flow is thus propelled by the systolic and diastolic phases of the rapid reversal of hydraulic (silicone) fluid. Because of the gentle, undulating movement of the hydraulic fluid (vs. the more vigorous, jerking pusher plate mechanisms previously used in HeartMate I), less turbulence is observed, which theoretically translates to lower hemolysis and increased durability of the device. It should be emphasized that the left and right ventricles pump alternatively with auto-controlled pump force to ensure full ejection, avoiding stasis and thrombus formation. Flow autoregulation is accomplished with pressor sensors that detect preload. A high preload leads to the acceleration of pump beat rate and flow (Fig. 28.3). Ultrasound sensors detect membrane position to ensure full ejection with every beat. Mathematical models have demonstrated a complete washout of the ventricles with minimal stress and hemolysis. Clinically, this was confirmed with no degradation of Von Willebrand Factor (VWF), platelet activation, thrombus formation, or gastrointestinal bleeding seen in patients in a small sample of patients [17]. The entire device is partially enclosed within the flexible polyurethrane compliance membrane containing the hydraulic fluid. A percutaneous driveline (diameter: 8 mm) exits the abdomen, connecting to the controller and batteries for energy sources. A key advantage of this device is the low incidence of thromboembolic complications, for which systemic anticoagulation is not required in the long term [21, 22].

The PIVOTAL study was a European Multicenter Study aimed at evaluating the safety and performance of the Carmat TAH that was initialed in 2016 (ClinicalTrials.gov Identifier: NCT02962973). In an interim analysis of this study, 73% of the first enrolled 11 patients achieved the primary endpoint of the study, corresponding to 6-month survival with the bioprosthesis or a successful transplant within six months after device implants achieved the primary objective of the study (compared to Syncardia t-TAH 54–67%; BiVAD 46–68% and LVAD 90–92%) [23]. Major adverse complications were relatively low, with no cerebrovascular (CVA), gastrointestinal bleeding, drive line infection, and 36% bleeding complications. These results enabled CARMAT to obtain a European Conformity marking in December 2020.

Nuketa et al. reported an initial experience of HTx in patients with CARMAT-TAH with seven HTx-eligible patients with end-stage biventricular failure (all men, mean age = $52.4 \pm 9.7$ years, and body surface area = $2.06 \pm 0.16$ m$^2$) enrolled in the PIVOTAL study. Three of them suffered from ischemic cardiomyopathy, and four patients had non-ischemic cardiomyopathy. One patient was in INTERMACS II, while the rest were in INTERMACS Profile III. Five patients

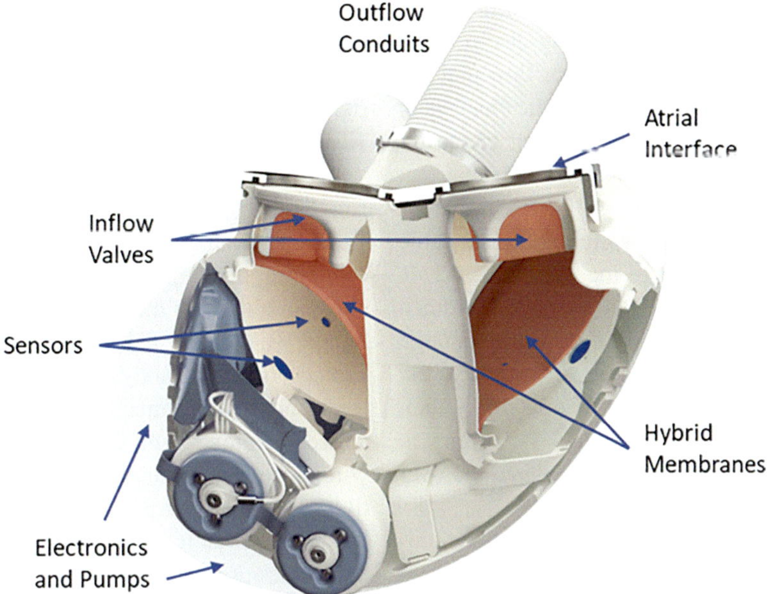


**Fig. 28.3** The Aeson (CARMAT SA) Total Artificial Heart. Reused from Vincentelli A, Pya Y, Netuka I, Haneya A, Schmitto J, Kindo M, et al. Implantation Technique for the Aeson Total Artificial Heart. Operative Techniques in Thoracic and Cardiovascular Surgery. 2024;29(2):149–67

were transplanted successfully; one-year post-transplant survival was 80% [24].

In the United States, the Carmat TAH Early Feasibility trial (NCT04117295) for a bridge-to-transplant enrolled 4 (out of 10 planned) patients, and due to quality issues, the study was suspended in 2021 [25, 26]. The EFICAS study is ongoing in France, and 50% of the anticipated 52 device implants has been achieved [27].

Overall, by the end of 2023, 50 patients have received the Carmat Aeson without CVA or gastrointestinal bleeding since 2013, and the company has built a second plant capable of manufacturing up to 500 units/year [28].

## BiVACOR TAH

The BiVACOR TAH combines a rotary blood pump using full magnetic levitation technology (Fig. 28.4). This unique design utilizes a contact-free spinning disc that simultaneously

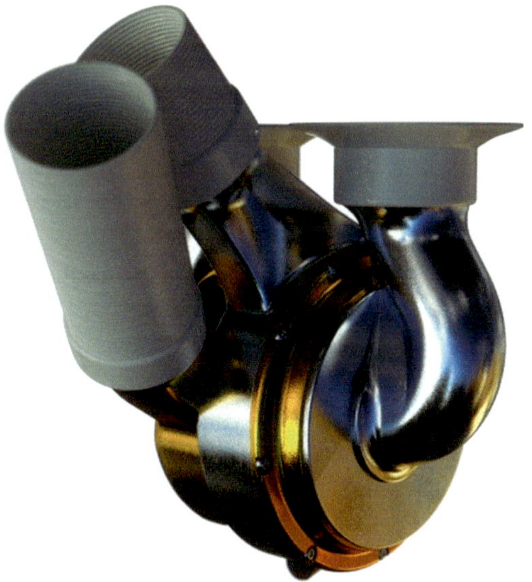

**Fig. 28.4** Bivacor total artificial heart. Reused with permission from Arabía FA, Murray CF. The total artificial heart: where have we been, where are we now, where are we going? Indian J Thorac Cardiovasc Surg. 2023;39(Suppl 1):198–205

provides systemic and pulmonic blood flow with a single moving part. The rotating disc reliably and efficiently provides continuous flow that can be made pulsatile by rapid and cyclic changes in pump speed. The system is powered electronically by a small, external portable controller that connects to the pump via a single 5 mm percutaneous driveline. A pair of lithium rechargeable batteries provide power to the device [29]. Due to its compact design, it can be used in women and most children. Yet, it is powerful enough to physiologically respond to the needs of an exercising adult male. The BiVACOR system, initially designed by Dr Daniel L Timms in Australia, has undergone several iterations over the past two decades [29, 30].

The BiVACOR TAH was designed to eliminate the majority of shortcomings of current and prior devices. It provides a durable, reliable, and physiologically responsive system that is small enough to accommodate women and most children (BSA > 1.45) yet powerful enough to meet the demands of a large adult male during exercise (flow 4–10 L/min). By incorporating a single moving part (rotor) suspended completely by magnetic levitation, it is completely contactless. The large gaps further minimize trauma to red blood cells, markedly reducing the risk of thrombosis and hemolysis. The valves and diaphragms that are utilized in volume displacement pumps are no longer required in a continuous flow system, which greatly enhances the longevity and durability of the BiVACOR system. By extending its durability and reducing long-term adverse events, this device can now be considered for long-term biventricular support, enhancing its role as a potential alternative to HTx (destination therapy). Power requirements are also minimized, promoting longer battery times. The driveline has been miniaturized, and it is completely silent, lightweight, and extremely portable. Internal sensors autoregulate rotor speeds and balance pulmonary and systemic flow with minimal mixing of circulations. The BiVACOR TAH was designed to exploit the success of a continuous flow LVAD system. The hope is that serious adverse effects, namely stroke, infection, bleeding, or device thrombosis (< 35% of LVAD patients are free of these complications at one year), are significantly reduced with this device. Certainly, it will help mitigate right heart failure associated with the poor survival seen with BIVAD currently in use.

Animal studies have been pioneered at Texas Heart Institute in Houston, TX. The BiVACOR TAH has been implanted in over 30 animals, supporting life for up to 3 months [30]. In a preclinical study of 5 calves supported for 30 days by the BiVACOR device, The calves demonstrated normal hemodynamics, end-organ function, and hemocompatibility. Despite minimal anticoagulation, significant thrombi were noted within the device or major organs at explanation [31]. The device received Early Feasibility Study approval from the U.S. Food and Drug Administration in December 2023 [25]. The first-in-human implantation of the BiVACOR TAH was completed in July 2024 at Baylor St. Luke's Medical Center in the Texas Medical Center [32].

## The Total Artificial Heart: Indications, Contraindications, and Complications

Ideally, a TAH must respond to demands and activities to provide adequate blood flow and maintain blood pressure in various physiologic situations to be effective. Other important qualifications include durability, reliability, hemocompatibility (thrombosis/embolic risk), size parameters, power source requirements, and portability of external components. To minimize wear and tear and device failure, the design of the TAH should be simple and have as few moving parts as possible. Although teleologically, the flow should be pulsatile, long-term durability may necessitate a continuous flow mechanism to be considered, particularly if support is to be 'permanent' for non-transplant candidates. Despite multiple TAH devices that have been trialed, only the SynCardia t-TAH is FDA-approved and commercially available.

As with many advances in MCS, selecting the right patient, condition, and timing of intervention is often the key to a successful outcome. Preop evaluation of advanced HF candidates for a TAH includes a thorough history looking specifically for the severity of advanced HF to satisfy the need for this device and to ensure that they are not suitable candidates for an LVAD, revascularization, medical management, or bridge directly to HTx with temporary percutaneous VADs [33]. It is critical that the patient be evaluated for underlying malignancies, bleeding or coagulopathies, renal, hepatic, vascular, and pulmonary diseases that would markedly increase morbidity and mortality. Other diagnostic studies typically required during the evaluation process include an echocardiogram, left/right heart catheterization, cardiopulmonary exercise test, gastrointestinal work-up, renal assessment, coagulation parameters, history of heparin-induced thrombocytopenia /bleeding/thrombotic, genetic complications along with caregiver support, patient sophistication and acceptance of technology and insurance coverage (i.e., MediCal does not cover TAH in California).

Indications for t-TAH include severe, irreversible, bi-ventricular HF, massive myocardial infarction with ventricular septal defect/free wall or impending rupture, severe restrictive/infiltrative (amyloidosis) or hypertrophic cardiomyopathy, refractory ventricular tachycardia, primary cardiac malignancy, congenital heart disease, s/p LVAD with refractory right ventricular failure and refractory transplant rejection or severe cardiac allograft vasculopathy.

Contraindications include non-transplant candidates, reversible cardiomyopathies, advanced age (i.e., >70 yo-center specific), size limitations with BSA < 1.65 $m^2$/<10 cm at T-10 (50 ccs available), multisystem or irreversible organ failure, uncontrolled bleeding diathesis or infection/sepsis, recent intracranial bleed, significant CVA and malignancy. Psychosocial issues and lack of adequate caregivers or stable residences may also preclude candidacy. While there are no absolute upper body mass index cutoffs in many programs, morbidly obese patients pose an increased risk for postoperative complications, including bleeding, poor wound healing, and physical recovery.

Major complications related to t-TAH use include driveline infections, device endocarditis, gastrointestinal bleeding, post-operative mediastinal bleeding, pneumonia, dysphagia, embolic events/CVA, device thrombosis, device malfunction, driveline fracture, diaphragmatic rupture, pneumatic driver failure, pump stoppage, and renal failure. A number of our patients have had hardening and fractures of their drivelines with leakage, requiring emergency taping and revision.

## Perioperative Management

The management of post-operative TAH implants is critical to short and long-term outcomes. Bleeding is the most frequent early issue, and emphasis on meticulous surgical attention to hemostasis and correction of thrombocytopenia/coagulopathy prior to leaving the operative room cannot be overemphasized. Some centers advocate delayed sternal closure for 24–48 h for closer visualization/monitoring of mediastinal bleeding, but infectious risk must be considered, and post-op antibiotics may be necessary. While tamponade is much less frequent with the non-compressible TAH, vascular structures can still be affected, and transesophageal echocardiography may be required to help make the diagnosis. Volume management is also important in maintaining adequate device flow, and frequent adjustments of pump speed, filling suction, and dP/dT are essential in early postop management. Central venous pressure is often helpful in assessing volume along with an hourly assessment of monitored parameters of the TAH console. A key recommendation is that only one team or individual (i.e., cardiothoracic surgeon) with close communication/consultation with intensivists and MCS service make TAH parameter adjustments to avoid confusion and discordant management. Anemia is seen in the majority of TAH recipients, but it is not necessary to maintain normal Hgb/Hct in these patients. In fact, due to the more favorable viscosity at lower hemoglobin, running levels of 7–9 with good oxygen delivery d/t higher flows would not be unusual. Inotropes are typically unnecessary, although IV vasoconstrictors are often utilized to maintain systemic vascular tone in vasoplegic conditions. Renal failure perioperatively is also a common complication requiring CRRT/HD, but with reasonable perfusion pressure and avoidance of nephrotoxic agents, many patients will demonstrate significant recovery over time. The usual attention to good pulmonary toilet and airway protection is important. Systemic anticoagulation is begun as soon as hemostasis is achieved, usually with chest tube output < 20 cc/hr in the form of IV heparin on postop day 2–4 (without bolus) and subsequently transitioned to PO coumadin with typical INR goal of 2–3. We have often utilized the thromboelastogram to gain a better understanding of the clotting cascade and platelet aggregation pathway. This appears particularly enlightening when there is a discordance between the INR and clinical coagulation/bleeding tendencies. Ambulation around the unit with a Companion 2 pneumatic driver system is often possible within the first week. Transition to the Freedom II portable driver usually occurs on the floor prior to discharge. Education of patients and family members is an ongoing process. The typical period of postoperative management prior to discharge is in the range of 3–4 weeks [34].

Patient complaints include excessively loud driver noise levels, frequent battery changes, the need for systemic anticoagulation, large bore/diameter drivelines, a chronically tethered existence, and the need for a caregiver 24 × 7.

## Clinical TAH Outcomes

In 2004, Dr Jack Copeland reported his outcome of the then CardioWest t-TAH in the New England Journal of Medicine [14]. Between January 1993 and September 2002, 81 TAHs were implanted at five centers in a non-randomized, prospective study using historical controls. There was a 79% survival to HTx on TAH support, with a 1-year survival on TAH support of 70% Compared with a 1-year survival for controls of 31%. The 1 and 5-year survival of transplant patients bridged with the TAH were 86 and 64%, respectively. Matched patients transplanted without TAH support had 69 and 34% survival, respectively. Coyan et al. reported outcomes following TAH as a BTT from the UNOS database for the years 2004 and 2020, with waitlist mortality being 7.4%, with 375 patients (86.6%) ultimately being transplanted. The authors cited age, CVA, functional status, and ventilator dependence as risk factors for waitlist mortality. One-year survival following successful BTT was 80% [35].

## Summary and Future Directions

Current technology for durable MCS is limited to the HeartMate III LVAD and Syncardia t-TAH devices. The latter device, while effective in providing biventricular support, is based on rather primitive technology and has many drawbacks. The most important include poor long-term durability, need for systemic anticoagulation, persistent thromboembolic/infectious complications, and user-unfriendly design. Is there a promising future device available to overcome many, if not all, of these drawbacks/limitations of the Syncardia t-TAH? Although the only non-tethered TAH ever implanted in man, the Abiomed AbioCor device is no longer available; the BiVACOR TAH appears to have the most desirable features ever found in a single device.

The last frontier in developing an ideal TAH would be a fully implantable system with an internal power source or possibly energy transmission across the skin to provide a non-tethered existence. It is truly unlikely that a perpetual internalized power source, such as nuclear energy, would ever be developed or approved due to potential disasters and prior incidents. Solar and radiofrequency energy transmission is unlikely to be a reliable enough energy source. TET technology has previously attempted to transfer energy across the skin using an internal capacitor (LionHeart, AbioCor). Still, due to the rigors of daily life, the proximity of the external and internal transmission devices is so critical that the reliability of this technology has been a logistical challenge. However, TET technology is currently our best option for powering a TAH, such as the BiVACOR, which has a fairly low baseline energy requirement and automatic physiological response to activity. We remain hopeful for a future TAH that we can utilize for long-term support both as BTT and destination therapy.

## References


1. Heidenreich PA, Bozkurt B, Aguilar D, Allen LA, Byun JJ, Colvin MM, et al. 2022 ACC/AHA/HFSA guideline for the management of heart failure. J Card Fail [Internet]. 2022;28(5):e1-167. https://doi.org/10.1016/j.cardfail.2022.02.010.
2. Members WC, Bozkurt B, Ahmad T, Alexander KM, Baker WL, Bosak K, et al. Heart failure epidemiology and outcomes statistics: a report of the Heart Failure Society of America. J Card Fail. 2023;29(10):1412.
3. Fang JC, Ewald GA, Allen LA, Butler J, Canary CAW, Colvin-Adams M, et al. Advanced (stage D) heart failure: a statement from the Heart Failure Society of America Guidelines Committee. J Card Fail. 2015;21(6):519–34.
4. Reich H, Ramzy D, Moriguchi J, Dimbil S, Levine R, Passano E, et al. Acceptable post–heart transplant outcomes support temporary MCS prioritization in the new OPTN| UNOS heart allocation policy. In: Transplantation proceedings. Elsevier; 2021. p. 353–7.
5. Mehra MR, Goldstein DJ, Cleveland JC, Cowger JA, Hall S, Salerno CT, et al. Five-year outcomes in patients with fully magnetically levitated vs axial-flow left ventricular assist devices in the MOMENTUM 3 randomized trial. JAMA. 2022;328(12):1233–42.
6. Arabía FA, Cantor RS, Koehl DA, Kasirajan V, Gregoric I, Moriguchi JD, et al. Interagency registry for mechanically assisted circulatory support report on the total artificial heart. J Heart Lung Transplant. 2018;37(11):1304–12.
7. Sade RM. A surprising alliance: two giants of the 20th century. Ann Thorac Surg. 2017;103(6):2015–9.
8. Khan S, Jehangir W. Evolution of artificial hearts: an overview and history. Cardiol Res. 2014;5(5):121.
9. Cooley DA. The amazing adventures of a heart surgeon [postscript]. Tex Heart Inst J. 2007;34:395.
10. Utah and the Artificial Heart: Impact and Reflections 40 Years Later|University of Utah Health | University of Utah Health [Internet]. https://uofuhealth.utah.edu/notes/2023/01/utah-and-artificial-heart-impact-and-reflections-40-years-later. Accessed 22 Sept 2024
11. SynCardia. Syncardia Total Artificial Heart (STAH) [Internet]. https://www.syncardia.com/syncardia-total-artificial-heart-stah.html. Accessed 1 Oct 2024
12. Chung JS, Emerson D, Megna D, Arabia FA. Total artificial heart: surgical technique in the patient with normal cardiac anatomy. Ann Cardiothorac Surg. 2020;9(2):81.
13. Arabía FA. SynCardia total artificial heart opportunities and challenges moving forward. Artif Organs. 2019;43(11):1051–2.
14. Copeland JG, Smith RG, Arabia FA, Nolan PE, Sethi GK, Tsau PH, et al. Cardiac replacement with a total artificial heart as a bridge to transplantation. N Engl J Med. 2004;351(9):859–67.
15. Carrier M, Moriguchi J, Shah KB, Anyanwu AC, Mahr C, Skipper E, et al. Outcomes after heart transplantation and total artificial heart implantation: a multicenter study. J Heart Lung Transplant. 2021;40(3):220–8.
16. Copeland JG, Copeland H, Gustafson M, Mineburg N, Covington D, Smith RG, et al. Experience with more than 100 total artificial heart implants. J Thorac Cardiovasc Surg. 2012;143(3):727–34.
17. Shah KB, Thanavaro KL, Tang DG, Quader MA, Mankad AK, Tchoukina I, et al. Impact of INTERMACS profile on clinical outcomes for patients supported with the total artificial heart. J Card Fail. 2016;22(11):913–20.
18. Chen Q, Chan J, Akhmerov A, Roach A, Emerson D, Megna D, et al. Heart transplantation after total artificial heart bridging—outcomes over 15 years. Clin Transplant. 2022;36(11):e14781.
19. Samak M, Fatullayev J, Sabashnikov A, Zeriouh M, Rahmanian PB, Choi YH, et al. Past and present of total artificial heart therapy: a success story. Med Sci Monit Basic Res. 2015;21:183.
20. Dowling RD, Gray LA Jr, Etoch SW, Laks H, Marelli D, Samuels L, et al. Initial experience with the AbioCor implantable replacement heart system. J Thorac Cardiovasc Surg. 2004;127(1):131–41.
21. Mohacsi P, Leprince P. The CARMAT total artificial heart. Eur J Cardio-Thorac Surg. 2014;46:933–4 Oxford University Press.
22. Schroder JN, McCartney SL, Jansen P, Plichta R, Katz JN, Smadja DM, et al. The first autoregulated total artificial heart implant in the United States. Ann Thorac Surg Short Reports. 2023;1(1):185–7.
23. Carmat. CARMAT: the feedback after 6 years and 8 months of cumulative support shows a constant improvement in the clinical outcomes of patients in the PIVOTAL study - Carmat: Carmat [Internet]. https://www.carmatsa.com/en/news/carmat-feedback-6-years-8-months-cumulative-

support-shows-constant-improvement-clinical-outcomes-patients-pivotal-study/#_ftnref2. Accessed 29 Sept 2024

24. Netuka I, Ivak P, Konarik M, Pya Y, Bekbossynova M, Gustafsson F, et al. Initial bridge to transplant experience with a bioprosthetic autoregulated artificial heart. J Heart Lung Transplant. 2020;39(12):1491–3.
25. Dual SA, Cowger J, Roche E, Nayak A. The future of durable mechanical circulatory support–emerging technological innovations and considerations to enable evolution of the field. J Card Fail. 2024.
26. Carmat SA. Study Details|Carmat TAH Early Feasibility Study|ClinicalTrials.gov [Internet]. https://clinicaltrials.gov/study/NCT04117295#study-record-dates. Accessed 27 Sept 2024
27. Half of enrolments targeted in the EFICAS study reached by CARMAT - Carmat: Carmat [Internet]. https://www.carmatsa.com/en/news/half-of-enrolments-targeted-in-the-eficas-study-reached-by-carmat/. Accessed 27 Sept 2024
28. Carmat. About Carmat - Carmat: Carmat [Internet]. https://www.carmatsa.com/en/about-carmat/. Accessed 27 Sept 2024
29. BiVACOR. BiVACOR, Inc. – Replacing hearts. Restoring lives. [Internet]. https://bivacor.com/. Accessed 29 Sept 2024
30. Kleinheyer M, Greatrex N, Nestler F, Timms DL. bivacor total artificial heart and future concepts. In: Mechanical circulatory support. Springer; 2023. p. 1–17.
31. Timms DL, Greatrex N, Nestler F, Wu E, Kleinheyer M, Cohn W, et al. (127) Preclinical evaluation of the bivacor total artificial heart. J Heart Lung Transplant. 2023;42(4):S66.
32. BiVACOR. The Texas Heart Institute Implants BiVACOR® Total Artificial Heart – BiVACOR, Inc. [Internet]. https://bivacor.com/the-texas-heart-institute-implants-bivacor-total-artificial-heart/. Accessed 29 Sept 2024
33. Arabia FA, Moriguchi JD. Machines versus medication for biventricular heart failure: focus on the total artificial heart. Future Cardiol. 2014;10(5):593–609.
34. Yaung J, Arabia FA, Nurok M. Perioperative care of the patient with the total artificial heart. Anesth Analg. 2017;124(5):1412–22.
35. Coyan GN, Huckaby LV, Diaz-Castrillon CE, Miguelino AM, Kilic A. Trends and outcomes following total artificial heart as bridge to transplant from the UNOS database. J Card Surg. 2022;37(5):1215–21.

# Xenotransplantation

# 29

Emily Newman, Indranee Rajapreyar, Yevgeniy Brailovsky, and Howard J. Eisen

**Abstract**

Following decades of experiments in animal models, the world's first genetically modified pig-to-human heart transplant took place in January 2022. In this chapter, we will discuss several considerations and challenges in xenotransplantation, including anatomic and physiologic differences between pig and human hearts: immunological response and rejection, organ overgrowth, infections, and ethical dilemmas. We also describe the clinical course of the first genetically modified heart xenotransplant.

**Keywords**

Advanced heart failure · Mechanical circulatory support · Total artificial heart · Heart transplantation

E. Newman · H. J. Eisen (✉) · Y. Brailovsky
Thomas Jefferson University,
Philadelphia, PA, USA
e-mail: howardeisen56@gmail.com

I. Rajapreyar
Tufts Medical Center,
Philadelphia, PA, USA

## Clinical Pearls

- Clustered, regularly interspaced short palindromic repeats (CRISPR)-Cas9 genome editing has helped mitigate several immunological challenges in xenotransplantation.
- Xenotransplant recipients require specialized immunosuppression and are at risk for infections similar to human transplant recipients but are also at risk for zoonotic infections.
- The use of genetically modified porcine organs as a source for organ transplants would greatly enlarge the pool of organs available to treat patients with end-stage cardiac disease and could result in a reduction in transplant waitlist times. However, xenotransplant brings its own set of ethical concerns.
- Before expanding xenotransplantation activities, several important hurdles must be overcome, including Xenograft rejection, zoonotic infections, and ethical considerations.

## History of Xenotransplantation

Xenotransplantation has been studied for decades, starting with Tulane University performing a number of chimpanzee-to-human kidney transplants in the early 1960s [1]. However, patients only survived for days to months. The first cardiac xenotransplant was performed in



J. Kobashigawa (ed.), *Clinical Guide to Heart Transplantation*, https://doi.org/10.1007/978-3-031-88290-6_29

1964, also using a chimpanzee donor; the heart was too small to support human circulation, and the graft failed after several hours due to antibody-mediated rejection [1]. In 1984, at Loma Linda University, an infant with hypoplastic left heart syndrome received a baboon heart transplant and survived for 21 days before death from rejection [1]. Initially, non-human primates were studied as organ donors, given the close evolutionary relationship with humans. Since the 1990s, attention has shifted to pigs, given that they have cardiac size and structure similar to human adults, shorter reproductive time, larger litter sizes, and rapid sexual maturity [1, 2]. Subsequent experimental attempts using pig hearts were limited in survival to less than 24 h primarily due to hyperacute rejection. Following decades of experiments in animal models, the world's first genetically modified pig-to-human heart transplant took place on January 7, 2022, followed by a second case in September 2023. In this chapter, we are going to discuss several considerations and challenges in xenotransplantation, including anatomic and physiologic differences between pig and human hearts: immunological response and rejection, organ overgrowth, infections, and ethical dilemmas. We also describe the clinical course of the first genetically modified heart xenotransplant (Fig. 29.1).

## Anatomical and Physiological Differences Between the Pig and Human Heart

Although pig hearts are markedly similar to human hearts, subtle anatomical differences exist. Compared to humans, the diameter of the great vessels in pigs is proportionally smaller, particularly for the ascending aorta and pulmonary artery [2]. In addition, the length of the great vessels proximal to major branches is proportionally shorter in pigs. In contrast, the suprahepatic inferior vena cava (IVC) is longer in pigs [2]. A pig heart has 5–7 pulmonary veins instead of 4, and the inferior vena cava and superior vena cava drain into the right atrium at right angles in the pig. The porcine azygous vein drains into the coronary sinus [3]. Several differences in coronary anatomy have been identified and are clinically relevant to cardiac catheterization after cardiac xenotransplantation. Such as the orientation of the right and left coronary ostia, arising from the aortic root (Pigs: at 90° vs. Humans: 120–140°) and the positioning of the left anterior descending artery (Pigs: Rightward to the left ventricle vs. Humans: overlying the left ventricle) [2]. Functionally, a healthy porcine heart has cardiac output, stroke volume, and heart rate similar to that of a healthy human [3]. While blood pressure and systemic vascular resistance are lower in pigs than in humans [4].

## Xenograft Rejection

Surface glycan antigens on porcine cells pose a risk of immune reactions in the human recipient. In addition, the absence of inhibitory natural killer (NK) cell ligands in porcine cells may potentially trigger human NK-cell-mediated responses. Clustered regularly interspaced short palindromic repeats (CRISPR)-Cas9 genome editing allowed to address these immunological challenges [5]. Overall, 10 genes were edited in the first genetically modified human xenotransplant, which included knocking out three genes that enable pigs to synthesize these cell surface antigens. Furthermore, six human genes were edited into the pig, including two anti-inflammatory genes, two genes that prevent blood vessel damage, and two regulatory protein genes that help suppress the antibody response. One final gene modification was done to prevent overgrowth of the pig heart, which will be discussed later in this chapter. However, the unusual immunological situation in a Xenotransplanted heart necessitates an adequate immunosuppression that may differ from conventional postoperative immunosuppressive regimens and prevent rejection. Therefore, it's essential to overcome these immunological barriers.

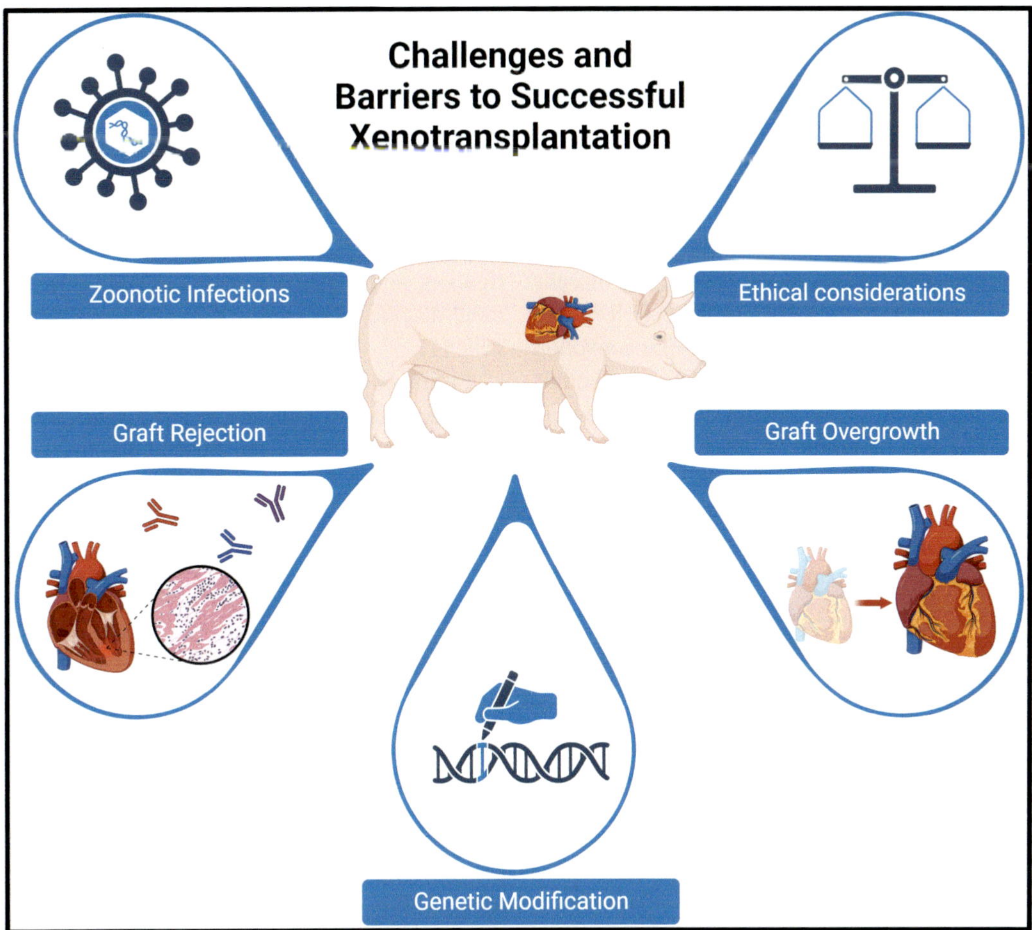


**Fig. 29.1** Challenges and barriers to xenotransplantation

## Hyperacute Rejection

Hyperacute rejection is a humoral response that starts within minutes to hours of transplant and is driven by preformed antibodies from the recipient that react to antigens on the donor organ. These antibodies bind to the endothelial lining of graft blood vessels and cause complement activation. This causes rapid destruction of the graft [4, 6]. In porcine xenotransplantation these preformed antibodies are against ∝-Gal (galactose-∝ 1,3-galactose) antigens from porcine cells [6]. Depleting these antibodies in baboons receiving porcine xenotransplants prevented hyperacute rejection [6]. Subsequent studies using pigs deficient in ∝-Gal similarly prevented hyperacute rejection in baboon cardiac xenotransplant [1]. Subsequent studies identified two further antigens, b1,4-N-acetylgalactosyltransfer-ase and CMP-N-acetylneuraminic acid hydroxylase as contributing to a delayed hyperacute rejection reaction and porcine organs genetically modified to remove these three antigens improved hyperacute rejection responses [1].

## Complement Activation

Complement activation also contributes to hyperacute rejection and can be activated through the classical or alternative pathways. Antigens other than α-Gal, b1,4-N-acetylgalactosyltransferase, and CMP-N-acetylneuraminic acid hydroxylase can activate complement through the classical pathway. Ischemia–reperfusion injury can activate complement through the alternative pathway (without antibody-antigen interaction) [7]. Both classic and alternative complement pathways result in the formation of the membrane attack complex, which leads to the destruction of cells [8]. Complement regulatory proteins (CRPs) are membrane-bound proteins that prevent activation of the complement systems to protect the body's own tissues from destruction by complement [8]. The incorporation of three of the human CRPs, CD55, CD46, and CD59, into the donor pig genome reduces hyperacute rejection from complement activation [1]. CD55 promotes the dissociation of C3 convertases and inhibits NK cells cytotoxic functions. CD59 inhibits the formation of the membrane attack complex by binding C8 and C9. CD46 blocks the formation of C3 convertase, which is required for the classic and alternative pathways. Additionally, CD55 and CD46 regulate T-cell activation [7].

## Acute Humoral Rejection

The acute humoral rejection or acute vascular rejection occurs from days to weeks after transplant and involves both humoral and cellular immune responses. Recipient antibodies react with graft antigens in the small arteries. NK cells and macrophages activate and adhere to the endothelium with subsequent platelet activation and clot formation [1]. Efforts to reduce acute vascular rejection target several cells involved. Altering class I MHC receptors has been shown to be beneficial. Incorporating human leukocyte antigen E and human CD46 into graft cells reduces NK cell cytotoxicity, and incorporation of human CD47 reduced phagocytosis by macrophages [1].

## Acute Cellular Rejection

Acute cellular rejection involves activated T cells, B cells, NK cells, macrophages, and neutrophils. It occurs within days to weeks of transplant [9] and occurs less frequently than acute humoral rejection in xenotransplanted nonhuman primates. Acute cellular rejection is primarily activated by CD8 and CD4 interaction with MHC I and II complex on graft cells. The use of gene editing to reduce the expression of class II leukocyte antigen in pigs is under investigation, and pigs have shown normal development despite reduced levels of CD8 and CD4 T cells [1].

Plasmapheresis and knockout pigs for the immunogenic antigens are used to reduce rejection but do not eliminate hyperacute and acute humoral rejection requiring immunosuppression, also required for cellular rejection [4].

## Graft Overgrowth

In addition to rejection, porcine xenotransplanted hearts are at risk for graft overgrowth after insertion into human and non-human recipients. The grafts can increase to 4 × their original size and cause diastolic heart failure and lung compression. This is not fully understood, but the higher baseline blood pressure of recipients compared to pigs is thought to contribute to this phenomenon. Lowering the blood pressure in baboon trials reduced post-operative hypertrophy. Other strategies included growth hormone receptor knockout pigs and early transition from steroid therapy to temsirolimus, which inhibits the effect of growth hormone [1].

## Infections

Xenotransplant recipients require immunosuppression and are at risk for infections similar to human transplant recipients but are also at risk for zoonotic infections. Viral infections, such as porcine cytomegalovirus (PCMV), porcine lymphotropic (PLHV) herpesvirus and porcine endogenous retroviruses (PERV), are particularly concerning in nonhuman trials because they can survive within and destroy the xenograft without need for human cells to replicate.

PCMV has not been shown in vivo to infect human cells but has been demonstrated in high doses in vitro. In vitro studies of antivirals against HHV-6 to treat PCMV found cidofovir reduced PCMV viral load, and foscarnet and cidofovir had better prophylactic effects than ganciclovir. PHLV is of uncertain significance as a pathogen to immunosuppressed humans, although it is associated with lymphoproliferative disorder in immunosuppressed pigs. There are no treatments for PLHV. PERV A and B can infect human cells, while PERV C infects only pigs. Pigs with genetic knockout of PERV retroviral elements have been developed to reduce transmission of PERVs to humans. Timing on infectious screening and prophylaxis protocols for xenotransplant recipients remains undetermined [10].

## Ethical Considerations

The use of genetically modified porcine organs as a source for organ transplants would greatly enlarge the pool of organs available to treat patients with end-stage cardiac disease and could result in a reduction in transplant waitlist times [11]. However, xenotransplant brings its own set of ethical concerns. There are cultures that do not use animal products in general or pigs in particular, and these groups may be excluded from this treatment option [12]. Some groups may be opposed to animals raised exclusively for the purpose of organ procurement or may be opposed to the isolating conditions required to raise animals free from disease. The possibility of zoonotic spread of disease from an immunosuppressed patient to the public raises further concerns about xenotransplant [4].

Patient selection for early xenotransplant trials also needs to be chosen with care. It may not be ethical to offer xenotransplantation to patients who are candidates for human organ transplant, which is the current standard of care, until we have more robust data. On the other hand, if we only offer xenotransplantation to patients who are too medically complicated for human organ transplants, it may result in data that is not translatable to the general transplant population. Additionally, patients denied from human organ transplant may feel coercion to enroll if the research trial as it is the only alternative to palliative care if they are not candidates for durable mechanical circulatory support [13].

Ethics around how xenotransplant is studied is also relevant, including when to transition from animal studies to trials involving human subjects. In 2021, New York University transplanted porcine kidneys into two humans who were dead by neurological criteria. The organs and urine output were monitored for over two days before the experiments were concluded [14]. Similarly, in 2022, researchers from the University of Alabama at Birmingham reported kidney xenotransplant on a human declared brain dead. The use of neurologically deceased subjects to evaluate xenotransplants can bridge the gap between animal studies and human trials but would need further regulation. How to obtain authorization for these procedures from family decision-makers, as well as how long a deceased body can ethically be monitored for scientific purposes and how remains would be returned to the family would need to be defined. Current research regulatory boards are only responsible for living humans, not those declared dead.

## First Genetically Modified Human Xenotransplant

The first genetically modified porcine xenotransplant in a human was performed at the University of Maryland in 2022 on a 57-year-old man with nonischemic cardiomyopathy [15, 16]. He initially presented with a heart failure exacerbation and had an LVEF of 10%. He advanced through inotropic support and required an intra-aortic balloon pump on hospital day 11. He had multiple ventricular arrhythmias and cardiac arrests and became dependent on venoarterial extracorporeal membrane oxygenation (ECMO) by hospital day 23. He was not a candidate for allotransplant or other advanced therapies due to nonadherence to treatment and was declined allotransplant from multiple centers before he was offered xenotransplant. The patient's competency and capacity were evaluated by three institutional evaluations and an external psychiatric evaluation. His hospital course pre procedurally was complicated by mild hypoxemia intermittently requiring supplemental oxygen, adrenal insufficiency, gastrointestinal bleeding, drug-induced leukopenia, and resolved bacteremia.

At the time of xenotransplant, the explanted graft was supported with a cardiac perfusion system. The patient was weaned from ECMO support postoperatively and had normal xenograft function. The postoperative course was complicated by peritonitis requiring abdominal washouts, poor feeding with weight loss, and continued thrombocytopenia. On day 43, he had somnolence requiring intubation, hypotension, and infiltrates on chest X-ray concerning viral or fungal infection. He received IVIG for hypogammaglobulinemia, and weekly infectious screening indicated a rise in PCMV DNA levels as the source, which was confirmed on tissue samples. Ganciclovir prophylaxis was switched to cidofovir with clinical improvement and extubation. On postoperative day 49, he had cardiogenic shock with failure of the graft and increased graft size. Atypical antibody-mediated rejection was suspected, and treatment was initiated with plasma exchange, IVIG, and complement and B cell inhibition. Repeat biopsy had ISLHT grade 1 antibody-mediated rejection with 40% myocardial necrosis without cellular rejection. He was unable to be weaned from ECMO support due to irreversible graft injury, and he ultimately died on post-op day 60 after life support was withdrawn [15, 16].

The graft heart was obtained from a pig with ten gene edits. It was knockout for galactose-$\alpha$ 1,3-galactose, Sda blood group antigen, and N-glycolylneuraminic acid to reduce hyperacute rejection. The organism was knocked out for growth hormone to reduce the risk of xenograft overgrowth. Human CD46 and DAF were inserted to reduce the risk of antibody-dependent complement activation. Human thrombomodulin and endothelial cell protein C receptor were expressed to improve activation of protein C. Human anti-inflammatory proteins CD47 and heme oxygenase 1 were also expressed in the donor [15, 16].

The post-transplant immunosuppressive strategy was based on protocols in nonhuman primate trials, and the patient's leukopenia and thrombocytopenia required intermittent dosing of some therapies. Rituximab, anti-thymocyte globulin, and complement C1 esterase inhibitor were used to inactivate B cells, T cells, and complement. CD40 was blocked using a humanized monoclonal antibody (KPL-404) for costimulation blockade of the rejection cascade. A pulse dose of methylprednisolone was given on the day of the transplant and then tapered. Mycophenolate mofetil and KPL-404 were used for maintenance immunosuppression. Mycophenolate was held on day 21 due to neutropenia, and tacrolimus was started on day 35 due to the inability to tolerate mycophenolate. The donor was genetically modified to not carry PERV-C and was tested every three months for potential zoonotic disease, including PERV A, B, C, PCMV, and PHSV. The host was screened for infections after the transplant. The initial infectious prophylaxis regimen included ganciclovir, isavuconazole, and atovaquone [15, 16].

There were several features of this case to learn from in order to proceed with future xenotransplantation [15]. Diastolic heart failure began on postoperative day 47. At postoperative day 50, the endomyocardial biopsy revealed damaged capillaries with interstitial oedema, red cell extravasation, rare thrombotic microangiopathy, and complement deposition. Increased anti-pig xenoantibodies, mainly IgG, were detected after IVIG administration for hypogammaglobulinaemia and during the first plasma exchange. Endomyocardial biopsy on postoperative day 56 showed fibrotic changes consistent with progressive myocardial stiffness. Microbial cell-free DNA testing indicated increasing titers of PCMV/PRV cell-free DNA. Post-mortem single-cell RNA sequencing showed overlapping causes. Potential mediators of the observed endothelial injury were identified.

First, widespread endothelial injury indicates antibody-mediated rejection. Second, IVIG bound strongly to donor endothelium, possibly causing immune activation. Finally, reactivation and replication of latent PCMV/PRV in the xenograft possibly initiated a damaging inflammatory response. The findings point to specific measures to improve xenotransplant outcomes in the future [15].

A second cardiac xenotransplant using genetically modified porcine hearts was performed at the University of Maryland and rejection has been mentioned as the cause of death (after 42 days). The patient received anti-CD154 monoclonal antibodies (more effective than anti-CD40) and complement-inhibition drugs (a C1-esterase inhibitor followed by a C5 inhibitor, eculizumab); full details on that case are pending publication [17].

More recently a patient at Massachusetts General hospital received a renal transplant from a pig and another patient at NYU underwent left ventricular assist device implantation accompanied by a xenotransplant kidney transplant from a pig. These exciting developments open doors for potential alternatives for patients with advanced cardiac disease and multiorgan failure [18].

In summary, organ shortage remains a major problem worldwide, with patients with end-stage organ dysfunction having prolonged wait times and needlessly suffering from increased complications and mortality without suitable organs. Xenotransplantation may offer an exciting solution to an otherwise unsolvable problem of organ shortage. However, before expanding xenotransplantation activities, there are still several important hurdles that must be overcome, including Xenograft rejection, graft overgrowth, zoonotic infections, and ethical considerations.

## References

1. Boulet J, Cunningham JW, Mehra MR. Cardiac xenotransplantation. JACC Basic Transl Sci. 2022;7(7):716–29.
2. Shah A, Goerlich CE, Pasrija C, Hirsch J, Fisher S, Odonkor P, et al. Anatomical differences between human and pig hearts and their relevance for cardiac xenotransplantation surgical technique. Case Reports. 2022;4(16):1049–52.
3. Reichart B, Cooper DKC, Längin M, Tönjes RR, Pierson RN, Wolf E. Cardiac xenotransplantation: from concept to clinic. Cardiovasc Res. 2023;118(18):3499–516.
4. Carrier AN, Verma A, Mohiuddin M, Pascual M, Muller YD, Longchamp A, et al. Xenotransplantation: a new era. Front Immunol. 2022;9:13.
5. Kobashigawa J. Pig-to-human heart transplantation: culmination of technology and ingenuity. Ann Thorac Surg. 2022;113(3):711.
6. Lin SS, Kooyman DL, Daniels LJ, Daggett CW, Parker W, Lawson JH, et al. The role of natural anti-galα1–3gal antibodies in hyperacute rejection of pig-to-baboon cardiac xenotransplants. Transpl Immunol. 1997;5(3):212–8.
7. Miyagawa S, Maeda A, Toyama C, Kogata S, Okamatsu C, Yamamoto R, et al. Aspects of the complement system in new era of xenotransplantation. Front Immunol. 2022;14:13.
8. Zhou H, Hara H, Cooper DKC. The complex functioning of the complement system in xenotransplantation. Xenotransplantation. 2019;26(4):e12517.
9. Zhou Q, Li T, Wang K, Zhang Q, Geng Z, Deng S, et al. Current status of xenotransplantation research and the strategies for preventing xenograft rejection. Front Immunol. 2022;28:13.
10. Mehta SA, Saharia KK, Nellore A, Blumberg EA, Fishman JA. Infection and clinical xenotransplantation: Guidance from the Infectious Disease Community of Practice of the American Society of Transplantation. Am J Transplant. 2023;23(3):309–15.
11. Mehra MR. Cardiac xenotransplantation: rebirth amidst an uncertain future. J Card Fail. 2022;28(5):873–4.
12. Sade RM, Mukherjee R. Ethical issues in xenotransplantation: the first pig-to-human heart transplant. Ann Thorac Surg. 2022;113(3):712–4.
13. Caplan A, Parent B. Ethics and the emerging use of pig organs for xenotransplantation. J Heart Lung Transplant. 2022;41(9):1204–6.
14. Montgomery RA, Stern JM, Lonze BE, Tatapudi VS, Mangiola M, Wu M, et al. Results of two cases of pig-to-human kidney xenotransplantation. N Engl J Med. 2022;386(20):1889–98.
15. Mohiuddin MM, Singh AK, Scobie L, Goerlich CE, Grazioli A, Saharia K, et al. Graft dysfunction in compassionate use of genetically engineered pig-to-human cardiac xenotransplantation: a case report. The Lancet. 2023;402(10399):397–410.
16. Griffith BP, Goerlich CE, Singh AK, Rothblatt M, Lau CL, Shah A, et al. Genetically modified porcine-to-human cardiac xenotransplantation. N Engl J Med. 2022;387(1):35–44.
17. Cooper DKC, Cozzi E. Clinical pig heart xenotransplantation—where do we go from here? Transpl Int. 2024;37:12592.

18. First-Ever Combined Heart Pump & Gene-Edited Pig Kidney Transplant Gives New Hope to Patient with Terminal Illness|NYU Langone News [Internet]. https://nyulangone.org/news/first-ever-combined-heart-pump-gene-edited-pig-kidney-transplant-gives-new-hope-patient-terminal-illness. Accessed 17 Oct 2024

# Part VII
# Ethical Considerations In Heart Transplantation

# Quality-of-Life After Heart Transplantation

# 30

Jignesh Patel and Michelle M. Kittleson

**Abstract**

The typical heart transplant (HTx) recipient often endures a poor quality of life prior to transplantation due to the sequelae of heart failure. A principal aim of transplantation is to attain an improved quality of life in addition to prolonging survival. Potential improvements in quality of life are frequently assessed when evaluating end-stage heart failure patients for transplantation. Quality-of-life can be measured both qualitatively and quantitatively. This chapter will explore aspects of quality of life in HTx, including assessing quality of life, physical well-being, functional status, employment, operating vehicles, mental health, social functioning, and reproductive health.

**Keywords**

Quality-of-life · Heart transplant · Psychosocial outcome

J. Patel (✉) · M. M. Kittleson
Cedars-Sinai Smidt Heart Institute, Los Angeles, CA, USA
e-mail: jignesh.patel@cshs.org

M. M. Kittleson
e-mail: Michelle.kittleson@cshs.org

## Clinical Pearls

- In general, quality of life following heart transplantation has been acceptable.
- Fear of rejection, dealing with hospitalizations from infections, and persevering with lifelong medication can affect patients' mental status and, therefore, impact their perceptions of their physical status.
- There are issues that prevent complete physiologic exercise recovery, including immunosuppressive medications, cardiac denervation, and deconditioning.
- Patients should be encouraged to keep their jobs for as long as possible pre-operatively and that returning to work should be proactively facilitated by a healthcare professional
- Social functioning may largely be dependent on support personnel, while sexual intimacy may be affected by both psychological and physiological factors.
- Successful pregnancy is possible in carefully selected patients following HTx.

## Introduction

Patient outcomes after heart transplantation (HTx) have historically been quantified with measures such as survival, freedom from infection, and rates of rejection. In today's era of increased survival, quality-of-life is now



J. Kobashigawa (ed.), *Clinical Guide to Heart Transplantation*, https://doi.org/10.1007/978-3-031-88290-6_30

appropriately recognized as an important outcome measure. The World Health Organization defines quality-of-life as, "an individual's perception of their position in life in the context of the culture and value systems in which they live and in relation to their goals, expectations, standards and concerns" [1]. In the context of cardiac transplantation, quality-of-life may be interpreted as the patient's perception of their heart failure, including any therapies, on their ability to live a satisfying life. HTx recipient often endures a poor quality-of-life prior to transplantation due to the sequelae of heart failure. A principal aim of transplantation is to attain an improved quality-of-life in addition to prolonging survival. Potential improvements in quality-of-life are frequently assessed when evaluating end-stage heart failure patients for transplantation. Quality-of-life can be measured both qualitatively and quantitatively, as will be discussed in this chapter.

## Aspects of Quality-of-Life

### Assessing Quality-of-Life

Quality-of-life is assessed across various domains, which are often subjective and involve considerable overlap. Physical wellbeing, functional status, mental health, and social standing are all established markers of quality-of-life in the post-transplant population. There are numerous methods for both assessing and presenting quality-of-life data. Often, a questionnaire is submitted to the patient and a score is generated from the answers given. The topics covered in a questionnaire may be generic to all individuals or focus on the patient's particular disease and therapies—in this case heart failure, HTx, and immunosuppression. Questions will often range from the overtly objective, such as whether a patient is currently in paid employment, to the subtly subjective, such as how many days he or she has felt depressed in the past month. Although the patient is the primary source for quality-of-life data, caregivers and relatives can be useful for supplementing or validating responses.

The hallmark of a good question is one that yields answers that are reliable, valid, and sensitive. Reliability refers to the frequency with which the same response is given, by the same patient, at different times. Validity means that a question evokes a response that correlates with the outcome measure. Sensitivity is the likelihood of a question discovering an outcome attributable to the patient. After constructing a questionnaire, subjects are selected. Care is needed to ensure that the sample is representative of the population. Those declining a questionnaire on the basis of being too unwell or too preoccupied represent important parts of the quality-of-life spectrum. Being unwell may refer to a hospitalization or it may refer to depression or anxiety. Conversely, being preoccupied may be due to a patient having regained employment or enjoying leisure activities. Every effort must be made to recruit a broad spectrum of patients for quality-of-life studies.

Determining whether variables are dependent on one another and establishing risk factors for outcome variables is a challenging task in the setting of quality-of-life. Studies often employ multivariate analysis. This means looking at the collective relationships between measured variables and outcomes. For example, determining whether a transplant recipient has returned to work or whether a patient is depressed, may depend on many other factors or even be co-dependent. A patient may not return to work because he or she is depressed or may be depressed because he or she cannot return to work. In turn, a patient may not be able to return to work because of health issues. These relationships can be subtle, but identifying the determinants of outcomes is important to allow patients to attain the highest possible quality-of-life.

### Physical Wellbeing

For the majority of HTx recipients who are free of serious complications, there is a universal improvement in physical status for after transplantation, particularly when compared with that of end-stage heart failure. The NYHA Heart

Failure scale mentioned in Chap. 1 serves as the traditional measure of functional status in heart failure. After transplantation, over 90% of patients self-classify themselves as NYHA class I [2], in stark contrast to the NYHA Class III-IV, which is the typical indication for transplantation evaluation and listing. In theory, these patients can return to their "normal" lives. In reality, however, the patient's psyche may be tainted by the harrowing experience of transplantation. Fear of rejection, dealing with hospitalizations from infections, and persevering with lifelong medication can weigh gravely on the patient's mind and thus on their perceptions of their own physical status.

In quality-of-life studies assessing physical status, patients have consistently reported substantial improvement [3]. Symptoms of heart failure are dramatically reduced in nearly all patients. A prospective study demonstrated that 90% of patients reported minimal or no symptoms of heart disease [4]. Furthermore, exercise capacity as measured by oxygen uptake, maximum heart rate, and anaerobic threshold significantly improves post-transplant [5], although it rarely returns to normal due to denervation and physiologic derangement. As addressed previously, the greatest improvements typically occur during the first-year post-transplantation [5]; however, rehabilitation programs and targeted exercise protocols are often able to achieve further incremental gains [6, 7].

## Functional Status

A HTx recipient's functional standing encompasses all the activities of daily living, such as grooming, mobilizing freely, performing domestic chores, participating in paid employment, attending school and partaking in leisure activities. Patients report improvements in all functional areas after transplantation. While on the waitlist, only 8% of patients classify their quality-of-life as high, and 84% of patients complain of difficulties at work or at school [8]. This compares with two-thirds of patients who report a high quality-of-life after transplantation. However, half of patients still report being unable to perform one or more work or school-related tasks [4]. Although there is a marked improvement in all the functional areas post-transplantation, a significant proportion of patients report a deficit of some kind in one or several of the areas. Two-thirds of patients complain of limitations to desired physical activities [4]. As time since transplantation increases, functional impairment is derived from the chronic use of immunosuppressive therapy. Patients can suffer from muscle atrophy, myalgia, osteopenia, or the sequelae associated with renal impairment. These complications can deter patients from activities involving physical exertion.

## Employment

Returning to work benefits patients and society at large. Individuals who resume employment not only gain financial independence but also increase their self-esteem, allow personal goals to be attained, and improve socialization [9]. Several factors influence a patient's likelihood of returning to work. These include age at time of transplant, education, length of disability, and the patient's perception of their own health [9–11]. Recipients who are younger, have a higher level of education, feel confident in their health, and are encouraged by their physicians have a higher chance of gaining employment. The number of patients who return to work varies widely across centers, ranging from 22 to 86% of HTx recipients [10–14]. These figures come from centers across the world. Large studies in the United States show rates of approximately 45% [9, 10, 12]. This contrasts with 69% of patients 1 year after transplantation in the UK [11]. One possible explanation for this difference is that a large proportion of those who did not return to work in the US was "insurance disabled". "Insurance disabled" refers to transplant recipients who would have liked to return to work and were medically fit enough to do so. They could not, however, because working would have resulted in a loss of Medicare health insurance, and private medical insurance was either unobtainable or prohibitively expensive. One study [14] found that 36% of patients fell into this category. Legislative changes such as lifelong Medicaid funding for immunosuppression, the Social Security Administration's "Ticket to Work" program, and the Affordable Care Act, may allow HTx recipients to more easily gain employment postoperatively. Therefore, future studies could show higher numbers of patients returning to work.

A dilemma facing transplant patients is the loss of disability benefits that may occur upon returning to work. Some patients will lose disability compensation upon starting a paid job. This is often anxiety-provoking since many are concerned that their health is in a fragile state and a sudden deterioration could put them in financial difficulties. Self-perception plays a significant role in employment rates amongst transplant patients. Paris et al. [10] found that of the 61% of HTx recipients who were unemployed, a mere 13% were deemed medically unable to work by their physicians.

More patients who have office jobs return to work than patients who have jobs involving manual labor prior to transplantation [15]. Other jobs, such as operators of heavy machinery or airline pilots, require health certification. Unfortunately, concerns over CAV and sudden death often mean patients fail health checks and, therefore, are denied employment.

The ISHLT guidelines [16] recommend that returning to work should be discussed HTx as a goal of post-operative rehabilitation. The guidelines advise that patients should be encouraged to keep their jobs for as long as possible pre-operatively and that returning to work should be proactively facilitated by a healthcare professional.

Although there is scope for improving the employment rate for HTx recipients, it should be noted that the rate is significantly higher when compared with employment rates for those on the waitlist. Patients who did find employment worked more hours, missed fewer days and had a higher performance rating than before their surgeries. These outcomes highlight the positive effects of HTx for society as a whole as well as for the patient.

## Operating Vehicles

In the initial postoperative period, sternotomy precautions must be taken. The motion of turning a steering wheel can impede healing, and therefore, a minimum 6- to 8-week abstention from driving is needed. Patients should be pain-free, ideally. When riding as a passenger in a car with airbags, patients should refrain from sitting in the front during the first postoperative weeks. Actual driving laws vary by geographic region. If a patient has had any episodes of syncope, then they must not drive until they have been free from an episode for a minimum of 6 months. A full neurological assessment should be done, looking for tremors, adequate visual acuity, and a stable gait. In addition, symptomatic bradycardia requires a permanent pacemaker to be implanted before driving is permissible. Piloting aircraft comes under heavy scrutiny from most aviation authorities owing to the high incidence of cerebrovascular accidents and the potential for sudden death.

## Mental Health

Patients suffer psychological sequelae as part of their end-stage heart failure and while awaiting transplantation. Anxiety, feelings of hopelessness about the future, a loss of control, and an increased dependency on others are frequently experienced by the patient [17–21]. Although physical symptoms abate quickly after transplantation, anxiety and depression often persist. Psychiatric morbidity has been reported in 39% of patients assessed for transplantation [21]. Patients with a longer duration of illness and patients who are unemployed are more likely to have pre-transplant morbidities. Major depressive disorder was most common, followed by generalized anxiety disorder. Sexual dysfunction, mostly in men, is also prevalent.

In the post-transplant population, there is actually an increase in the number of patients suffering from depression and anxiety during the first postoperative year [20]. Some patients report feelings of euphoria, guilt, and changes in body image [19]. It is known that corticosteroids, as part of the immunosuppression regimen, contribute to anxiety and mood swings. Patients who suffer from postoperative complications experience anger and resentment. Psychiatric morbidities usually resolve after the first-year post-transplantation. Interestingly, patients who have psychiatric disorders pre-transplantation also show a resolution of symptoms [18]. Depression and anxiety should, therefore, not be a contraindication to listing a patient. They are usually the result of chronic illness and do not normally progress to post-operative adjustment disorders. Unfortunately, patients who do show persistent signs of psychological morbidities have a reduced quality-of-life and more physical morbidities [22].

After the 5th year post-HTx, recipients generally have good psychological outcomes. Depression and anxiety are lessened or absent, body image improves, and overall quality-of-life measures are higher [23]. The levels of stress and the ability to cope with stress do not decrease over time. Clinicians should be aware of this and consider therapies focusing on stress management for the long term.

## Social Functioning

Although there are significant improvements in many areas of a patient's life, social relationships tend to suffer. Immediate family members often endure financial hardships and act as caregivers. Increased stress and anxiety from the patients can also strain relationships further. The physical and psychological sequelae of end-stage heart disease often prevent social relationships outside the family unit from being maintained. Family members should be acknowledged as an important part of the transplant process. Healthcare professionals should be mindful of making family members feel included where permissible by the patient themselves [24].

Support networks are important for the patient. Recipients with strong relationships are more likely to be compliant with their long-term management plans. Measures of socialization increase during the first 5 years after transplantation [5]. Relationships are an important part of the quality-of-life. Support should be given to assist in maintaining these interpersonal bonds.

## Reproductive Health

With improved survival and decreased morbidities, HTx patients may contemplate conception [25]. The data on pregnancy after HTx are limited, with most clinical guidelines derived from studies relating to kidney and liver recipients. There are important genetic and ethical considerations, particularly for patients with hereditary heart disease. Male patients frequently suffer from erectile dysfunction after transplantation. Psychological causes should be excluded before commencing medical therapy. Initially medical therapy with a phosphodiesterase (PDE) 5 inhibitor can be attempted. As with the general population, concomitant use of nitrates is contraindicated. If PDE inhibitors are ineffective or contraindicated, then a referral to an ED specialist with a view to administering intracavernous injections of prostaglandin E1 can be considered [16].

Sexually active patients should have routine monitoring for sexually transmitted infections (STIs). A sexual history is useful, particularly in adolescent patients. If warranted, ano-genital exams may also be included in the routine follow up to screen for lesions indicative of HSV, HPV and molluscum contagiosum. Female transplant candidates should receive the HPV vaccine preoperatively. There are no contraindications to postoperative administration, but the effectiveness is unproven.

The conceptive method of choice for HTx recipients is intrauterine devices (copper-containing IUD and levonorgestrel-releasing IUD), which offer long-term, highly effective, reversible contraception [26–28]. Immunosuppression is not a contraindication to IUD use [29, 30]. IUDs are considered the only acceptable sole method of contraception in transplant recipients taking mycophenolate mofetil, which is teratogenic and must be stopped at least 6 weeks prior to planned conception. IUDs are considered preferable to other forms of birth control in transplant recipients because of their low failure rate, ability to remain in place for several years, lack of required daily adherence for effectiveness, lack of drug-drug interactions, and straightforward removal to reverse contraception.

Depo-medroxyprogesterone acetate administered every 3 months is a highly effective form of contraception, but it is associated with delayed return to fertility after cessation and decreased bone mineral density and weight gain [31], which may be significant in transplant recipients who are also exposed to long-term corticosteroid therapy [32]. Thus, depo-medroxyprogesterone acetate is not routinely recommended as a long-term contraceptive option [16].

Use of combined hormonal contraceptives should be considered carefully in patients with CAV or hypertension, and their use is contraindicated in patients with an increased risk of thrombosis, liver disease, or estrogen-sensitive malignancies [26]. Combined hormonal contraceptives portend increased risk in patients with prior myocardial infarction, stroke or deep venous thrombosis, hypertension, migraine with aura, and liver disease [32]. Furthermore, due to the inhibition of the cytochrome P450 3A4 pathway with these drugs, additional monitoring of immunosuppression blood levels is required after initiation. Progestin-only pills are not routinely recommended as their efficacy is strongly dependent on consistent timing of administration due to the short half-life, and thus the effectiveness will diminish with non-adherence.

Barrier methods are not recommended as a sole method of contraception, given their relatively high failure rates. They should be used, in combination with another reliable form of birth control, for protection against sexually transmitted infection when indicated.

Patients wishing to have children should receive adequate counseling to discuss genetic and ethical considerations. Although survival has improved, it is still significantly lessened when compared to those of reproductive age in the normal population. Patients should be aware of the distinct possibility that children will have lost a natural parent by their teenage years. For female patients, a multidisciplinary team of cardiologists, fetal medicine specialists, anesthesiologists, neonatologists, geneticists, and psychiatrists is needed for a full evaluation.

HTx recipients should wait at least 1-year post-HTx before pursuing pregnancy. Before planned conception, recipients should have stable heart function (LVEF > 45% without significant allograft vasculopathy or donor-specific antibodies), no rejection in the past 12 months, stable doses of maintenance immunosuppression safe in pregnancy, and no acute infection. Non-adherence with medical therapy, poorly controlled hypertension, diabetes, and renal dysfunction (eGFR < 30 ml/min/1.73 $m^2$) are considered contraindications to pregnancy.

The pre-transplant diagnosis may have an impact on the risk for pregnancy: (1) those with PPCM have worse post-transplant outcomes compared to those without PPCM, (2) there is a risk of recurrence of congenital heart disease (CHD) in the offspring of those with CHD, and (3) heritable cardiomyopathies may be passed on to the fetus.

During pregnancy, clinical evaluation and echocardiography form the cornerstone of rejection surveillance; echocardiogram should be performed at least every trimester but ideally every 1–2 months until 24 weeks of gestation and then monthly until delivery. Noninvasive assessment of rejection with donor-derived cell-free DNA cannot be used as current assays cannot distinguish fetal from donor DNA. Pregnant lung transplant and HTx recipients should be screened for gestational diabetes at 24–28 weeks of gestation.

Important pregnancy-related comorbidities include diabetes, hypertension, and CMV infections. Treatment of diabetes during pregnancy in transplant recipients, in conjunction with consultation with endocrinology or maternal–fetal-medicine, requires non-pharmacological strategies (daily exercise, diet, self-monitoring of blood glucose) and pharmacological measures (insulin or metformin as cornerstone treatments; other oral agents such as sulfonylureas, GLP-1 receptor agonists, and SGLT-2 inhibitors are not recommended due to lack of safety data). Hypertension is common in pregnant transplant recipients and should be managed to reduce the risk of preeclampsia and preterm delivery; nifedipine, amlodipine, labetalol, hydralazine, and methyldopa can be used safely during pregnancy. As CMV infection poses risks to the fetus, transplant recipients should be periodically tested for CMV viremia and CMV-seronegative patients are advised to adopt specific behaviors to minimize the risk of primary infection. The premature delivery rate has been reported to be up to 30%, and the surgical delivery rate up to 33% in transplant patients [33]. While low levels of immunosuppressive agents may be detected in breast milk, the risk is considered low, and breastfeeding while on corticosteroids and calcineurin inhibitors is considered safe.

In general, the quality-of-life following HTx has been acceptable. Mental and physical health appears to improve over time but can be affected by post-transplant complications and medications. Social functioning may largely be dependent on support personnel, while sexual intimacy may be affected by both psychological and physiological factors. Finally, successful pregnancy is possible in carefully selected patients following HTx.

## References


1. WHOQOL - Measuring quality of life|The World Health Organization [Internet]. https://www.who.int/tools/whoqol. Accessed 12 Sept 2024
2. Taylor DO, Edwards LB, Aurora P, Christie JD, Dobbels F, Kirk R, et al. Registry of the International Society for Heart and Lung Transplantation: twenty-fifth official adult heart transplant report—2008. J Heart Lung Transplant. 2008;27(9):943–56.
3. Bunzel B, Grundböck A, Laczkovics A, Holzinger C, Teufelsbauer H. Quality of life after orthotopic heart transplantation. J Heart Lung Transplant. 1991;10(3):455–9.
4. Evans RW. The national cooperative transplantation study; 1991.
5. Carter R, Al-Rawas OA, Stevenson A, Mcdonagh T, Stevenson RD. Exercise responses following heart transplantation: 5 year follow-up. Scott Med J. 2006;51(3):6–14.
6. Kobashigawa JA, Leaf DA, Lee N, Gleeson MP, Liu H, Hamilton MA, et al. A controlled trial of exercise rehabilitation after heart transplantation. N Engl J Med. 1999;340(4):272–7.
7. Dall CH, Gustafsson F, Christensen SB, Dela F, Langberg H, Prescott E. Effect of moderate-versus high-intensity exercise on vascular function, biomarkers and quality of life in heart transplant recipients: a randomized, crossover trial. J Heart Lung Transplant. 2015;34(8):1033–41.
8. Buxton M. Costs and benefits of the heart transplant programmes at Harefield and Papworth Hospitals. Vol. 12. HM Stationery Office; 1985.
9. Paris W, Woodbury A, Thompson S, Levick M, Nothegger S, Hutkin-Slade L, et al. Social rehabilitation and return to work after cardiac transplantation—a multicenter survey 1. Transplantation. 1992;53(2):433–7.
10. Paris W, Woodbury A, Thompson S, Levick M, Nothegger S, Arbuckle P, et al. Returning to work after heart transplantation. J Heart Lung Transplant. 1993;12(1 Pt 1):46–53.
11. Kavanagh T, Yacoub MH, Kennedy J, Austin PC. Return to work after heart transplantation: 12-year follow-up. J Heart Lung Transplant. 1999;18(9):846–51.
12. Harvison A, Jones BM, McBride M, Taylor F, Wright O, Chang VP. Rehabilitation after heart transplantation: the Australian experience. J Heart Transplant. 1988;7(5):337–41.
13. Rosenblum DS, Rosen ML, Pine ZM, Rosen SH, Borg-Stein J. Health status and quality of life following cardiac transplantation. Arch Phys Med Rehabil. 1993;74(5):490–3.
14. Meister ND, McAleer MJ, Meister JS, Riley JE, Copeland JG. Returning to work after heart transplantation. J Heart Transplant. 1986;5(2):154–61.
15. White-Williams C, Jalowiec A, Grady K. Who returns to work after heart transplantation? J Heart Lung Transplant. 2005;24(12):2255–61.
16. Velleca A, Shullo MA, Dhital K, Azeka E, Colvin M, DePasquale E, et al. The International Society for Heart and Lung Transplantation (ISHLT) guidelines for the care of heart transplant recipients. J Heart Lung Transplant. 2023;42(5):e1-141.
17. Rideout E, Montemuro M. Hope, morale and adaptation in patients with chronic heart failure. J Adv Nurs. 1986;11(4):429–38.
18. Deshields TL, McDonough EM, Mannen RK, Miller LW. Psychological and cognitive status before and after heart transplantation. Gen Hosp Psychiatry. 1996;18:62–9.
19. Shapiro PA, Kornfeld DS. Psychiatric outcome of heart transplantation. Gen Hosp Psychiatry. 1989;11(5):352–7.

20. Dew MA, Simmons RG, Roth LH, Schulberg HC, Thompson ME, Armitage JM, et al. Psychosocial predictors of vulnerability to distress in the year following heart transplantation. Psychol Med. 1994;24(4):929–45.
21. Trumper A, Appleby L. Psychiatric morbidity in patients undergoing heart, heart and lung, or lung transplantation. J Psychosom Res. 2001;50(2):103–5.
22. Dew MA, Kormos RL, DiMartini AF, Switzer GE, Schulberg HC, Roth LH, et al. Prevalence and risk of depression and anxiety-related disorders during the first three years after heart transplantation. Psychosomatics. 2001;42(4):300–13.
23. Jones BM, Chang VP, Esmore D, Spratt P, Shanahan MX, Farnsworth AE, et al. Psychological adjustment after cardiac transplantation. Med J Aust. 1988;149(3):118–22.
24. Haugh KH, Salyer J. Needs of patients and families during the wait for a donor heart. Heart Lung. 2007;36(5):319–29.
25. Kittleson MM, DeFilippis EM, Bhagra CJ, Casale JP, Cauldwell M, Coscia LA, et al. Reproductive health after thoracic transplantation: an ISHLT expert consensus statement. J Heart Lung Transplant. 2023;42(3):e1-42.
26. Rajapreyar IN, Sinkey RG, Joly JM, Pamboukian SV, Lenneman A, Hoopes CW, et al. Management of reproductive health after cardiac transplantation. J Matern Fetal Neonatal Med. 2021;34(9):1469–78.
27. Curtis KM. US medical eligibility criteria for contraceptive use, 2016. MMWR Recomm Reports. 2016;65.
28. Curtis KM. US selected practice recommendations for contraceptive use, 2016. MMWR Recomm Reports. 2016;65.
29. Krajewski CM, Geetha D, Gomez-Lobo V. Contraceptive options for women with a history of solid-organ transplantation. Transplantation. 2013;95(10):1183–6.
30. Gordon C, Harken T. Controversies in family planning: intrauterine device placement in solid organ transplant patients. Contraception. 2019;100(3):250–2.
31. Sims J, Lutz E, Wallace K, Kassahun-Yimer W, Ngwudike C, Shwayder J. Depo-medroxyprogesterone acetate, weight gain and amenorrhea among obese adolescent and adult women. Eur J Contracept Reprod Health Care. 2020;25(1):54–9.
32. Estes CM, Westhoff C. Contraception for the transplant patient. In: Seminars in perinatology. Elsevier; 2007. p. 372–7.
33. Wagoner LE, Taylor DO, Olsen SL, Price GD Sr, Rasmussen LG, Larsen CB, et al. Immunosuppressive therapy, management, and outcome of heart transplant recipients during pregnancy. J Heart Lung Transplant. 1993;12(6 Pt 1):993–9.

# 31 Patient Selection in the Context of Organ Scarcity

Jignesh Patel and Yael Peled

**Abstract**

In the context of organ scarcity, judicious use of available organs is crucial. In this chapter we discuss the foundational principles that create the ethical framework for listing a patient for heart transplantation, optimizing donor & recipient risk matching, as well psychosocial and financial considerations. While each patient's case must be evaluated on its own merits, the broader goal is to maximize the overall benefit of transplant programs and ensure the fair distribution of donor hearts.

**Keywords**

Heart failure · Heart transplantation · Ethics · Scarcity · Disparities

J. Patel (✉)
Cedars-Sinai Smidt Heart Institute, Los Angeles, CA, USA
e-mail: jignesh.patel@cshs.org

Y. Peled
Leviev Heart and Vascular Center, Sheba Medical Center, Tel Hashomer, Ramat Gan, Israel
e-mail: yael.peled-potashnik@sheba.health.gov.il

Y. Peled
Faculty of Medical and Health Sciences, Tel Aviv University, Tel Aviv, Israel

## Clinical Pearls

- Utility, respect for patient autonomy, non-maleficence, and justice are the foundational principles that create the ethical framework for listing a patient for heart transplantation.
- Infections, renal disease, and malignancy are potential post-transplant hazards that must be kept in mind when considering heart transplantation candidacy, especially when comorbidities exist that introduce competing risks of non-cardiac death.
- Efforts to minimize bias within transplant selection committees through transparency and systemically through critical appraisal of organ allocation policies are vital.
- Accepting borderline-quality donors for lower-risk recipients may enhance organ utilization without impacting post-transplant survival.
- Intellectual disabilities or psychiatric disorders should not be absolute contraindications to transplantation, and a thorough assessment of the patient's functional capacity, support systems, and ability to manage self-care should guide decision-making.
- In patients with history of substance abuse, structured rehabilitation programs, pharmacotherapy, and social contracts may provide a pathway to heart transplant eligibility.


J. Kobashigawa (ed.), *Clinical Guide to Heart Transplantation*, https://doi.org/10.1007/978-3-031-88290-6_31

## Introduction

In patients with advanced heart failure (AHF), guideline-directed medical therapies may not be sufficient for all patients, and advanced treatments may be required [1]. Heart transplant (HTx) evaluation is frequently requested in patients with AHF. The patient selection committee of the transplant center determines the suitability of candidates for transplantation. Decisions of the committee are made by consensus. Committees should be open and include members from multiple disciplines. Often led by AHF and transplant cardiologists, and cardiothoracic surgeons, the team reviews the clinical and psychosocial findings from the evaluation to determine whether the patient meets the criteria for HTx. They determine if the patient will reasonably expect to receive a substantial improvement in quantity and quality of life after an HTx and can be expected to adhere to a long-term disciplined medical regimen following transplantation. If there is no contraindication to HTx, the patient will be accepted by the committee for listing for transplant. Complete details of the medical considerations behind transplantation listing are found in Chaps. 3 and 4.

Currently, in 2024, there are approximately 3400 patients waiting for a HTx in the United States, according to data from the Organ Procurement and Transplantation Network (OPTN). According to the Eurotransplant annual report, more than 1000 patients were active on the HTx waiting list. By the end of 2023 [2]. In countries across Asia, including India and Japan, HTx waiting lists also comprise several thousand patients. In the rest of the world, like Latin America, Africa, and the Middle East, data availability varies significantly, but the number of patients is generally lower due to fewer transplant centers and less frequent organ donation [3–5]. Overall, the global number of patients waiting for an HTx is estimated to be in the range of 10,000–15,000. This figure is likely underestimated the true demand due to less developed healthcare systems in some regions. According to data from the Global Observatory on Donation and Transplantation, 8,988 HTx were performed in the year 2022. The number of HTx in the Americas Region continued to increase over the years, reaching a peak of 4,996 transplants in 2022, while 2,444 transplants were performed in the European region that same year [6].

## Ethical Principles

Utility, respect for patient autonomy, non-maleficence, and justice are the foundational principles that create the ethical framework for listing a patient for HTx. Donor hearts are a scarce resource and are gifts made to the community for patients in need, heightening the responsibility of the transplant team and requiring the team to adhere to a higher standard to ensure the heart is allocated in a way that is likely to result in significant benefit to the recipient (representing the principle of utility). Respect for patient autonomy requires that patients be fully informed about their disease and treatment options, empowering them to refuse or consent to proposed interventions. In the current era, well-selected left ventricular assist device (LVAD) recipients receiving the HeartMate III device (Abbott, United States) demonstrate approximately 80% two-year survival [7], but LVAD recipients demonstrate lower likelihood of HTx, particularly after the 2018 United States allocation change [8]. This can make discussions around therapies ethically complex when trying to preserve patient autonomy for patients with preferences toward transplant over LVAD but who may be medically appropriate for durable mechanical circulatory support. Efforts are currently underway to improve LVAD technology to make devices less intrusive for patients with fewer complications and thus improve quality of life, as well as to evolve the HTx allocation system to a continuous rather than 6-tier allocation that may be more focused on medical urgency and less reliant on treatment modality [9, 10]. The principle of non-maleficence also comes to the forefront when considering HTx. While

**Table 31.1** Sample ethical questions regarding patient selection in the context of organ scarcity

| |
|---|
| • How should transplant teams approach the selection of patients who have previously rejected organ transplants due to poor adherence or lifestyle factors, knowing that organs are a limited resource? |
| • Should patients who refuse certain medical interventions, such as blood transfusions for religious reasons, be considered for heart transplants? |
| • How should marijuana substance use be viewed by transplant committees, given recent legalization in certain areas? |
| • What are the ethical implications of matching a donor with a recipient who has donor-specific antibodies when there are others in the donor pool who are unsensitized with a decreased risk of rejection? |
| • Should there be an absolute age limit beyond which heart transplantation should not be considered? |

transplantation is the gold standard therapy for end-stage heart disease, it is a disease-exchanging therapy given the lifelong immunosuppression patients necessitate, potentially leading to infections, renal disease, and malignancy. These potential hazards must be kept in mind when considering HTx candidacy, especially when comorbidities exist that introduce competing risks of non-cardiac death. Finally, the ethical principle of justice emphasizes the fair allocation of donor hearts. There are known disparities in outcomes of certain groups of patients, including racial minorities [11], adult congenital heart disease patients [12], and those who are highly sensitized [13]. Geographic disparities based on region also persist [14]. Efforts to minimize bias within transplant selection committees through transparency and systemically through critical appraisal of organ allocation policies are vital. Table 31.1 outlines several ethical questions regarding patient selection in the context of organ scarcity.

## Optimizing Donor and Recipient Risk Matching

HTx recipients have become older over the last three decades, with the median age at the time of transplant exceeding 55 years [15], but recipient age has consistently been shown to be a risk factor for mortality after transplant. Similarly, re-transplantation has been shown to have worse outcomes compared to primary HTx [16, 17], though the very sick patients presenting with primary graft dysfunction may be driving these results. Nevertheless, given the scarcity of donor organs, candidate selection and matching must be optimized. Though there are some advocates who suggest that high-risk recipients should be matched with higher-risk donors (such as an older candidate being matched with an older donor heart), there has been evidence to suggest that accepting borderline-quality donors for lower-risk recipients could enhance organ utilization without negatively impacting recipient survival [18].

## Psychosocial Considerations

Psychosocial factors are an essential but often controversial aspect of HTx eligibility. Patients with cognitive or functional impairments, substance abuse histories, or psychiatric conditions may be considered poor candidates due to concerns about their ability to adhere to post-transplant care, including strict medication regimens and lifestyle changes. While these concerns are valid, they must be weighed against the ethical principle of justice, ensuring that vulnerable populations are not unfairly excluded from life-saving treatments.

Recent guidelines suggest that conditions such as intellectual disabilities or psychiatric disorders should not be absolute contraindications to transplantation [19]. Instead, a thorough assessment of the patient's functional capacity, support systems, and ability to manage self-care should guide decision-making. For patients with a history of substance abuse, structured rehabilitation programs, pharmacotherapy, and social contracts may provide a pathway to eligibility, ensuring that these individuals are not automatically denied based on past behavior [20].

Additionally, patients without adequate support systems are at higher risk for non-adherence and poor outcomes, making social support a key consideration in transplant eligibility [21]. However, ethical concerns arise when patients are excluded solely based on their lack of social resources, as this may disproportionately affect those from disadvantaged backgrounds.

## Financial Considerations

HTx is an expensive procedure, with costs extending well beyond the surgery itself to include lifelong medical care, medications, and regular follow-ups. The financial burden on patients, their families, and the healthcare system is substantial. In some cases, patients may be denied transplantation due to inadequate insurance coverage or financial resources, raising significant ethical concerns.

From an ethical standpoint, denying transplantation based on financial considerations poses a challenge to the principle of justice. However, it is also necessary to consider the sustainability of healthcare systems and the equitable distribution of resources. Financial counseling and assistance programs may help mitigate these issues, but in the context of organ scarcity, difficult decisions may still need to be made regarding the allocation of limited healthcare resources.

## Balancing Individual and Societal Interests

Ultimately, HTx in the context of organ scarcity requires a balance between individual patient interests and societal needs. While each patient's case must be evaluated on its own merits, the broader goal is to maximize the overall benefit of transplant programs and ensure the fair distribution of donor hearts. Ethical decision-making in this area involves balancing compassion for individual patients with a responsibility to manage scarce resources wisely, ensuring that as many lives as possible are saved through the judicious use of available organs.

## References

1. Kobashigawa JA. The future of heart transplantation. Am J Transplant. 2012;12(11):2875–91.
2. Eurotransplant Annual Report 2023.https://www.eurotransplant.org/wp-content/uploads/2024/06/ETP_AR2023_LowRes.pdf
3. Bader F, Manla Y, Ghalib H, Al Matrooshi N, Khaliel F, Skouri HN. Advanced heart failure therapies in the Eastern Mediterranean Region: current status, challenges, and future directions. Curr Probl Cardiol. 2024;49(7):102564.
4. Uribe-Buritica FL, Olaya P, Rivera EL, Cimbaro JP, Barisani JL, Schwartzmann P, et al. Advancing cardiac care: a registry of heart transplantation in Latin America (1968–2022). In: Transplantation proceedings. Elsevier; 2024.
5. Bader F, Manla Y, Hammouri M, Attallah N. Organ donation in the Eastern Mediterranean region. Transplantation. 2021;105(1):6–9.
6. GODT. Those [2023] data are based on the Global Observatory on Donation and Transplantation (GODT) data, produced by the WHO-ONT collaboration.
7. Mehra MR, Cleveland JC Jr, Uriel N, Cowger JA, Hall S, Horstmanshof D, et al. Primary results of long-term outcomes in the MOMENTUM 3 pivotal trial and continued access protocol study phase: a study of 2200 HeartMate 3 left ventricular assist device implants. Eur J Heart Fail. 2021;23(8):1392–400.
8. Truby LK, Garan AR, Givens RC, Takeda K, Takayama H, Trinh PN, et al. Ventricular assist device utilization in heart transplant candidates: nationwide variability and impact on waitlist outcomes. Circ Heart Fail. 2018;11(4):e004586.
9. Zhang KC, Narang N, Jasseron C, Dorent R, Lazenby KA, Belkin MN, et al. Development and validation of a risk score predicting death without transplant in adult heart transplant candidates. JAMA. 2024;331(6):500–9.
10. Continuous distribution - OPTN [Internet]. https://optn.transplant.hrsa.gov/policies-bylaws/a-closer-look/continuous-distribution. Accessed 17 Sept 2024.
11. Breathett K, Spatz ES, Kramer DB, Essien UR, Wadhera RK, Peterson PN, et al. The groundwater of racial and ethnic disparities research: a statement from circulation: cardiovascular quality and outcomes. Circul Cardiovasc Qual Outcomes Am Heart Assoc. 2021;14:e007868.
12. Nguyen VP, Dolgner SJ, Dardas TF, Verrier ED, McMullan DM, Krieger EV. Improved outcomes of heart transplantation in adults with congenital heart disease receiving regionalized care. J Am Coll Cardiol. 2019;74(23):2908–18.
13. Kransdorf EP, Kittleson MM, Patel JK, Pando MJ, Steidley DE, Kobashigawa JA. Calculated panel-reactive antibody predicts outcomes on the heart transplant waiting list. J Heart Lung Transplant. 2017;36(7):787–96.

14. Hess NR, Seese LM, Sultan I, Wang Y, Hickey GW, Kilic A. Geographic disparitics in heart transplantation persist under the new allocation policy. Clin Transplant. 2021;35(11):e14459.
15. Khush KK, Cherikh WS, Chambers DC, Harhay MO, Hayes D, Hsich E, et al. The International Thoracic Organ Transplant Registry of the International Society for Heart and Lung Transplantation: thirty-sixth adult heart transplantation report—2019; focus theme: donor and recipient size match. J Heart Lung Transplant. 2019;38(10):1056–66.
16. Zhu Y, Shudo Y, Lingala B, Baiocchi M, Oyer PE, Woo YJ. Outcomes after heart retransplantation: a 50-year single-center experience. J Thorac Cardiovasc Surg. 2022;163(2):712–20.
17. Lund LH, Edwards LB, Kucheryavaya AY, Benden C, Christie JD, Dipchand AI, et al. The registry of the International Society for Heart and Lung Transplantation: thirty-first official adult heart transplant report—2014; focus theme: retransplantation. J Heart Lung Transplant. 2014;33(10):996–1008.
18. Moayedi Y, Rodenas-Alesina E, Mueller B, Fan CPS, Cherikh WS, Stehlik J, et al. Rethinking donor and recipient risk matching in Europe and North America: using heart transplant predictors of donor and recipient risk. Circ Heart Fail. 2023;10(5):e009904
19. Dew MA, DiMartini AF, Dobbels F, Grady KL, Jowsey-Gregoire SG, Kaan A, et al. The 2018 ISHLT/APM/AST/ICCAC/STSW recommendations for the psychosocial evaluation of adult cardiothoracic transplant candidates and candidates for long-term mechanical circulatory support. Psychosomatics. 2018;59(5):415–40.
20. Peled Y, Ducharme A, Kittleson M, Bansal N, Stehlik J, Amdani S, et al. International society for heart and lung transplantation guidelines for the evaluation and care of cardiac transplant candidates. J Heart Lung Transplant. 2024.
21. Mollberg NM, Farjah F, Howell E, Ortiz J, Backhus L, Mulligan MS. Impact of primary caregivers on long-term outcomes after lung transplantation. J Heart Lung Transplant. 2015;34(1):59–64.

# Diversity and Access in Heart Transplantation

# 32

Andriana P. Nikolova

**Abstract**

This chapter will summarize significant racial, ethnic, and gender disparities in heart failure and heart transplant care in the United States of America and further underline shortcomings in expanding access to heart transplantation, the impact of socioeconomic stressors on transplant-related outcomes, and the implications of the new allocation system for improving access to transplantation for racial minority communities. Additionally, the chapter will outline future directions aimed at addressing these persistent disparities in care.

**Keywords**

Racial disparities · Diversity · Heart failure · Heart transplant · Diversity · Access to care · Minorities · Social determinants of health

## Clinical Pearls

- Significant racial and ethnic disparities in heart failure and heart transplant outcomes, particularly among black patients, exist across the United States of America.
- One of the major shortcomings in expanding heart transplant access is the availability of public health insurance.
- Social determinants of health have a profound impact on access to and outcomes following heart transplantation.
- The new allocation system has improved transplantation rates for minorities, but the improvement remains disproportionate compared to the growing prevalence of end-stage heart failure in these communities.
- Compared to men, women have less access to advanced heart failure therapies, increased risk of allosensitization and post-transplant rejection.
- Given the limited supply of donor hearts, it is imperative to dissect the factors leading to disparities among different patient groups to achieve equitable access to heart transplantation and improve patient outcomes.

A. P. Nikolova (✉)
Cedars-Sinai Smidt Heart Institute, Los Angeles, CA, USA
e-mail: andriana.nikolova@csmc.edu

 
J. Kobashigawa (ed.), *Clinical Guide to Heart Transplantation*, https://doi.org/10.1007/978-3-031-88290-6_32

## Map of Racial Disparities in Heart Failure Prevalence and Access to Advanced Therapies

There is a significantly higher prevalence of heart failure (HF) among racial and ethnic minorities and those impacted negatively by the social determinants of health [1]. Black adults have a 20-fold higher incidence of HF before age 50 years, and they exhibit the highest rates of HF hospitalizations, readmissions, and 5-year mortality risk after incident HF diagnosis [1]. However, the statistics on the medical care available for and offered to such patients are sobering. Black and Hispanic adults less often receive needed care by a cardiologist when admitted for HF and are less likely to be referred to HF specialists or considered for advanced HF therapies [2, 3]. Additionally, black patients with left ventricular assist devices (LVAD) awaiting heart transplant (HTx) are less likely to be transplanted and more likely to be delisted [4]. Similarly, there is a disproportionately lower five-year post-HTx survival in Black recipients compared to other minority groups [5]. These racial and ethnic disparities in HF and HTx-related mortality are non-homogenously present across the USA. A study using data from the United Network for Organ Sharing and Centers for Disease Control and Prevention Wide-ranging Online Data for Epidemiological Research (CDC Wonder) provides a geographical map of such disparities in outcomes over the period 2016–2018 [6]. The primary outcome examined in the study was the HTx to HF mortality rate ratio. Ratios were calculated for each race/ethnicity in the United States and by state as the number of HTs per 100,000 population divided by the age-adjusted HF mortality rate per 100,000 population [6]. The authors regarded the HTx to HF mortality ratio for White patients as the expected ratio for the other racial groups. Compared with White patients, the HTx/HF mortality ratio was lower than expected at 0.67 for African American patients and as expected at 0.92 for Hispanic patients on a national level [6]. Among the 30 states included for African American patients, States with the lowest ratios (≤0.50, Michigan, Wisconsin, Illinois, and Minnesota) were clustered in the upper Midwest [6]. Among the 11 states included for Hispanic patients, states with the lowest ratios (≤0.50, Colorado and New Mexico) were both Southwestern states; however, Arizona, another Southwestern state, had a higher-than-expected ratio [6]. The reasons at play in these alarming statistics are complex, multifactorial, and still poorly understood. Potential explanations include differences in access to care embedded in the societal structure, patient preference, and implicit provider bias. Ongoing research on the intersection of these different factors is direly needed. The following sections explore some of the existing evidence on the topic.

## Insurance Status and Access to Transplantation

Adequate healthcare insurance is a prerequisite for access to HTx, given the high costs associated with peri-HTx care and long-term follow-up [7]. Underinsurance is a major factor in the inequalities in HTx allocation among minorities, and historically, racial/ethnic minorities have had the highest rates of uninsurance. Approximately 43% of HTx patients have public insurance, with the majority of them (30%) having Medicaid. The trends in listing patterns for racial minorities have mirrored the trends in access to insurance. For example, HTx listings increased by 30% among Black patients following the implementation of the Affordable Care Act in 2014. These statistics were driven by the states that adopted the Affordable Care Act policy, where Medicaid coverage gains were highest for Black and indigenous people of color aged<64 years [8]. Overall, uninsured rates for Hispanic adults, Black adults, and American Indian adults decreased from 32.6 to 19.1%, from 19.9 to 10.7%, and from 32.0 to 22.0%, respectively, between 2010 and 2016 [8]. Uninsured rates in Asian and White adults also decreased, from 16.7 to 7.1% and from 13.1 to 7.1%, respectively, over the same interval [8]. An analysis shows that fewer than 15% of all listed candidates of any demographic group were noted to be working for income. As political tides turn, the availability of low-cost insurance to people of limited income fluctuates. As the above findings demonstrate, the availability of public health insurance has a considerable impact on expanding HTx access, particularly in financially disadvantaged communities, and is a vital tool to bridge the disparities gap.

## Socioeconomic Stressors and Heart Transplant-Related Outcomes

The social determinants of health play an important role in the observed high mortality after HTx for racial minorities. These factors have been nicely examined in multiple analyses. Suarez-Pierre et al. evaluated the impact of the social vulnerability index (SVI) on outcomes after HTx among 23,700 patients undergoing HTx between 2012 and 2021 and found lower 5-year survival, higher incidences of 5-year hospital readmission, and graft rejection among individuals living in highly vulnerable communities (SVI ≥ 75%) compared to those living in less vulnerable communities (SVI < 75%) [9]. In a study of 32,494 adult HTx recipients from 2005 to 2020, in which the authors performed a detailed analysis of ZIP code-level socioeconomic disadvantage using the Distressed Communities Index, which includes parameters such as educational level, poverty, unemployment, housing vacancies, median income and business growth [5]. Comparing HTx recipients from distressed communities (n = 5,043) with all others (n = 27,451), the authors found that, not surprisingly, recipients from the most distressed communities were more likely to be of racial minorities, had lower educational levels and were more likely to have public insurance [5]. Such disadvantaged patients received HTx at lower-volume centers and lived farther away from their transplant centers. Furthermore, HTx recipients from distressed communities suffered from acute rejection at higher rates before discharge from the index hospitalization and also had higher 1-year readmission rates and worse 5-year survival [5]. This study illustrates how the comprehensive burden of social and financial stressors interplay in their impact on post-HTx outcomes. Similar to the above study, analyses of racial and ethnic groups over the span of 3 decades have consistently identified Black patients to be at higher risk of mortality after cardiac transplantation [10, 11]. Apart from the social determinants of health, other contributing factors have been hypothesized, including racial and ethnic differences between the donor and recipient and immunologic and genetic mismatch. Given the limited supply of donor hearts, it is imperative to dissect the factors leading to disparities among different patient groups to achieve equitable access to HTx and improve patient outcomes.

## The New Allocation System and Its Impact on Improved Access to Transplantation for Racial Minorities

The primary directive of the United Network for Organ Sharing (UNOS) is the Final Rule: equitable allocation of organs. Various iterations of the organ allocation system have occurred through the years, striving to mitigate the inherent inequalities in access to transplantation resulting from arbitrary geographical boundaries. The older geographic sharing methodology created longer wait times for patients in diverse, highly populated regions, potentially affecting minority recipients more. In a previous study of trends, Liu et al. demonstrated that the proportion of racial and ethnic minorities increased from 1987 to 2009, and by 2005 to 2009, accounted for nearly one-third of all transplants [12]. In 2018, UNOS revised the organ allocation system from three tiers to six tiers, incorporating broader regional sharing for the sickest patients, thus aiming to remedy geographic inequities. An analysis by Chouairi et al. based on a decade of data from the UNOS registry examines HTx outcomes and trends among 32, 353 patients who self-identified as Black, Hispanic, and White pre- and post-the-new allocation system [13]. Over the span of a decade, the study reports an increased proportion of self-identified Black and Hispanic patients who were listed for HTx (from 21.7 to 28.2% and from 7.7 to 9.0%, respectively, from 2011 to 2020) [13]. Similarly, the proportion of Black candidates transplanted has increased steadily from 20.8 to 27.3%. However, the improved transplantation rates for minorities appear to be proportionately less compared to the rising rates in the prevalence of end-stage HF in these communities [13]. The study by Chouairi et al. also found an increased likelihood of transplantation among all racial/ethnic groups after the change in the allocation system [13]. However, Black candidates were still significantly less likely to be transplanted after allocation amendments, despite similar acuity and listed status [13]. On the other hand, the likelihood of transplantation among Hispanic and White candidates was similar after the 2018 policy changes [13]. Although such efforts to improve access to HTx for vulnerable groups are fruitful, much work still remains to be done.

## Gender Disparities

It has been well established that the prevalence of HF in women is higher than in men, and yet, women are less likely to be referred to or receive HTx and LVAD [14]. However, the exact denominator of the women afflicted with this condition is still unknown. Alarmingly, women account for 54% of HF-related deaths, but only comprise 21% of LVAD recipients and 25% of HTx waitlist candidates [15, 16]. In a multicenter analysis of patients referred for advanced HF therapies at nine centers in the United States, only 26.6% were women, corroborating the under-utilization of advanced HF therapies in female patients [17]. Factors that could account for the lower access to needed therapies for women include social determinants of health, frailty burden, higher rates of allosensitization, and others [16]. However, recent studies shed light on the conscious and unconscious biases that might be at play in these observed referral patterns. In an analysis using identical patient vignettes, HF specialists tended to consider that the same level of available social support was adequate for men but not for women [18]. The same study showed that having children was considered a liability for women, particularly Black women, but not for men [18]. Another single-center analysis from Emory University found that women were less likely to be considered eligible for advanced therapies than men despite similar social support and SIPAT (Stanford Integrated Psychosocial Assessment for Transplantation, a comprehensive psychosocial assessment tool) scores [19]. In terms of patients already listed for HTx, data indicate that women suffer from higher waitlist mortality, particularly at the highest acuity tiers, compared to men. In the previous 3-tiered heart allocation system, women had an adjusted hazard ratio (aHR) of 1.20 of waitlist mortality compared to men, even after adjustment for relevant clinical characteristics [20]. These sex disparities in mortality rates unfortunately remain in the current 6-tiered allocation system [20]. Of candidates waiting for HTx as Status 1, women have a significantly lower rate of HTx compared with men after adjustment for clinical characteristics (aHR: 0.74 [95% CI: 0.62–0.88]; $P<0.0001$) and a significantly higher rate of delisting for death or clinical deterioration (aHR: 1.48 [95% CI: 1.05–2.09]; $P=0.026$) [20]. Possible factors that negatively impact women's waitlist outcomes include vascular access barriers for temporary mechanical circulatory support (tMCS) devices due to smaller caliber vessels in women, as well as complications from MCS devices [16, 20]. More data are needed on the safety and adverse events associated with tMCS devices in women. Other postulated barriers to transplantation in female and Black patients are immunologic factors, such as higher rates of allosensitization [21]. The presence of anti-HLA antibodies limits the donor pool size, increases waitlist mortality, and leads to increased post-HTx rejection rates [22]. In women, in particular, a history of pregnancy is an important risk factor for allosensitization that uniquely disadvantages them. There is a lack of large, multicenter studies on sex differences in response to desensitization therapies, listing practices, and transplant outcomes. Studies have shown that among sensitized HTx candidates, women with a history of pregnancy are at higher risk of antibody-mediated rejection (AMR) than recipients without a history of pregnancy [23]. A study reported that, on average, women experienced more episodes of acute rejection than men and also tended to have higher rates of moderate to severe rejection on biopsies performed within the first year post-HTx [23]. Another single-center study similarly showed that women had a greater risk of developing AMR than men at 1-year follow-up [23]. In that study, AMR treatment response was similar between the sexes, and there was no difference in rejection-related mortality [23]. However, calculated panel reactive antibody levels do not completely account for the increased risk of delisting or waitlist mortality observed in women, nor did the use of extracorporeal membrane oxygenation [20].

## Future Directions

Solutions to address these racial and gender disparities are direly needed but not easy to implement as they affect the root structure of our society. A recent statement from the American Heart Association highlights structural racism is a foundational element of these disparities in care [24]. This structural racism is pervasive—in the quality of housing, the neighborhood environments, the opportunities for educational and economic advancement, etc. A fulcrum point of such change can be the fair inclusion of minorities in clinical trials, access to affordable public insurance, and the creation of bridges between academic institutions and local community hospitals and medical centers. A guiding force in these changes should be fair societal policies that address the very mechanisms underlying the disparities in cardiovascular care.

## References


1. Khariton Y, Nassif ME, Thomas L, Fonarow GC, Mi X, DeVore AD, et al. Health status disparities by sex, race/ethnicity, and socioeconomic status in outpatients with heart failure. JACC Heart Fail. 2018;6(6):465–73.
2. Breathett K, Liu WG, Allen LA, Daugherty SL, Blair IV, Jones J, et al. African Americans are less likely to receive care by a cardiologist during an intensive care unit admission for heart failure. JACC Heart Fail. 2018;6(5):413–20.
3. Glynn P, Lloyd-Jones DM, Feinstein MJ, Carnethon M, Khan SS. Disparities in cardiovascular mortality related to heart failure in the United States. J Am Coll Cardiol. 2019;73(18):2354–5.
4. Lui C, Fraser CD III, Zhou X, Suarez-Pierre A, Kilic A, Zehr KJ, et al. Racial disparities in patients bridged to heart transplantation with left ventricular assist devices. Ann Thorac Surg. 2019;108(4):1122–6.
5. Chen Q, Malas J, Emerson D, Megna D, Catarino P, Esmailian F, et al. Heart transplantation in patients from socioeconomically distressed communities. J Heart Lung Transplant. 2024;43(2):324–33.
6. Breathett K, Knapp SM, Carnes M, Calhoun E, Sweitzer NK. Imbalance in heart transplant to heart failure mortality ratio among African American, Hispanic, and White patients. Circulation. 2021;143(24):2412–4.
7. Pagani FD. Insurance coverage and heart transplant outcomes. Circul Cardiovasc Qual Outcomes Am Heart Assoc. 2016;9:501–3.
8. Breathett K, Allen LA, Helmkamp L, Colborn K, Daugherty SL, Khazanie P, et al. The Affordable Care Act Medicaid expansion correlated with increased heart transplant listings in African-Americans but not Hispanics or Caucasians. JACC Heart Fail. 2017;5(2):136–47.
9. Suarez-Pierre A, Iguidbashian J, Kirsch MJ, Cotton JL, Quinn C, Fullerton DA, et al. Importance of social vulnerability on long-term outcomes after heart transplantation. Am J Transplant. 2023;23(10):1580–9.
10. Kilic A, Higgins RSD, Whitson BA, Kilic A. Racial disparities in outcomes of adult heart transplantation. Circulation. 2015;131(10):882–9.
11. Allen JG, Weiss ES, Arnaoutakis GJ, Russell SD, Baumgartner WA, Conte JV, et al. The impact of race on survival after heart transplantation: an analysis of more than 20,000 patients. Ann Thorac Surg. 2010;89(6):1956–64.
12. Liu V, Bhattacharya J, Weill D, Hlatky MA. Persistent racial disparities in survival after heart transplantation. Circulation. 2011;123(15):1642–9.
13. Chouairi F, Fuery M, Clark KA, Mullan CW, Stewart J, Caraballo C, et al. Evaluation of racial and ethnic disparities in cardiac transplantation. J Am Heart Assoc. 2021;10(17):e021067.

14. Morris AA, Khazanie P, Drazner MH, Albert NM, Breathett K, Cooper LB, et al. Guidance for timely and appropriate referral of patients with advanced heart failure: a scientific statement from the American Heart Association. Circulation. 2021;144(15):e238-50.
15. Hsich EM, Blackstone EH, Thuita L, McNamara DM, Rogers JG, Ishwaran H, et al. Sex differences in mortality based on united network for organ sharing status while awaiting heart transplantation. Circ Heart Fail. 2017;10(6):e003635.
16. DeFilippis EM, Nikolova A, Holzhauser L, Khush KK. Understanding and investigating sex-based differences in heart transplantation: a call to action. Heart Fail. 2023;11(9):1181–8.
17. Herr JJ, Ravichandran A, Sheikh FH, Lala A, Chien CV, Hsiao S, et al. Practices of referring patients to advanced heart failure centers. J Card Fail. 2021;27(11):1251–9.
18. Breathett K, Yee E, Pool N, Hebdon M, Crist JD, Yee RH, et al. Association of gender and race with allocation of advanced heart failure therapies. JAMA Netw Open. 2020;3(7):e2011044–e2011044.
19. Steinberg RS, Nayak A, Burke MA, Aldridge M, Raja Laskar S, Bhatt K, et al. Association of race and gender with primary caregiver relationships and eligibility for advanced heart failure therapies. Clin Transplant. 2022;36(1):e14502.
20. DeFilippis EM, Masotti M, Blumer V, Maharaj V, Cogswell R. Sex-specific outcomes of candidates listed as the highest priority status for heart transplantation. Circ Heart Fail. 2023;16(6):e009946.
21. Morris AA, Cole RT, Veledar E, Bellam N, Laskar SR, Smith AL, et al. Influence of race/ethnic differences in pre-transplantation panel reactive antibody on outcomes in heart transplant recipients. J Am Coll Cardiol. 2013;62(24):2308–15.
22. Kransdorf EP, Kittleson MM, Patel JK, Pando MJ, Steidley DE, Kobashigawa JA. Calculated panel-reactive antibody predicts outcomes on the heart transplant waiting list. J Heart Lung Transplant. 2017;36(7):787–96.
23. Nguyen LS, Coutance G, Salem JE, Ouldamar S, Lebreton G, Combes A, et al. Effect of recipient gender and donor-specific antibodies on antibody-mediated rejection after heart transplantation. Am J Transplant. 2019;19(4):1160–7.
24. Churchwell K, Elkind MSV, Benjamin RM, Carson AP, Chang EK, Lawrence W, et al. Call to action: structural racism as a fundamental driver of health disparities: a presidential advisory from the American Heart Association. Circulation. 2020;142(24):e454-68.

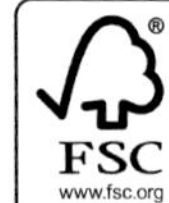


MIX
Papier aus verantwortungsvollen Quellen
Paper from responsible sources
FSC® C105338

If you have any concerns about our products,
you can contact us on
**ProductSafety@springernature.com**

In case Publisher is established outside the EU,
the EU authorized representative is:
**Springer Nature Customer Service Center GmbH**
**Europaplatz 3, 69115 Heidelberg, Germany**

Printed by Libri Plureos GmbH
in Hamburg, Germany